3RD EDITION

Introduction to Communication Disorders

A Lifespan Perspective

ROBERT E. OWENS, JR.

State University of New York at Geneseo

DALE EVAN METZ

State University of New York at Geneseo

ADELAIDE HAAS

State University of New York at New Paltz

PEARSON

Boston   New York   San Francisco
Mexico City   Montreal   Toronto   London   Madrid   Munich   Paris
Hong Kong   Singapore   Tokyo   Cape Town   Sydney

Executive Editor and Publisher: Stephen D. Dragin
Series Editorial Assistant: Meaghan Minnick
Marketing Manager: Tara Kelly
Production Editor: Joe Sweeney
Editorial Production Service: Walsh & Associates, Inc.
Composition and Manufacturing Buyer: Megan Cochran
Electronic Composition: Publishers' Design and Production Services, Inc.
Interior Design: Denise Hoffman
Cover Designer: Linda Knowles

For related titles and support materials, visit our online catalog at www.ablongman.com

Between the time website information is gathered and then published, it is not unusual for some sites to have closed. Also, the transcription of URLs can result in typographical errors. The publisher would appreciate notification where these errors occur so that they may be corrected in subsequent editions.

Library of Congress Cataloging-in-Publication Data

Owens, Robert E.
    Introduction to communication disorders : a lifespan perspective / Robert E. Owens, Jr., Dale Evan Metz, Adelaide Haas.—3rd ed.
        p.   cm.
    Includes bibliographical references and index.
    ISBN 0-205-48787-4
    1. Communicative disorders.   I. Metz, Dale Evan.   II. Haas, Adelaide.
III. Title.
RC423 095 2006
616.85'5—dc22   2005058659

Printed in the United States of America

10 9 8 7 6 5 4 3 2   09 08 07 06

Kurt Haas, Ph.D.
Husband, Educator, Friend
We miss your dry wit, keen intellect, mischievous smile, knowing look,
and ever-insightful comments.
You made us all a little better for knowing you.

Contents

CHAPTER 3

ANATOMY AND PHYSIOLOGY RELATED TO SPEECH, HEARING, AND LANGUAGE   53

CHAPTER 4

ASSESSMENT AND INTERVENTION   65

CHAPTER 5

CHILDHOOD LANGUAGE IMPAIRMENTS   91

CHAPTER 9

THE VOICE AND VOICE DISORDERS   245

CHAPTER 10

DISORDERS OF ARTICULATION AND PHONOLOGY   269

CHAPTER 11

Cleft Lip and Cleft Palate   311

CHAPTER 12

NEUROGENIC SPEECH DISORDERS   343

CHAPTER 15

AUGMENTATIVE AND ALTERNATIVE COMMUNICATION

Preface

We hope this book will serve as a good introduction to the fields of speech-language pathology and audiology. Our goals have been to be informative and interesting, to provide enough information without overwhelming the reader, and to be scholarly in our production of a challenging text. Unlike edited texts, we have attempted to speak with one voice and to provide an overview, not to force-feed the reader with our pet approaches to assessment and intervention. This does not mean that our text is without perspective. It has been our objective to follow models of good practice and approaches that represent the best of our own clinical experience.

Within each chapter, we have attempted to describe a specific disorder and related assessment and intervention methods. In addition, we have included lifespan issues to provide the reader with added insights. Each disorder is also illustrated by the personal story of an individual with that disorder. Reader interest and reflection are stimulated by thought questions placed throughout each chapter and by margin notes. Further knowledge can be gained by the suggested readings and the Internet locations provided at the conclusion of each chapter.

Students will find the accompanying CD-ROM helpful as a learning device and study tool. Many disorders are also presented in sound and video format on this disk. In addition, self-study questions follow the outline of each chapter and highlight important information.

This new edition of *Introduction to Communication Disorders: A Lifespan Perspective* has many new features that strengthen the existing text and make it more readable. In addition to updates from clinical research, you'll find new focus and a more attention to lifespan issues. Let's discuss some of these exciting changes.

First, we have been guided by evidence-based practice in all the therapeutic approaches that we cite. This level of accountability in the fields of speech-language pathology and audiology is a welcome one.

Second, we have reorganized the book to reflect the needs of students in introductory courses. The amount of information in the anatomy and physiology chapter has been modified to provide just the amount needed to understand the disorders that follow. Sections on physical development have been moved to the appropriate chapters, improving the flow of information in those chapters and supplying developmental information when it's needed.

Third, the communication development chapter has been divided and placed in the chapters with disorders, improving the flow of information in those chapters as well and supplying developmental information again when and where it's needed. Again, the amount of information on development has been modified to reflect the needs of beginning students.

Fourth, a new chapter targets literacy impairments with sections on reading, writing, and related skill areas. As with other chapters, this one follows a lifespan perspective.

Fifth, the lifespan perspective throughout the text has been strengthened. In addition to the changes mentioned above, more emphasis has been placed on lifespan issues within each chapter.

Finally, the audiology and augmentative and alternative communication (AAC) chapters have been revamped. The audiology chapter reflects renewed interest by both audiologists and speech-language pathologists in the area of aural rehabilitation and discusses issues related to cochlear implants and central auditory processing. The AAC chapter also reflects current knowledge and developments in that area.

We hope that you'll agree with us when we claim that this is a more user-friendly and informative text than the previous editions. Please feel free to contact us with suggestions for further strengthening our work.

ACKNOWLEDGMENTS

ROBERT OWENS

I would like to thank the faculty of the Department of Communicative Disorders and Sciences at State University of New York at Geneseo for their forbearance and assistance with this book. Ms. Wendy Metz and Dr. Kathlyn Jones, who both have taught introductory courses, were especially helpful in their review of the manuscript and their insistence that the text adhere to high standards of inclusiveness and content coverage. A clinical perspective, especially with young children, was provided by Ms. Linda Deats and Ms. Irene Belyakov. Finally, my and Dr. Metz's chair, Dr. Linda House, has been extremely helpful both with her expertise and her understanding of the magnitude of our writing task. She has provided a genial atmosphere in which to create. A very special thanks to Jesse Anzalone and Laura Gillespie for compiling the website and PowerPoint information, respectively.

My most personal thanks goes to my partner, who supported and encouraged me and truly makes my life fulfilling and happy. I'm looking forward to our life together.

DALE EVAN METZ

I gratefully acknowledge Dr. Donald Warren, University of North Carolina, Chapel Hill, for the photographs of children with cleft lip and palate, and Dr. Robert Orlikoff, Memorial Sloan-Kettering Cancer Center, New York City, for the photographs of laryngeal pathology and for the audio samples of voice disorders. I also greatly appreciate Dr. Bright Russell for contributing the CD-ROM video segments of vocal fold behavior.

Ms. Janice Masterson kindly contributed video fluoroscopic samples of swallowing, which can be seen on the book's CD-ROM. Kelly Julian and

Julie Klejdys were invaluable to the development of the book's CD-ROM and they also, along with Shanna Wiech, were significant contributors to selected tracks of the CD-ROM. We are especially appreciative of the videotape segments supplied for the CD-ROM by the Prentke-Romich Company of Wooster, Ohio, a developer of augmentative and alternative communication equipment.

Kay Elemetrics, Inc., Pine Brook, New Jersey, kindly provided pictures of some of their clinical instruments, and we thank them for their cooperation. I deeply appreciate the efforts of my wife, Wendy, for her tireless reading of this book at all stages of development and for her love and boundless forbearance with me.

ADELAIDE HAAS

I wish to thank former and current members of the Department of Communication Disorders State University of New York at New Paltz; Anne Balant, Wendy Bower, Gretchen Brassard, Wendell Brooks, James Dembowski, Helen Hook, Patricia Mullins, Stella Turk, Sandy Vayo, Robert Volin, and Donald Wildy. They each offered assistance within their own areas of expertise. Professor Phillip Schneider of Queens College, City University of New York, remains a steady source of inspiration. Hong Lee dos Reis was helpful in defining sociolinguistic and multicultural issues. Professor Loek Helminck of North Carolina State University, Tony dos Reis and Linda Smith of SUNY New Paltz, and Joseph M. Haas and Carma Haas were consistently available to solve computer problems. Librarians and staff of the Sojourner Truth Library at SUNY New Paltz extended every courtesy to help me obtain needed source material. I am indebted to speech-language pathologist Nadine Rod, who permitted me to follow her in her work with clients with dysphagia, and to Cathy Augello, who shared information regarding her work with prescholers. Professor Emerita Susan L. Puretz and Michael Lecesse offered encouragement and insights at various stages of the project. Suggestions and recommendation from students in my classes who used the *first edition* as a text are incorporated in this *second edition*. Thanks go to SLPs Louisa Finn, Andrea Thompson, and John Trembley for arranging for tapes of their clients for the CD-ROM.

My beloved late husband Kurt, who enticed me to collaborate with him on a textbook many years ago and honed my writing skills, receives my special thanks. Our adult children Ruth and Joseph, both teachers themselves, listened, encouraged, and advised as I strove to make complex material accessible to introductory-level students.

The following reviewers of this edition diligently questioned chapter organization and content in conscientious detail and offered many fine suggestions for improving the manuscript. Their efforts are sincerely acknowledged: Ellyn Arwood, Brigham Young University; Jennifer E. Kent-Walsh, University of Central Florida; and Kenneth J. Logan, University of Florida.

Finally, we appreciate Steve Dragin's positive appraisal of our abilities and the energetic work of the entire Allyn and Bacon team that helped to make this book a reality.

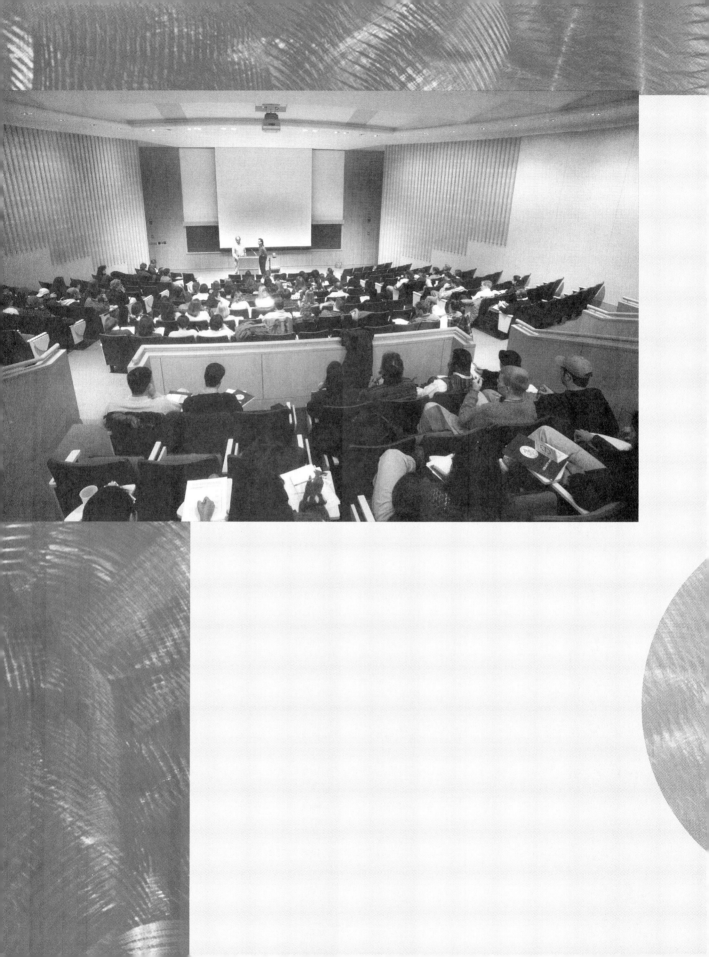

A Journey: From Student to Professional

1

CHAPTER
LEARNING
GOALS

When you have finished this chapter, you should be able to:

- Describe the roles of audiologists, speech-language pathologists, and speech, language, and hearing scientists

- Explain the process of going from student to professional in the field of communication disorders

- Identify the functions of the American Speech-Language-Hearing Association

- Outline the history of changing attitudes toward individuals with disabilities over the centuries and especially legislation over the past several decades

Can you imagine life without communication? No talking, no listening, no interacting with others? Communication is part of what makes us human. Even minor or temporary problems with communication, such as laryngitis, are often frustrating.

Many individuals who choose to study communication disorders have experienced a problem in speaking or listening at some time in their lives, or someone close to them is in this situation. Perhaps your impetus in reading this book is largely personal: to better understand yourself, a friend, or a relative. On the other hand, you may be embarking on a first step toward a possible career objective of becoming a speech-language pathologist or audiologist.

For all readers, we hope to offer some insights into the nature of **communication disorders**. In this first chapter, we take you on a journey from student to professional, outlining the steps for becoming an audiologist, speech-language pathologist, or speech scientist. We'll also explore other professional team members, where speech-language pathologists and audiologists work, and what they do.

You will learn about the various types of credentials that are needed in different employment settings and about the organizations through which professionals can address issues, learn, and advocate for the people they serve. This first chapter also provides a historical perspective and outlines the laws that mandate appropriate care for those in need. Along the way, we'll find out why people choose these careers.

HELPING OTHERS TO HELP THEMSELVES

Why do people decide to become speech-language pathologists or audiologists? It is mostly because of the satisfaction that they receive from helping others to live a fuller life. Box 1.1 contains excerpts from student applications to communication disorders programs. Many students cite a personal or family encounter with a communication disorder. Almost all write about a desire to be useful to society.

Box 1.1

Reasons for Selecting a Major in Communication Disorders

Students who applied to major in communication disorders were asked to write a brief essay explaining their motivation. Some excerpts from these essays follow:

Erika B.: When I was a little girl, I can painfully remember being picked on by the other children about the way I spoke. My once cute lisp was no longer cute at 8. I was told that "I talked like a baby" or sometimes the kids would mimic what I said in an exaggerated way. At age 10, my family moved to a new school district. A speech-language pathologist there worked with me on my lisp and other articulation problems. People who meet me today can hardly believe that I ever had a problem! I want to help people who are in similar situations. I know the

Box   1.1

(Continued)

hurt that accompanies the humiliation of being teased because you can't communicate properly.

Dana C.: One of my best friends was born with a complete bilateral cleft lip and palate. After thirteen operations and over nine years of speech therapy, a stranger would never know that my friend ever had a communication problem. I want to have the opportunity to help to make a similar difference in someone's life.

Victoria F.: All of her life, my cousin Jackie's family had been told that she had a common disfluency problem and that she would outgrow it. However, Jackie was a teenager and continued to be dysfluent. Finally Jackie's parents took her to a speech-language pathologist in private practice. The speech therapy resulted in transforming Jackie from a shy child with a reluctance to speak to a gregarious adolescent. At her Sweet 16 party, Jackie took the microphone and read her own speech of thanks and recognition and everyone cried. That's when I realized that I wanted to be a speech pathologist.

Tara F.: My interest in speech science began soon after I graduated from our local community college with a business degree. I knew this would result in a monotonous desk job, and I wanted my career path to take a different direction but I did not yet know what. That August my grandmother had quadruple heart bypass surgery and a stroke followed. I entered the world of speech science three days after she slipped into a semi-coma. When she awoke, she couldn't speak at all. I went to my library and checked out a book about strokes and read it cover to cover that night. I learned that even though she couldn't express herself through spoken word, she might be able to do so in writing, and she did. Each day was frustrating, but my grandmother improved and was soon able to grunt. From grunting, she moved to words like "No!" and she laughed aloud. Often words would come out, but they did not make sense. It was as though she was speaking a foreign language. She eventually recovered, but not fully. Although she regained her ability to speak, she speaks more slowly and more thought is required than before the stroke. My grandmother is the moti-

vation behind my anticipated speech pathology career choice.

Denise F.: I had always considered attending college after completing my high school education, but due to unfortunate financial circumstances at that time, I was unable to do so. I took a job with an insurance agency and through eighteen years of employment developed a satisfying career. About twelve years ago, at the age of 2, my oldest son was classified as Speech Impaired and Learning Disabled. He is now in the ninth grade and has made tremendous progress. He is mainstreamed for all subjects with only minimal Resource Room time. He is no longer classified as Speech Impaired. Although I tried to help him at home, I know my son would never have made the progress that he has without the professional services of special educators. I want the opportunity to provide these services and benefits to other families and their children.

Devon T.: My mother is hard-of-hearing. She has less than 50 percent hearing in each ear. Growing up was a little bit different because of this. I had to repeat myself most of the time while talking to her. I had to speak clearly, and most of all, I could not cover my mouth. My mother reads lips. Whenever the phone rings in my house, a lamp in my mother's room lights up. My mother bought her first hearing aid several years ago and cried all night. The only thing I could think of was how amazing that this little machine could help her hear better. I loved looking at it, and I admired my mother for overcoming her hardships and handicap.

John T.: I am a 40-year-old successful pastry chef. Since I have a family, a career change took lots of planning and the beginning of a dream being fulfilled. When my son was 3 years old, he still was only babbling. His doctor was wonderful, but from Korea and did not see any problems with Jimmy's speech. Since my wife and I were worried, we had Jimmy evaluated by a speech-language pathologist. He was diagnosed with language and articulation difficulties. We took him to the clinic at St. John's University. The therapy made a difference in my son's life. It also crystallized my desire to work with children in a helpful and meaningful way.

THE PROFESSIONALS

Opportunities for speech-language pathologists and audiologists include serving individuals of all ages from infancy through the aged with varied disorders, from mild to profound, in a wide assortment of settings.

Today, professionals who serve individuals with communication disorders come from several disciplines. They often refer clients to one another or work together to provide optimal care. Specialists in communication disorders are employed by preschools, schools, colleges and universities, hospitals, independent clinics, nursing care facilities, research laboratories, and home-based programs. Many are in private practice. Speech-language pathologists and audiologists receive similar basic training but in their advanced study concentrate on one profession or the other.

AUDIOLOGISTS

Audiologists are specialists who measure hearing ability and identify, assess, manage, and prevent disorders of hearing and balance. They use a variety of technologies to measure and appraise hearing in people from infancy through old age. In addition, audiologists evaluate and assist individuals with **central auditory processing disorders (CAPD)** and select, fit, and dispense hearing aids and other amplification devices and provide guidance in their care and use. They work within educational settings to improve communication and programming for people with hearing disabilities. Audiologists also contribute to the prevention of hearing loss by recommending and fitting protective devices and by consulting to government and industry on the effects and management of environmental noise. Licensed audiologists are independent professionals who practice without a prescription from any other health care provider (ASHA, 2001b). Box 1.2 contains an audiologist's comments on some of the challenges and rewards of the profession. As you will note, being a good detective, or problem solver, is one of the skills that is needed.

Box **1.2**

An Audiologist Reflects

Stella T.: I love the detective work of diagnostic procedures and the closure of rehab. I am given the clues from case history and my test findings. My job is to quickly and efficiently come up with an accurate diagnosis, recommendations, and rehabilitative plan. I have to be able to explain these in terms my patients can understand. I have to have completed all of this in less than one hour before moving on to save the rest of the world. I get closure by being able to measure the success of my rehabilitative plan within a relatively short span of time (a few weeks) and make adjustments in my plan as needed. I love making another person's life a little easier.

Credentials for Audiologists

At the present time, the entry-level requirement for audiologists is a master's degree. Prospective audiologists study hearing science, the assessment and remediation of hearing loss, anatomy and physiology, and related subjects and obtain supervised clinical experience (see Table 1.1: Steps to becoming a speech-language pathologist).

Beginning in the year 2012, individuals wishing to work as audiologists will need three to five years of education beyond the bachelor's degree. Their studies will culminate in a doctoral degree that may be an audiology doctorate (Au.D.), doctor of philosophy degree (Ph.D.), or doctor of education degree (Ed.D.). Preparation will include additional emphasis on hearing science and disorders, as well as assessment, treatment, and professional issues. The number of hours and types of settings used for preprofessional clinical experience will also increase.

After a person has earned either a master's degree (prior to 2012) or a doctorate (after 2012), obtained the required preprofessional as well as paid clinical experience, and passed a national examination, she or he is eligible for the Certificate of Clinical Competence in Audiology (CCC-A) awarded by the American Speech-Language-Hearing Association (ASHA). ASHA CCC-A (sometimes referred to as ASHA "Cs") is the generally accepted standard for most employment opportunities for audiologists. In addition, most states require audiologists to obtain a state license. The requirements tend to be the same or very similar to the ASHA standards (ASHA, 2001 b,c).

> Beginning in the year 2012, a doctorate degree will be required for professional employment as an audiologist.

SPEECH-LANGUAGE PATHOLOGISTS

Speech-language pathologists (SLPs) are professionals who provide an assortment of services that relate to communicative disorders. The distinguishing role of the SLP is to identify, assess, treat, and prevent communication disorders in all modalities (including spoken, written, pictorial, and manual) both receptively and expressively. This includes attention to physiological, cognitive, and social aspects of communication. Speech-language pathologists also provide services for disorders of swallowing and may work with individuals who choose to modify a regional or foreign dialect. Like audiologists, licensed speech-language pathologists are independent professionals who practice without a prescription from any other health care provider (ASHA, 2000a, b, c). Box 1.3 contains reflections by two speech-language pathologists; the first one has been in private practice as a clinician for about twenty-five years. Although sometimes frustrated by the lack of support within his work setting, he believes in setting his imagination free and not giving up in the challenge to help others. The other SLP notes the detective-like work and satisfaction of helping others.

Credentials for Speech-Language Pathologists

With technology, the task of the SLP is changing. The technology for digital speech recording and analysis are now readily available, as are new and exciting assistive technologies for those with great difficulty communicating

Table 1.1
Steps to becoming a speech-language pathologist

I. Graduate degree from a regionally accredited institution of higher education.

II. Completion of a program of study (a minimum of 75 semester credit hours overall, including at least 36 at the graduate level) that includes:

A. At least one course in each of the following areas: biological sciences, physical sciences, social/behavioral sciences, and mathematics.

B. Demonstrated knowledge of
1. Basic human communication and swallowing processes, including their biological, neurological, acoustic, psychological, developmental, and linguistic and cultural bases; and the ability to integrate information pertaining to normal and abnormal human development across the life span, including basic communication processes and the impact of cultural and linguistic diversity on communication.
2. The nature of speech, language, hearing, and communication disorders and differences and swallowing disorders, including the etiologies, characteristics, anatomical/ physiological, acoustic, psychological, developmental, linguistic, and cultural correlates. Specific knowledge must be demonstrated in articulation, fluency, voice and resonance including respiration and phonation, receptive and expressive language, hearing including the impact on speech and language, swallowing, cognitive and social aspects of communication, and communication modalities including augmentative and alternative communication techniques and assistive technologies.
3. The principles and methods of prevention, assessment, and intervention for people with communication and swallowing disorders, including consideration of anatomical/physiological, psychological, developmental, and linguistic and cultural correlates of the disorders.
4. Standards of ethical conduct.
5. Processes used in research and the integration of research principles into evidence-based clinical practice.
6. Contemporary professional issues.
7. Certification, specialty recognition, licensure, and other relevant professional credentials.

III. Completion of a curriculum of academic and clinical education that follows an appropriate sequence of learning including:

A. Supervised clinical experiences sufficient in breadth and depth to achieve the following skills outcomes:
1. Evaluation:
   a. Conduct screening and prevention procedures (including prevention activities)
   b. Collect case history information and integrate information
   c. Select and administer appropriate evaluation procedures
   d. Adapt evaluation procedures to meet client/patient needs
   e. Interpret, integrate, and synthesize all information to develop diagnoses and make appropriate recommendations for intervention

Table 1.1
(Continued)

        f. Complete administrative and reporting functions

        g. Refer clients/patients for appropriate services

   2. Intervention:

        a. Develop setting-appropriate intervention plans with measurable and achievable goals that meet clients'/patients' needs

        b. Implement intervention plans

        c. Select or develop and use appropriate materials and instrumentation for prevention and intervention

        d. Measure and evaluate clients'/patients' performance and progress

        e. Modify intervention plans, strategies, materials, or instrumentation as appropriate to meet the needs of clients/patients

        f. Complete administrative and reporting functions necessary to support intervention

        g. Identify and refer clients/patients for services as appropriate

   3. Interaction and personal qualities:

        a. Communicate effectively, recognizing the needs, values, preferred mode of communication, and cultural/linguistic background of the client/patient, family, caregivers, and relevant others

        b. Collaborate with other professionals in case management

        c. Provide counseling regarding communication and swallowing disorders

        d. Adhere to the ASHA Code of Ethics and behave professionally

        e. Demonstrate skill in oral and written or other forms of communication sufficient for entry into professional practice.

  B. A minimum of 400 clock hours of supervised clinical experience in the practice of speech-language pathology. Twenty-five hours must be spent in clinical observation, and 375 hours must be spent in direct client/patient contact. At least 325 of the 400 clock hours must be completed while the applicant is engaged in graduate study.

  C. Supervision must be provided by individuals who hold the Certificate of Clinical Competence in the appropriate area of practice. No less than 25 percent of the student's total contact with each client/patient and must take place periodically throughout the practicum.

  D. Supervised practicum must include experience with client/patient populations through the lifespan and from culturally/linguistically diverse backgrounds and with various types and severities of communication and/or related disorders, differences, and disabilities.

IV. Passing the national examination adopted by ASHA for purposes of certification in speech-language pathology.

VI. Successful completion a Speech-Language Pathology Clinical Fellowship (SLPCF), consisting of the equivalent of 36 weeks of full-time clinical practice. The mentoring speech-language pathologist and Clinical Fellow will establish outcomes and performance levels to be achieved and engage in periodic assessment.

Box   **1.3**

Two Speech-Language Pathologists Reflect

Phillip S.: Gladys was 12 when I met her. She had NO voice, no laugh, no cry, no moan, no words, and no song. The administrators of the school for multiply handicapped children said not to work with her because she could not be helped—after all, she had no voice. Why? Why no voice? Why no way to help? Why such pessimism? Against the will of the institution, we began to explore, and she sang in the school show five months later. It was not until the following fall that she began to speak normally, as though she had been doing it all her life. It was experiencing the birth of Gladys's voice that sent me back to school for my doctoral studies. Was this a miracle? I guess a miracle is when something is possible, and does happen, but it was beyond your imagination. In our work we must first see something that is not yet there and believe in it long enough to become a partner in making it come about.

Robert O.: For me, the exciting part of my job is the problem solving and the satisfaction of helping others. Similar to a fictional detective who collects all the clues, synthesizes the information, and deduces the guilty party, I evaluate each client and determine the best course of intervention. The more severe the impairment, the greater the challenge, and I love a challenge. How can I help a young man who attempted suicide and is now brain injured to access the language within him? How can a young child with autism begin the road through communication to language? How can I help parents communicate with their infant who has deafness, blindness, and cerebral palsy? When is the best time to introduce signing with a nonspeaking client? These are all challenges for me and the children and adults I serve. We work together as I try to solve each communication puzzle and propose and implement possible intervention strategies. Sometimes I'm very successful and sometimes I have to reevaluate my methods, but as I said, I love a challenge.

via speech (Ingram, Bunta, & Ingram, 2004). Speech-language pathologists have a master's or doctoral degree and have studied typical communication and swallowing development; anatomy and physiology of the speech, swallowing, and hearing mechanisms; phonetics; speech and hearing science; and disorders of speech, language, and swallowing.

Three types of credentials are available for speech-language pathologists:

1. Public school certification normally stipulates basic and advanced coursework, clinical practice within a school setting, and a satisfactory score on a state or national examination. At the least, prospective school SLPs need a bachelor's degree, although in most states, a master's degree either is the entry-level requirement or is mandated after a certain number of years of employment. The exact requirements to become a school SLP vary from state to state. The American Speech-Language-Hearing Association encourages the same standards for SLPs in all employment settings, as described in the following paragraph.

2. The American Speech-Language-Hearing Association issues a Certificate of Clinical Competence in Speech-Language Pathology (CCC-SLP) to individuals who have obtained a master's degree or doctorate in the field with at least 25 hours of clinical observation and 375 clock hours of supervised clinical practicum. In addition, certificate

holders must have a year of paid professional experience and have passed a national examination. Ongoing professional development must be demonstrated through any of a variety of continuing education options (ASHA, 2000a). As of 2004, the United States, United Kingdom, Australia, and Canada allow mutual recognition of certification in speech-language pathology (Boswell, 2004).

3. Many states have licensure laws for speech-language pathologists, audiologists, and other professionals that are independent of the state's department of education school certification requirements. A license might be needed if you plan to engage in private practice or work in a hospital, clinic, or other setting apart from a public school. Most states accept a person with ASHA CCC-SLP as having met licensure requirements, although you will need to check with your state licensing board on the specifics.

Table 1.2 shows the credentials that are needed in the professions of audiology and speech-language pathology.

The professions of speech-language pathology and audiology require lifelong learning. Clinicians need to be able to intelligently use relevant research findings in their practice.

SPEECH, LANGUAGE, AND HEARING SCIENTISTS

Individuals who are employed as speech, language, or hearing scientists typically have earned a doctorate degree, either a Ph.D. or an Ed.D. They are employed by universities, government agencies, industry, and research centers to extend our knowledge of human communication processes and disorders. Some may also serve as clinical speech-language pathologists or audiologists.

What Speech, Language, and Hearing Scientists Do

Speech scientists may be involved in basic research exploring the anatomy, physiology, and physics of speech-sound production. Using various tech-

Table 1.2
Credentials for speech-language pathologists and audiologists

Credentialing Organization	Speech-Language Pathologist	Audiologist
American Speech-Language-Hearing Association	Certificate of Clinical Competence in Speech-Language Pathology (CCC-SLP)	Certificate of Clinical Competence in Audiology (CCC-A)
State department of education	Certification as Teacher of Students with Speech and Language Disabilities*	–
State professional licensing board	License as Speech-Language Pathologist	License as Audiologist

*The title for the school-based speech-language pathologist varies from state to state.

nologies, these researchers strive to learn more about typical and pathological voice and articulation. Their findings help clinicians to improve service to clients with speech disorders. Recent advances in knowledge of human genetics provide fertile soil for continuing investigation into the causes, prevention, and treatment of various speech impairments. Some speech scientists are involved in the development of computer-generated speech that may be used in telephone answering systems, substitute voices for individuals who are unable to speak, and many new purposes. Box 1.4 contains some observations by a speech-language scientist who enjoys the interdisciplinary nature of his work. His current research involves the study of tongue placement in the production of speech sounds.

Language scientists, also called **linguists,** may investigate the ways in which children learn their native tongue. They may study the differences and similarities of different languages. Over the past half a century or so, the United States has become increasingly linguistically and culturally diverse; this provides an excellent opportunity for cross-cultural study of language and communication. Some language scientists explore the variations of modern-day English (dialects) and how the language is changing. Others are concerned with language disabilities and study the nature of language disorders in children and adults. An in-depth knowledge of typical language is critical to understanding language problems.

THOUGHT QUESTION

W hat language and cultural groups were represented in your elementary and high school? Were issues regarding bilingualism or cultural diversity raised? What important research might a language scientist conduct in this environment?

Box **1.4**

A Speech-Language Scientist Reflects

James D.: What I like best about speech-language science is the way it combines disciplines. When I was in high school, my favorite subjects were English and biology. Studying speech-language science is like studying English and biology at the same time. To be a good speech-language scientist, or a good speech-language pathologist, or a good neurolinguist, you have to know about BOTH language and physiology. It is not enough to be just a linguist or just a physiologist. And you have to know how these two things, one primarily a product of the "mind" (however one chooses to define that) and the other a function of the body, interact. Furthermore, the physiology of speech and language encompasses a broad range of

bodily systems, including the neurologic, respiratory, laryngologic (or phonatory), and upper vocal tract articulatory. As if that wasn't enough in itself, you must know something about the physics of sound to really understand speech and its production. If you choose to explore speech modeling or have a clinical interest in augmentative communication systems, you could even touch on areas that we normally think of as associated with engineering. Thus, the study of speech-language science is a truly interdisciplinary study, in any number of ways. In that respect, it is a continual challenge, intellectually, and provides an opportunity to interact with a tremendously broad range of other professionals.

Hearing scientists investigate the nature of sound, noise, and hearing. They may work with other scientists in the development of equipment to be used in the assessment of hearing. They are also involved in the development of techniques for testing the hard-to-test, such as infants or those with severe physical or psychological impairments. Hearing scientists develop and improve assistive listening devices such as hearing aids and telephone amplifiers to help people who have limited hearing. In addition, hearing scientists are concerned with conservation of hearing and are engaged in research to measure and limit the impact of environmental noise.

> Paraprofessionals usually have an associate's or bachelor's degree; they work closely with and are supervised by professionals with more training and experience.

Professional Aides

Professional aides, sometimes referred to as paraprofessionals or speech-language pathology or audiology assistants, are individuals who work closely with SLPs or audiologists. The title, educational requirements, and responsibilities of these individuals vary from state to state.

Speech-language pathology assistants (SLPAs) typically participate in screenings. They often engage in routine therapy tasks that have been structured by an SLP. They may engage in clerical tasks and assist the SLP in the preparation of assessment and treatment materials. SLPAs may work in any of the settings in which a fully credentialed SLP is found. Audiology assistants may conduct screenings, participate in calibration of audiological instrumentation, and engage in a variety of clerical tasks.

Support personnel may work only with supervision and are not permitted to perform such tasks as interpretation of test results, service plan development, family/client counseling, or determination of when to discharge a client from treatment (ASHA, 1995b; Paul-Brown & Goldberg, 2001).

RELATED PROFESSIONS: A TEAM APPROACH

Specialists in communication disorders do not operate in a vacuum. They work closely with family members, regular and special educators, psychologists, social workers, doctors and other medical personnel, occupational, physical, and music therapists. They may collaborate with physicists and engineers. Box 1.5 contains a speech-language pathologist's schedule, showing a tremendous amount of teamwork.

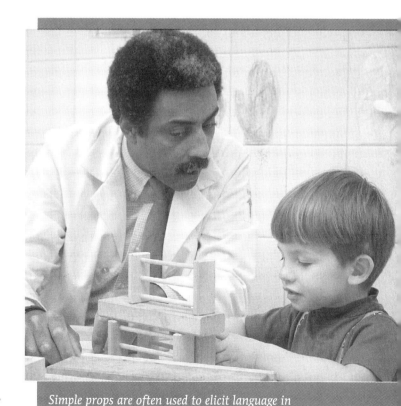

Simple props are often used to elicit language in a nonthreatening way.

Box **1.5**

A Team Approach

Alicia is the senior speech-language pathologist in a community-based rehabilitation center in New York state. During the mornings, Alicia works with infants, preschoolers, and school-age children at the center. In the afternoons, she directs the Augmentative/Alternative Communication Program and assists severely impaired individuals of all ages to improve their communication abilities. The schedule outlined below has a bit more collaboration than is normally found in any one day, but it suggests the kinds of activities that are typical within a workweek.

8:30 A.M.	Education staff meeting for preschool children: classroom teacher, psychologist, social worker, occupational therapist, physical therapist.
9:00	Preschool class activity: eight children ages 3–4, one classroom teacher, two aides.
10:00	Individual half-hour therapy sessions with children in the preschool and school programs.
11:30	Combined physical and speech therapy for Jeramy, age 4, diagnosed with spastic cerebral palsy; work with physical therapist.
noon	Lunch
12:30 P.M.	Prepare for the afternoon.
1:00	Consult with engineer on wheelchair switch for Lucretia, age 7, who is multiply handicapped.
1:30	Outpatient, David, aged 24, had been in a motorcycle accident and experiences some speech and language difficulties.
3:00	Conference with Sally Brown, Bettina's foster mother, and Barbara Sloane, the social worker for the family.
3:30	Communication Disorders Department Meeting. Malcolm, an audiologist, reports on three-hour course he took on Saturday on cochlear implants.
4:30	The workday is officially over, but Alicia stays until 5:00 to read the professional journal *Language, Speech, and Hearing Services in the Schools*, which arrived today. Alicia is especially interested in the article about using children's books in working with preschoolers and photocopies it to share with other staff members.

SERVICE THROUGH THE LIFESPAN

Individuals with communication disorders may be of any age, and professionals address their needs from birth through old age. Infants may be screened for hearing loss and a host of other disabilities soon after birth. About 2 percent of all children born in the United States have some disabling condition, and hearing loss occurs more often than any other physical problem (U.S. Census Bureau, 1997). Babies and toddlers may exhibit developmental delay and mental retardation. They may have physical problems including those involving movement, hearing, and vision. These disabilities may be due to a wide range of causes, discussed later in this text, and may impact the youngster's communication and feeding abilities. An interdisciplinary approach is necessary in the assessment and treatment of young children, and an Individualized Family Service Plan (IFSP), developed for each child treated, must be directed at the entire family with sensitivity to its language and culture. Early intervention has been demonstrated to be highly valuable in facilitating optimum results and potentially preventing later difficulties.

Preschoolers with communication difficulties must also be identified and helped. For some, services begun earlier may now be handled by different agencies. The youngster may be placed in a special preschool; professionals may continue to assist the family in addressing the child's needs.

Almost half of all speech-language pathologists are employed by school systems. They work with youngsters in all grades, addressing a full range of communication and swallowing problems. These are described in the chapters that follow. School-age children with communication difficulties often also suffer academically and socially, thereby adding additional urgency to the work of communication experts.

Some young adults such as those who were identified earlier as being developmentally delayed or with physical disabilities may continue to receive certain services until they are 21 years old. At this point some of these women and men may enter day-treatment programs, and/or find employment in workshops where speech-language pathologists and audiologists may be available to serve their needs.

Other individuals may find themselves in need of communication services for the first time later in life. More than 5 million Americans are reported to have suffered traumatic brain injury (see Chapters 5 and 7) stemming from bicycle, motorcycle, or car accidents or from falls. As a result, they may have cognitive and/or motor problems that interfere with their ability to communicate and/or eat normally. The speech-language pathologist may play an important role in rehabilitative efforts.

Among those over age 65, stroke, neurological disorders, and dementia may interfere with effective communication and swallowing. Hearing loss may affect at least one in four, creating a need for assessment and treatment. Speech-language pathologists and audiologists work directly with older people. They often also work with spouses and children, as well as staff members of nursing homes and other adult facilities in providing counseling and guidance directed at improving quality of life in these later years (Lubinski & Masters, 2001)

PROFESSIONAL ORGANIZATIONS

AMERICAN SPEECH-LANGUAGE-HEARING ASSOCIATION

The American Speech-Language-Hearing Association (ASHA) is a nonprofit organization of speech-language pathologists, audiologists, and speech and hearing scientists that was founded in 1925. In 2005, it had 115,000 members and affiliates from throughout the United States and the world. It is the largest association for those concerned with communication disorders. ASHA's mission is to "promote the interests of and provide the highest quality services for professionals in audiology, speech-language pathology, and speech hearing science, and to advocate for people with communication disorders" (ASHA, 2002). Toward these ends, ASHA promotes scientific study, encourages quality clinical services, supports high ethical principles, and advocates for those with communicative disorders.

Scientific Study of the Processes and Disorders of Human Communication

ASHA encourages study of typical and disordered communication by mandating a curriculum of study for prospective speech-language pathologists and audiologists. This is outlined in Table 1.1. In addition, ASHA provides financial grants to individuals who are engaged in research that furthers our knowledge of communication and assessment, treatment, and prevention of pathologies. ASHA works closely with governmental agencies that may sponsor relevant scientific investigation.

Students who join the National Student Speech-Language-Hearing Association (NSSLH) receive professional journals, attend conferences at reduced rates, and pay less for their initial ASHA certification and membership.

To dispense knowledge among professionals, ASHA publishes several scholarly periodicals: *Journal of Speech, Language, and Hearing Research; Language, Speech, and Hearing Services in Schools; American Journal of Speech-Language Pathology: A Journal of Clinical Practice;* and *American Journal of Audiology: A Journal of Clinical Practice*. ASHA also holds an annual convention at which members and others share information and learn through scientific sessions, exhibits, seminars, and short courses. Additional institutes, workshops, conferences, and teleseminars are held throughout the year. Continuing education for professionals is fostered through these activities.

Clinical Service in Speech-Language Pathology and Audiology

Programs that provide clinical services to people with communicative disorders may be accredited by ASHA. This means that representatives of ASHA will review the procedures that are used in diagnosis and treatment. A site visit will ensure that equipment, materials, and record keeping adhere to the highest professional standards. Clinical service will be the responsibility of individuals who meet ASHA standards for the CCC-SLP or CCC-A (see Table 1.1).

Maintenance of Ethical Standards

To ensure that the highest moral and ethical principles are followed within the professions of speech-language pathology and audiology, ASHA provides a code of ethics, which is in the appendix to this chapter. The basic principles are as follows:

Ethical questions pervade our lives as individuals and professionals. At all times, it is up to each individual to know the code of ethics and to seek consultation in assuring adherence to the highest possible standards.

1. The welfare of the persons served by communication disorders specialists is paramount.

2. Each professional must achieve and maintain the highest level of professional competence. The ASHA Certificates of Clinical Competence (CCC) are considered the minimal achievement for independent professional practice. Clinicians should provide service only within their own areas of competence. Professional development and continuing education should be ongoing. New technology requires that speech-language pathologists and audiologists continually update their skills so as to safely and accurately address patient needs.

3. Professionals must promote understanding and provide accurate information in statements to the public.

4. Professionals are responsible for assuring that ethical standards are maintained by themselves, colleagues, students, and members of allied professions. All members of ASHA are responsible for the monitoring and maintaining of ethical standards throughout the profession (ASHA, 2001a).

Why must clinical supervisors consider the welfare of their clients of primary importance? Does this impinge on student learning?

THOUGHT QUESTION

Advocacy for Individuals with Communicative Disabilities

The American Speech-Language-Hearing Association is active in encouraging members of Congress and state legislatures to pass legislation that provides for appropriate services for communication-impaired individuals. Bills such as the Individuals with Disabilities Education Act and the Americans with Disabilities Act became law in part because of the extensive promotional activities of organizations such as ASHA.

The needs and characteristics of people with speech, language, and hearing disabilities are clarified and publicized by ASHA on radio, on television, and through print media. In May, which is "Better Speech and Hearing Month," you are especially likely to hear public service announcements that advocate for understanding, prevention, and treatment of communication disorders.

RELATED PROFESSIONAL ASSOCIATIONS

Although ASHA is the largest organization for communication disorder professionals, other groups are also active and worthwhile. Some speech-language pathologists and audiologists belong to several associations. Table 1.3

Table 1.3

Selected professional associations relevant to communication disorders

Academy of Dispensing Audiologists	American Auditory Society	National Hearing Conservation Association
Academy of Rehabilitative Audiology	American Speech-Language-Hearing Association	National Student Speech-Language-Hearing Association
American Academy of Audiology	Audiology Foundation of America	Orton Dyslexia Society
American Academy of Otolaryngology–Head and Neck Surgery	Canadian Association of Speech-Language Pathologists	Stuttering Foundation of America
	Council on Education of the Deaf	

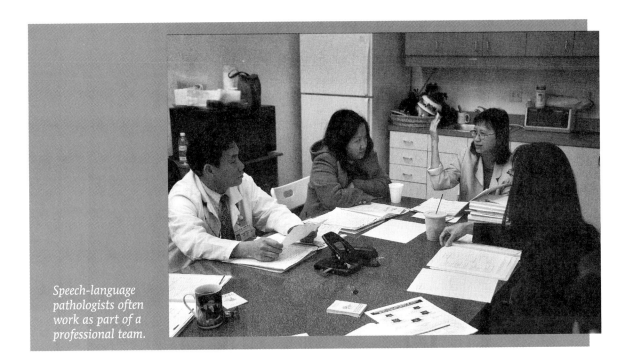

Speech-language pathologists often work as part of a professional team.

lists some of those most closely affiliated. Prospective speech-language pathologists and audiologists are advised to take courses in biology, psychology, and sociology in order to better understand their clients and to work more effectively with professionals from other disciplines.

COMMUNICATION DISORDERS IN HISTORICAL PERSPECTIVE

Handicaps of any type were viewed harshly by early humans. Society was built on a survival-of-the-fittest mentality, and less able individuals were shunned. Children who were malformed were often abandoned, and the aged who could no longer contribute were sometimes abandoned, deprived of food, or even killed.

Over the centuries attitudes changed somewhat and by the late 1700s in some parts of the world, societal efforts were being made to help those who were unable to care for themselves. Individuals began to be classified and grouped according to their disorder. Special residences for individuals with deafness, blindness, mental illness, and intellectual limitations were established, although most were little more than warehouses providing no services other than what was necessary to keep the residents alive (Karagiannis, Stainback, & Stainback, 1996).

The first U.S. "speech correctionists" were educators and others in the helping or medical professions who took an interest in speech problems (Duchan, 2002). These were accompanied by a few "quacks" who promised curing therapies or drugs. The more legitimate therapists came from already established professions. Among them were Alexander Melville Bell and his father, Alexander Graham Bell, of telephone fame. Other Americans trained with famous "speech doctors" in Germany and Austria or became interested in speech correction because of their own difficulties, often with stuttering. The first professional journal, *The Voice*, appeared in 1879 and focused primarily on stuttering research and intervention.

Early interest groups were formed primarily among teachers within the National Education Association and among physicians and academics belonged to the National Association of Teachers of Speech. The latter group formed the American Academy of Speech Correction in 1925, a precursor to the ASHA, and attempted to promote scientific inquiry and to set standards for training and practice. ASHA has had varying names over the years, finally settling on the American Speech-Language-Hearing Association in 1978.

The profession of audiology originated in the 1920s when *audiometers* were first designed for measuring hearing. Interest surged in the 1940s when returning World War II veterans exhibited noise-induced hearing loss due to gunfire or to prolonged and unprotected exposure to noise. Others had psychogenic hearing loss as a result of trauma. The Veterans Administration provided hearing testing and rehabilitation.

Gradually, ASHA was able to establish professional and educational standards and to advocate for the rights of individuals with disabilities. During the 1960s in the United States and elsewhere, intense energy was directed toward the advancement of civil rights for all people. Just as the rights of women, ethnic minorities, gays, and lesbians have been and are being recast, the status of individuals with disabilities has been reevaluated, and bold reforms initiated. The American Coalition of Citizens with Disabilities was created in 1974; legislative action on behalf of all Americans with handicapping conditions began in earnest around the same time. In many cases, people with disabilities occupied leadership roles in the push for change. As a result of this work, providing opportunities for individuals with disabilities to develop to their full potential was no longer simply an ethical position. It became federally mandated through a series of laws.

Congress enacted the Education for All Handicapped Children Act (EAHCA) as Public Law Number 94-142 in 1975. It mandated that a free and appropriate public education must be provided for all handicapped children between the ages of 5 and 21. Several years later, Public Law 99-457 extended the age of those served to cover youngsters between the ages of birth and 5. In 1990, Congress reauthorized the original law and renamed it the Individuals with Disabilities Education Act (IDEA). IDEA addressed the multicultural nature of U.S. society. The needs of individuals with limited English proficiency and those from racial and ethnic minorities were targeted for special consideration. Reauthorized in 2004, IDEA established birth-to-six programs and established new early intervention services. ASHA has been a vital advocacy agency throughout this long legislative process. Table 1.4 summarizes major federal legislation that has implications for individuals with communication disorders.

A series of laws passed by the United States Congress over the past fifty years mandate appropriate treatment for individuals with disabilities.

Table 1.4

It's the law: Major provisions of important federal legislation affecting people with communicative disabilities

1965: *Elementary and Secondary Education Act (Public Law 89-10)*
- States were provided federal funds so that students with special needs, including the gifted, would be evaluated and educated.

1966: *Handicapped Children's Early Education Act (Public Law 90-247)*
- Model programs for educating children with disabilities were federally funded.

1973: *Section 504 of the Vocational Rehabilitation Act (Public Law 93-112)*
- Forbids discrimination of services or employment to people with disabling conditions.

1975: *Education of All Handicapped Children Act (EAHCA) (Public Law 94-142)*
- All school-age children with disabilities must be provided a free, appropriate public education in the least restrictive environment.
- All related services (including speech-language therapy, physical therapy, and occupational therapy) that are needed for the child to benefit from the education must be provided.
- To benefit from this law, children must be evaluated and found to have a disabling condition as defined in the law.
- An Individual Education Plan (IEP) must be written for each child and must stipulate:
  Present level of performance
  Annual long-term goals and short-term objectives
  Designated instruction, services, and placement
  Date services are to be initiated and anticipated duration of services
- A Committee on Special Education (CSE) composed of the child's parents (or person designated by them), school administrator, and relevant educators and teachers must meet to review and endorse the IEP.
- Parents must agree to the initial evaluation in writing and approve and sign the IEP.
- The IEP must be reviewed each year.

1986: *Education of the Handicapped Amendments (Public Law 99-457)*
- Federal funds were provided to states that want

to develop programs for disabled infants and toddlers from birth through age 2.

1986: *Education of the Handicapped Amendments (continued)*
- The provisions of P.L. 94-142 were extended to disabled children between the ages of 3 and 5 years.
- Services must be provided by qualified personnel who meet the criteria for licensure stipulated by the state. (The intent was to end the double standard with one set of requirements needed to provide services in a school setting and another set needed to work in hospitals or private agencies.)
- An Individualized Family Service Plan (IFSP) must be written for each child with special needs that may include home-based instruction and therapy and parent education.

1988: *Technology-Related Assistance for Individuals with Disabilities (Public Law 100-407)*
- Included funding for centers to serve children and adults who may benefit from augmentative and alternative communication (AAC).
- Additional technological support became available.

1990: *Individuals with Disabilities Education Act (IDEA)*
- Reauthorized and renamed the 1975 EAHCA.
- Recognized and made provisions for increasing diversity of U.S. population.

1990: *Americans with Disabilities Act (ADA) (Public Law 101-336)*
- Mandated improved access to buildings and facilities that provide goods or services to the public through provision of ramps, parking facilities.
- Mandated accessible rest rooms.
- Provided for effective communication with people with disabilities, including use of interpreters, appropriate signage; and telecommunication devices for the deaf (TDDs).
- Included reasonable modifications of policies and practices that may be discriminatory.

Sources: Rosenfeld (1999), U.S. Department of Justice (2000), Zantal-Wiener (1988).

SUMMARY

Speech-language pathologists, audiologists, and other specialists work together to assist those with communicative impairments. They work in a variety of settings and with people of all ages. They are rewarded by contributing to the well-being of others. Professionals who are engaged in clinical service for those with communication disorders have a minimum of a master's degree and supervised clinical experience. They generally have earned the American Speech-Language-Hearing Association Certificate of Clinical Competence (ASHA-CCC) in their area of specialization.

Services are provided to individuals from birth through old age. The American Speech-Language-Hearing Association (ASHA) is the largest organization of professionals working with communication disorders. ASHA's missions include the scientific study of human communication, provision of clinical service in speech-language pathology and audiology, maintenance of ethical standards, and advocacy for individuals with communication disabilities. As a result, federal legislation currently mandates services for people with disabilities.

REFLECTIONS

- What do speech-language pathologists and audiologists do?
- What do speech, language, and hearing scientists do?
- What are the requirements for becoming a professional in the fields of communicative disorders?
- What services might be needed for individuals at different ages?
- What are the missions of the American Speech-Language-Hearing Association?
- How have attitudes toward people with disabilities changed through the centuries?

SUGGESTED READINGS

Nicolosi, L., Harryman, E., & Kresheck, J. (1996). *Terminology of communication disorders: Speech, language, hearing* (4th ed.). Baltimore: Williams & Wilkins.

Nolan, C. (1987). *Under the eye of the clock: The life story of Christopher Nolan.* New York: St. Martin's Press.

Peterson's Guides. (Ed.). (2000). *Peterson's graduate & professional programs 2001: An overview.* Princeton, NJ: Peterson's (published annually).

Singh, S. (Ed.). (2000). *Singular's illustrated dictionary of speech-language pathology.* San Diego: Singular.

ⓞNLINE RESOURCES

http://www.acoustics.org/   Acoustical Society of America.
Of special interest to hearing scientists and audiologists.

http://www.audiology.org/   American Academy of Audiology.
Consumer and professional information regarding hearing and balance disorders as well as audiological services.

http://professional.asha.org/   American Speech-Language-Hearing Association.
Information for professionals, students, and others who are interested in careers in speech-language pathology, audiology, or speech, language, or hearing science.

http://nidcd.nih.gov/   National Institute on Deafness and Other Communication Disorders (NIDCD).
The U.S. governmental agency site containing relevant health and research information.

http://iiswinprd01.petersons.com/   Peterson's Guide to Graduate and Professional Education.
Links to a list and descriptions of institutions offering programs in communication disorders.

Code of Ethics

Last Revised January 1, 2003

PREAMBLE

The preservation of the highest standards of integrity and ethical principles is vital to the responsible discharge of obligations by speech-language pathologists, audiologists, and speech, language, and hearing scientists. This Code of Ethics sets forth the fundamental principles and rules considered essential to this purpose.

Every individual who is (a) a member of the American Speech-Language-Hearing Association, whether certified or not, (b) a nonmember holding the Certificate of Clinical Competence from the Association, (c) an applicant for membership or certification, or (d) a Clinical Fellow seeking to fulfill standards for certification shall abide by this Code of Ethics.

Any violation of the spirit and purpose of this Code shall be considered unethical. Failure to specify any particular responsibility or practice in this Code of Ethics shall not be construed as denial of the existence of such responsibilities or practices.

The fundamentals of ethical conduct are described by Principles of Ethics and by Rules of Ethics as they relate to the conduct of research and scholarly activities and responsibility to persons served, the public, and speech-language pathologists, audiologists, and speech, language, and hearing scientists.

Principles of Ethics, aspirational and inspirational in nature, form the underlying moral basis for the Code of Ethics. Individuals shall observe these principles as affirmative obligations under all conditions of professional activity.

Rules of Ethics are specific statements of minimally acceptable professional conduct or of prohibitions and are applicable to all individuals.

PRINCIPLE OF ETHICS I

Individuals shall honor their responsibility to hold paramount the welfare of persons they serve professionally or participants in research and scholarly activities and shall treat animals involved in research in a humane manner.

Rules of Ethics

A. Individuals shall provide all services competently.

B. Individuals shall use every resource, including referral when appropriate, to ensure that high-quality service is provided.

C. Individuals shall not discriminate in the delivery of professional services or the conduct of research and scholarly activities on the basis of race or ethnicity, gender, age, religion, national origin, sexual orientation, or disability.

D. Individuals shall not misrepresent the credentials of assistants, technicians, or support personnel and shall inform those they serve professionally of the name and professional credentials of persons providing services.

E. Individuals who hold the Certificates of Clinical Competence shall not delegate tasks that require the unique skills, knowledge, and judgment that are within the scope of their

Source: American Speech-Language-Hearing Association. (2001a, December 26) Code of ethics (revised). *ASHA Leader*, 6(23), p. 2.

profession to assistants, technicians, support personnel, students, or any nonprofessionals over whom they have supervisory responsibility. An individual may delegate support services to assistants, technicians, support personnel, students, or any other persons only if those services are adequately supervised by an individual who holds the appropriate Certificate of Clinical Competence.

F. Individuals shall fully inform the person they serve of the nature and possible effects of services rendered and products dispensed, and they shall inform participants in research about the possible effects of their participation in research conducted.

G. Individuals shall evaluate the effectiveness of services rendered and of products dispensed and shall provide services or dispense products only when benefit can reasonably be expected.

H. Individuals shall not guarantee the results of any treatment or procedure, directly or by implication; however, they may make a reasonable statement of prognosis.

I. Individuals shall not provide clinical services solely by correspondence.

J. Individuals may practice by telecommunication (for example, telehealth/e-health), where not prohibited by law.

K. Individuals shall adequately maintain and appropriately secure records of professional services rendered, research and scholarly activities conducted, and products dispensed and shall allow access to these records only when authorized or when required by law.

L. Individuals shall not reveal, without authorization, any professional or personal information about identified persons served professionally or identified participants involved in research and scholarly activities unless required by law to do so, or unless doing so is necessary to protect the welfare of the person or of the community or otherwise required by law.

M. Individuals shall not charge for services not rendered, nor shall they misrepresent services rendered, products dispensed, or research and scholarly activities conducted.

N. Individuals shall use persons in research or as subjects of teaching demonstrations only with their informed consent.

O. Individuals whose professional services are adversely affected by substance abuse or other health-related conditions shall seek professional assistance and, where appropriate, withdraw from the affected areas of practice.

PRINCIPLE OF ETHICS II

Individuals shall honor their responsibility to achieve and maintain the highest level of professional competence.

Rules of Ethics

A. Individuals shall engage in the provision of clinical services only when they hold the appropriate Certificate of Clinical Competence or when they are in the certification process and are supervised by an individual who holds the appropriate Certificate of Clinical Competence.

B. Individuals shall engage in only those aspects of the professions that are within the scope of their competence, considering their level of education, training, and experience.

C. Individuals shall continue their professional development throughout their careers.

D. Individuals shall delegate the provision of clinical services only to: (1) persons who hold the appropriate Certificate of Clinical Competence; (2) persons in the education or certification process who are appropriately supervised by an individual who holds the appropriate Certificate of Clinical Competence; or (3) assistants, technicians, or support personnel who are adequately supervised by an individual who holds the appropriate Certificate of Clinical Competence.

E. Individuals shall not require or permit their professional staff to provide services or conduct research activities that exceed the staff member's competence, level of education, training, and experience.

F. Individuals shall ensure that all equipment used in the provision of services or to conduct research and scholarly activities is in proper working order and is properly calibrated.

PRINCIPLE OF ETHICS III

Individuals shall honor their responsibility to the public by promoting public understanding of the professions, by supporting the development of services designed to fulfill the unmet needs of the public, and by providing accurate information in all communications involving any aspect of the professions, including dissemination of research findings and scholarly activities.

Rules of Ethics

A. Individuals shall not misrepresent their credentials, competence, education, training, experience, or scholarly or research contributions.

B. Individuals shall not participate in professional activities that constitute a conflict of interest.

C. Individuals shall refer those served professionally solely on the basis of the interest of those being referred and not on any personal financial interest.

D. Individuals shall not misrepresent diagnostic information, research, services rendered, or products dispensed; neither shall they engage in any scheme to defraud in connection with obtaining payment or reimbursement for such services or products.

E. Individuals' statements to the public shall provide accurate information about the nature and management of communication disorders, about the professions, about professional services, and about research and scholarly activities.

F. Individuals' statements to the public—advertising, announcing, and marketing their professional services, reporting research results, and promoting products—shall adhere to prevailing professional standards and shall not contain misrepresentations.

PRINCIPLE OF ETHICS IV

Individuals shall honor their responsibilities to the professions and their relationships with colleagues, students, and members of allied professions. Individuals shall uphold the dignity and autonomy of the professions, maintain harmonious interprofessional and intraprofessional relationships, and accept the professions' self-imposed standards.

Rules of Ethics

A. Individuals shall prohibit anyone under their supervision from engaging in any practice that violates the Code of Ethics.

B. Individuals shall not engage in dishonesty, fraud, deceit, misrepresentation, sexual harassment, or any other form of conduct that adversely reflects on the professions or on the individual's fitness to serve persons professionally.

C. Individuals shall not engage in sexual activities with clients or students over whom they exercise professional authority.

D. Individuals shall assign credit only to those who have contributed to a publication, presentation, or product. Credit shall be assigned in proportion to the contribution and only with the contributor's consent.

E. Individuals shall reference the source when using other persons' ideas, research, presentations, or products in written, oral, or any other media presentation or summary.

F. Individuals' statements to colleagues about professional services, research results, and products shall adhere to prevailing professional standards and shall contain no misrepresentations.

G. Individuals shall not provide professional services without exercising independent professional judgment, regardless of referral source or prescription.

H. Individuals shall not discriminate in their relationships with colleagues, students, and members of allied professions on the basis of race or ethnicity, gender, age, religion, national origin, sexual orientation, or disability.

I. Individuals who have reason to believe that the Code of Ethics has been violated shall inform the Board of Ethics.

J. Individuals shall comply fully with the policies of the Board of Ethics in its consideration and adjudication of complaints of violations of the Code of Ethics.

Typical and Disordered Communicaton

2

When you have finished this chapter, you should be able to:

- Explain the role of culture and environment in communication

- Describe what is involved in human communication

- Demonstrate how communication disorders may be classified

- Name some types of communication disorders

- Discuss and estimate the frequency of occurrence of communication disorders

Human COMMUNICATION

THE SOCIAL ANIMAL

Possibly the worst punishment that can be given to a prisoner is to be sentenced to isolation. Discipline for a teenager might include limitations on telephone or email use. These restrictions are punitive because we humans are social beings. We have powerful drives to be with and to communicate with others.

What is **communication?** In general, we can say that communication is an exchange of ideas between sender(s) and receiver(s). It involves message transmission and response or feedback. "Someone does or says something, and others think or do something in response to the action or the words as they understand them" (Beebe, Beebe, & Redmond, 1996, p. 6). We communicate to make contact, to reach out to others. We communicate to satisfy our needs, to reveal feelings, to share information, and to accomplish a host of purposes. If your mother ever said, "Talking to you is like talking to the wall," you recognized that she was unhappy because you did not respond. Communication is interactive; it is a give-and-take. The importance of effective communication is highlighted in Box 2.1.

> It is axiomatic to say, "We cannot *not* communicate" (Watzlawick, Beavin, & Jackson, 1967, p. 48). Even a lack of response to someone sends a message to "leave me alone."

THOUGHT QUESTIONS

If you speak and no one listens, has communication occurred? What reasons can you think of for communicating? Have you ever spoken for no reason at all?

Box 2.1

Mundo Pax

Mundo pax means "world peace" in Latin. A school superintendent we know uses this as his email address. As an educator, he deeply believes that peace on earth comes through education. As communication specialists, we suggest that the key element of education that may lead to peace is effective communication. Visualize a 2-year-old child, whom we'll call Donna. Unable to use language well enough to express her needs, she will push, hit, cry, grab, and engage in temper tantrums. If Donna were older and had words to ask for what she craved, all that fussing might have been avoided. This might be especially true if she had the words "please" and "thank you" to open opportunities for her. If what Donna wants was possessed by another child who was not easily swayed by polite requests, Donna, if able to use sophisticated language, could trade, negotiate, or bargain. She could offer a toy that she had in exchange for the one she wanted, or she might suggest taking turns or playing together. Now picture nations that are greedy for wealth, building up military might to enable them to attack to obtain what they desire. Could improved communication skills spare us warfare? Can effective communication lead to mundo pax?

Several variables affect communication and its success or failure. These include cultural identity, setting, and participants. The study of these influences on communication is called **sociolinguistics.**

Cultural Identity

Each of us is a member of a language community. The more you understand about your own culture and that of the people with whom you communicate, the more effective your interaction will be. If this text were written in perfectly good Mandarin Chinese and you could not read that language, it would communicate nothing meaningful to you. Speakers and listeners must share competence in a common language if they are to communicate fully.

Perhaps you have traveled to a country in which a language that you did not know was spoken. You might have been able to communicate by gesture and pantomime; however, you would have to agree that while you could exchange some meaning, it fell far short of optimal communication. Even when two people come from the same language background, "perfect" communication is rare. This is because successful communication depends on related factors such as age, socioeconomic status, geographical background, ethnicity, and gender.

Babette and John were college sweethearts; however, they recognized significant differences in ways of relating. When Babette was growing up, her family openly discussed issues and disagreements, often to the point of forceful argumentation and yelling. These heated discussions sometimes led to tears, but eventually they typically terminated in hugs. John's family was more reserved. When two people did not agree, it was considered polite to keep your thoughts to yourself. In her relationship with John, Babette soon learned that she could not criticize him without his becoming sullen and hurt. On the other hand, she often wished that he would comment more frankly on decisions she was making. They both recognized that each would have to make major adjustments if their future marriage was to succeed.

How do the sociolinguistic factors that describe you influence your communication? What variations in communication may be due to age, gender, and ethnicity? Are these differences perfectly predictable?

THOUGHT QUESTIONS

Setting and Participants

The location of communication influences its nature. Where you interact affects how and what you'll say. You communicate differently at home, in school, in a noisy restaurant, and at a ballgame. Similarly, you might speak quite differently to your best friend, your mother, your father, your boss, your grandmother, and large audiences.

How might your speech change as you communicate with different people, in different settings, and with large or small groups? How might you communicate with someone who stutters or has another type of communication disorder?

MEANS OF COMMUNICATION

Communication takes many forms. It can involve any or a combination of our senses including sight, hearing, smell, and touch. We often think of good communication skills as a sign of intelligence: Humans have used this premise to search for life beyond the earth. Long the province of science fiction, this question has been investigated by physicists and astronomers since 1960. The Search for Extraterrestrial Intelligence (SETI) League has major search sites around the United States and in Australia, Canada, Argentina, Puerto Rico, and Russia, where optical and radio telescopes hooked to supercomputers scan the skies for intelligent signals.

What are they looking for? Researchers admit that they are not really sure, but the basic task is to find patterns or signals that go beyond random noise. Whether the signals are deliberate messages from aliens trying to contact us or signs of an environment that has been altered by intelligent beings, the search goes on (Owen, 2001).

If you were to send messages into the cosmos for intelligent beings to receive, what form would they take? What do you think a signal from space might be like? How would you judge the effectiveness of the communication?

Language

The primary vehicle of human communication is **language.** Language may be defined as "a socially shared code or conventional system for representing concepts through the use of arbitrary symbols and rule-governed combinations of those symbols" (Owens, 2005, p. 470). Some characteristics of language follow:

- Socially shared tool
- Rule-governed system
- Arbitrary code
- Generative process
- Dynamic scheme

Parents often assume that their infant's earliest "ma ma" or "da da" are uttered in reference to themselves. These sound combinations are not considered true words unless there is evidence that they are used meaningfully.

Language is a tool for relating to others and for accomplishing a variety of objectives. As we pointed out earlier, others must share the code if communication is to occur. When an infant utters, "ga da da ka," we cannot call this language, since this "code" is not shared.

Many people are so accustomed to their own language that they fail to recognize its arbitrary nature. Is there anything in the sound combination or the written letters of the word "water" that resembles the wet stuff? Is the French word "l'eau" or the Italian "l'acqua" any more or less moist? A comparison of different languages rapidly confirms this very arbitrary nature. The equivalent of the English word "butterfly" is "farfalla" in Italian, "mariposa" in Spanish, and "Schmetterling" in German—four very different renditions of that graceful creature. Some words have no equivalent in other languages.

Each language, in addition to being composed of arbitrary but agreed upon words, consists of rules that dictate how these words are arranged in sentences. In English, an adjective precedes a noun; for example, we say, "brown cow." In French, as in many other languages, this sequence is reversed, and they say, "le vache brun" ("the cow brown"). The rules of a language make up its **grammar.** Interestingly, you do not have to be able to explain the rules to recognize when they have been broken. Take, for example the sentence, "The leaves of the maple green tree in the breeze swayed." Most American students will simply know that the sentence is wrong and say, "It doesn't sound right." This recognition of "wrong" and "right" grammar is called **linguistic intuition** and is possessed by native speakers of a language.

Language is **generative;** this means that each utterance is freshly created. We do not just quote or repeat what has been heard. We paraphrase and modify and present our own ideas in an individual way. Imagine a conversation if all we could do was imitate one another.

Languages are also **dynamic;** they change over time. The famous Academie Française has tried to keep French "pure" and true to its origins. The Academie still attempts to keep "foreign" words from infiltrating French. For example, it has tried to ban the English words "jet" and "drugstore." But "le jet" is apparently easier to use than the French "l'avion de reaction," and so it stays. No academy, no school, no law, and no army can keep languages from being modified. In American English, we add five or six new words each day. Pronunciation, grammar, and ways of communicating also change.

In what ways has English changed since your grandmother was a child? Do you use words that she doesn't understand?

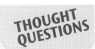
THOUGHT QUESTIONS

All human languages consist of similar basic ingredients. The primary components have been labeled form, content, and use (ASHA, 1993; Bloom, 1970).

Form   Form consists of phonology, morphology, and syntax. The sound system, or **phonology,** of English consists of about forty-three phonemes (unique speech sounds). Although different languages use many of the same phonemes, variations exist. Spanish and German, to name only two, do not use the English "th." As a consequence, since this sound is not learned as a child, it is difficult for some nonnative English speakers to produce.

Phonotactic rules specify how sounds may be arranged in words. Like rules of grammar, phonotactic rules are not universal. For example "k" and "n" cannot be blended in spoken English, though this combination is acceptable in German. For this reason the "k" in "knife" and "Knoxville" is silent for native English speakers but might be pronounced by Germans speaking English as a second language.

THOUGHT QUESTIONS

Which of the following nonsense words violates a phonotactic rule of English: sprell, framble, ngopi? Do you know what rule was broken? Can you make up some "acceptable" nonsense words?

Morphology involves the structure of words. A **morpheme** is the smallest grammatical unit within a language. Words contain both **free morphemes** and **bound morphemes.** A free morpheme may stand alone as a word. For example, "cat," "go," "spite," "like," and "magnificent" are all free morphemes. If you attempt to break them into smaller units, you lose the meaning of the word. On the other hand, "cats," "going," "spiteful," "dislike," and "magnificently" each contain one free and one bound morpheme. The bound morphemes (-s), (-ing), (-ful), (dis-), and (-ly) change the meanings of the original words by adding their own meanings but can be used only as attachments to free morphemes.

Syntax pertains to how words are arranged in a sentence. In an English declarative sentence, the subject comes before the verb: "John is going to the opera." When we reverse the order of the subject and the auxiliary or helping verb, we change the meaning of the sentence and end up with a question: "Is John going to the opera?" In the sentence "Mary was kissed by John," who is doing the kissing? Even though "John" comes after the verb, he is the actor because this sentence is in the passive voice. Although you probably don't consciously know and can't recite the rules for active and passive sentences, your linguistic intuition makes it easy for you to comprehend their meaning (Chomsky, 1965).

In addition to phonemes, morphemes, and syntactic units, language form also contains **suprasegmental** features such as loudness, rate, and intonation. "Supra-" means above or beyond, so suprasegmental features go beyond individual speech sound segments and are applied to whole phrases or sentences. Suprasegmentals, gestures, facial expression, and other **nonverbal** (meaning nonword) aspects of communication will be discussed later in this chapter.

Content   Since language is used to communicate, it must be about something, and that is its content, meaning, or **semantics. Semantic features** are the pieces of meaning that come together to define a particular word. For example, "girl" and "woman" share the semantic features of *feminine* and *human,* but *child* is generally considered a feature in "girl" and not in "woman." You'll notice that we said "generally" because, while most of us think of a "girl" as being young, it is common among some groups of people to refer to any woman as a "girl." Each word has multiple meanings, as you can quickly verify by looking in the dictionary. It is the other aspects of language, such as use and form, that determine the appropriate definition in context.

If you are beginning to think that this is complicated, you are right. As we said earlier, social and cultural factors influence the way language is used. The more two people know about one another, the more effectively they will be able to communicate.

Use   Use, or **pragmatics,** is the driving force behind all aspects of language. We speak for a reason. It is the purpose of our utterance that primarily determines its form and content. For example, if you are with a friend and are hungry, you might say, "Let's get something to eat." If function was a simple biological drive, then "eat" grunted out might suffice. But who and where you are, whom you are with, and the time of day also influence what you say. If you are at your home and you have invited the friend to dinner, you might say, "Dinner is ready." If you are working with someone as noon approaches, you might suggest, "Let's break for lunch."

Pragmatic rules of communication have been identified (Grice, 1975), some of which vary with culture (Gumperz & Hymes, 1972). For example, in the United States, business meetings tend to be very task oriented. Very little time is spent on social exchanges; the work to be done has center stage. On the other hand, in Saudi Arabia when two people meet for the first time for business purposes, they might spend the entire session talking about family and friends and not get to the meat of the business until the second meeting. The rules for business conversations in each of these societies are different. A few general rules for speakers of American English are presented in Table 2.1.

> While all are important, it is the use or purpose of communication that dictates form and content.

Speech

Speech may be defined as spoken language. Language also may be expressed in writing or in sign. When speech is used, interconnected features such as articulation, fluency, and voice influence the final product.

Articulation   Articulation refers to the way in which speech sounds are formed. How do we move our tongue, teeth, and lips in order to produce the specific phonemes of a language? How do we combine these individual sounds to form words? After all, we don't speak in a series of isolated sounds such as "h-e-ll-o" or we'd sound like robots. Chapter 10 explains the nature of speech sound production and describes the problems that may occur.

Fluency   Fluency is influenced by the rhythm and rate of speech. Every language has its own rhythmic pattern; we often think of rhythm as timing. Do

> ### Table 2.1
> #### A sampling of pragmatic rules for speakers of American English
>
> 1. Only one person speaks at a time. Each person should contribute to the conversation.
> 2. Speakers should not be interrupted.
> 3. Each utterance should be relevant.
> 4. Each speech act should provide new information.
> 5. Politeness forms reflect the relationship of the speakers.
> 6. Topics of conversation must be established, maintained, and terminated.
> 7. The speaker should be sensitive to successfully communicating the message, avoiding vagueness and ambiguity.
> 8. The listener should provide feedback that reflects comprehension of the message.

we pause after each word that we speak? Do we pause after each sentence? If we do, how long do the pauses last? What is our phrasing? You'll note that timing is not an isolated feature of speech. A word or syllable that is held tends to be emphasized and said more loudly. A skilled storyteller uses pauses and rhythmic variations for dramatic effect.

The speed at which we talk is our **rate.** Overall rate can reveal things about us. It may provide clues as to where we come from. For example, people from New York usually speak more rapidly than those from Georgia. On the other hand, if you habitually speak very quickly, it may suggest that you are in a hurry, are impatient, or have a great deal to say. By contrast, slow speech may connote a relaxed or casual personality.

The rate and rhythm of speech are sometimes referred to as vocal **prosody.** When it is smooth and relatively free of disruptions, we say that the speech is **fluent.**

Although most of the time we attempt to use a clear, sufficiently loud voice, sometimes our meaning may be more effectively communicated by a whisper, a whine, or a throaty rasp. When you are upset, your voice might sound angry to the point where someone says, "Don't use that tone of voice with me." Clearly, tone communicates information.

THOUGHT QUESTION

What different meanings can you convey by saying the sentence "I love you," with varying suprasegmental features?

Voice can reveal things about the speaker as well as about the message. A woman with a hoarse voice might (correctly or not) communicate to others that she smokes. A person with a soft, high-pitched voice might be communicating youth or immaturity. A deep, throaty voice might connote masculinity or authority.

Both the overall level of loudness and the loudness pattern within sentences and words are important. A generally loud voice may communicate strength, while a soft one may suggest timidity. By stressing different words within a sentence, you are also conveying different meanings. Say the following sentence in each of the ways listed below, with the emphasis or increased loudness on the underlined word. Notice how the meaning changes.

I got an "A" on my Physics final.

I got an "A" on my Physics final.

I got an "A" on my Physics final.

I got an "A" on my Physics final.

Placing the stress on different syllables within certain words also changes the meaning. Contrast the following:

record/record

recess/recess

present/present

You might have noticed that as you vary the stress, the pitch, rhythm, and pronunciation of different speech sounds may also change. The pitch tends to go up as the loudness is increased. Similarly, you are likely to prolong the syllable that receives stress. The first vowel in the noun "record," meaning a log or old-fashioned musical platter, is usually pronounced /ɛ/, as in "bed," while in the verb "record," as in the act of jotting something down or making a tape or CD, that "e" is more likely a schwa, /ə/, the first sound in "above," or an /ɪ/, as in "bid."

> The symbols /ɛ/, /ə/, and /ɪ/ represent phonemes or speech sounds to be described in more detail in Chapter 10, "Disorders of Articulation and Phonology."

THOUGHT QUESTIONS

What are the different meanings of the words "recess" and "present" with the stress patterns suggested above? Can you think of other words that have a single spelling but change in meaning with variations in stress?

Pitch is a listener's perception of how high or low a sound is; it can be physically measured as frequency or cycles per second, called hertz. **Habitual pitch** is the basic tone that an individual uses most of the time. Women usually have higher pitched voices than men, and children have higher voices than adults of both sexes. So our habitual pitch tells something about who we are.

Pitch movement within an utterance is called **intonation.** A rising intonation turns a statement into a question. First say the following sentence

> Some adolescent boys are eager for their voices to lower so that they will sound more grown up.

by bringing your pitch down for the last word, then say it by raising your pitch at the end:

> I want to do the dishes.

You'll notice that intonation influences meaning. You should also observe that as you alter intonation, your rhythm and loudness patterns also change.

Nonverbal Communication

Although most humans rely heavily on spoken communication, some researchers report that about two-thirds of human exchanges of meaning take place nonverbally (Zeuschner, 1997). The term *nonverbal* encompasses both the suprasegmental aspects of speech that we described in the previous section and the **nonvocal** (without voice) message exchange that we present in the following paragraphs.

Artifacts   The way you look and the way you have decorated your personal environment communicate something about you. Even the car that you drive can deliver a message. One young man we know impressed a woman on their first date by correctly selecting her car out of thirty in a parking lot. He did this by evaluating the make and year as well as the items on the seat and dashboard. If you walk into the best hotel in your area dressed in a business suit and ask for the restroom, you will be treated better than if you were wearing shabby jeans and looking unkempt. Assumptions are made about our personalities and trustworthiness on the basis of our possessions, clothing, and general appearance.

Music, art, architecture, and furniture are also artifacts that communicate. They communicate messages from the artists who designed and produced them and also from the people who purchase, patronize, or in some way support them.

*P*unctuation and font type and size may contribute to the meaning of an email. A century ago, perfumed letter paper modified the written word.

---

*W*hat might the music you listen to communicate about you?

THOUGHT QUESTION

Kinesics   **Kinesics** refers to the way we move our bodies, or *body language*. This includes overall body movement and position as well as gestures and facial expression. While there is some overlap with signing, gesturing typically lacks **explicit** (clearly defined) movements. In signing, the meanings of particular movements are well specified. For example, in American Sign Language (ASL), a thumb stroke down the cheek means "girl." Kinesics tend to be more general, subtle, or **implicit.** While gestures such as a "brush-off" have explicit meanings, they support and contribute to the larger speech system. By contrast, signing is a primary means of communication that is used by many people who are deaf. ASL is described in greater detail in Chapter 14, "Audiology and Hearing Loss," and Chapter 15, "Augmentative and Alternative Communication."

*A*re there some conversations that you would rather have in person than over the telephone? Why? What can a person's facial expression or body movement tell us?

Space and Time   The study of the physical distance between people as it affects communication is called **proxemics.** Proxemics not only reflects the relationship between people, but is also influenced by age and culture. Infants, children, people from Middle Eastern and Latin cultures, and those with strong emotional attachments, such as lovers, tend to interact in intimate or close proximity, very near one another. One young U.S. student we know reported feeling "backed into a corner" by an exchange student from Spain whom she had just met at a social gathering. It is likely that the Spanish woman felt that the American was "too distant."

Tactiles are touching behaviors. Who touches whom and how and where on the body the touch occurs can reveal a great deal. For example, some friends hug and kiss, others shake hands, and still others simply greet with a smile and a nod. Children in our society learn that touching others is usually not appropriate and are told early on to "keep your hands to yourselves." In contrast, infants' earliest interactions normally include considerable parental and caretaker touch.

Chronemics is the effect of time on communication. Again, cultural and age factors influence this nonvocal aspect of communication. People from German and Scandinavian backgrounds tend to be exactingly prompt, while those from Latin and African cultures may permit greater time flexibility. When two individuals come from cultures with different time rules, conflicts can easily arise. Status and context also affect chronemics (Poyatos, 1983). You might be kept waiting at the doctor's office, but your doctor does not expect to have to wait for you. Promptness is part of the U.S. work ethic. If you are routinely late to class or to a job, you've violated a chronemic norm and might have to pay a price in terms of a lowered grade or lost employment.

Young children operate in the here and now. When infants cry to be fed, they do not accept "Dinner will be ready in half an hour." Most toddlers do not normally patiently wait to have their needs and desires fulfilled. During these years, their communication is also only about the present. With increasing maturity, youngsters learn to tell time, to wait, and to talk about past, future, and nonpresent events, people, and things.

Age, sex, education, and cultural background influence every aspect of communication. These variations in communication are not impairments. Differences reflect regional, social, cultural, or ethnic identity and are not a disorder of speech or language (ASHA, 1993). Table 2.2 offers a sampling of typical communication features at different life stages. We describe communication impairments in the next section.

S peech-language pathologists recognize the heterogeneous nature of the U.S. population and strive to be sensitive to both verbal and nonverbal variations.

*D*o you think a person can have a disorder of chronemics? If so, what might be some symptoms and implications?

Table 2.2
A lifespan view of typical communication

Age Range	Receptive Communication — Language: Form	Expressive Communication — Language: Form	Language: Content	Language: Use	Speech: Articulation	Speech: Fluency	Voice	Artifacts	Nonverbal Communication — Kinesics	Nonverbal Communication — Space/Time
Infancy	Quiets/turns to human voice; Distinguishes speech sounds	Prelinguistic sound-making	No "true" speech; vocalizations, body movement focus on here and now	Obtain assistance; imitate; respond to others	Gurgles, coos, babbles	Rhythm and rate begin to resemble that of surrounding language toward end of year	Varies volume, rate, pitch	Toys, materials given to child, may "give" objects to others	Gestures precede meaningful spoken language	Close proximity/immediacy
Toddler	Responds to some verbal commands	Vocabulary growth from 4 to 300 words; moves from single word to short utterances	Familiar names, actions	Imitate, greet, protest, question	Simplified phonology		High (childish) pitch, more variability than adults	Toys, begins to construct things, start of imaginary play	Gestures slowly take second place to spoken language	Proximity decreases, begins to comprehend "now" and "later"
Preschool	Comprehension far exceeds expression; enjoys stories, books; follows increasingly complex commands; comprehends simple humor	Vocabulary grows from 1,000 to more than 2,000 words; uses complete sentences	Immediate to imaginary, includes past, present, and future	Greet, request, protest, inform, pretend, entertain	Almost all speech sounds correctly produced by the end of this period	Part-word, whole word, and phrase repetition not uncommon	Adjusts to listener; often used effectively to enhance verbal communication	Tremendous variability, reflects social/cultural background	Gestures used to enhance verbal communication	Begins to understand personal space

Age Group										
School-Age	Reading skills improve; receptive language grows to 50,000 words by sixth grade, 80,000 words end of high school; comprehension becomes adult-like	Vocabulary grows to 25,000-30,000 words; slang important; written language more complex than spoken language	Very broad, includes distant as well as near and abstract concepts	Many enjoy talking, sharing thoughts, raising and answering personal as well as abstract questions; narrative skills expand	Speech sounds correctly produced	Rate may be rapid, fluency is good	Pitch drops to adult levels with puberty, voice used to supplement verbal message	Clear indication of what is wanted, reflect peer group, gender	Gestures used in wide array of means to supplement speech	Becomes territorial, mature understanding of space and time
Early and Middle Adulthood	Comprehension increases	Education and occupation may be reflected in vocabulary	Full range of topics; written language continues in importance and sophistication	Instructing, directing others may be added if not there earlier	Mature articulation	Use of rhythm and rate to enhance message	Mature pitch, full-bodied vocal quality	Tremendous variety dependent on sociocultural and individual variables	Body movement and gesture continue to supplement verbal communication	Space may reflect relative "importance" in environment as well as cultural factors
Old Age	Comprehension may decrease	Vocabulary may reflect "older" generation	May focus more on past than future	May have limited communication partners, speech may be major way to achieve companionship	Normally not impaired	Rate may slow	Pitch may increase, vocal quality become "thinner"	Old/familiar items may become increasingly treasured	Body movement may be less forceful	May crave touch, as significant others become less available

Sources: Owens, (2001), Shadden & Toner (1997).

Note: This is a sampling of communication behaviors. Variability within each age group is the norm.

COMMUNICATION THROUGH THE LIFESPAN

The most complex and challenging task newborns face is learning the abstract code called language that those around them use to communicate. To do this, infants must first learn the rudiments of communication and begin to master the primary means of language transmission, called speech. The early establishment of communication between children and their caregivers fosters the development of speech and language, which in turn influences the quality of communication. This intricate pattern is further complicated by physical, cognitive, and social development as children mature. We can go even further to suggest studies in several languages that reveal that language proficiency is critical to development of higher cognitive skills, even nonverbal ones (Oller, Kim, & Choe, 2001).

Communication is established very early between the child and caregiver.

THOUGHT QUESTION

Are newborns totally helpless? Next time you're with one, observe the things the child can do and try to make a mental list of the abilities of a newborn.

Every person's speech and language continue to change until the end of life. Communication reflects the changes occurring in us and around us. Even the means of communication can change. Your great-grandparents might have begun life without a telephone and had to learn this new means of communication. Your grandparents probably began life without television. We, the authors, had to learn to use computers to communicate when we were well into our adult lives. You, on the other hand, grew up with the Internet.

Languages change too. New words and phrases have entered American English within your lifetime, such as *Internet, compact disc, disco, rollerblade, clap skate, rap,* and *European Union.* Other cultures and languages have contributed *mullah, sushi, mensch, salsa,* and *tsunami.* The competent communicator continues to adapt to changes in the language and in the communication process.

Children become communicators because we treat them as if they already are.

THOUGHT QUESTIONS

Have you become dependent on email to communicate with your friends? Do you routinely use the Internet to chat or explore areas of interest? Only a few years ago, neither was available to college students. (How did they survive?)

The key to becoming a communicator is being treated as one. While both speech and language are dependent on physical and cognitive maturation, neither is sufficient to account for the rapid developments in children's communication. Most linguists would also agree that language has strong biological underpinnings, although this too is an insufficient explanation in itself of the language learning process.

The process of learning speech and language is a social one that occurs through interactions of children and the people in their environment. Speech and language are learned within routines and familiar activities that shape children's days and within conversations about food, toys, and pets and later about school, social life, and the like. As listeners, we use a variety of lexical, syntactic, and stress-pattern cues flexibly to break continuous speech into more readily interpretable chunks (Sanders & Neville, 2000).

In different cultures, the type of child-caregiver interaction, the model of language presented to the child, and the expectations for the child differ, but each is sufficient for the learning of language. Learning to become an effective communicator is a dynamic and active process in which children in our culture become involved in the give-and-take of conversations. Even the more formal educational processes of learning to read and write are initially social and occur within book-reading activities in the home involving children and caregivers.

COMMUNICATION IMPAIRMENTS

Now that we have an idea of the complexity and varied nature of communication, it should be easy to see that much can go wrong. The American Speech-Language-Hearing Association (ASHA) defines communication and related disorders as disorders of speech (articulation, voice, resonance, fluency), orofacial, myofunctional patterns, language, swallowing, cognitive communication, hearing, and balance" (ASHA, 1997, p. I-64iii). You will notice that this definition does not confine itself to speech and hearing; also included are reading and writing, as well as manual and other communication systems, in addition to processes such as swallowing and balance that share anatomy and physiology with parts of the communication mechanism. Communication disorders may be categorized on the basis of whether reception, processing, and/or expression is affected. Is the problem primarily one of hearing, comprehending and manipulating language, or speaking? In fact, the three dimensions may be intertwined, reflecting the "interaction and interdependence among the processes of speech, language, and hearing" (ASHA, 2001b, Standard 3.4). Table 2.3 various presents systems for categorizing communication disorders.

Etiology, the cause or origin of the problem, may be used to classify a communication problem. Disorders may be due to faulty learning, neurological impairments, anatomical or physiological abnormalities, cognitive deficits, hearing impairment, or damage to any part of the speech system.

Sometimes a dichotomy is made between **congenital** and **acquired** problems. Congenital disorders are present at birth; acquired ones are the result of illness, accident, or environmental circumstances anytime later in life. Finally, disorders may range from borderline or mild to profoundly severe.

Table 2.3
Possible classification of speech communication disorders

Reception	Expression	Etiology	Time of Onset
Hearing Acuity:	*Speech:*	Neuromotor	Congenital
Conductive	Articulation	abnormalities	Acquired
Sensorineural	Fluency	Hearing impairment	
Mixed	Voice	Environmental/	*Severity*
Central Auditory	*Language:*	learning factors	Borderline
Processing:	Form	Cognitive deficits	Mild
Decoding	Phonology	Anatomical or	Moderate
Integration	Morphology	physiological	Severe
Organization	Syntax	impairments	Profound
Understanding speech	Content		
under adverse	Lexicon		
conditions	Use		
Short-term memory	Pragmatics		
Multiple categories			

Variations in communication are not impairments. Communication **dialects** are differences that reflect a particular regional, social, cultural, or ethnic identity and are not disorders of speech or language (ASHA, 1993).

In this text, we provide a **holistic** approach to diagnosis and treatment of people with communicative impairments. While we have separate chapters that discuss speech characteristics such as voice, fluency, and phonology, we also provide chapters that are organized on the basis of etiology such as neurogenic and craniofacial disorders. Within each chapter, we examine the interconnectedness of age, time of onset, social and cultural factors, and cause on the presenting disorder. We observe that it is common for an individual who demonstrates difficulties with one aspect of communication to be affected in other areas as well. We demonstrate that differences and dialects do not constitute disorders, and we examine the sometimes perplexing contrast between "typical" and "impaired."

Speech-language pathologists are concerned with both verbal and nonverbal disorders of communication.

LANGUAGE DISORDERS

Disorders of Form

As we explained earlier, the form of language includes phonology, morphology, and syntax. We speak in sounds (phonemes) that are combined into words (morphemes), which in turn are combined into phrases and sentences (based on syntactical rules). Errors in sound use, such as not producing the ends of words ("hi shi i too sma" for "his shirt is too small), constitutes a disorder of phonology. Incorrect use of past tense or plural markers ("the girl wented home" for "the girls went home") is an example of a disorder of morphology. It should be noted that these patterns are sometimes a reflection of a particular speech dialect. The SLP must distinguish between dialectal variations, which do not signify impairment, and disorders (see Chapter 4, "Assessment and Intervention"). Syntactical errors include incorrect word order and run-on sentences (for example, "I want to go mall and go skate and buy peanuts and you come with me 'cause I want you to but not Jimmy 'cause he's not big enough to go skate"). These errors in school-age children may affect academic achievement and social well-being.

Disorders of form may be due to many factors, including sensory limitations such as hearing problems or perceptual difficulties such as learning disabilities. Limited exposure to correct models may also handicap a child's language development. For many children who are delayed in their production of mature language forms, the cause is not apparent.

*W*hat type of error has occurred when a 6-year-old child says, "John and Mary is my best friends"? What might be the cause?

THOUGHT QUESTION

Disorders of Content

Children and adults with limited vocabularies, those who misuse words, and those with word-finding difficulties may have disorders of content or semantics. Similarly limited ability to understand and use abstract language as in metaphors, proverbs, sarcasm, and some humor suggests semantic difficulties. A persistent pattern of avoiding naming objects and referring instead to "the thing" is another indication of a disorder of content. Limited experience or a concrete learning style may contribute to this problem in youngsters. Among older people, cerebrovascular accidents (strokes), head trauma due to accidents, and certain illnesses may result in word-retrieval problems and other content-related difficulties.

Disorders of Use

Disorders of use, or pragmatics, involve inappropriate or inadequate communication. From the birth cry through the first few months of cries, coos, smiles, and awkward movements, the responsibility for communication rests primarily with people other than the infant. As children mature, the responsibility for communicating their intention through speech and nonverbal means becomes increasingly theirs.

Pragmatic language problems may stem from poor or in some way unacceptable conversational, social, and narrative skills; limited spoken vocabulary; and/or immature or disordered phonology, morphology, and syntax. The group affiliations, setting, and participants that we described earlier in this chapter play a major role in judgments of pragmatic competence.

SPEECH DISORDERS

Disorders of speech may involve articulation (the production of speech sounds), **fluency** (rhythm and rate), or **voice** (vocal tone and resonance).

*I*t is not uncommon for an individual to have an impairment in more than one aspect of communication.

They may affect people of all ages, be congenital or acquired, be due to numerous causes, and reflect any degree of severity.

Disorders of Articulation

Production of speech requires perception and conceptualization of the speech sounds in a language as well as motor movements to form these sounds in isolation and in context. You must have both a mental/auditory image of the sound you are going to say and the neuromuscular skills to produce the sound. The cognitive and theoretical concepts of the nature, production, and rules for producing and combining speech sounds in language is known as phonology. The actual production of these sounds is called **articulation.**

It is not always possible to determine whether an individual's speech-sound errors indicate an impairment of phonology or articulation. To sort this out, speech-language pathologists (SLPs) identify the phonemes that are incorrectly produced and look for error patterns that may point to phonological disturbances. The sound system of a language is usually fully in place by age 7 or 8. Children with multiple speech-sound errors past age 4 may have *phonological* difficulties. The causes are often not known but may be the result of faulty learning due to illness, such as ear infections, hearing or perceptual impairments, or other problems in the early years.

The SLP also assesses the client's ability to move the structures needed in speech, such as the tongue and lips; poor coordination may suggest articulatory difficulties. The causes for articulation disorders include neuromotor problems such as cerebral palsy, physical anomalies such as cleft palate, and faulty learning. When paralysis, weakness, or poor coordination of the muscles for speech result in poor speech articulation, the disorder is called **dysarthria.** Speech **apraxia** is similarly poor articulation due to neuromotor difficulties; however, the difficulty appears to be in programming the speech mechanism while muscle strength is normal. Dysarthria and apraxia can affect children as well as adults. Assessment and treatment of phonological and articulatory disorders are described in Chapter 10, "Disorders of Articulation and Phonology."

Disorders of Fluency

As we described earlier, fluency refers to the rate and rhythm of language. Certain types of fluency disruptions are fairly common at different ages. For example, many 2-year-olds repeat words: "I want-want-want a cookie." Around age 3, youngsters often make false starts and revise their utterances: "Ben took . . . he broked my crayon." Because these speech patterns are so common, they are sometimes referred to as **developmental disfluency.** Typically fluent adults occasionally use **fillers** ("er," "um," "ya know," and so on), **hesitations** (unexpected pauses), **repetitions** ("g-go-go"), and **prolongations** ("wwwwell"). However, when these arhythmic patterns exceed or are qualitatively different from the norm or are accompanied by excessive tension or struggle behavior, they may be identified as **stuttering.** Appropriate diagnosis and intervention when warranted are the task of the SLP (Yairi, Watkins, Ambrose, et al., 2001).

Fluency disorders are generally first noticed before 6 years of age. If remediation efforts are not made or are unsuccessful, this condition might continue and even worsen by adulthood. Adult onset of disfluency also occurs. Advancing age, accidents, and disease can all disrupt the normal ease, speed, and rhythm of speech. The causes of nonfluent speech are typically unclear; this is explored further in Chapter 8, "Fluency Disorders."

Speech-language pathologists use several indices to differentiate developmental disfluency from early stuttering.

Voice Disorders

As in other areas of speech, voice matures as the child gets older. From uncontrolled cries to carefully modulated whispers, shouts, and variations in pitch, the development of voice follows a predictable pattern. Although occasionally children are born with physiological problems that interfere with normal voice (such as a congenital laryngeal web; to be described in Chapter 9, "The Voice and Voice Disorders"), more common is the pattern of **vocal abuse.** It is characterized by excessive yelling, screaming, or even occasional loud singing that results in **hoarseness** or another voice disorder.

Habits such as physical tension, yelling, coughing, throat clearing, smoking, and alcohol consumption can disrupt normal voice production. These behaviors may result in pathology to the vocal folds such as polyps, nodules, or ulcers. Disease, trauma, allergies, and neuromuscular and endocrine disorders may also affect voice quality. For example, individuals with Parkinson's disease, a progressive neurological disorder, often have a soft voice with limited vocal variety.

HEARING DISORDERS

According to ASHA, a hearing disorder "is the result of impaired auditory sensitivity of the physiological auditory system" (ASHA, 1993, p. 40). It may affect the ability to detect sound, to recognize voices or other auditory stimuli, to discriminate between different sounds, such as mistaking the phoneme /s/ for /f/, and to understand speech.

Deafness

When a person's ability to perceive sound is limited to such an extent that "the primary sensory input for communication [is] other than the auditory channel," the individual would be considered deaf (ASHA, 1993, p. 41). Deafness may be congenital or acquired.

Total communication, including sign, speech, and speechreading, is often considered the most effective intervention. **Assistive listening devices, cochlear implants,** and **auditory training** may be helpful. These are explained in Chapter 14.

Many hospitals have instituted universal neonatal hearing screening. In this way, congenital deafness can be identified and addressed very early.

What differences might you expect in someone who was born deaf compared to someone who lost hearing at an older age? Why?

THOUGHT QUESTION

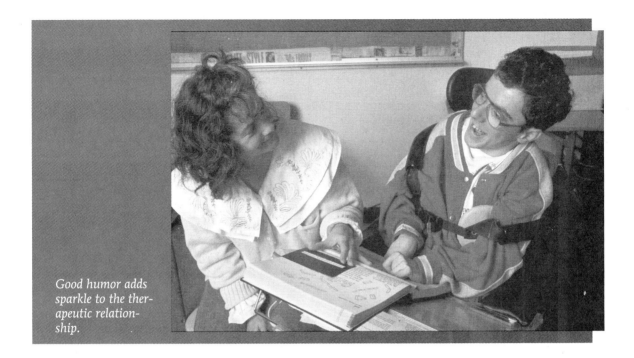

Good humor adds sparkle to the therapeutic relationship.

Hard of Hearing

A person who is hard of hearing, in contrast to one who is deaf, depends primarily on audition for communication. Hearing loss may be temporary due to an illness, such as an ear infection, or permanent, caused by disease, injury, or advancing age. Hearing loss is usually categorized in terms of severity, laterality, and type. The severity of a hearing loss may range from mild to severe. It may be **bilateral,** involving both ears, or **unilateral,** affecting primarily one ear. Finally, the loss may be **conductive, sensorineural,** or **mixed.** A conductive loss is caused by damage to the outer or middle ear; people with this type of loss usually report that sounds are generally too soft. A sensorineural loss involves problems with the inner ear and/or auditory nerve; this type of damage is likely to affect a person's ability to discriminate and consequently understand speech sounds, although they may "hear" them. A typical pattern is that of older people who report that they hear just fine but wish others would not mumble. Mixed hearing loss, as the name implies, is a combination of both conductive and sensorineural loss (see Chapter 14 for further discussion).

THOUGHT QUESTIONS

Do you know anyone with a hearing loss? How does he or she cope with this situation? Is that person's speech affected? How do you modify your communication when speaking with him or her?

CENTRAL AUDITORY PROCESSING DISORDERS

An individual with a central auditory processing disorder (CAPD) may have normal hearing but still have difficulty understanding speech. People with CAPD may have difficulty keeping up with conversation, understanding speech under varying conditions, and integrating what they hear with nonverbal aspects of communication (Stecker, 1998). These problems are sometimes traced to tumors, disease, or injury to the brain, but more often the cause is unknown. CAPD can be present in both children and adults, and special tests are required in its diagnosis. Often implicated in speech, language, and learning disabilities, CAPD may co-occur with attention deficit hyperactivity disorder (ADHD).

HOW COMMON ARE COMMUNICATION DISORDERS?

Before we attempt to estimate the numbers of people who have disorders of communication, we examine the concepts of normalcy and patterns of disability.

What Is "Normal"?

A recent cartoon showed an empty room and a sign reading "Meeting of Members of Functional Families." The implication was that there are no functional or "normal" families. Likewise, we could ask, "Is anybody normal?" If anything, variability is the norm. We humans are remarkable in our diversity. Just as no two snowflakes are identical, no two individuals, even twins, are exactly alike. Our faces, fingerprints, and manner of communication are unique.

The bell-shaped normal curve graphs measurements that are used to distinguish those who are average from those who perform above and below others of the same population (see Figure 2.1). Many language tests use a scoring system comparable to IQ scores. Most people (a little over 68%) of those tested will have IQ scores between 85 and 115. Higher or lower scores are above or below average. An individual who performed in the lowest 5 to 10 percent achieved a score that is significantly below average (Haynes & Pindzola, 1998).

Does being like your peers make you "normal"? If everyone on a boat, including you, is seasick, is this normal or does everyone have a problem? If fifty students in your Intro to Communication Disorders class take an exam and only one person gets more than 65 percent of the questions correct, should all but that one person fail? Do you believe that exams should be graded on a curve? Why or why not?

THOUGHT QUESTIONS

Since the word "normal" suggests "without problems," we prefer to use the term "typical" when we mean "like most others of the same age and

Figure 2.1

The normal curve, percentile equivalents, and IQ scores.

Source: Adapted from Nuttall, E. V., Romero, I., & Kalesnik, J. (1992).*Assessing and screening preschoolers.* Boston: Allyn and Bacon and Wiig, E. H., & Secord, W. A. (1991). *Measurement and assessment.* Chicago: Riverside Publishing Co.

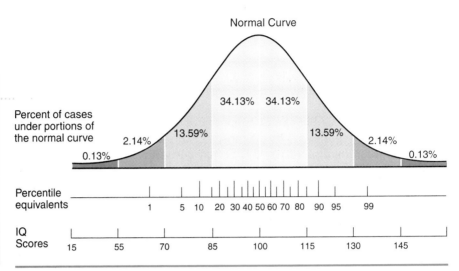

group." Classifying people on the basis of a bell curve, using a statistical percentage cutoff, may be little more than disability "by decree" (Lubker, 1997, p. 4). A more valid approach requires clear definitions of speech and language disorders. We discuss this further in Chapter 4, "Assessment and Intervention."

Communication Disorders as Secondary to Other Disabilities

Most communication disorders are secondary to other disabilities. For example, children with a cleft palate will have physical health problems as well as voice and articulation disorders. People with cerebral palsy have motor deficits beyond speech. Children with learning disabilities are especially likely to have language difficulties but may also have articulation, voice, fluency, and/or hearing deficits (Gibbs & Cooper, 1989). In addition, they experience academic and social difficulties.

Estimates of Prevalence

Prevalence refers to the number or percentage of people within a specified population who have a particular disorder or condition at a given point in time. If you determined the prevalence of stuttering in the entire U.S. population, among first-grade children, among college seniors, among U.S. males, or among U.S. females, you would get different prevalence figures in each case. For this reason, prevalence statistics must specify the population on which they are based.

The terms *incidence* and *prevalence* are often confused. Incidence refers to the number of *new* cases of a disease or disorder in a particular time period. Prevalence is the number of *new and old* cases in a particular time period.

Current estimates suggest that about 17 percent of the total U.S. population have some communicative disorder. About 11 percent have a hearing loss, and approximately 6 percent have a speech, voice, or language disorder. Many of those with hearing losses also have speech, voice, or language disorders. Six to ten million Americans (about 3% of the population) have a disorder of swallowing (Castrogiovanni, 1999b, c), and many of these individuals also have a communicative impairment. While these figures are rel-

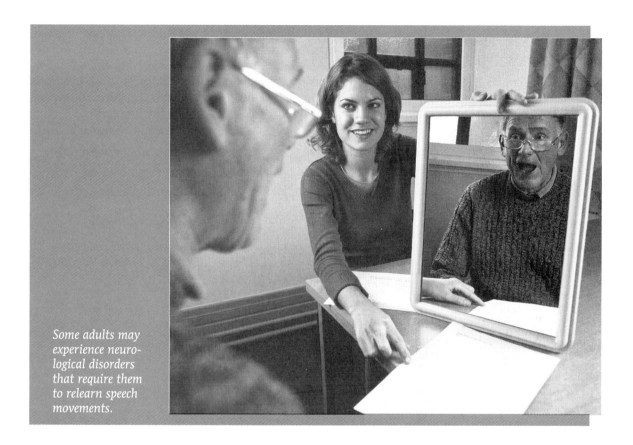

Some adults may experience neurological disorders that require them to relearn speech movements.

atively low, it is likely that more, generally mild, cases are not reported (Tierney, McPhee, & Papadakis, 2000).

What is the prevalence of communication disorders in your Communication Disorders class? How does it compare with national figures? What could explain any differences?

THOUGHT QUESTIONS

The percentage of people with hearing loss increases with age. Between 1 percent and 2 percent of people under 18 years of age have a chronic hearing loss, compared with approximately 32 percent of those over age 75. Exposure to noise has contributed to the hearing loss in about one-third of those affected (Castrogiovanni, 1999a).

Impairments of speech-sound production and fluency are more common in children than adults and more common among males than females. Speech disorders due to neurological disorders or brain and spinal cord injury occur more often among adults. It has been estimated that anywhere between 3 percent and 10 percent of Americans have voice disorders; this percentage is greater among school-age children and people over age 65 (Castrogiovanni, 1999b).

Communication disorders also vary with gender. For example, certain disorders, such as autism spectrum disorder, are four times as prevalent in males.

Language disorders occur in 8 to 12 percent of the preschool population; the prevalence decreases through the school years. Language deficits in older adults may be associated with stroke or dementia. It is likely that 5 to 10 percent of people over age 65 experience language disabilities related to these disorders (Bello, 1994; Castrogiovanni, 1999b). Table 2.4 highlights some communication disorders that may appear through the lifespan.

Table 2.4
Communication disorders that may manifest themselves through the lifespan

Age Range	Disorders	Receptive Communication	Expressive Communication	Swallowing
Infancy	Hearing impairment Fetal alcohol or drug-exposure syndrome Parental neglect/abuse Cerebral palsy	Limited response to sound/speech Limited response to others Atypical physical postures and movement	Atypical birth and other early cries Deaf infants vocalize normally for first 6 mos. Others may have little vocalization Passivity	May have difficulties with breast or bottle; later problems with solid foods
Toddler	Autism/Pervasive developmental disorder may be identified (hyper-sensitive to stimuli) Mental retardation not suspected earlier may now become apparent Brain injury due to falls	Comprehension of spoken language limited	Delay in first spoken word Utterances limited May use objects ritualistically	Rigid food preferences/dislikes Caution needs to be taken to prevent putting small objects in mouth that may be swallowed/choked on
Preschool	Delays that were suspected earlier may become more pronounced Fluency difficulties may emerge Specific language disabilities Middle ear problems common	Interactions with peers and others may be difficult	Inappropriate use of toys/objects Vocabulary may be limited, utterances short Alternative/augmentative communication may be recommended Excessive dysfluency; delayed phonology and grammatical development	Food preferences may be more entrenched

Table 2.4
(Continued)

Age Range	Disorders	Receptive Communication	Expressive Communication	Swallowing
School-Age	Language learning problems Hyperactivity/ Attention deficit disorder Brain injury due to falls and other accidents	Difficulties attending, following directions, speech and reading comprehension	Narrative and other pragmatic skills may be affected	Inappropriate eating habits may become established
Young Adulthood	Brain injury due to bike, motorcycle, car, and other accidents most prevalent in these years	Comprehension affected, generalized confusion, abstract thinking impaired	Pragmatic skills affected Life plans altered Dysarthria and apraxia may affect speech intelligibility	Neuromotor injury may impact on swallowing
Middle Adulthood	Hearing often starts to decline Life-threatening illnesses such as cancer may be diagnosed Neurogenic problems may appear; multiple sclerosis, ALS, Parkinson's, and Alzheimer's diseases; stroke (aphasia)	Speech in noise may be hard to comprehend Aphasia and Alzheimer's may result in comprehension difficulties	Illness-related depression may affect expressive communication Dysarthria and apraxia may impair speech intelligibility Alzheimer's and aphasia cause language impairments	Eating/swallowing not usually impaired in early stages
Old Age	Hearing deficits common Neurogenic problems become progressively worse	Difficulty understanding speech may cause "tuning out"	Voice may be weak Word-finding problems Inappropriate speech Perseveration	Disinterest in food; swallowing impairments may lead to aspiration pneumonia

Sources: Owens (2004); Shadden & Toner (1997).

Note: This is a sampling of problems that may be seen. Variability within each age group is the norm.

SUMMARY

Communication is an exchange of ideas; it involves message transmission and response. Human communication is remarkable and may take many forms. It is strongly influenced by culture and environment. Not only do people speak different languages, but within language groups, age, gender, socioeconomic status, geographical background, ethnicity, and other factors influence our communication.

The primary vehicle of human communication is language. It may be spoken, written, or signed and has been described in terms of form, content, and use. Form refers to the sound system, or phonology; word structure, or morphology; and syntax, or how the words are arranged in sentences. Content is semantics or meaning, and use is the purpose or pragmatics of the communication. Communication is also transmitted by nonverbal behaviors and characteristics.

A breakdown can occur in any aspect of communication. When communication is unimpaired, we tend to take it for granted, but when it fails us, we may feel frustrated and isolated. About 17 percent of the U.S. population currently experience some limitation of hearing, speech, and/or language.

REFLECTIONS

- How do social and cultural aspects of human beings influence communication?
- In what ways can disorders of communication be described and classified?
- What communication disorders are likely to be diagnosed in different age groups?
- How are estimates made regarding the number of people with communication disorders?

SUGGESTED READINGS

Axtell, R. E., & Fornwald, M. (Illustrator). (1998) *Gestures: The do's and taboos of body language around the world.* New York: John Wiley & Sons.

Hamaguchi, M. P. (1995). *Childhood speech, language, and listening problems: What every parent should know.* New York: John Wiley & Sons.

Hirsh-Pasek, K., & Golinkoff, R. M. (1999). *The origins of grammar: Evidence from early language.* Cambridge, MA: MIT Press.

Morrison, T., Conaway, W. A., et al. (1995). *Kiss, bow, or shake hands: How to do business in 60 countries.* Avon, MA: Adams Media Corp.

Ruben, B. D., & Stewart, L. P. (1998). *Communication and human behavior* (4th ed.). Boston: Allyn and Bacon.

Winner, E. (1997). *The point of words: Children's understanding of metaphor and irony.* Cambridge, MA: Harvard University Press.

ONLINE RESOURCES

http://asha.org American Speech-Language-Hearing Association.
Information for the general public concerning communication disorders.

http://www.nonoise.org The Noise Pollution Clearinghouse.
A national nonprofit organization with extensive online noise-related resources. Its goal is to raise awareness about and combat noise pollution.

Anatomy and Physiology Related to Speech, Hearing, and Language

3

CHAPTER LEARNING GOALS

When you finish this chapter, you should be able to:

- Explain the respiratory processes for quiet breathing and for speech breathing
- Explain the phonation process
- Describe the cavities of the articulation/resonance system
- Explain the articulatory and resonating processes for human speech

Speech production is generally taken for granted as a biological function that takes care of itself; your thoughts and ideas are expressed with little or no apparent effort. But for all its apparent simplicity, the production of speech requires an incredibly complex coordination of biophysical events involving hundreds of muscles and millions of nerves. It is paradoxical that such complex physiological behavior appears to be so effortless. This natural paradox, however, is probably necessary. If we had full conscious comprehension of what we are doing when we speak, we would probably be unable to utter a single word. Monitoring all the nerves and muscles, the tone of the voice, facial expression, and word order would be an impossible intellectual feat (Thomas, 1979).

For many individuals, however, speech production is anything but effortless. Sometimes abnormalities of anatomical structures and physiological systems that support speech interfere greatly with speech production. Thus, knowledge of the anatomy and physiology of the speech mechanism is fundamental to understanding many different communication disorders that are evaluated and treated by speech-language pathologists. Successful treatment of voice and swallowing disorders, laryngectomy (the surgical removal of the larynx), and cleft palate requires a thorough understanding of the anatomy and physiology of the speech mechanism.

THE PHYSIOLOGICAL SUBSYSTEMS SUPPORTING SPEECH

Anatomy is the study of the structures of the body and the relationship of these structures to one another. **Physiology** is a branch of biology and is defined as a science concerned with the functions of organisms and bodily structures.

Harvard neuroscientist Steven Pinker says, "One easy way to understand speech sounds is to track a glob of air through the vocal tract into the world, starting in the lungs." (Pinker, 1995, p. 163). Obviously, the production of speech is more complicated than Pinker's musing, but speech production does require control of air pressure and air flow from your lungs through your vocal tract into the atmosphere. Three physiological subsystems are involved with speech production: (a) the **respiratory system** provides the driving force for speech by generating positive air pressure values beneath the vocal folds; (b) the vocal folds, anatomical structures in the **laryngeal system** or **larynx,** vibrate at high rates of speed, setting air molecules in the vocal tract into multiple frequencies of vibration; and finally, (c) the **articulatory/resonating system** acts as an acoustic filter allowing certain frequencies to pass into the atmosphere while simultaneously blocking other frequencies. In this chapter, we will briefly consider how each of these physiological subsystems supports the production of speech and how this process changes through the lifespan.

THE RESPIRATORY SYSTEM

The primary biological functions of your respiratory system are to supply oxygen to the blood and to remove excess carbon dioxide from the body. This process is automatic and controlled by the respiratory centers located within the brain stem of the central nervous system. Although the primary function of respiration is to sustain life, it also serves as the generating source for speech production. Through the respiratory system, air is inhaled into your lungs to become the potential energy source for sound production. The air is then expelled in a controlled manner, to be modified by your vocal folds and/or articulators to generate speech sounds.

The Physiology of Quiet Breathing and Speech Breathing

Quiet breathing is breathing to sustain life. As you are reading this chapter, you are using quiet breathing. The rate and depth of breaths taken during quiet breathing are determined by your body's oxygen needs and the amount of carbon dioxide in the blood. Contraction of inhalation muscles causes the thorax, and in turn the lungs, to expand. Expansion of the lungs results in an increase of lung volume, and air pressure within the lungs drops below atmospheric pressure. Air rushes into the lungs, equalizing lung pressure with atmospheric pressure. Approximately one-half liter of air is inhaled when you are sitting and breathing quietly. Such breathing is also called **tidal breathing.**

Muscles of inhalation cease contracting at the end of an inhalation, your rib cage is elevated, and your lungs expand. As exhalation begins, the size of your thorax decreases, reducing lung volume. Air pressure within the lungs elevates to levels that are above atmospheric pressure and air rushes out of your lungs.

Exhalation during quiet breathing does not require active contraction of expiratory muscles. Gravity acting on the elevated rib cage and the elasticity of lung tissue help to return your thorax and lungs to their relaxed state, ready to begin the next respiratory cycle. A respiratory cycle is defined as one inhalation followed by one exhalation. During quiet breathing, inhalation and exhalation are approximately equal in duration.

Speech breathing is the kind of breathing you do when speaking aloud, and it differs from quiet breathing in a number of ways. First, during speech breathing, inhalations occur only at major linguistic boundaries such as the end of phrases or sentences. One would never inhale in the middle of a word or phrase.

*S*ay the word "baseball" normally. Now say it again, but take a breath between "base" and "ball." What happened to the normal flow of your speech?

THOUGHT QUESTION

During speech breathing, the time spent inhaling is shortened greatly, and the time spent exhaling is increased greatly. Additionally, you may inhale as much as 2 liters of air during speech breathing, depending on the specific demands of the utterance. Speaking is usually begun at lung levels above tidal breathing. In contrast to quiet breathing, speech breathing frequently requires active muscle contraction during exhalation. At the beginning of an utterance, muscles of inhalation may be active, controlling the descent of the rib cage, whereas at the end of an utterance, muscles of exhalation may be active to sustain lung pressure for longer utterances.

Your respiratory system's primary role during speech breathing is to control vocal intensity. The loudness of your voice is directly proportional to the amount of air pressure your lungs apply to the inferior aspects of the vocal folds. This air pressure is called **subglottal pressure.**

THOUGHT QUESTIONS

Have you ever heard a heavy smoker complain of shortness of breath? How does the shortness of breath affect speech breathing patterns?

THE LARYNGEAL SYSTEM

The larynx is the organ of the laryngeal system. Although the larynx is the principal sound generator for speech production, it has several important primary biological functions. As the superior termination of the trachea, the larynx is a protective organ that prevents foreign objects from entering the trachea and lungs. Additionally, the larynx can impound air for forceful ex-

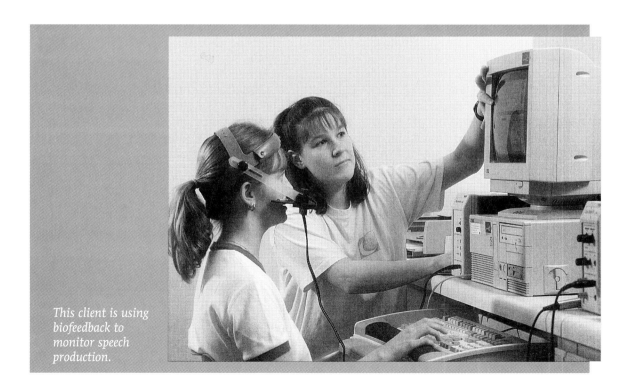

This client is using biofeedback to monitor speech production.

Figure 3.1

Stroboscopic film images of the vocal folds during one complete vibratory cycle. (Photograph courtesy of Robert Orlikoff, Ph.D., Memorial Sloan-Kettering Cancer Center, New York, NY)

pulsions of foreign objects or coughing if those objects threaten the lower airways.

The Vocal Folds

When viewed from above, the paired vocal folds appear to be ivory-colored bands of tissue. Vocal fold vibration produces the human voice, and voice production will be discussed later in this chapter. Figure 3.1 pictures the human vocal folds during a single vibratory cycle. Sustained vocal fold vibration is shown on the book's CD-ROM.

Some of the significant developmental changes that affect the larynx and the vocal folds over the life span are discussed in "The Voice and Voice Disorders" (Chapter 9).

THE ARTICULATORY/RESONATING SYSTEM

The articulatory/resonating system comprises the **pharyngeal cavity** or neck, the **oral cavity,** and the **nasal cavity.** Collectively, these three cavities

Figure 3.2

Schematic of the human vocal tract.

form your vocal tract, which is a resonant acoustic tube where all the sounds of spoken English are formed. Structures important for speech production such as the teeth, tongue, and soft palate are housed within these three cavities. Figure 3.2 illustrates the relationship of these three cavities.

THE SPEECH PRODUCTION PROCESS

The production of speech begins with the sound produced by vocal fold vibration, or **phonation.** Phonation is initiated by approximating or adducting the vocal folds and closing the glottis or opening. Once the vocal folds are closed, air pressure generated by the respiratory system increases beneath the vocal folds. The air pressure that builds beneath the vocal folds is called subglottic pressure.

Figure 3.3

Anterior view of the voice folds during one cycle of vibration. Air from the lungs creates a pressure beneath the vocal folds (1, 2, and 3). This pressure causes the vocal folds to separate (4). Decreased pressure in the glottis and elastic recoiling of vocal fold tissue cause the vocal folds to begin to close (5 and 6). The vocal folds close the glottis to end the cycle, and the next cycle begins (7).

As subglottic air pressure increases, vocal fold tissue is displaced in a lateral or sideward and superior or upward direction (frames 1, 2, and 3 of Figure 3.3), and the vocal folds are literally blown apart once the subglottic pressure reaches a critical value, as illustrated in frame 4. No abductory muscle activity is associated with vocal fold opening during phonation. Air rushing through the glottis increases in velocity. This increase in velocity produces a negative pressure (partial vacuum) between the medial edges of the vocal folds, which tends to pull the vocal folds toward one another, closing the glottis (frames 5, 6, and 7).

Two other forces bring the vocal folds back to an adducted state during phonation. The first force is the natural elasticity of the vocal folds, which acts to restore them to their original adducted state. The second force is the contraction of adductory intrinsic laryngeal muscles.

Each time the vocal folds open and close, one complete vibratory cycle, the air in the vocal tract is set into vibration, producing sound. The sound that results from vocal fold vibration is complex, containing a **fundamental frequency,** or the lowest frequency component that is directly related to how fast the vocal folds are opening and closing, and approximately forty additional higher frequencies called **harmonics.** Figure 3.4 is a stylized spectrum of the complex sound that is produced by vocal fold vibration. A spectrum represents the frequencies of a complex sound along the horizontal axis, and their relative intensity is represented on the vertical axis. Note the relationship of the harmonic frequencies to the fundamental frequency. The harmonic frequencies are whole-number multiples of the fundamental frequency. For example, when the fundamental frequency is 100 Hz, the second harmonic is 200 Hz, the third is 300 Hz, and so on. Note that the relative intensity decreases systematically with increases in harmonic frequency.

The vocal tract is an acoustic resonator that will modify the quality of the sound produced by your larynx. In any acoustic resonator, some frequencies are reduced or attenuated and other frequencies are enhanced dependent upon certain physical aspects of the resonator.

Figure 3.4

Spectrum illustrating a fundamental frequency of 200 Hz and related harmonics (a) and a spectrum of a fundamental frequency of 100 Hz and related harmonics (b).

THOUGHT QUESTIONS

You are drinking soda from a bottle. After you have taken a few sips, you blow air across the opening on the top of the bottle, and a sound is produced. After taking a few more sips, you again blow across the opening. Was the sound different the second time you blew across the top of the bottle? The bottle is a resonator. What characteristics of the resonator changed and how did those changes influence the sound that was produced?

Air-filled cavities are acoustic resonators. The frequency or frequencies at which a filled cavity will resonate are determined by the volume of the cavity, the area of the opening of the cavity, and the length of the opening of the cavity.

Movement of the tongue, lips, and larynx will change the shape of the vocal tract and in turn modify the sound emanating from the larynx. Produce the vowels /i/ (as in the word "bee") and /u/ (as in the word "boot"). Try to sense how your tongue and lips change position for the production of these two vowels. Changes in the position of your lips and tongue in turn change certain physical characteristics of the vocal tract that directly affect the quality of the sound that emanates from your mouth.

Figure 3.5 represents how changes of vocal tract shape influence which frequencies are enhanced and which are attenuated. A complex sound is produced by vocal fold vibration (a), and the vocal tract acts as a filter attenuating some frequencies and enhancing others (b). The sound that emanates from the mouth during vowel production (c) is related directly to the general shape of the vocal tract determined largely by tongue position. Note that for the /u/ vowel, low frequencies are enhanced, whereas high frequencies are somewhat attenuated. For the /i/ vowel, low frequencies are somewhat attenuated, whereas high frequencies are enhanced.

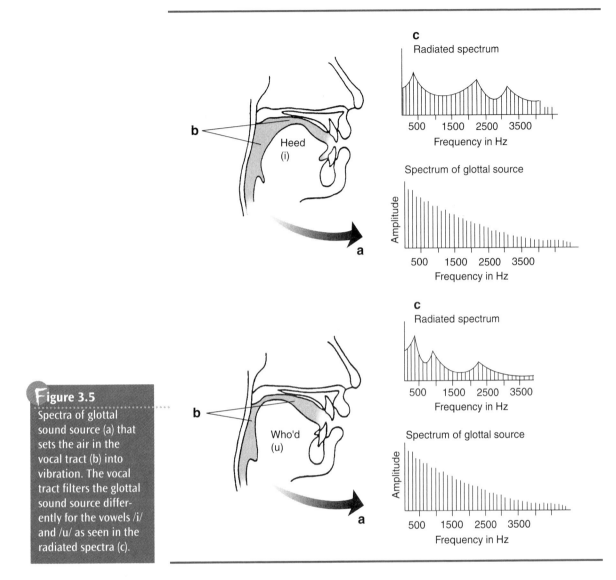

Figure 3.5
Spectra of glottal sound source (a) that sets the air in the vocal tract (b) into vibration. The vocal tract filters the glottal sound source differently for the vowels /i/ and /u/ as seen in the radiated spectra (c).

During consonant production, your tongue is sometimes used to momentarily occlude your vocal tract for the production of stop sounds such as /t/, /d/, /k/, and /g/. Production of sounds such as /s/ and /sh/ require your tongue to form a constriction in the vocal tract that will produce frication noise when air is passed through the constriction.

ANATOMICAL AND PHYSIOLOGICAL CHANGES TO THE SPEECH MECHANISM THROUGH THE LIFESPAN

The way we generate and control the pressure and flow of air from the lungs to the atmosphere changes with age. Anatomical changes in the physiological subsystems supporting speech production have significant consequences on how speech is produced across the life span.

THE RESPIRATORY SYSTEM

At birth, you had a breathing rate at rest between thirty and eighty breaths per minute. By 3 years of age, this tidal breathing decreases to between twenty and thirty breaths per minute. The rate changes because a newborn has very few alveoli, the gas-exchange areas in the lungs, while adults have several million (Zemlin, 1998). Watch a preschool child speak. Note the more frequent and deeper inhalations compared to adult speakers.

As a child develops, the respiratory system's structures increase in size, and lung capacities increase. Maximum lung capacities are reached in early adulthood and remain fairly constant until middle age. Respiratory function is affected by exercise, health, gender, age, and smoking. It is estimated that smoking in older people could result in a 500 milliliter (approximately 1 pint) cumulative loss in pulmonary function every ten years (Kent, 1997).

THE LARYNGEAL SYSTEM

The laryngeal system also goes through significant changes as a function of age. First, at birth the larynx is very small and it is positioned very high in the pharynx or throat. The vocal folds are approximately 3.0 mm long in newborns and, as a function of age, they increase in length equally in both boys and girls up to the time of puberty. During puberty, boys' vocal folds grow larger than those of girls. Subsequent to puberty, adult male vocal fold length is approximately 17 to 21 mm and adult female vocal fold length is approximately 11 to 15 mm (Sapienza, Ruddy, & Baker, 2004). The sex difference in adult vocal fold length accounts for the fact that men normally have lower pitched voices than females.

THE ARTICULATORY/RESONATING SYSTEM

Dentition or teething begins to emerge at about 6 months of age. Your first teeth are temporary and are usually referred to as primary or deciduous dentition. Emergence of the primary dentition is usually complete by 3 years of age. At approximately 5 years of age, you began losing your primary teeth, and your permanent or secondary teeth began to appear. The emergence of the secondary teeth is usually complete by 18 years of age.

The tongue of a newborn is large enough to occupy most of the oral cavity (Kent, 1997). As the infant grows during the first several years, the posterior portion of the tongue descends into the pharyngeal cavity, and the tongue reaches its mature size at about 16 years of age. In general, the growth of the tongue is similar to the growth of the lower jaw or mandible and to the lips (Kent, 1997).

Finally, as one ages, the length and volume of the oral cavity increases. This anatomical change influences the general resonance properties of the vocal tract in both sexes by lowering the frequencies at which the vocal tract naturally resonates (Xue & Hao, 2003).

SUMMARY

This chapter has been a brief overview of the anatomy and physiology of the speech and voice mechanism. The study of the structures that are used to produce speech and their function is extensive and complex. It is important to remember that although anatomy is static, these structures are capable of dynamic movement that can result in the unique human processes of speech.

The study of anatomy and physiology is essential for the speech-language pathologist. Knowledge and understanding of this topic will assist in the evaluation and treatment of clients whose communication disorder is the direct or indirect result of a breakdown within these systems.

REFLECTIONS

- Explain the respiratory processes for quiet breathing and for speech breathing.
- Explain the phonation process.
- Describe the vocal tract cavities.
- Explain the articulatory and resonating process for human speech.

SUGGESTED READINGS

A.D.A.M.® Animated Dissection of Anatomy for Medicine. Atlanta, GA: A.D.A.M. Software, Inc.

Kent, R. D. (1997). *The speech sciences.* San Diego, CA: Singular Publishing Group.

The Respiratory System (CD-ROM). New York: Insight Media.

Thomas, L. (1979). *The medusa and the snail: More notes of a biology watcher.* New York: Viking.

Zemlin, W. R. (1998). *Speech and hearing science anatomy and physiology* (4th ed.). Boston: Allyn and Bacon.

ONLINE RESOURCES

http://www.madsci.org/~lynn/VH/ Animated anatomical images of the three major body planes and more.

http://www.uchsc.edu/sm/chs/ Anatomical views of various body structures.

http://faculty.washington.edu/chudler/introb.html Excellent information about the nervous system.

4

Assessment and Intervention

CHAPTER LEARNING GOALS

When you have finished this chapter, you should be able to:

- Describe the communication continuum of differences, dialects, and disorders

- Explain the purposes and procedures involved in assessment of communication disorders

- Explain how targets are selected for clinical remediation

- Describe some of the basic procedures in treatment and intervention

The human communication process is remarkable but not flawless. Each of us has experienced frustration at not remembering someone's name or faltering when trying to express ourselves clearly. We also know that sometimes a friend speaks to us, and we don't fully understand what she or he is trying to say. The reverse happens, too, when we know that someone else misinterprets what we say. But when do these often minor annoyances constitute a problem? How do we determine that a communication disorder exists? And how do we categorize its nature? In this chapter, we provide an overview of assessment procedures. We also examine principles and techniques for assisting people who have communication disorders.

DIFFERENCES, DIALECTS, DISORDERS

Age influences all aspects of communication; however, considerable variation exists within each age group.

We learned in Chapter 2 that communication takes place within a social context. We communicate with other people. Our own culture and that of others influence the nature and success of this interaction. Ordered and disordered communication can be described only within cultural standards. It is obvious that the communication skills of a 4-year-old generally will be less sophisticated than those of a 12-year-old. Age, therefore, is one determiner of communicative proficiency. But factors such as gender, ethnicity, geographical region, language background, and socioeconomic status also contribute to the ways in which we communicate. The speech-language pathologist must recognize that variety is typical, and she or he must be able to distinguish differences from disorders.

A COMMUNICATION CONTINUUM

Everyone in Carol's family, including Carol, speaks rapidly; sometimes their words come out so fast they are hard to understand. Peter comes from a family of slow and deliberate speakers; occasionally, such a long lag time appears between Peter's words that one wonders whether he's going to complete his sentence. Carol and Peter represent different ends of the speech rate continuum. While they are clearly not speakers you might encounter every day, you might wonder whether they are different enough to have disordered speech. To make this determination, consider the following:

1. Does the speaker feel embarrassed or uncomfortable?
2. Do listeners react negatively?
3. Is the intent of the speaker communicated?

THOUGHT QUESTIONS

Does either Peter or Carol have a communication disorder? On what basis did you make your judgment?

DIALECTS

Dialects are variations of a language used by all speakers of a language. Whereas languages typically, but not always, represent the political boundaries of a country, dialects usually represent less formal geographical distinctions. We can usually distinguish people from Boston and Dallas by their distinctive ways of speaking. Ethnicity may also result in a dialect as in African American English or Black English. Foreign language background contributes to dialect, too. Within each region, ethnicity, and language background, additional variations exist. Not all Bostonians or African Americans share a common dialect. Similarly, speakers of Spanish (or French or any language) from different countries and regions are not identical in their communicative patterns. For example, the French of a person from Quebec is distinct from that of someone from Haiti, which is different from that of a Parisian. Women and men, too, often differ in their manner of communication, giving rise to **genderlect,** or gender-based dialect.

Individuals who use a particular dialect belong to the same **speech community** and "share knowledge of the communicative constraints and options governing a significant number of social situations" (Gumperz, 1972, p. 16). Speech communities may differ from one another in specifics of vocabulary, grammar, pronunciation, rate and rhythm of speech, topics of communication, body language, and pragmatic rules.

Pragmatic dialect differences are not always obvious. For example, narrative or storytelling styles of schoolchildren may reflect their ethnic background. European American youngsters, like their elders, tend to build a story to its climax and then provide a resolution. Algonquin and Chinese American children typically develop a story to its high point and then stop. From the European American viewpoint, the Algonquin and Chinese tales may appear incomplete, but to someone from these cultures, this might be seen as a positive technique for leaving the listener in the midst of the story (Crago, Eriks-Brophy, Pesco, & McAlpine, 1997).

Everyone uses a dialect. People with a dialect that differs from yours do not have a disorder of communication. It is important to recognize that dialects are normal variations; they are not pathological.

W hat pragmatic differences can you think of that distinguish female from male speakers?

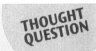
THOUGHT QUESTION

In summary, dialects are variations of Standard American English. Because we all speak some dialect, none should not be considered "substandard" or "wrong." Table 4.1 highlights a few dialect differences.

In addition to dialect, we must consider **idiolect,** which is an individual's unique way of speaking based on an interaction of such things as age, education, personality, family, geographical background, and linguistic background. Not everyone in your hometown sounds the same. Some people will use one or two aspects of a dialect, such as vocabulary (even just a few words) or grammar, and others will use different aspects such as pronunciation. Many people are bidialectal or multidialectal; they are competent in

Table 4.1
A few examples of possible dialect differences

Although features can be identified as characteristic of a particular dialect, you should recognize that each dialect contains variations. For example, Latino English is spoken by people from Spain, Mexico, Puerto Rico, and many parts of South and Central America, and their linguistic patterns are not identical. In addition, individual speakers may use some or none of the features listed below. It must be emphasized that dialects are not "wrong," they are rule-based modifications of the standard. The examples that follow are a small sample of differences based on ethnicity and language background.

SAE = Standard American English, AAE = African American English, ME = Mandarin English, LE = Latino English.

Grammar

Past tense

(SAE) I talked to her yesterday.

(AAE) I talk to her yesterday.

(ME) I talk to her yesterday.

(LE) I talk to her yesterday.

Possession

(SAE) That is Mary's dress.

(AAE) That is Mary dress.

(ME) That is dress of Mary.

(LE) That is dress of Mary.

Negation

(SAE) She doesn't like him.

(AAE) She don't like him.

(ME) She don't no like him.

(LE) She no like him.

Phonology

Substitutions, Omissions

(SAE) "feet" "it"

(AAE) "fee-" "i-"

(ME) "fit" "eat"

(LE) "fit" "eat"

Pragmatics

Direct eye contact

(SAE) Sign of respect and that attention is being paid

(AAE) Used by speaker but may be considered disrespectful when used by listener

(ME) Generally avoided

(LE) Generally avoided

Laughter/giggling

(SAE) Response to humor

(AAE) Sign of friendliness

(LE) Response to humor

Source: Adapted from Owens (2001) and Paul (1995).

more than one dialect. They will choose the dialect that is appropriate to the setting and conversational partners.

THOUGHT QUESTION

Do you think someone who speaks with a foreign dialect has a communication disorder? Why? Why not?

DISORDERS

Communication disorders may affect language processing and/or transmission, that is, any aspect of speech, hearing, listening, reading, or writing. The American Speech-Language-Hearing Association (ASHA) defines a communication disorder as "an impairment in the ability to receive, send, process, and comprehend concepts or verbal, nonverbal and graphic symbol systems" (ASHA, 1993, p. 40). The exact nature and degree of impairment will vary from individual to individual. It is the task of the speech-language pathologist or audiologist to describe the problem clearly and identify its extent.

Some clinicians object to the term "disorder," especially when it is used simply to report test results that are below average. They suggest that differences make us distinct as human beings and that we should redirect our attention toward people's strengths (Miller, 1993). While we agree, we also recognize, as do other specialists, that terminology is needed to identify people who are in need of speech, language, or hearing services, and to state that a person has an impairment, disability, or disorder should not carry with it negative stigma. It is important to recognize that an individual with a communication disorder is not a disordered person. We do not label a person as a "stutterer" or a "lisper" but rather "a person who stutters or lisps." The person is primary; the disorder is simply one aspect of the individual.

THOUGHT QUESTIONS

How do you react to the words "disability," "disorder," "handicap," "impairment," "atypical," and "abnormal"? Are the words loaded? Can you propose a solution to this dilemma? What is your opinion of the concept of so-called politically correct terms such as "communicatively challenged"?

IS THERE A PROBLEM?

Not everyone is assessed for communication disorders. When there is a possibility of a problem, recognition of this precedes formal assessment. Selection for assessment may come from either referral or screening.

REFERRALS

Individuals at any age may be referred from various sources for an evaluation for a communication disorder. An infant in a hospital neonatal intensive care unit who has feeding or other oral difficulties may be referred to the speech-language pathologist (SLP) for evaluation and management of these problems.

A pediatrician may refer a toddler. Sometimes a parent, grandparent, neighbor, or friend observes that a young child is not communicating as well as others of the same age. This person might take appropriate steps so that an assessment will occur. A phone call to an area speech and hearing center, school system, rehabilitation program, or to a clinician in private practice might lead to a formal evaluation of the youngster's hearing and speech. For

Specialists in communication disorders may encourage referrals from other professionals and concerned individuals by publicizing the nature of the services that they provide.

children enrolled in a preschool or regular school, it is common for a teacher to express a concern about a child's speech and recommend an assessment by an SLP or audiologist.

Adults may refer themselves if they feel they have a communication disorder. Sometimes a person might feel handicapped professionally and/or socially because of hearing or speech limitations. Often a family member takes the initiative in seeking help. Frequently, a physician refers an individual who has had an accident or a medical problem such as a stroke.

SCREENING

The legislation in IDEA (see Table 1.4) mandates that *all* children from birth to age 20 be given the opportunity to receive special services if needed. To ensure this, departments of health and welfare and departments of education throughout the country must provide a system for identifying at-risk individuals at no personal expense. Children between the ages of birth and 36 months may be brought to special centers for screening for speech, language, hearing, motor, and other functions. Older children are screened in preschools and schools.

Several states in the United States have passed legislation requiring that hearing screening tests be given to infants at their birthing facility or as soon after birth as possible. Babies who are identified as being at risk for hearing loss are then assessed more fully, and steps toward appropriate intervention are initiated. It is likely that universal infant hearing screening will be soon mandated throughout the United States.

Some SLPs devise and use their own speech and language screening test; others use commercially available ones such as the *Fluharty Speech and Language Screening Test-2* (Fluharty, 2000) or the *Adolescent Language Screening Test* (Morgan & Guilford, 1984). Figure 4.1 is an example of a screening test developed by SLPs who work together in the same school district.

DEFINING THE PROBLEM

Assessment of communication disorders is the systematic process of obtaining information from many sources, through various means, and in different settings to verify and specify communication strengths and weaknesses, identify possible causes of problems, and make plans to address them. If a problem is identified, a speech-language pathologist may make a **diagnosis,** which distinguishes an individual's difficulties from the broad range of possible problems. Although a diagnosis includes a label such as "harsh voice," it should also contain a more complete description of this disorder that reflects the person's ability to communicate, variability of symptoms, severity, and possible causes (Haynes & Pindzola, 1998).

ASSESSMENT GOALS

The goals of assessment are listed in Table 4.2 and explained in the paragraphs that follow. The procedures that are used in meeting these objectives are described later in this chapter.

Figure 4.1
Clinician-developed speech and language screening test.

Student's Name _____   Date _____

Age _____   Grade _____   Pass _____   Refer _____

Comments: _____
_____

Articulation
Errors: _____

Oral-motor: _____

WNL: _____

Auditory Skills
Digit Memory: 4-3-3 _____   5-4-2 _____   7-1-6 _____

                    2-7-3-3 _____   6-3-5-1 _____   8-2-9-3 _____

Wh- Questions: "One night Sally brought pizza to John's house. Sally and John ate the pizza and drank orange soda. They were so full that they couldn't eat the last piece."

Who ate pizza? _____   What did they drink? _____

Where did they eat the pizza? _____

How many pieces were left? _____

Definitions
bird   _____

apple   _____

brown   _____

ice   _____

bed   _____

cow   _____

Informal Language Sample (+ 2)

| | Simple | Compound |
MLU _____   sentences _____   sentences _____

Pragmatics:

Use _____   Topic maintenance _____   Turn taking _____

Syntax _____

Semantics: Expressive vocabulary _____   Word finding _____

(Continued)

Figure 4.1
(Continued)

Concepts (_____ /20 correct)

top _____	over _____	side _____	through _____
bottom _____	nearest _____	first _____	right _____
inside _____	farthest _____	last _____	left _____
around _____	next to _____	same _____	front _____
under _____	middle _____	different _____	back _____

Voice

WNL* _____   Questionable _____

Fluency

WNL* _____   Questionable _____

Grammar: Evoked Sentences	*Articulation*
	circle if incorrect
1. Susan saw a mouse and a lizard.	s z
2. They thanked her mother for the cloth.	θ
3. The little boy wants a yellow balloon.	l
4. The treasure chest was not in the usual place.	ʒ
5. Karl had a cookie and some cake after school.	k
6. He was wearing his red suspenders.	r
7. Biff laughed when he caught the fish.	f
8. She wished for a dish of ice cream with syrup.	ʃ
9. John couldn't budge the heavy chair, could he?	ʤ
10. Charlie didn't watch television because he wanted to play checkers.	tʃ

Error score _____

Suggested cut-offs: Kindergarten—12 errors; Second Grade—5 errors; Fifth Grade—4 errors

*Within Normal Limits

Source: Adapted from Speech & Language Department, Marlboro Central School, NY. Used with permission.

Verification of Communication Problems

The primary goal of assessment is to determine the presence or absence of a problem. A secondary goal is the diagnosis, determining exactly what is wrong. Sometimes **diagnostic therapy** is suggested. This means that the SLP will work with the client for a time and will obtain a clearer picture of the person's communication abilities and limitations in the process.

Description and Quantification of Deficits and Strengths

We have previously learned that communication impairments may involve hearing, speech, language, and/or processing or, more likely, some combination of these. During assessment, specifics of all of these are probed. Both the client's communicative strengths and limitations are noted. Techniques that the client uses for overcoming difficulties are observed. The SLP provides data reporting the consistency of behaviors and, where appropriate, indicates how the client compares with peers. In short, assessment must provide detailed information about all aspects of the client's communicative disabilities and abilities, recognizing the interrelatedness of speech, language, and hearing.

A person who has been identified during screening as having a communication disorder is likely to have a problem. However, a screening is not a diagnostic evaluation. Screenings simply suggest which individuals should receive further evaluation.

What are the differences between screening, evaluation, and diagnosis? Are the goals and outcomes different?

Statement of Severity

If a problem exists, you will want to know how serious it is. At a general level, the SLP will determine whether the disorder is profound, severe, moderate, mild, or borderline. Individuals with a profound impairment have very little functional speech communication. A person with a severe disorder would require a great deal of intervention and support. Moderate disorders also require significant treatment and accommodation. A mild or borderline communication problem might not be readily apparent to the individual himself or herself or to others; however, even subtle communication problems can have a negative impact on social, academic, and professional success. Exactly what determines a particular severity rating varies with each disorder.

Published tests often suggest severity ratings depending on a client's performance scores. These must be used with caution. The clinician must be aware that there is always a range of typical communication behavior and also that a single test should not be overly relied upon.

Clinicians may differ in their judgments of the severity of a disorder. Use of objective criteria ensures more consistency in this determination.

How would you feel if your ability were determined on the basis of a single test such as the SAT or GRE? What information is missing from this measure?

Table 4.2
Goals of assessment

The communication disorders specialist is charged with answering the following questions when assessing an individual:

1. Does a communication problem exist?
2. What is the diagnosis?
3. What are the deficit areas? How consistent are they?
4. What are the individual's strengths?
5. How severe is the problem?
6. What are the probable causes of the problem?
7. What recommendations should be made?
8. What is the prognosis (likely outcome) without and with intervention?

Source: Adapted from Lund & Duchan (1993).

Etiology

Etiology is the study of cause. The SLP must try to ascertain the reason(s) for the communication deficit. Three categories of cause may be identified. A **predisposing cause** describes the underlying factor that led to the problem, for example something genetic. A **precipitating cause** is a factor that triggered the disorder, such as a stroke. A **maintaining** or **perpetuating cause** is something that keeps the problem going. In the case of Sally M. that follows, the SLP formed hypotheses concerning all three categories of etiology.

Sally M., age 7, had multiple articulation, phonological, and morphological errors in her speech. The SLP learned that Sally had frequent ear infections during her second and third years of life. The SLP hypothesized that inability to hear adequately during this period may have interfered with mastery of the sound system of English. Sally was ill so much that she may not have had the energy to focus on learning speech. The SLP observed that Sally's mother laughed good-naturedly at Sally's way of speaking. The SLP reported that the likely predisposing cause of Sally's communication difficulties was a tendency toward ear infections. The precipitating cause may have been the history of middle ear infections (otitis media). Possible maintaining factors were the attention and "rewards" Sally received from her immature speech.

Causality is sometimes viewed from another perspective. The terms **organic/somatogenic** and **functional/psychogenic** may also be used in describing etiology. An organic disorder has an identifiable physical cause; for example, cleft palate, cerebral palsy, and cancer of the larynx all are likely to result in communicative difficulties. The term "somatogenic" means coming from the body, and it therefore indicates a physical basis.

When no physical cause can be identified, the disorder is considered functional. Functional disorders may be due to psychogenic (psychological) factors; for example, in elective mutism, an individual has no physiological reason for not being able to speak but decides not to talk, perhaps as retaliation toward an abusive parent (Haynes & Pindzola, 1998).

It is helpful to remember that the causes of communication problems are often elusive; sometimes we simply cannot figure out what they are. In these cases, clinicians report that the etiology is unknown. The mystery may be partly because original causes do not always persist; for example, Sally M.'s ear infections are no longer apparent at age 7. Furthermore, we have no way of knowing why Sally was especially vulnerable to getting ear infections in the first place. Finally, causality is often complex, with many factors coming together to result in the development of a particular disorder.

Do you think the etiology of Sally's communication problems is organic/somatogenic or functional/psychogenic? Could it be a combination? What are the limitations of this terminology? Why is it important to attempt to determine the cause(s) of communication problems?

THOUGHT QUESTIONS

The Treatment Plan

Recommendations for addressing the client's communicative deficiencies are often the most read portion of an assessment report. In making a plan, the first decision is whether any intervention at all is warranted. If it is, then its nature must be described. Should the client be enrolled in speech and language therapy? Where? How frequent and how long should therapy sessions be? Would the client benefit more from individual or group work? What specific targets should be addressed initially? What style of therapy might be optimal? Some options include high or low structure, client or clinician directed, behavioral or cognitive, direct or indirect, pull-out or push-in. These are described later in this chapter in the section on treatment procedures. The plan should also indicate referrals for other services such as psychological or medical evaluation. Treatment recommendations provide a basis for a "working hypothesis" (Haynes & Pindzola, 1998, p. 11); the initial recommendations may need to be altered as intervention proceeds. Assessment continues throughout treatment, and one affects the other in a circular fashion (see Figure 4.2).

Prognosis

A **prognosis** is an informed prediction of the outcome of a disorder. For example, a parent of a 5-year-old with very disfluent speech will want to know what will happen if this is left untreated and whether therapy will prevent the child from stuttering later in life.

In communication disorders, the SLP makes a prognosis regarding whether the problem will persist if no intervention occurs and what the likely outcome is if a course of therapy or other treatment plan is followed.

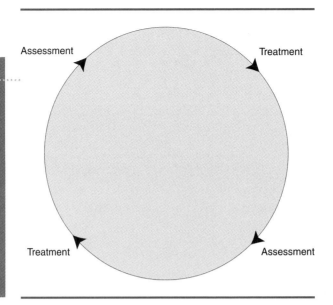

Figure 4.2

The assessment/treatment cycle.

Assessment is an ongoing process. The initial assessment determines the treatment plan. A thorough assessment includes trial therapy. As treatment proceeds, the client's functioning is monitored (assessed) and modifications in treatment are made.

Family members and clients are often eager to know the prognosis. They will ask questions such as "Will my child outgrow this problem?" "How long will it take to correct this disorder?"

The SLP must consider the nature and severity of the disorder; the client's responsiveness to trial therapy during assessment; and the client's overall communicative, intellectual, and personal strengths and weaknesses. The client's environment is also important. Are family members able and willing to help? Is support available within the school or through other agencies involved with the client?

ASSESSMENT PROCEDURES

Assessment may take many forms. Ideally, the clinician should sample a broad variety of communication skills through multiple procedures in several settings. The focus should be on the collection of **authentic data,** that is, actual real-life information, in sufficient quantity to be able to make meaningful and accurate decisions (Damico, 1997). Several aspects of a typical evaluation are presented on the accompanying CD-ROM.

Case History

The written **case history** provides background information that helps the SLP to prepare for an evaluation. Most speech-language pathologists require that histories be completed before the client's first visit. Normally, one form is tailored for adult clients, and a comparable one is for a parent or other responsible person to use with regard to a child.

Although the written case history is a valuable tool, its reliability may be limited for various reasons. The respondent might not have understood all the questions. She or he might not know the answers to many questions and might guess or recall incorrectly. Cultural differences can influence the manner of response to some items (Shipley & McAfee, 1998).

Opening Interview

Once the SLP has the completed case history form, additional background information is obtained through an interview. The basic purposes of the initial interview are (1) to learn more about the client that might be relevant to his or her communication and (2) to answer questions and provide reassurance and support for the client and/or family. Open-ended questions are used to encourage the respondent to provide adequate detail. In addition, the respondent must be given the opportunity to express concerns. The clinician must be sure to listen openly and nonjudgmentally. Experienced SLPs are able to guide the interview so that the objectives are met in a supportive, natural way within the allotted time frame.

The SLP obtains background information about a client from a written case history completed by the client, parent, or significant other; an interview; and reports from other professionals.

Systematic Observation/Sampling

Watching the client in more than one setting and with different people can provide considerable insight into the individual's communicative skills. One 5-year-old client stuttered severely with his gruff 60-year-old father but very little with the SLP.

Clinicians often begin their observation when the client and a family member are in the waiting room. Some children are very talkative with a parent but become silent with a stranger. Classroom and recess or lunchtime observations for school-age children can be revealing. Hospitalized clients should be observed with significant others when possible.

Most clinicians use a **speech** and/or **language sampling** technique when assessing the communication of both children and adults. Guidelines

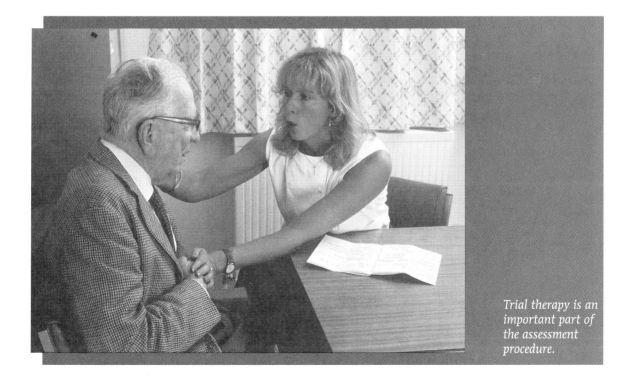

Trial therapy is an important part of the assessment procedure.

for sample collection and analysis are described in Chapter 5, "Childhood Language Impairments," and Chapter 10, "Disorders of Articulation and Phonology."

Hearing Screening

Hearing is routinely screened in most communication evaluations. Since hearing is so important to speech, the SLP needs to ascertain that the client's hearing is normal for speech purposes.

Oral-Facial Examination

An **examination of the peripheral speech mechanism** is commonly part of the overall assessment process. The purpose is to determine that the physical structures involved in speech are not impaired and that they function adequately. During this procedure, the face, jaw, lips, teeth, tongue, pharynx, and hard and soft palates are evaluated at rest and while the client engages in specified nonspeech and speech movements.

Standardized Testing

Literally hundreds of published tests exist that can be used to assess overall speech and language or specific components such as articulation and syntax. Most of these instruments are **norm referenced.** In other words, they yield scores that compare a particular client with a sample of individuals of the same sex and similar age. They may be used to justify a particular educational or other placement and to obtain funding from the government or private insurance companies. Other published tests are **criterion referenced.** They provide a systematic method for evaluating a client's strengths and weaknesses with regard to particular skills. Many tests yield both norm- and criterion-referenced information. Table 4.3 contains examples of the kinds of items you would find in some published tests.

Is a driving test norm referenced or criterion referenced? What about the SATs? Why do you think these types of assessments were chosen for these tests?

Can different data be collected from systematic observation and formal testing? What are the relative advantages and disadvantages of each type of information gathering?

Consolidation of Findings: Making the Diagnosis

It is axiomatic to say that professionals must treat the "whole person" and not just the disorder. After the speech-language pathologist has obtained information about the client from various sources, it is necessary to summa-

Table 4.3

Examples of types of items found on published tests

Articulation Test for Children

Ask child to name the following objects:

shoe, hat, ring, letter, pencil, book, cookie, telephone, chair, scissors

Complex Phonological Naming Task

Ask client to name pictures of the following:

elephants, encyclopedia, valentine, television, telescope, library, photograph

Grammatical Understanding

Ask client to point to the correct picture when give a choice of three:

The boy is getting dressed. The boy is dressed. The boy is getting undressed.

The lady is hiding from the boy. The boy is hiding from the lady. The boy and the lady are hiding.

Grammatical Production

Ask client to complete the sentence:

Clinician: This is a picture of one shoe. This is a picture of two _____.

Clinician: The boy is putting on his sock. The boys are putting on _____.

Pragmatic Language Use

Ask the client what you would say under various conditions:

A person gave you a present.

You meet a friend.

You are offered food by a friend, but you do not want any.

Functional Communication Test for Adults

The clinician must observe the client on a minimum of three occasions. On the basis of these observations, the clinician records whether the client does the following readily, with minimal assistance, with moderate assistance, with maximal assistance, or not at all:

- Refers to people by name.
- Exchanges information on the phone.
- Understands facial expressions.
- Knows what time it is.
- Expresses feelings.

The SLP makes a determination about a client's current functioning and the nature of the problem from multiple sources and clinical intuition.

rize the results and make connections between the findings. For example, background information may give insights into presenting behavior. Scores from norm-based tests need to be reconciled with observations by the SLP and other important people in the client's life. The client's communicative limitations must be viewed in the context of strengths, such as motivation and family or other support. Often an individual is more capable in some aspects of communication, while other features are weak. For example, a child's speech might be easy to understand (readily intelligible), although he or she has a limited expressive vocabulary. The SLP must attempt to obtain a well-rounded picture of the person who is being assessed.

THOUGHT QUESTION

Can you think of a situation in which a parent, a teacher, and a speech-language pathologist would each have a different perception of a child's communicative competence? (Do you know the story of the blind men and the elephant?)

Closing Interview

The client and/or family will want to know the outcome of the evaluation as soon as possible. When and how this information is shared may depend on whether the setting is a hospital, private clinic, university center, or public school. In addition, each facility will establish its own set of policies.

In general a brief conference is held immediately after the formal assessment. The SLP will probably indicate that all of the information gathered about the client has not yet been analyzed, so more complete recommendations will appear in the diagnostic report. The SLP might suggest another meeting to discuss this report.

Report Writing

Effective writing skills are required to accurately convey assessment information to the client, the client's family, and other professionals.

The diagnostic report is a summary of the client's history and a record of what transpired during the assessment. The implications of the findings should be clearly stated and thoughtfully justified. The report is normally the springboard for intervention and treatment. It may be sent to other professionals who will be working with the client. It is also available to the client or client's family. The report must be carefully written. If technical terms are used, they should be explained. Speech-language pathologists may develop individual styles of writing, but most reports follow a similar format and contain comparable information.

INTERVENTION WITH COMMUNICATION DISORDERS

Intervention for individuals with communication disorders is influenced by the nature and severity of the disorder, the age and status of the client, and environmental considerations, as well as personal and cultural characteristics of both client and clinician. Despite this, some general principles and procedures can be identified.

Before discussing some general clinical intervention strategies, we will consider briefly some new initiatives being developed by ASHA that are designed to link research and clinical practice.

EVIDENCE-BASED PRACTICE

Recently, ASHA has taken a proactive position stressing the need to integrate research and clinical practice (Katz, 2003; Ramig, 2002; Wambaugh & Bain, 2002). ASHA's Code of Ethics requires clinicians to "provide services that are based on careful, professional reasoning" (Apel & Self, 2003, p. 6). Evidence-based practices ensure that "clinicians abide by these ethical codes while best serving their clients." (Apel & Self, 2003, p. 6).

Evidence-based practice (EBP) is the integration of high-quality scientific clinical research evidence with individual clinical expertise to ensure ethical and optimal client management (Dollaghan, 2004; Sackett, Straus, Richardson, Rosenberg, & Haynes, 2000). Dollaghan (2004, p. 12) suggests that ". . . EBP offers us a framework and a set of tools by which we can systematically improve in our efforts to be better clinicians, colleagues, advocates, and investigators . . . ." ASHA has recently established the National Center for Treatment Effectiveness in Communicative Disorders and is currently coordinating a National Institutes of Health funded effort to promote clinical research that will support EBP.

Evidence-based practice is hardly unique to communicative disorders (Poggi, 2003). Physicians diagnosing patients, lawyers advising clients, and educators teaching children are all now expected to base their practices on evidence that demonstrates proven results. The No Child Left Behind Act of 2001 relies so strongly in the use of scientifically based research that it is referenced over 100 times in the legislation.

Despite the widespread acclaim for EBP, there is a fundamental issue that confronts clinicians who wish to establish an EBP: locating relevant, germane sources of clinical evidence in a timely fashion. No SLP has the time to scour hundreds of journals and textbooks for clinical evidence. EBP proponents suggest using "high-yield sources" that are easily accessible via the Internet (Dollaghan, 2004; Schlosser, 2004). For example, the Agency for Healthcare Research and Quality supports a website (www.guideline.gov) that is a compilation of clinical evidence reviews from a large number of disciplines and a wide variety of topics. Several additional high-yield source websites are listed at the end of this chapter (Dollaghan, 2004).

OBJECTIVES OF INTERVENTION

Regardless of the specific nature of the problem, intervention in speech-language pathology has as its overriding goal the improvement of the client's communication skills.

1. The client should show improvement not just in a clinical setting; progress should generalize to his or her real-world environments, such as home, school, and work.

2. The client should not have to think about what has been learned; in large part, it should be **automatic.**

3. The client must be able to **self-monitor.** Although modifications should be automatic, they will still require monitoring. The client

should be able to listen to and observe himself or herself and make corrections as needed without the therapist's being present.

4. The client should make optimum progress in the minimum amount of time.

5. Intervention should be sensitive to the personal and cultural characteristics of the client.

TARGET SELECTION

The assessment report should provide recommendations for long-term goals and short-term objectives for communication intervention. The clinician, however, will have to decide which specific targets should be addressed and in what sequence. The client's personal needs and the potential for generalization are most relevant in making meaningful choices. Likely success of mastery and typical behavior of others of the client's age and gender might provide additional insights.

Client Needs

Each client has individual needs. The SLP must attempt to determine which are paramount at this time and then develop a plan to meet these needs.

The client's individual needs are paramount in target selection. For example, Johnny M. is a 6-year-old boy with numerous articulation and grammatical errors in his speech. When asked his name, he is reluctant to answer, but he may be coaxed to say, "Doddy." According to Mrs. M., people tease him about his pronunciation of his name, and this is a great source of anxiety for the child. Because of this, the phonemes /ʤ/ ("J" in Johnny) and /n/ are very important to this child and should be considered for early targeting.

How the Target Will Generalize

Generalization refers to the use of the trained target with different people in varied environmental settings and linguistic contexts. If what has been learned in therapy is in conflict with patterns found in the home environment, generalization may be difficult.

Ease of Mastery

A careful assessment includes diagnostic or trial therapy. In the case of Johnny M., the clinician observed that he could correctly say /n/ and "knee" when these were modeled and he was asked to repeat what he heard; in other words, Johnny was stimulable for the /n/ sound. Johnny was not successful in producing /ʤ/ even though the clinician used a variety of techniques to elicit this sound; he was not stimulable for /ʤ/. On the basis of this information, Johnny will more quickly acquire /n/ than /ʤ/. However, recent research has concluded that once learned, nonstimulable phonemes prompt greater generalization than those that were stimulable (Gierut, 1998). For this reason, both /n/ and /ʤ/ are appropriate targets.

Age Appropriateness

Knowledge of normal development provides insights into which communication forms and functions are typical at different ages. For example, /n/ is generally mastered by age 2, and /ʤ/ is customarily correctly produced by age

4 (Stoel-Gammon & Dunn, 1985). This information confirms the decision to select the production of the phonemes /n/ and /ʤ/ as first objectives for Johnny.

In summary, target selection requires consideration of several variables. The clinician must make a decision that is appropriate for the particular client's needs.

*M*r. Brown had a stroke at age 75. He is able to say a few words, but these are often garbled, and the speech sounds are not correctly produced. He becomes frustrated when he tries to talk. He can accurately point to things around the room to express basic wants and needs. Using the criteria above, which is probably a better early communication target: (1) correctly pointing to pictures to express himself or (2) learning to produce the sounds (phonemes) of English?

BASELINE DATA

Before beginning a program of intervention, SLPs obtain **baseline data;** that is, they try to elicit the target behavior(s) multiple times, under multiple conditions, and record the accuracy of the client's responses. This gives them information about the client's starting point. Baselines are essential to determine the client's progress and the success of the treatment program.

Unlike a sample and standardized tests used in the initial assessment, baselines specifically probe the communication behavior that will be the focus of therapy. Let's return to Johnny M. The speech-language pathologist has decided that the phoneme /n/ is a first target. The child pronounces his name as "Doddy" and says "do" for "no" and "dife" for "knife." The SLP knows that Johnny can correctly imitate the sound /n/ and the word "knee." In baseline testing, the SLP may obtain ten pictures of objects beginning with /n/ and ten of objects ending with /n/. The SLP asks Johnny to name the objects. The percentage of correct /n/ productions in each of these positions is Johnny's baseline for the phoneme /n/. These data provide a starting point both for planning therapy and for measuring progress.

Formal test results during assessment differ from baseline data. During formal testing, a wide range of communicative skills are evaluated. Baseline data reveal an individual's performance level with regard to a few selected potential targets.

BEHAVIORAL OBJECTIVES

Once the clinician has obtained baseline data, short-term objectives are developed. These are the targets for each treatment session or for several sessions. A behavioral objective is a statement that specifies the target behavior in an observable and measurable way. To do this requires that the clinician identify what the client is expected to do, under what conditions, and with what degree of success. The letters ABCD might help you to remember the format for writing behavioral objectives:

A. Actor. Who is expected to do the behavior?

B. Behavior. What is the observable and measurable behavior?

C. Condition. What is the context or condition of the behavior?

D. Degree. What is the targeted degree of success?

Returning to Johnny M., the SLP has decided that she or he wants Johnny to experience early success and establishes the following as one behavioral objective for the first session:

A. Johnny

B. will produce the phoneme /n/ correctly

C. in the initial and final position of one-syllable words when modeled by the clinician

D. in 60 percent of the opportunities presented.

This seems a reasonable goal, since Johnny was accurate in this condition 50 percent of the time during baseline testing.

Behavioral objectives may be used for a broad range of teaching targets. Table 4.4 lists ten objectives written by student clinicians. Read each one to

Table 4.4
Test yourself: Behavioral objectives

Which of the following is NOT a well-written behavioral objective and why? (Answers are at the bottom of the table, upside down.)

1. The client will understand the words "over" and "under" when they are said to him in 90 percent of the opportunities presented.

2. The client will answer "What" questions using sentences that are 5 words in length in response to 4 of 5 questions.

3. The client will use a rate of speech of no more than 150 wpm when reading aloud from the local newspaper for 5 minutes.

4. The client will correctly name 8 of 10 farm animals when shown cards with their pictures.

5. The client will correctly use the plural form.

6. The client will appropriately respond to the clinician's greeting at the beginning of the therapy session.

7. The client will follow two-part directions given by the clinician in 90% of the opportunities presented.

8. The client will improve vocal quality while reading sentences aloud.

9. The client will distinguish between the phonemes /s/ and /z/ when produced by the clinician.

10. The client will sustain the phoneme /a/ for 20 seconds at a loudness level of 50 decibels.

Answers: 1. No, can't observe or measure "understand." 2. Yes. 3. Yes. 4. Yes. 5. No, in what situation and how often? 6. No, how often? Just today? What is meant by "appropriate"? 7. Yes. 8. No, "improve" is not measurable, also no degree is given. 9. No, degree is not given. 10. Yes.

see whether it is a valid objective. Use the ABCD criteria. If the instructional objective for this task for readers of this text is 80 percent accuracy, did you meet it?

CLINICAL ELEMENTS

Direct Teaching

Traditional clinical sessions begin with the SLP's explaining or reviewing the target. The amount and complexity of the explanation vary with the training target and the client's age and cognitive ability. A behavior modification approach is widely used after the client has been prepared.

Behavior modification training programs have been shown to be successful for a broad variety of communication disorders (Hegde, 1993). Behavior modification is a systematic method of changing behavior. Before training, the SLP establishes a target and collects baseline data. During training, the SLP attempts to evoke the desired response from the client by providing a **stimulus.** The client is expected to *respond,* and the clinician **reinforces** this response. The SLP records the accuracy of the client's response. After training, the SLP counts the percentage of accurate responses and determines the next target response. Table 4.5 is a general format for a therapy session.

Even young and relatively low-functioning individuals are more responsive to therapy when they understand the goals.

Incidental Teaching

Behavior modification follows a highly structured format and is directed by the speech-language pathologist. The SLP has a well-thought-out plan and works to guide the client through the stages required for mastery of the target.

Sometimes a low-structured or more client-led approach is used. The SLP follows the client's lead but teaches along the way. This is referred to as **incidental teaching.** For this to be effective, planning is also necessary so that targets are reached. The SLP manipulates the environment so that communication should occur naturally. For example, imaginary play with a young child or a cooking or an art project with one who is older may serve as situations in which therapy occurs. The approach is described further in Chapter 5, "Childhood Language Impairments."

Counseling

In addition to direct work with the client on the communication problem, the SLP can provide a supportive environment for the client and other key people in the client's life. A person with a communication disorder may experience a host of feelings, including embarrassment, anger, depression, and inadequacy. Family members may have similar emotions regarding the client's communication and may also feel guilty, perhaps blaming themselves for the problem.

Family and Environmental Involvement

An individual might spend two hours a week with a speech-language pathologist and 110 awake hours alone and with other people. Very young language-delayed children are sometimes bombarded with questions at home.

Table 4.5

A possible format for a therapy session

A. Introduction

   Greetings

   Review previous sessions' targets and/or activities

   Summarize format for current session

B. Teach concept

   Explain

   Provide example

   Demonstrate (model)

   Provide strategy

   Define

C. Practice concept

   Game

   Worksheet

   Books/magazines

   Hands-on activity

D. Assess learning

   Ask specific questions

   Prompt problem solving

   Ask for paraphrasing

E. Summary/conclusion

   How does this skill affect daily life?

Notes

1. Steps A through E are appropriate for most individual or group sessions.
2. The specific techniques listed under each step are suggestions and will vary.
3. When possible, use more than one modality. For example, use visual, verbal, and tactile stimuli.
4. Use teachable moments to review previously learned skills unrelated to target concept.
5. In working with groups, recognize that there will be a variety of targets and skill levels.
6. Be sensitive to clients' cultural backgrounds.
7. Consider how to maintain high levels of motivation.
8. Recognize that details will need to be tailored to the needs of the individual client and will change as the client progresses in therapy.

Source: Adapted from scheme developed by D. Moneymaker, Beacon Central School System, NY. Used with permission.

Others may have older siblings who do the talking for them. In Johnny's case, described earlier in this chapter, it might be recommended that the younger sibling with highly unintelligible speech also receive therapy. This would benefit both youngsters.

When children are seen for speech or language therapy, SLPs often ask that a parent observe the sessions on a regular basis. Depending on the family circumstances, family members may be asked to help the child with specific homework assignments. For individuals with multiple or severe handicaps, the speech-language pathologist must coordinate efforts with other specialists such as the physician, physical and occupational therapist, and psychologist.

Families and friends may learn ways of helping adults with communicative impairments. A spouse may be critical in assisting therapy for an adult who had a stroke or has a voice problem due to recent accident or illness. The SLP must recognize the significant others in the client's life, from infancy through old age, and engage them in productive ways. **Support groups** consisting of individuals who have similar difficulties often provide an avenue to practice what has been learned in therapy, to share feelings related to the disability, and to maintain communication skills once formal treatment has been terminated.

Whatever approaches are used, the client's interests and strengths should be utilized. For example, some individuals learn more easily when shown diagrams and pictures, whereas others profit more from a verbal approach. Some are quicker to grasp concepts; others learn more rapidly from drill. Some have families who can provide strong support; some must look elsewhere for this. Ongoing assessment helps the SLP to determine the most useful procedures for individual clients.

Intervention for communication disorders occurs in many settings. Broadening the base for treatment helps to ensure that what is learned in a clinical setting is transferred to a variety of real-world contexts.

MEASURING EFFECTIVENESS

The speech-language pathologist determines readiness for dismissal from therapy largely by assessing its effectiveness. Did the client meet the long-term goals and short-term objectives? SLP-designed **post-therapy tests** similar to those used to determine baselines are normally used to answer this question. In addition, it is essential that the client has gained a degree of *automaticity* in the use of the communication target. If he or she has to stop and think each time, overall communication will be impaired, and the targets will not have been fully mastered. Errors will occur, however, and the client should be able to *self-monitor* and self-correct when needed. If therapy has been effective, the client has been successful in *generalizing* learned skills to the out-of-clinic world. This might require the SLP to observe the client in different settings, such as home or school. More often, the SLP depends on reports from others to assess this type of generalization.

FOLLOW-UP AND MAINTENANCE

After a client has been dismissed from therapy, the SLP must take steps to ensure that the progress that was achieved is not lost. This is done in two ways: Upon dismissal, the client or family should be encouraged to return when anyone feels a need. More reliable is the establishment of a regular follow-up schedule. The client may be contacted by telephone or letter every six months for a period of two years or so after the termination of therapy. At this time, retesting may be suggested, and **booster treatment** may be provided if needed. In **follow-up testing,** the SLP evaluates the client's communication skills to see that they are at least at dismissal level. This usually consists of a combination of conversational interaction and systematic probing of therapy targets. During booster treatment, the SLP reintroduces the therapy targets and addresses them again. Often different and abbreviated procedures are used, and the client returns to the dismissal level of accomplishment relatively quickly.

SUMMARY

Assessment of communication disorders requires an understanding of communication in context. Dialects as a result of geography, ethnicity, foreign language background, and other factors contribute to our communicative individuality. The SLP recognizes that dialects and differences do not constitute disorders. Communication behaviors, as much of life, can be viewed as occurring on a continuum.

Referrals and screenings are the primary ways in which individuals are selected for assessment. During assessment, the SLP verifies and defines the client's problem, identifies deficits and strengths, probes causality, makes a treatment plan, and provides a prognosis for improvement. This is achieved through multiple techniques, including sampling of communicative behaviors in several settings.

Assessment and treatment function in a cyclical fashion, with one influencing the other. In many ways, an SLP is assessing the client each time the client is seen in therapy. Successful intervention often uses a team approach that involves family members as well as professionals. Provisions for follow-up ensure that the gains made in therapy are maintained. In the chapters that follow, techniques for assessment and treatment of specific communication disorders will be described.

REFLECTIONS

- What is meant by the continuum connecting communication differences, dialects, and disorders?
- What are the basic goals of communicative assessment?
- Why is it important to obtain information about a client from several sources?
- What are some differences you might expect to find as a result of systematic observation and formal testing?

- How does a speech-language pathologist decide what to target for intervention?
- How is the success of speech and language therapy determined?

SUGGESTED READINGS

Bliss, L. S. (2002). *Discourse impairments: Assessment and intervention applications.* Boston: Allyn and Bacon.

Coleman, T. J. (2000). *Clinical management of communication disorders in culturally diverse children.* Boston: Allyn and Bacon.

Hamayan, E. V., & Damico, J. S. (1991). *Limiting bias in the assessment of bilingual students.* Austin, TX: Pro-Ed.

Haynes, W. O., & Pindzola, R. H. (1998). *Diagnosis and evaluation in speech pathology* (5th ed.). Boston: Allyn and Bacon.

Klein, H. B., & Moses, N. (1999). *Intervention planning for children with communication problems: A guide for clinical practicum and professional practice* (2nd ed.). Boston: Allyn and Bacon.

Roth, F. P., & Worthington, C. K. (1996). *Treatment resource manual for speech-language pathology.* San Diego, CA: Singular.

Shipley, K. G., & McAfee, J. G. (1999). *Assessment in speech-language pathology. A resource manual* (2nd ed.). San Diego, CA: Singular.

ONLINE RESOURCES

http://professional.asha.org/resources/multcultural/reading_6.cfm
American Speech-Language Hearing Association Multicultural Issues Board: Service delivery with multicultural populations. Includes references to cross-cultural differences in beliefs about health and disorder, strategies for professionals, and relevant statistics.

http://professional.asha.org/resources/multcultural/reading_4.cfm
American Speech-Language Hearing Association Multicultural Issues Board: Intervention with multicultural populations. Includes references to guidelines for determining the most appropriate language of intervention, cultural factors that impact on intervention, and selecting culturally sensitive materials and activities.

Childhood Language Impairments

5

CHAPTER LEARNING GOALS

When you have finished this chapter, you should be able to:

- Characterize language impairment
- Describe the disorders associated with language impairment
- Explain the process of assessment in language impairment
- Describe the overall design of language intervention

Language impairments are a complex group of diverse disorders and delays with a wide range of characteristics, levels of severity, and causes. Some children may exhibit disorders in which language is inappropriate, inefficient, or ineffectual while others exhibit language that is seemingly immature.

The term **language impairment** applies to a heterogeneous group of developmental and/or acquired disorders and/or delays that are principally characterized by deficits and/or immaturities in the use of spoken or written language for comprehension and/or production purposes that may involve the form, content, and/or function of language in any combination. Let's take this definition apart and examine it.

1. Children and adolescents with language impairment will be very different. The impairment may occur at any time within the lifespan of the individual and may vary in symptoms, manifestations, effects, and severity over time and as a consequence of context, content, and learning task.

2. The impairment may be the result of developmental abnormalities; may be acquired as the result of accident, injury, or other environmental factors; and/or may be delayed.

Case Study 5.1

Case Study of a Child with Language Impairment: Kassandra

Kassandra, an active 5-year-old, is an engaging child and an enthusiastic kindergartner. Born one month preterm and weighing only slightly over four pounds, she was kept in the hospital for postnatal care and observation for several weeks. The team of specialists who worked with Kassandra in the hospital recommended to her parents that she receive early intervention services, first in the home and later at a local clinic. The team was concerned because Kassandra was at risk of having later developmental problems.

By 18 months, Kassandra was not talking and the team recommended to her parents that she attend a special language-intensive preschool where she would receive both individual and group intervention services. Working together, the speech-language pathologist, developmental specialist, and classroom teacher conducted a thorough evaluation of Kassandra's early communication behaviors, motor skills, and cognitive abilities. Although Kassandra's speech and language were delayed, she appeared to have motor and cognitive abilities that were close to that of typical children.

The speech-language pathologist worked closely with both the classroom teacher and Kassandra's parents to ensure that there was consistency across different communication environments in the way the others interacted with the girl and in the communication requirements. Kassandra's program was individualized to include words and phrases for entities in her environment. Once she began to use single words, Kassandra quickly learned to combine them into longer and longer phrases. When she entered kindergarten, she demonstrated language abilities in the low normal range.

As you read the chapter, think about

- Possible explanations for Kassandra's delay.
- Possible evaluative procedures that could be used to measure Kassandra's language.
- Possible targets that the intervention team might choose to help Kassandra develop and use language.

3. Deficits and/or immaturities may exist in one or more means of communication, such as listening/speech or reading/writing, and may affect receptive and/or expressive language. For example, preschoolers with language impairments are often less able to recognize and copy letters and less likely to write and draw every day, to pretend to read, and to ask questions during parental reading (Marvin & Wright, 1997). In short, young children with language impairments are at risk for literacy difficulties when they later attend school (Nathan, Stackhouse, Goulandris, & Snowling, 2004).

4. One or more aspects of language—form, content, and use—may be affected. For example, as a group, children with language impairment have shorter, less elaborated sentences than typical children their age (Greenhalgh & Strong, 2001).

Box 5.1 presents an example of the somewhat scrambled language that we might find exhibited by children with language impairment. It is unclear whether most children with language impairment exhibit impairments in other areas of development as well, but language deficits persist at least through the primary school years for many children (Casby, 1997; Tomblin, Zhang, Buckwalter, & O'Brien, 2003). In the classroom and even on the playground, children with language impairments, especially boys and those with severe receptive language deficits, may be reticent to speak and may lack social maturity and exhibit behavioral problems (Hart, Fujiki, Brinton, & Hart, 2004; Huaqing Qi & Kaiser, 2004).

Box 5.1

Example of Conversation with a Language-Impaired Child

Teacher: Does your family have a pet?

Child: Yeah.

Teacher: Tell me about this pet.

Child: Got a pet.

Teacher: Um-hm, tell me about the pet.

Child: Got a pet.

Teacher: Yes, and I really want to hear about him.

Child: Go with my . . . ah, go with my . . . Dad go with . . .

Teacher: Your dad walks the pet.

Child: No, me.

Teacher: Oh, you and your dad walk the pet.

Child: No, me.

Teacher: Oh, just you walk the dog.

Child: No, me.

Teacher: I'm confused.

Child: Me dog.

Teacher: Oh, it's your dog. Who walks your dog?

Child: With one of them things, you know.

Teacher: What things? Who walks your dog?

Child: With them things like this.

Teacher: Yes, you use a leash.

Noticeably absent from our definition of impairment are language differences, such as those found in some dialectal speakers and in **limited English proficient** individuals learning English as a second language. Differences do not in themselves constitute language impairments and do not require clinical intervention by a speech-language pathologist, although elective intervention is possible at the client's request.

How's your Urdu or Farsi? Few Americans know these languages, which are spoken in parts of India and in Iran, respectively. If you don't speak either, do you have a language disorder? Of course not. But if you moved to Pakistan or Iran, you would need time to learn these languages or any of the others spoken there.

Theoretically, all speakers of a language should be able to communicate. Some differences are so great as to impair communication, but these differences still do not qualify as a disorder.

To guide you through this complicated topic, we'll first look at typical language development followed by a discussion of the major disorders associated with language impairment. Of necessity, this discussion will be an overview.

LANGUAGE DEVELOPMENT THROUGH THE LIFESPAN

As you already know, language is complex; thus any attempt to describe its development will be, of necessity, very complicated. In the following section, we will cover only the highlights and relate these to some of the disorders to be discussed later in the chapter. An outline of language development is presented in Table 5.1.

PRE-LANGUAGE

Children become communicators because they are treated as if they are communicators.

Much of the first year of life is spent learning to be a communicator. Caregivers talk to newborns as if these children understand what the adults are saying. Later on, as children begin to comprehend language in limited ways, caregivers will modify their style of talking to maximize comprehension and participation by the child. Listen to the caregiver-child conversations on the accompanying CD-ROM.

As a speech-language pathologist, should you treat your clients as you treat infants even if they are adults but are unable to speak or to use language?

Shortly after birth, you become actively involved in a reciprocal process with your caregivers. Infants are especially responsive to their caregivers' voices and faces. By as early as two weeks, infants are able to distinguish their caregivers from strangers.

TABLE 5.1
Language development through the lifespan

Age	Accomplishments
3 months	Responds vocally to partner.
8 months	Begins gesturing.
12 months	First word spoken. Words fill intentions previously signaled by gestures.
18 months	Begins combining words on the basis of word-order rules.
2 years	Begins adding bound morphemes. Average length or mean length of utterance (MLU) is 1.6–2.2 morphemes.
3 years	More adultlike sentence structure. MLU is 3.0–3.3 morphemes.
4 years	Begins to change style of talking to fit conversational partner. MLU is 3.6–4.7 morphemes.
5 years	Ninety percent of language form learned.
6 years	Begins to learn visual mode of communication with writing and reading.
Adolescence	Able to competently participate in conversations and telling of narratives.
	Knows multiple meanings of words and figurative language.
	Uses a gender style, or genderlect, when talking.
Adult	Vocabulary has expanded to 30,000–60,000 words.
	Specialized styles of communicating with different audiences and for diverse purposes.

Sources: Klee, Schaffer, May, Membrino, & Mougey, 1989; Miller, 1981; Scarborough, Wyckoff, & Davidson, 1986; Wells, 1985.

To maintain attention, caregivers exaggerate their facial expressions and voice and vocalize more often. In turn, infants respond. Developmental changes affect the dynamic relationship between child and caregiver behaviors and the context (Sameroff & Fiese, 1990).

For some children with communicative impairment, the caregiver-child interaction is disrupted. For example, a child with either mental retardation or autism might not respond in the expected manner.

How would you respond to a child who went limp or stiff when held and would not make eye contact? Or a child who was more interested in objects than in people?

THOUGHT QUESTION

Early on, pre-language dialogues become important. Infants are full partners, and their behavior is influenced by the communication behavior of their caregivers. Turn taking by adults benefits infant sound making. Babbling becomes more speechlike and mature, containing syllables rather than individual sounds.

Eye gaze is very important in these early dialogues. Infants are more likely to begin and to continue looking if their caregivers are looking at them. In return, the caregivers' behavior becomes more social, and play interactions begin.

During the first three months, caregivers' responses teach children the "signal" value of specific behaviors and infants learn a stimulus-response sequence. If they signal, by crying, for example, caregivers will respond. In addition, they learn that a relatively constant stimulus or signal, such as the bottle, results in a predictable response.

Games and rituals share many characteristics with conversations.

By 3 to 4 months, rituals and game playing have emerged. Rituals, such as feeding and diaper changing, provide children with predictable patterns of behavior and speech. As they learn that interactions can unfold in predictable ways; they begin to form expectations of events. Games such as "peekaboo" and "I'm gonna get you" have many of the aspects of communication. There is an exchange of turns, rules for each turn, and particular slots for words and actions. Games, like communication, are also predictable.

At about 8 to 9 months, infants also develop **intentionality** in their interactions with their caregivers and the ability to share goals with others primarily through gestures. Children who are deaf and have been exposed to signing will begin to communicate meaningfully with immature signs at about this age. For the first time, a child considers the audience or other person when attempting a potentially communicative act. In this way, communicative behaviors, such as requesting, interacting, and attracting attention, are first fulfilled by prelinguistic communicative means and only later by language.

An intention to communicate is noted in gestures accompanied by eye contact with the child's communication partner, the use of consistent sound and intonational patterns for specific intentions, and persistent attempts to communicate. Children with autism may be so seemingly uninterested in communication that they do not even communicate with gestures.

Early intentions, such as attracting attention, are established in gestures and first words fill these same functions, often with the accompanying gesture.

Initially, gestures appear without vocalizations, but the two are gradually paired. Consistent vocal patterns, dubbed **phonetically consistent forms (PCFs),** accompany many gestures. PCFs are a transition to words in a highly creative developmental period when the child is also adept at employing gestures and intonation.

Around 12 months, you probably used your first meaningful word. Children's intentions become encoded in a language symbol or word. Real words are used with or without gestures to accomplish the functions previously filled by gestures. To develop spoken language, children must be able to store sounds, use this information for later comparison and identification, and relate these sounds to meaning.

Children "understand" or comprehend in a limited way on the basis of word sounds, nonlinguistic and paralinguistic cues, and context. Most words are probably not comprehended by sound alone. The exceptions may be the child's name and *no*.

The task of learning language and learning to represent and to symbolize is strongly related to cognitive abilities. **Representation** is the process of having one thing stand for another. For example, in play, a piece of paper might be used as a blanket for a doll. **Symbolization** is using an arbitrary symbol, such as a word or sign, to stand for something. Children with cognitive processing difficulties, such as learning disability, or limited cognitive abilities, such as mental retardation (MR), may have problems breaking the language code.

After repeated exposure to mom's face, an infant will smile in recognition upon reexposure. Soon, the mother's voice alone will be enough to recall her image. Her voice *represents,* or stands for, her image.

Later, an arbitrary symbol or word, such as *mama* or *mommy,* will be enough to recall the image or concept of mom. The symbol comes from the linguistic code that is used in the child's environment by caregivers. At about 18 months of age, by using the word, the child will be able to refer to mom even though she is not present. Later, the concept will be expanded to include a definition of mother. In this very simplified explanation, the symbol has come to represent the referent or to symbolize it.

TODDLER LANGUAGE

By 18 months, you probably could produce approximately fifty single words and began to combine two words in predictable ways. Within a few short months, three- and four-word combinations appeared. Accompanying the increases in utterance length and vocabulary is a decrease in the use of babbling.

Use

People who are unfamiliar with young children's language often think that children either imitate all first words or use them only to name. In fact, single words are used to make requests, comments, inquiries, and more.

Words are acquired first within the intentions that the child is able to express in previously acquired gestures. Several early intentions are presented in Table 5.2. Note all the uses or intentions expressed in the conversation presented in Box 5.2.

*T*ry altering a word's purpose or intention by changing the pitch contour and the gesture. Say the word "cookie" as a statement, as a question, and as a demand. A question has a rising intonation, implying "Is this a cookie?" A demand might employ a reach and a whining or insistent intonation. Intent can easily be inferred from these behaviors.

THOUGHT QUESTION

TABLE 5.2
Examples of early intentions of children

Intention	Example
Wanting demand	Says the name of the desired item with an insistent voice. Often accompanied by a reaching gesture.
Protesting	Says "No" or the name of the item while pushing it away, turning away, and/or making a frowning face.
Content questioning	Asks "What?," "That?," or "Wassat?" while pointing and/or looking at an item.
Verbal accompaniment	Speech accompanies some action, such as "whee-e-e" when swung or "Uh-oh" when something spills.
Greeting/farewell	Waves hi or bye with accompanying words.

Note: A fuller list can be found in Owens (2001).

Box **5.2**

Example of Toddler Language

Stacy and her mother are coloring and talking while they do. Note that the language concerns the task. Stacy's mom keeps her utterances short and cues Stacy to respond by asking questions. Stacy participates by talking about the task, often incorporating part of the previous utterance into her own.

Mom: What are you making?

Stacy: Doggie.

Mom: Are you making a doggie? Oh, that's nice, Stacy.

Stacy: Where more doggie?

Mom: Is there another doggie underneath?

Stacy: Yeah.

Mom: Where? Can you find the picture? Is that what you're looking for, the picture of the doggie? Where's a doggie?

Stacy: A doggie. Color a doggie.

Mom: Okay, you color the doggie.

Stacy: Mommy color crayon.

Mom: Mommy has crayons. Mommy's coloring. What's mommy making?

Stacy: Doggie.

Mom: A doggie.

Stacy: Okay.

Mom: All right, I'll make a doggie. Is this the doggie's tail?

Stacy: Doggie's tail. More.

Mom: More doggie?

Stacy: Okay.

Mom: Can Stacy color? Hum?

Stacy: More doggie there. More doggie daddy.

Mom: More doggie daddy?

Stacy: Want a more doggie. More doggie. Put more doggie there.

Mom: Okay, you color the doggie on this page. What color's your doggie?

Stacy: Blue. Color this page, mommy.

Content and Form

The second year is one of vocabulary growth and word combinations. Vocabulary growth is slow for the first few months, but then increases rapidly. By age 2, the toddler has an expressive vocabulary of about 150 to 300 words.

Each toddler has his or her own **lexicon,** or personal dictionary, with words that reflect that child's environment. In general, toddlers' definitions, based on each child's limited experience, are not the same as those of adults.

Early word combinations follow predictable word-order patterns based on semantic categories. For example, *agents,* which cause action, are placed before the *action,* which in turn precedes *objects,* which receive action. As a result, we hear *Daddy eat* and *Mommy throw,* plus *Eat cookie* and *Throw ball,* but only rarely the reverse, such as *Cookie eat.* Within a few months, short-term memory has increased, so the child can attempt a few longer constructions such as *Daddy eat cookie* or *Throw ball me.*

> Adult and toddler definitions are very different, toddler definitions being based almost exclusively on experience while adult ones are based more on meanings shared with others.

PRESCHOOL LANGUAGE

Most communication still occurs within the framework of conversations with caregivers. With increased memory, children expand their conversational skills to include recounting the past and remembering short stories. This memory and recall are aided by the child's increased language skills.

From interaction with others, children form hypotheses about the rules of language and use these hypotheses to produce ever more complex language. Caregivers in each child's environment provide feedback on the child's attempts and models for further growth. Through this process of further and further refinement, children's language increasingly reflects that used in their environment. Many interrelated variables, such as maternal education level and socioeconomic status (SES), affect the child's language development.

The process of language rule hypothesis building is evident in constructions such as *eated* and *goed* that are not found in adult speech but represent a rule in English: Verbs are made past tense by adding *-ed.* Some children and adults with severe mental retardation may have very limited ability to hypothesize about language rules inferred from the language they hear. Children with learning disabilities may be unable to perceive the subtle difference of adding a bound morpheme, such as *-ed,* to change word meaning.

> Language rule learning is a lengthy process that involves hypothesis testing and refinement.

Use

Within conversations with caregivers, preschool children introduce topics but maintain these topics for an average of only two to three turns. It is often easier for a preschool child to introduce a new topic than to continue an old one, as in the following example:

Child: I got a new bike.
Partner: What color is it?
Child: Red.

Partner: Did you ride it on your birthday?

Child: Mommy saw a spider.

Within conversations, preschool children begin to consider that the listener needs to know certain information and the amount of information needed and that there is a need to change conversational style when speaking to younger children. A typical preschool conversation is presented in Box 5.3. Another example is presented on the accompanying CD-ROM.

Style of talking is also reflected in role playing and narration or storytelling. Four-year-old children can tell simple sequential stories of their own or others' authorship.

Box   5.3

Example of Preschool Language

G and B are young 4-year-olds. They are playing with firefighter hats, dishes, and dolls. Notice how different this sample is from the toddler language in Box 5.2. Each child supports her portion of the conversation. The syntax seems adultlike, but the content is pure preschool. The rapid change of topics gives this sample a nonsensical quality. With no adult to maintain a cohesive topic structure, this is a free-for-all with only one or two turns on each topic before it shifts.

G: And I gonna wear both of these.

B: At the same time? No, I'm wearing this one.

G: I'm wearing this one.

B: And then I do this.

G: You wear this and I'll wear this.

B: Two colored cups. You drink out of this one. I drink out of the big one. I'm putting the box up there.

G: Okay, I will. I have this and you have this.

B: Stay up there.

G: She doesn't look too happy.

B: Uh-oh. Why did I spill it?

G: Mine will only stand.

B: Mine sat.

G: All done with supper. What kind of spoon is this?

B: A plastic one, what else? Now it's time for me to make my own dinner.

G: Time for me too. I have to use this. My baby has to go to bed now. We have to first change their diapers.

B: No we don't.

G: Come here, look.

B: There's a button. I want something to drink.

G: Okay, I'll give you some. Look at this. Watch this. I'm gonna try and make this stand. Do you think this is a girl or a boy?

B: A boy.

G: Oh, cause the boy has the pants on and the girl has the dress on.

B: Happy birthday to you.

G: Grab everythin' up. I'm grabbing most of the doll stuff.

Content

From a few words at age 1, children's expressive vocabularies grow to approximately 300 words by age 2, then mushroom to 900 and 1,500 at ages

3 and 4, respectively. Children may comprehend two or three times that many words in context.

Words are learned quickly through a process called **fast mapping** in which the child infers the meaning from context and uses the word in a similar manner. Fuller definitions evolve over time.

In addition to single words, preschool children acquire some relational words and phrases that are used to join other words and create longer units of language. Categories of relational words include locational terms such as *in, on,* and *under*; temporal terms such as *first* and *last*; quantitative terms such as *more than*; qualitative terms such as *bigger than*; familial terms such as *brother*; and conjunctions, such as *and, if, so, but,* and *because.*

> Adultlike forms of many sentences evolve during the preschool years.

In part, semantic development reflects cognitive development. For example, 4-year-olds demonstrate categorization skills that seem to indicate more advanced procedures for storage of learned information than are seen in younger children.

Form

During the preschool years, the emphasis in language development is on language form. The changes in language form are very dramatic.

Beginning with short, two- to four-word sentences at age 2, you probably acquired 90 percent of adult syntax by age 5. For English-speaking preschoolers, language becomes more complex as it becomes longer. We can describe children's language development by calculating the average or **mean length of utterance** (**MLU**) in morphemes. The calculation of MLU will be discussed later in this chapter. Some MLU values are presented in Table 5.1.

The simple word-order rules found in the utterances of 18- to 24-month-olds form the basis for a more elaborate grammar, and by age 3, most children's utterances contain both a subject and a verb. This basic structure is elaborated with the addition of articles, adjectives, auxiliary verbs, prepositions, pronouns, and adverbs.

In addition, adultlike negative, interrogative, and imperative sentence forms evolve. For example, the toddler negative consisting of a Negative + X form, as in *No cookie,* is modified by words such as *no, not, can't, don't,* and *won't* being placed between the subject and verb, as in *Mommy can't catch me.* Other negatives such as *wouldn't, couldn't, is not,* and *isn't* are added later.

Similarly, interrogatives or questions go from single words, such as *Doggie?* and *What?* or *Wassat?,* to more complex questions that ask *what* and *where,* followed developmentally by *who, which,* and *whose,* and finally *when, why* and *how,* and a more mature form in which the verb or auxiliary verb and subject are reversed, as in *Are you happy?*

By the end of preschool, children are joining two or more independent clauses together to form compound sentences. Late preschoolers can also attach dependent clauses to independent clauses to form complex sentences such as *I didn't liked the big dog that barked at grandpa last night.* These structures appear infrequently and will develop slowly and be refined throughout the school-age years.

Several bound morphemes are added during the preschool years. These include the progressive verb ending *-ing,* as in *jumping;* plural *-s,* as in *cats;* possessive *-'s* (or *-s'*), as in *mommy's;* and the past tense verb ending *-ed,* as in *talked.* As might be expected, it takes children some time to acquire the use of these morphemes, and it is not uncommon to hear words such as *eated, goed, sheeps,* and *foots.* Two samples of the speech and language of 3-year-olds is presented on the accompanying CD-ROM.

*L*et's be fair about this. You're a mature speaker, and you don't make mistakes with the plural ending. Is it simply adding an "s" sound? Say a few plural words. Can you figure out the three rules for saying the plural ending well enough to state them? It's not easy.

SCHOOL-AGE AND ADOLESCENT LANGUAGE

When children begin to attend school, they start the long process of establishing their identity independent of their family. Most communication now occurs in conversations outside the home. In part, the status of adolescents within their own social grouping is determined by communication skills. The child with a language problem, an inappropriate voice pitch, or disfluent speech may be unpopular and unhappy.

The means of communication change in school as children learn to read and write. In turn, this skill enables children to use computers and opens a whole new world of information.

Reading and writing development is related to metalinguistic skills. **Metalinguistic skills** enable the child to consider language in the abstract, to make judgments about its correctness, and to create verbal contexts, such as in writing. Younger children are unable to make such judgments, especially without a supporting nonlinguistic context. Children with poor oral language skills will most likely have difficulty with literacy.

*D*oes the possibility of difficulty reading in school justify early intervention with preschool children who have slow language development? When should we become concerned?

Five-year-olds use very adultlike language form, although many of the more subtle syntactic structures are missing. In addition, these children have not acquired some of the pragmatic skills that are needed to be truly effective communicators.

Over the next few years, language development slows and begins to stabilize, but it will be nonetheless significant. Many complex forms and subtle linguistic uses are learned in the adolescent period. The preschool emphasis on development of language form becomes less prominent, and semantic and pragmatic development blossoms.

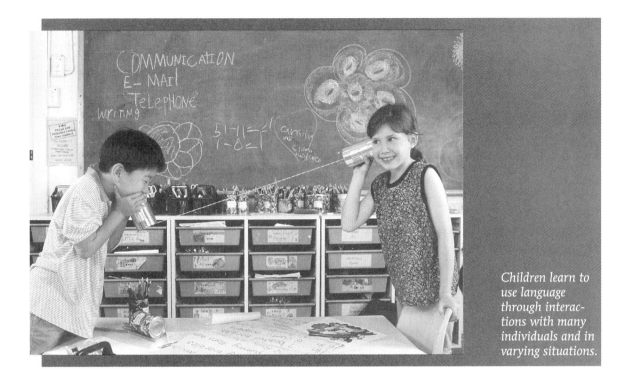

Children learn to use language through interactions with many individuals and in varying situations.

Conversation continues to be the primary locus of communication, and children and adolescents learn to be more effective and efficient communicators. Adolescents consolidate their self and personal identity through multi-tiered peer relationships and restructured family interactions. Slang is used within the peer group to distinguish adolescents from both children and adults. The equality of the peer group aids in this transition at the same time that the lessons of family relationships form a basis for the deepening relationships with peers (Whitmire, 2000).

Use

During the early school-age years, children's language use changes in two ways: Conversational skills continue to develop, and narratives expand and gain all the elements of mature storytelling. Children refine their conversational skills and learn effective ways to introduce new topics and to continue and to end conversations smoothly and appropriately. While in a conversation, they make relevant comments and adapt their roles and moods to fit the situation. In addition, school-age children learn to make even more and increasingly subtle assumptions about the level of knowledge of their listeners and to adjust their conversations accordingly.

> Even with the development of writing, conversation is still the predominant use for language.

Within conversation, teens demonstrate more affect and discuss topics infrequently mentioned at home. The number of turns on a topic increases greatly. Although interrupting increases, it has evolved into behaviors, such as asking pertinent questions, that serve to move the topic along (Larson & McKinley, 1998).

Narratives, both in conversation and in writing, gain the elements needed in our culture to be considered satisfying. English literate narratives contain an introductory setting statement and a challenge or challenges that the characters overcome. Events are organized both sequentially and by cause and effect.

Content

Vocabulary continues to grow but number of words is only the most superficial measure of semantic change. First graders have an expressive vocabulary of approximately 2,600 words but may understand as many as 8,000 root English words and possibly 14,000 when various derivations are included. Aided in school, this receptive vocabulary expands to approximately 30,000 words by sixth grade and to 60,000 words by high school. Multiple word meanings are also acquired.

Definitions become more dictionary-like, which means that they become less experiential or less based on individual experience and more shared, categorical, as in *An apple is a kind of fruit,* and more precise. The increasing size of children's vocabularies requires more precision and an organization into categories for easy retrieval.

School-age children also learn to understand and use **figurative language.** Unlike literal meanings, figurative language does not always mean what it seems to mean. For example, *idioms* are expressions that often cannot be justified literally, such as "hit the road" or "off the wall." Figurative language enriches communication but requires higher language functions of interpretion. Some forms are not comprehended until adulthood.

Form

Following the rapid development of language form in preschool, there is a gradual slowing, although development continues. Many forms will continue to develop into adolescence. Initially, children's speech is much more complex than their writing, but the relationship reverses permanently for most of us in late elementary school.

*I*f mastery of language form is a slow process during the school years, when do we decide that a child is having enough difficulty to require therapeutic intervention?

By age 5, children use most verb tenses with common verbs and auxiliary or helping verbs, such as *would, should, must,* and *might,* although they still have some difficulty with multiple auxiliary verbs, as in *should have been;* possessive pronouns (*his, her, your*); and the conjunctions *and, but, if, because, when,* and *so.* Five-year-old children also have limited use of the comparative *-er,* as in *bigger,* and superlative *-est,* as in *biggest;* relative pronouns used in complex sentences (I know *who* lives next door); gerunds (We go *fishing*); and infinitives (I want *to eat* now).

Many syntactic structures appear slowly, and children may struggle with acquisition well into the school years. During the school years, children gradually add passive sentences, such as *The cat is chased by the dog,* in which the entity performing the action is placed at the end rather than the beginning of the sentence; reflexive pronouns, such as *myself, yourself, himself,* and *themselves;* conjunctions, such as *although* and *however* and variations of compound and complex sentences.

It frequently takes the child several years of practice to gain complete control of these linguistic structures. As might be expected, children with perceptual problems, as in learning disability, frequently miss subtle differences of meaning.

Morphological development focuses on derivational suffixes—word endings that change the word class, such as adding *-er* to a verb to make a noun, as in *paint/painter*—and prefixes. Development of prefixes, such as *un-, ir-,* and *dis-* will continue into adulthood.

ADULT LANGUAGE

Language development continues through your lifespan, although at a much slower pace. Adults continue to add new words and to perfect grammatical forms, especially in the written mode. Specialized vocabulary and syntax will reflect your work environment, religion, hobbies, education level, and so on. As long as you remain free of any neuropathology, you should continue to improve into old age. And you will amaze yourself with your ability to express complicated ideas with equally complex syntax.

ASSOCIATED DISORDERS AND RELATED CAUSES

Language and its use are extremely complex. It stands to reason, then, that language impairment would be even more so. So many things can go wrong at so many junctures that each child with a language impairment represents a unique set of circumstances.

In this section, we discuss several disorders in which language impairment is a significant factor. Of necessity, we will be discussing groups of children under different categories of disorder. Categories are helpful for discussion of shared characteristics, but categories are not the same as individuals. Each individual is unique.

Has anyone ever said to you "Oh, you're so intelligent"—or athletic, good-looking, or some similar trait? Did you then feel that you had to act a certain way around that person? Did you feel that this person treated you differently?

THOUGHT QUESTION

The effect that any disorder has on communication and on language development will vary with the severity of the disorder and the age of the client. As individuals mature, the communicative requirements change.

We will not be discussing all children with language impairment. The largest group to be excluded are individuals with hearing impairments. These individuals will be discussed in Chapter 14, "Audiology and Disorder of Hearing." Children may also exhibit impairments such as aphasia, which are generally considered to be adult disorders. Aphasia is a loss of language as the result of localized brain injury and will be discussed in Chapter 7, "Adult Language Impairments."

MENTAL RETARDATION/DEVELOPMENTAL DISABILITIES

According to the American Association on Mental Retardation, **mental retardation (MR)** is characterized by the following:

1. Substantial limitations in present functioning
2. Significantly subaverage intellectual functioning
3. Concurrent related limitations in two or more of the following applicable adaptive skill areas: communication, self-care, home living, social skills, community use, self-direction, health and safety, functional academics, leisure, and work
4. Manifestation before age 18 (American Association on Mental Retardation, 1992)

Accounting for approximately 2.5 percent of the population, people with mental retardation/developmental disability vary based on causality and other factors such as the amount of home support, the living environment, education, mode of communication, and age.

Mental retardation means more than just a low IQ. Values such as IQ usually measure past learning only.

THOUGHT QUESTION

Could you ever become mentally retarded? No, according to the definition, because you're over 18. You might acquire some other problem that would impair your performance, such as a head injury, but MR is a developmental disorder and, by age 18, most of development is complete.

Severity classifications are usually based on the level of IQ and range from mild to profound. Ranges of severity and characteristics are presented in Table 5.3. However, a rating that is based only on IQ may reveal little about overall functioning. Each individual is different, and IQ is only one measure of overall functioning. For example, relatively high social skills may either mask or compensate for low intelligence. In addition, similar IQs in individuals with different ages will result in very different skill levels.

Causes of retardation are almost as varied as individuals. Two large categories of possible causal factors are biological and socioenvironmental, although for many individuals, the cause is unknown. These factors are

TABLE 5.3

Severities of mental retardation/developmental disability

Category	IQ Range	% of MR Population	Characteristics
Mild	52–68	89	Usually absorbed into the community where they work and live independently
Moderate	36–51	6	Capable of learning self-care skills and working within a sheltered environment; live semi-independently, with relatives, or in a community residence
Severe	20–35	3½	Capable of learning some self-care skills and are not totally dependent; often exhibit physical disabilities and deficits in speech and language
Profound	Below 20	1½	Capable of learning some basic living skills but require continual care and supervision; often exhibit severe physical and/or sensory problems

Source: Reprinted by permission from Owens, R. E. (1997). Mental retardation: Difference and delay. In D. K. Bernstein & E. Tiegerman (Eds.), *Language and Communication Disorders in Children* (4th ed.). Boston: Allyn and Bacon.

complicated by cognitive limitations that affect the processing of incoming and outgoing information. Biological factors include the following:

Genetic and chromosomal abnormalities

Maternal infections during pregnancy

Toxins and chemical agents

Nutritional and metabolic causes

Gestational disorders affecting development of the fetus

Complications from pregnancy

Complications from delivery

Brain diseases

Socioenvironmental factors include a stimulation-impoverished environment, poor housing, inadequate diet, poor hygiene, and lack of medical care. The effect of each of these factors varies with each child.

Information processing consists of four steps: attending, discriminating, organizing, and retrieving. In general, individuals with mild-moderate MR can sustain attention as well as mental-age-matched non-MR peers but have difficulty scanning and selecting stimuli to which to attend.

Individuals with mental retardation may process incoming sensory information differently from those without retardation.

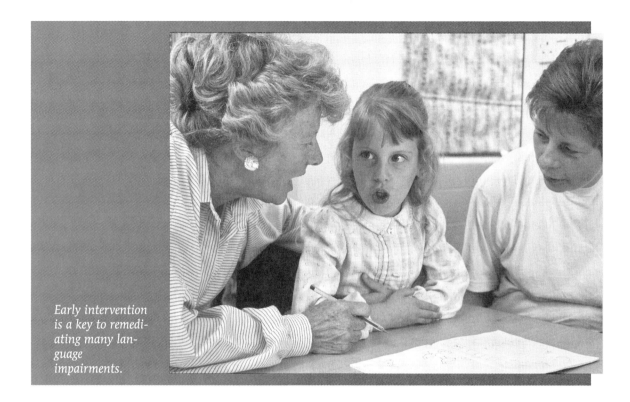

Early intervention is a key to remediating many language impairments.

The ability to discriminate likenesses and differences is related to the severity of mental retardation. The more severe the mental retardation, the more difficulty the person will have in discriminating. In general, individuals with MR are limited in their ability to identify relevant cues and attend to all dimensions of a task.

Organization or the categorizing of information for storage is especially challenging for individuals with MR. In short, they do not rely on strategies that link words and concepts to one another. Nor do they spontaneously rehearse information for easy retrieval.

Memory or retrieval of previously stored information is poor and operates more slowly within the MR population. Organizational deficits contribute to this performance. Humans generally retain information by rehearsal, but those with MR do not seem to use this strategy spontaneously. To some extent, memory is affected by the type of information (Kay-Raining Bird & Chapman, 1994). Individuals with MR have more difficulty with auditory input, especially linguistic, than with visual input.

Incoming linguistic information undergoes several types of decoding. Simultaneous synthesis occurs all at once and extracts overall meaning. Successive synthesis is more linear, occurring a piece at a time. Although individuals with MR exhibit some difficulty with both types, those with Down syndrome have much greater difficulty with successive processing, possibly reflecting poor short-term auditory memory.

Lifespan Issues

Some newborns and infants with MR will be identified early because of obvious physical factors, such as syndromes or anatomical anomalies, at-risk indicators such as low birthweight or poor physical responses, or delayed development. Intervention may begin at home or in special early intervention centers. It is best for the child if intervention begins as soon as possible. Early intervention will focus on sensorimotor skills, physical development, and social and communicative abilities. An Individualized Family Services Plan (IFSP) is written with specified services.

Some children with MR are not identified until age 2 or 3. These youngsters, along with those previously identified, will likely attend a special preschool. They may also receive some intervention services, such as physical therapy, special education, or speech-language therapy in the home.

Depending on the severity of a school-age child's mental retardation, she or he may attend a regular education class and receive special services. Some children will receive education in a self-contained, special classroom. Education and training will focus on academic skills, daily living and self-help activities, and vocational needs.

Only those children with the most profound MR accompanied by other disabilities are institutionalized. Generally, children who cannot reside at home live in community residences with eight to ten other children their age and houseparents.

Mike, a boy with profound MR and cerebral palsy, lived at home with his parents as an infant and preschooler. As he matured and his parents aged, Mike was placed in a community residence run by the Association for Retarded Citizens. He received daily care at this center and was able to continue his education at the same school. Most of his training involved daily living skills and use of a communication board to communicate.

In adulthood, living and working arrangements vary widely. People with milder retardation often live in the community and work competitively in minimally skilled jobs. More severely involved individuals may live with family or in community residences containing a small group of similar adults. They may work in a special workshop or be enrolled in a day treatment program in which education and training continue to be the focus.

Language Characteristics

For many individuals with MR, language is the single most important limitation. For 50 percent of the MR population, language comprehension and/or production is below the level of cognition (Miller, Chapman, & MacKenzie, 1981). This might be indicative of cognitive processing problems that accompany MR. For example, children with Down syndrome exhibit auditory short-term memory deficits (Seung & Chapman, 2000).

In initial language development, individuals with MR follow a similar but slower developmental path than that of typically developing children. Even so, children with MR produce shorter, less elaborated utterances—a quantitative difference. Individuals with MR use more immature forms (Boudreau & Chapman, 2000). In later development, the paths begin to dif-

Very few individuals with mental retardation live in large institutions. Beginning in the 1970s, a philosophy called deinstitutionalization has been responsible for the movement of individuals with MR into small community residences.

fer more qualitatively. All areas of language exhibit some delay and disorder in children with MR.

LEARNING DISABILITIES

The National Joint Committee on Learning Disabilities (1991) defines *learning disabilities (LD)* as follows:

> a generic term that refers to a heterogeneous group of disorders manifested by significant difficulties in the acquisition and use of listening, speaking, reading, writing, reasoning, or mathematical abilities. These disorders are intrinsic to the individual and are presumed to be due to *central nervous system dysfunction*. Even though a learning disability may occur concomitantly with other handicapping conditions or environmental influences, it is **not** the direct result of those conditions or influences. (p. 19)

Approximately 15 percent of children with LD have their major difficulty with motor learning and coordination, while more than 75 percent primarily have difficulty learning and using symbols (Miniutti, 1991). This latter group is said to have a **language-learning disability.**

Approximately 3 percent of all individuals have LD, but the severity varies widely. Learning disabilities affect males four times as frequently as they do females.

The characteristics of LD fall into six categories: motor, attention, perception, symbol, memory, and emotion. Few children will exhibit all of the characteristics described. Motor difficulties may include either hyperactivity or hypoactivity. Hyperactivity or overactivity is more prevalent, especially among boys. This results in difficulty attending and concentrating for more than very short periods. Children with hypoactivity may be deficient in their sense of body movement, definition of handedness, eye-hand coordination, and space and time conceptualization.

Attentional difficulties include a short attention span, inattentiveness, and distractibility. Irrelevant stimuli may capture the child's attention, and overstimulation easily occurs. Some children become fixed on a single task or behavior and repeat it, a process called *perseveration*.

Those who have hyperactivity and attentional difficulties but do not manifest other characteristics of LD may be labeled as having **attention deficity hyperactivity disorder (ADHD).** Children with ADHD have an underlying neurological impairment in executive function that regulates behavior; as a result, they are impulsive. Although these children have difficulty using language socially and educationally, they may be missed on language testing that ignores pragmatics (Oram, Fine, Okamoto, & Tannock, 1999).

Perceptual difficulties involve interpretation of incoming stimuli, but this is not a sensory disorder, such as deafness or blindness. Children with perceptual disabilities often confuse similar sounds, similar-sounding words, and similar-looking printed letters and words. In addition, children with LD may have difficulty both in determining where to focus their attention and in integrating sensory information from different sources, such as vision and hearing. Those children having particular difficulty in comprehending

> Children with language learning disabilities have difficulty learning and using symbols for speaking, listening, reading, and writing.

printed symbols may be labeled *dyslexic*. **Dyslexia** is characterized by word recognition and/or reading comprehension problems. Children who have difficulty producing written symbols are said to have **dysgraphia.** Both will be discussed in more detail in Chapter 6, "Developmental Literacy Impairments."

Memory difficulties affect short-term retrieval, as in remembering directions, and long-term retrieval as in recalling names, sequences, and words. Some children also will exhibit word-finding problems. The resultant blocks and the use of fillers ("Ah, ah, you know . . .") or circumlocutions ("Oh, it's that thing that does that stuff that goes round . . .") may resemble similar behaviors in stutterers, discussed in Chapter 8 (German & Simon, 1991).

Emotional problems are usually an accompanying factor, not a causal factor. They are a reaction to the frustration that these children feel. Although most children with LD have normal intelligence, they perform poorly on language-based tasks and are told that they are not trying or that they're lazy or stupid. Emotional behavior may result in children being described as aggressive, impulsive, unpredictable, withdrawn, and/or impatient. These youngsters may exhibit poor judgment, unusual fears, and/or poor adjustment to change.

> Learning disabilities are not caused by emotional disorders; rather, the emotional problems result from misperception and from frustration.

The fact that LD occurs more frequently in families with a history of the disorder and in children who had a premature or difficult birth suggests possible biological causal factors. The central nervous system dysfunction mentioned in the definition may involve a breakdown along the neural pathways that connect the midbrain with the frontal cortex, an area that is responsible for attention, regulation, and planning of cognitive activity (Bass, 1988).

Socioenvironmental factors may account for at least some of the behaviors. For example, misperceptions by the child affect interactions, which influence the child's development, especially language. Language difficulties, in turn, affect the child's interactions.

Processing difficulties are characterized by an inability to use certain strategies or to access certain stored information. In general, children with LD exhibit poor ability to attend selectively, concentrating on inappropriate or unimportant stimuli (Levine, 1987). They have difficulty deciding on the relevant information to which to attend. As we have seen, discrimination is extremely difficult because children with LD are not sure of the relevant aspects of a stimulus that make it similar or dissimilar to another.

Are you able to attend to lectures? Are you sometimes distracted by competing stimuli, such as the hum of the lights, the sniffling of the person next to you, or the noise outside? Imagine what it would be like if you couldn't screen these out.

Information that is poorly attended to and poorly discriminated will be poorly organized. The cognitive organization of children with LD reflects this confusion. In short, the organization is too inefficient for easy retrieval, so memory is less accurate and retrieval is slower.

Lifespan Issues

As preschoolers, children with LD may exhibit little interest in language or even in books. When a child reaches school, the linguistic demands of the classroom are often well above her or his oral language abilities. The result is often academic underachievement.

Most learning disabilities are not discovered until children go to school, although some children may be enrolled in special preschool programs or may receive therapy services because of poor motor coordination, hyperactivity, or a failure to develop language typically. When they reach school and its accompanying demand for language skills, many children with LD require the services of special educators, speech-language pathologists, and reading specialists. Some children might not be identified in early grades. Very bright children may "learn" to read by memorizing word shapes rather than using phonics-based word-attack skills.

Children with LD often receive special services while being included in regular classrooms. They can be successful if some adaptation, such as repeating instructions or allowing for a quiet work space, is made by the teacher to accommodate their needs. Case Study 5.2 tells the story of one child with language learning disability.

Some children with LD seem to outgrow their disability. Hyperactivity seems to fade in adolescence. Some adolescents succeed well enough to continue their education and graduate from college. We know adults with learning disabilities who are chemists, engineers, teachers, and speech-language pathologists, although some have lingering vestiges of LD.

Other adults continue to have difficulty. Matt received special services throughout his school years and finished high school. His language difficulties were complicated by a volatile temper and frequent misinterpretations of the communicative intentions of others. After being fired from a series of jobs, he hit upon the idea of informing his new boss that he was "partially deaf" and needed all instructions and feedback repeated while he watched the speaker. He no longer flies off the handle when given a simple directive by his supervisor.

Language Characteristics

All aspects of language, spoken and written, usually are affected in children with language-learning disabilities (Wallach & Butler, 1995). These children experience difficulty with the give-and-take of conversation and with the form and content of language. Synthesizing of language rules is particularly difficult, resulting in delays in morphological rule acquisition and in the development of syntactic complexity. As a result, overall oral language development may be slow, and frequent communicative breakdown is possible (MacLachlan & Chapman, 1988). Word-finding problems may exist, resulting in greater time being needed to respond verbally.

Some children with LD experience disfluent speech that on the surface might seem like stuttering. Called **cluttering,** the behaviors are character-

Attentional, discriminatory, and memory deficits along with both receptive and expressive symbol use problems can result in many communication breakdowns.

ized by overuse of fillers and circumlocutions associated with word-finding difficulties, rapid speech, and word and phrase repetitions. Unlike the situation with stuttering, the child seems barely to recognize his or her disfluency, and no fear of words or speech situations seems to exist.

Case Study 5.2

Personal Story of a Child with Language Learning Disabilities

Darren's language learning disability went undetected until second grade. As a preschooler, he had some difficulty with speech sounds and displayed little interest in books, letters, or drawing. His mother considered his lack of interest and his overactivity to be a "boy thing." Darren received no preschool education. In first grade, he was slow to learn to read and write, as were several of his classmates.

When Darren still seemed to be struggling in second grade, his teacher suggested an evaluation to determine whether he had a learning disability. He was evaluated by the school psychologist, a reading specialist, a special education teacher, and a speech-language pathologist. It was found that Darren's mother had received little, if any, prenatal care and that Darren was born preterm, weighing only 4 pounds, 10 ounces. After a stay in the hospital of several days, Darren went home with his mother. The rest of his preschool years were uneventful, and he remained at home with his older sister and younger brother, experiencing the occasional middle ear infection or childhood illness. Although his sister exhibits no signs of a learning disability, Darren's younger brother does exhibit hyperactivity.

At age 11, Darren is a very active child who enjoys sports, especially soccer, which he plays with his best friend Carlos. Darren has great difficulty reading and writing, and letter and word reversal and transposition are common in both. He has great difficulty sounding out new words. His speech is characterized by word retrieval problems and a limited vocabulary, peppered with "Ya know," "thing," and "one," as in "An' I got that one, ya know, that thing that goes like this."

Darren has had some difficulty behaving in school. His attention easily wanders, and he fidgets in his seat often. If he is not kept busy, he bothers the other students and keeps them from working. He finds himself in frequent fights in school, usually because he has misunderstood some comment of another student. His temper flares easily, possibly because school can be very frustrating.

Although his schoolwork has improved somewhat, he is still well behind his classmates in his ability to read, write, and work independently. This deficit, in turn, has inhibited his ability to problem solve and to think critically in class. He continues to receive tutoring in reading and writing and to see the speech-language pathologist weekly to work on vocabulary, word retrieval, and language use skills.

SPECIFIC LANGUAGE IMPAIRMENT

Approximately 10 to 15 percent of middle-class U.S. children may be "late bloomers" whose early language development is delayed. Most outgrow it. Slightly fewer than half of these children will continue to have problems (Dale, Price, Bishop, & Plomin, 2003). These children are at risk for academic failure when they begin school because they will not have the basic language skills for reading and writing in first grade (Choudhury & Benasich, 2003). Affecting males more than females, the oral and written language deficits of SLI appear to be cross-generational in nature (Flax, Realpe-Bonilla, Hirsch, Brzustowicz, Bartlett, & Tallal, 2003).

These children exhibit significant limitations in language functioning that cannot be attributed to deficits in hearing, oral structure and function, general intelligence, or perception. In other words, no obvious anatomical, physical, intellectual, or perceptual cause seems to exist. When this occurs, these children are said to possess a specific language impairment (SLI).

Similar to those with LD, children with SLI exhibit language performance scores that are significantly lower than their intellectual performance scores on nonverbal tasks. The major distinction between those with LD and SLI is that those with SLI do not exhibit perceptual difficulties, the misinterpretation of incoming information.

Although mostly preschoolers, children with SLI are a very heterogeneous group, especially in their language skills. Because the disorder is characterized primarily by the exclusion of other disorders, some professionals doubt the very existence of the disorder (Kamhi, 1998). Still, there are many children with language impairment for whom no readily identifiable causal factors exist.

Causal factors are difficult to identify. Nonverbal intelligence, birth and delivery, hearing, and self-help and motor skills all seem to be within normal limits (Paul, 1991). There is an increased prevalence in families with a history *of speech and language problems.*

Biological factors point to possible brain asymmetry, in which language functions are located in different areas from those found in the majority of individuals (Aram & Eisele, 1994).

There is no single, obvious cause for specific language impairment.

Children with SLI do exhibit some information-processing problems with certain types of incoming sensory information, memory, and problem solving (Kamhi, 1998; Weismer & Hesketh, 1996). Short-term auditory sequential memory and problem solving in complex reasoning tasks are affected (Kamhi, Gentry, Mauer, & Gholson, 1990). Limits in verbal working memory suggest that children with SLI have a limited capacity for language processing (Deevy & Leonard, 2004; Marton & Schwartz, 2003; Weismer, Evans, & Hesketh, 1999). Brain imaging of children with SLI indicates brain symmetry in the left and right hemispheres unlike the usual asymmetry of left-side predominance in language processing regions (Ors, Ryding, Lindgren, Gustafsson, Blennow, & Rosén, 2005).

Lifespan Issues

Children with SLI are perceived negatively, even by other preschool children, because their communication skills do not match expectations (Segebart DeThorne & Watkins, 2001). In addition, children with SLI exhibit poor social skills (Conti-Ramsden & Botting, 2004).

Many children with SLI are later identified as having a language-learning disability. Lingering effects of SLI may result in reading difficulties that reflect difficulty with earlier language skills, such as rhyming, letter naming, and concepts related to print (Boudreau & Hedberg, 1999). In general, children with SLI exhibit slower and poorer processing of both linguistic and nonlinguistic material even in elementary school (Miller, Kail, Leonard, & Tomblin, 2001; Weismer, Tomblin, et al., 2000; Windsor & Hwang, 1999).

Long-term data on children with SLI are sparse. Studies have indicated later academic difficulties, especially with language-based activities.

Language Characteristics

In general, children with SLI have difficulty (1) extracting regularities from the language around them; (2) registering different contexts for language; and (3) constructing word-referent associations for lexical growth (Connell & Stone, 1992; Kiernan, Snow, Swisher, & Vance, 1997). As a result, these youngsters experience difficulty in morphological and phonological rule formation and application and in vocabulary development (Frome Loeb & Leonard, 1991; Oetting & Morohov, 1997; Redmond, 2003). Pragmatic problems seem to result from an inability to use language forms effectively, resulting in more inappropriate utterances (Brinton, Fujiki, & Powell, 1997). Although word-learning is difficult for children with SLI, comprehension seems to be easier than production (Gray, 2004).

Language comprehension and processing are active processes, yet children with SLI do not appear to employ them actively. Auditory processing problems may result in difficulties with morphological inflections, such as past tense -*ed,* function words such as prepositions and articles (e.g., *a, the*), auxiliary verbs, and pronouns. Children with SLI exhibit persistent problems with morpheme use regardless of the language (Bedore & Leonard, 2001; Dromi, Leonard, Adam, & Zadunaisky-Ehrlich, 1999; Redmond & Rice, 2001), and they are less efficient in using syntax to aid in the acquisition of lexical items (Rice, Cleave, & Oetting, 2000).

AUTISM SPECTRUM AND PERVASIVE DEVELOPMENTAL DISORDERS

Autism spectrum disorder (ASD) is at the more severe end of an impairment known as **pervasive developmental disorder (PDD).** Some children with PDD may have **hyperlexia,** an inordinate interest in letters and words, characterized by early ability to read but with little comprehension. Others have **semantic-pragmatic disorder,** characterized by limited vocabulary, concrete definitions, and poor conversational skills (Aram, 1997; Snowling & Frith, 1986). A milder form of PDD, called **Asperger's syndrome,** is characterized by normal intelligence and typical language development with deficits in social and communication skills.

Autism spectrum disorder is described as an impairment in reciprocal social interaction with a severely limited behavior, interest, and activity repertoire that has its onset before 30 months of age (American Psychiatric Association, 1987). It is characterized by disturbances in the following areas (Ritvo & Freeman, 1978):

- *Developmental rates and the sequence of motor, social-adaptive, and cognitive skills.* Development often proceeds in spurts and plateaus, rather than smoothly, and most areas of development are affected. Slightly more than half of the children with ASD have IQs below 50. The remainder are split evenly between IQs of 50–70 and IQs of 71 and above. These figures might not be accurate but rather represent our inability to test adequately.

- *Responses to sensory stimuli.* The same child may be both hypersensitive and hyposensitive in audition, vision, and tactile, motor, olfactory, and taste stimulation. The child may have preferences for

Few children are labeled as autistic. Usually, children are described as having "autisticlike" behavior or "autistic tendencies." More recently, children are described as having ASD or a severe form of PDD.

routines and become extremely upset with change. In addition, the child might engage in self-stimulatory behaviors, such as hand flapping, rocking, or spinning shiny objects.

- *Speech and language, cognition, and nonverbal communication.* Individuals with ASD may be nonspeaking, minimally verbal, echolalic, or nearly typical in their communication.

- *Capacity to appropriately relate to people, events, and objects.* As infants, children with ASD are described as either lethargic, preferring solitude and making few demands, or highly irritable, with sleeping problems and screaming and crying. As they age, they may exhibit little affection and inappropriate play behaviors.

At this point, you may be suffering from *characteristics overload.* Stop briefly and try to recall the differences between MR, LLD, SLI, and ASD.

THOUGHT QUESTIONS

Might the world seem very different to you if you could perceive stimuli differently? Suppose that you had a dog's sense of smell. Could sensory differences alone explain the behavior of children with ASD?

The primary causal factors in autism are probably biological (Schreibman, 1988). Approximately 65 percent of all individuals with ASD have neurological differences and 20 to 30 percent experience seizures. In addition, some researchers have found unusually high levels of serotonin, a neurotransmitter and natural opiate, and abnormal development of the cerebellum, which regulates incoming sensations, and of sections of the temporal lobe responsible for memory and emotions.

Neural studies suggest that the eye and face detection processing of children with autism may be delayed, explaining, in part, the early failure to bond with caregivers (Grice, Halit, Farroni, Baron-Cohen, Bolton, & Johnson, 2005). Additionally, infants with autism show no difference in brain response to familiar and unfamiliar faces, supporting the notion of facial processing impairment (Dawson et al., 2002).

The incidence of ASD is higher among males—by a 4:1 ratio to females—and among those with a family history of autism. The family pattern suggests a genetic basis for the disorder, although no specific single gene has been directly linked to the disorder.

Some causal factors relate to processing incoming information. Individuals with ASD experience difficulty in analyzing and integrating information. Their responding is often very overselective, resulting in a tendency to fixate on one aspect of a complex stimulus, often some irrelevant, minor detail. As a result, discrimination is difficult.

Overall processing by children with ASD has been characterized as a gestalt in which unanalyzed wholes are stored and later reproduced in identical fashion. The storage of unanalyzed wholes may account for the way in which individuals with ASD become quickly overloaded with sensory information. Storage of unanalyzed wholes also might hinder memory. It's difficult to organize information on the basis of relationships between stimuli if those stimuli remain unanalyzed. Lack of analysis would also hinder transferring or generalizing learned information from one context to another.

Lifespan Issues

Children with ASD are usually identified by the time they're 2 or 3 years of age. Parental concerns may involve lack of communication and/or lack of social skills. Toddlers may fail to begin gesturing or talking, seem uninterested in other people, lack vocal and verbal responding, or focus on an object intently even though parents interact with their children with ASD at the appropriate language level. These young children are generally involved in early intervention and special preschooling.

School-aged children and adolescents with ASD or PDD may be included in regular education classes or be in special classes, depending on the severity of the disorder. In some children, the severity of autism or ASD lessens with age. For example, as Jeffery became a teenager, his behavior seemed to be less disruptive, and there were fewer outbursts. Although he could engage in conversation easily, he continued to become annoyed and to begin flapping his hands if more than one person spoke at a time.

People with milder forms of the disorder may be able to live on their own and hold competitive employment. For example, Dr. Temple Grandin, an individual with ASD, is employed as a college professor. Unfortunately, the vast majority of people with ASD are not so successful and require supervision and care. Many have adult life patterns similar to those of adults with MR. Case Study 5.3 presents the story of a young man with ASD.

Language Characteristics

Communication problems are often one of the first indicators of possible ASD. Between 25 and 60 percent of individuals with ASD remain nonspeaking throughout their life. Those who speak often have a wooden or robotlike voice that lacks any musical quality. Many autistic children who use speech and language demonstrate some immediate or delayed echolalia, which is a whole or partial repetition of previous utterances, often with the same intonation. Mickey would say little during the day but store things said to him during the day and repeat them in sequence before he went to sleep at night. For some children, echolalia might either be a language processing strategy or signal agreement with the previous utterance. Even though echolalia may be outgrown, other problems, especially those related to pragmatics, persist in the child's language.

Pragmatics and semantics are affected more than language form (Lord, 1988). Syntactic errors seem to represent a lack of underlying semantic relationships. Prosodic phonology or suprasegmentals, such as stress, intonation, loudness, pitch, and rate, are often affected, giving the speech of children with ASD its sometimes mechanical quality. Individuals with ASD often have peculiarities and irregularities in their language, especially in the pragmatics of conversation. The range of intentions is often very limited and may consist solely of demands and seemingly self-entertaining gibberish. Some individuals incorporate entire verbal routines, called *formuli,* into their

> Pragmatics is a continuing problem for individuals with autism, even those with seemingly typical language.

communication. For example, a child might repeat part or all of a television commercial to indicate a desire for the item that had been in the advertisement. A formula represents the person's attempt to overcome the difficulty of matching the content and form of language to the communicative context. Adults with ASD who have good language skills might still misinterpret some of the subtleties of conversation.

Case Study 5.3

Story of a Young Man with Autism Spectrum Disorder (ASD)

During high school and well into college, literal thinking and little imagination governed how I took in a lot of information and interpreted much of the world. These factors also limited comprehension of what I read.

This was the central tenet of the larger picture: I suffered from autism. I was born with the disability. Compulsions and fixations changed with time, but varied little with intensity. My childhood was devoid of comfort, security, and pleasure; repetitive activities over which I exerted control filled a void. . . . For years I saw life's events in black and white, had a profound lack of imagination, and blocked out that which was not the compulsion of the moment.

My lack of imagination compounded my lack of self-esteem and other psychological problems that developed and fused as I got older. . . . I reacted angrily when someone inadvertently violated one of my arbitrary rules. I had a set notion of the order in which family members were to come to the breakfast table and where they should sit . . . My out-of-proportion anger when someone broke a rule that I could not articulate the need for caused . . . embarrassment. . . .

Numerous other life examples followed this pattern. I felt comfortable watching and being mesmerized by spinning objects such as a washing machine or a top. But a top's movement wasn't the only circular aspect of my autism. Later, the more severe my autistic behavior was, the more I alienated people; the more I alienated other kids, the more I withdrew. And the more I withdrew, the more my fragile self-esteem suffered, adding to the need to do repetitive activities for comfort.

All of this was my way of trying to relate to, and make sense of, a chaotic world. These behaviors provided short-term comfort and control. . . .

Unlike a fine wine, my life did not get better with age. Certain fixations disappeared over time, but were replaced with others. As a teenager, my speech, thinking, and relating to others was mechanical, rote, literal, and rigid. . . . [M]y most terrifying moments as a [h]igh [s]chool student occurred not in class, but between classes. My self-esteem was so low that when the halls exploded with 2,000 students, I felt on display. At times, I clung precariously to the wall's edge, holding on for dear life as I made my way to the next class. . . .

My slow recovery made me realize how much I missed and how much I didn't know. For years, I had little perspective about relationships; if people showed me positive attention, I would "absorb" them. . . . When I was flipping light switches off and on and doing numerous other compulsive activities, I wasn't bonding with other children. Years later, no sudden transformation took place that allowed me to naturally and spontaneously reach out to others. . . .

As my point of view expanded, I began to see how my behavior affected other people other than myself, and how socially inept I was. Soon, I began to turn years of unresolved anger and blame inward. . . . And I constantly feared I would one day regress. Such fears were "confirmed" whenever I reacted to stress in an autistic way. . . . Gradually, I reached a point where I could objectively discuss any aspect of my autism.

Unfortunately, not everyone will make a full recovery. Like most things in life, autism has varying degrees. . . . But I hope I've shown that there's nothing hopeless about it. . . . I'm free.

Source: From Barron, S. (2001, September 25). A personal story. *The ASHA Leader, 6*(17), 5, 7, 17. © American Speech-Language-Hearing Association. Reprinted by permission.

BRAIN INJURY

Brain injury can be confused with LD, MR, or emotional disorders, although individuals with these disorders are very different. Impaired brain functioning can result from **traumatic brain injury (TBI),** cerebrovascular accident or stroke, congenital malformation, convulsive disorders, or encephalopathy, such as infection or tumors. Among children, the most common form of injury is TBI. Cerebrovascular accidents will be discussed in Chapter 7, "Adult Language Impairments."

Approximately one million children and adolescents in the United States have experienced TBI, which is diffuse brain damage as the result of external force, such as a blow to the head in an auto accident. Individuals with brain injury differ greatly from one another as a result of the site and extent of lesion, the age at onset, and the age of the injury. In general, the smaller the damaged area, the better the chance of recovery. Some individuals recover fully; others remain in a vegetative state. People with TBI exhibit a range of cognitive, physical, behavioral, academic, and linguistic deficits, any of which may be long-term in nature (Zitnay, 1995).

Cognitive deficits include difficulties in perception, memory, reasoning, and problem solving. Deficits vary and may be permanent or temporary and may partially or totally affect functioning ability. Children with TBI tend to be inattentive and easily distractible. All aspects of organization—categorizing, sequencing, abstracting, and generalization—may be affected. Children with TBI seem unable to see relationships, make inferences, and solve problems. They have difficulty formulating goals, planning, and achieving their ends. Memory is also affected, although long-term memory before the trauma is usually intact.

Psychological maladjustment or "acting out" behaviors, called *social disinhibition,* may occur in which a person is incapable of inhibiting or controlling impulsive behavior. Other characteristics of TBI may include a lack of initiative, distractibility, inability to adapt quickly, perseveration, low frustration levels, passive-aggressiveness, anxiety, depression, fear of failure, and misperception.

Lifespan Issues

After the accident, an individual may be unconscious. The coma may last only a few minutes or much longer. Upon regaining consciousness, the individual usually experiences some disorientation and memory loss. Amnesia may involve only the time of the immediate accident or may be more extensive, including long-term memory. The disoriented individual might not recall what happened or understand the extent of his or her injuries or limitations. TBI may be accompanied by physical disability and personality changes.

Neural recovery over time is often unpredictable and irregular, and the variables that affect recovery of children with TBI are extremely independent. In general, a better recovery is signaled by a shorter, less severe period of unconsciousness following the injury, a shorter period of amnesia, and better posttraumatic abilities (Dennis, 1992; Russell, 1993).

Although the brains of younger children are more malleable or more adaptable, this does not mean that younger children will always recover more fully. In addition to recovering the language lost, younger children may still have much language to learn, a task that is possibly made more difficult by the brain injury.

The age of the injury can be an inaccurate predictor. In general, the older the injury, the less chance of change, although this can be complicated by the delayed onset of some deficits (Russell, 1993). For example, some neurological problems might not be manifested until later in recovery, making neural recovery unpredictable and irregular over time.

When stabilized, the individual with TBI begins a long recovery process that can take years. Within the first few months, she or he might experience spontaneous recovery when large gains in ability are made.

Young children often recover quickly but experience difficulties learning new information and may exhibit more severe and more long-lasting problems. Older children and adolescents have more to recover from their memory but less new information to learn.

Even individuals who have made a seemingly full recovery may lack subtle cognitive and social skills. For example, Mary was a college student who had suffered TBI. She was able to succeed with minimal modifications in the classroom. Her main difficulties were in sustained attending and shifting tasks. In an evaluation, we found an inability to change *cognitive set* quickly. When you solve problems, you go about it systematically. If the problem changes, you change your way of thinking or your cognitive set. You can go easily from defining words to adding numbers. Mary could not.

THOUGHT QUESTIONS

Do you think intervention would be different for brain injury with a child who is learning language and an adult for whom development is complete? Why or why not? If so, how?

Language Characteristics

Language problems are evident even after mild injuries. Some deficits, especially in pragmatics, will remain long after the injury even when general improvement is good. Overall, pragmatics seems to be the most disturbed aspect of language. The child may lose the central focus or topic (Chapman, Watkins, Gustafson, Moore, Levin, & Kufera, 1997). Utterances are often lengthy, inappropriate, and off topic, and fluency is disturbed.

Language comprehension and higher functions such as figurative language and dual meanings are also often impaired, although language form is relatively unaffected. Semantics, especially concrete vocabulary, is also relatively undisturbed, although word retrieval, naming, and object description difficulties may be present. Narration, especially maintaining story structure and providing enough information, may pose a problem (Chapman et al., 1997).

NEGLECT AND ABUSE

More than one million children are neglected or abused each year in the United States. Neglect and abuse are the outward signs of a dysfunctional family, the social environment in which these children learn language.

Although neglect and abuse are rarely the direct cause of communication problems, the context in which they occur directly influences the child's development. Medical and health problems among poor Americans also can contribute, although neglect and abuse are not limited to poor families. Poor maternal health, substance abuse, poor or nonexistent pediatric services, and poor nutrition can all affect brain development and maturation.

The quality of the child-mother attachment is a more significant factor in language development than is maltreatment (Carlson, Cicchetti, Barnett, & Braunwald, 1989). Maternal attachment can be disturbed by childhood loss of a parent; death of a previous child; pregnancy and/or birth complications; family, marital, or financial problems; substance abuse; maternal age; and/or illness. The result is a lack of support for the development of meaningful communication skills.

> Lack of maternal interaction rather than outright physical abuse accounts for much of the language impairment noted among children from abusive and neglectful environments.

Lifespan Issues

The affects of childhood abuse and neglect can remain with a child for life. There might be recurring physical, psychological, and emotional problems. Many children who have been abused abuse their own children later, thereby perpetuating this pattern with all its ill effects.

Language Characteristics

Although all aspects of language are affected, it is in pragmatics that children who have been neglected or abused exhibit the greatest difficulties. In general, they are less talkative and have fewer conversational skills than their peers. They are less likely to volunteer information or to discuss emotions or feelings. Utterances and conversations are shorter than those of their peers. In school, they have depressed oral and written language performance.

Why might an abused child have inappropriate pragmatics?

THOUGHT QUESTION

FETAL ALCOHOL SYNDROME AND DRUG-EXPOSED CHILDREN

Within the last twenty years, there has been an increase in the prevalence of **fetal alcohol syndrome (FAS)** and drug-exposed children. FAS accounts for one in every 500 to 600 live births. Infants have a low birthweight and exhibit central nervous system problems. Later, they demonstrate hyperactivity, motor problems, attention deficits, and cognitive disabilities (Mallette, 1994). As a group, their mean IQ is in the borderline MR range.

The effects of drugs on the fetus vary with the drug, the manner of ingestion, and the age of the fetus (MacDonald, 1992). Crack is especially destructive because it alters the fetus's neurochemical functioning. Like infants with FAS, those who are exposed to crack cocaine have low birthweight. They also have small head circumference and are jittery and irritable (Lesar, 1992).

Lifespan Issues

Preterm babies, especially those with FAS or early drug exposure, are more likely to die during infancy and to experience developmental difficulties. The drug-exposed child's poorly coordinated behaviors and motor delays may disrupt caregiver-infant bonding (Crites, Fischer, McNeish-Stengel, & Siegel, 1992). In addition, caregivers who are dependent on alcohol or drugs might not attend to or might reject the child. As a result, these children behave very much like children with learning disabilities. The limitations noted at birth remain with the child for life.

Language Characteristics

Children with FAS exhibit language problems characterized by delayed development of oral language, echolalia, and comprehension problems. Infants who were exposed to drugs have few infant vocalizations, inappropriate gestures, and language deficits. As preschoolers, they exhibit word-retrieval problems, short sentences, and inappropriate conversational turn taking and topic maintenance (Mentis & Lundgren, 1995). These difficulties persist and are compounded by problems with abstract meanings, multiple meanings, and temporal and spatial terms, such as *before* and *after, next* and *near, next to,* and *in front of.* Both children with FAS and those with fetal drug exposure are behind their peers in reading and other academic tasks.

> Children with FAS and drug exposure have many learning problems similar to those of children with learning disabilities.

CONCLUSION

There are so many disorders associated with language impairment that they probably all have begun to look similar to you. To help your memory, Table 5.4 presents the major characteristics of each disorder. In most cases, the child with a language impairment has other physical, cognitive, and psychological difficulties, too. In actual practice, speech-language pathologists treat each child as an individual, not as a member of a category. Of importance is each child's behavior and language features, not group characteristics.

While this section focuses on associated disorders, it does not address all of the factors that may be related to language impairment. Factors such as poverty, nutrition, child and maternal health, and maternal sensitivity to and stimulation of a child are also important. For example, most children and mothers living in homeless shelters exhibit language deficits (La Paro, Justice, Skibbe, & Pianta, 2004; O'Neil-Pirozzi, 2003).

ASPECTS OF LANGUAGE AFFECTED

In addition to the etiological categories we have just described, language impairments can also be characterized by the language features affected. For example, a child may have difficulty with word recall and conversational initiation or possess a limited vocabulary and seemingly nonstop talking. Another child may have poor syntax and very short sentences or withdraw from conversational give-and-take. Table 5.5 presents the most common language features associated with language impairments. A sample of a

TABLE 5.4

Summary of disorders associated with language impairment

Disorder Most Affected	Expected Deficit Area					Language Features		
	Developmental	Cognitive	Perceptual	Affective	Unknown	Form	Content	Use
Mental retardation		X				X	X	X
Language learning disability			X			X	X	X
Specific language impairment					X	X		
Autism				X				X
Traumatic brain injury		X		X				X
Neglect and abuse	X							X

school-aged child with a language impairment is presented on the accompanying CD-ROM. In an evaluation, speech-language pathologists assess many language features to determine where to begin intervention.

Assessment

Language assessment is a process of discovery and information gathering. As was noted in Chapter 4, good clinical practice requires that the boundary between assessment and intervention be permeable. A portion of any good assessment is attempting to determine possible avenues for intervention. In turn, each intervention session should contain some assessment of the client's current skill level.

Assessment should be sufficiently broad and deep so that all areas of possible concern are identified and described as accurately as possible. For example, assessment for semantics must include more than receptive understanding and expressive vocabulary size. A thorough examination might also include areas such as word learning abilities and word storage and retrieval (Brackenbury & Pye, 2005).

The nature and severity of some language impairments is such that an interdisciplinary team assessment is most appropriate. For example, an interdisclinary assessment that includes families as active participants and collaborators has been shown to be effective with young children with ASD (Prelock, Beatson, Bitner, Broder & Ducker, 2003)

Assessment and intervention overlap and are parts of the same process.

TABLE 5.5
Most common language characteristics of children with language disorders

Pragmatics

Difficulty answering questions or requesting clarification

Difficulty initiating, maintaining a conversation, or securing a conversational turn

Poor flexibility in language when tailoring the message to the listener or repairing communication breakdowns

Short conversational episodes

Limited range of communication functions

Inappropriate topics and off-topic comments; ineffectual, inappropriate comments

Asocial monologues

Difficulty with stylistic variations and speaker-listener roles

Narrative difficulties

Few interactions

Semantics

Limited expressive vocabulary and slow vocabulary growth

Few or decontextualized utterances, more here-and-now; more concrete meanings

Limited variety of semantic functions

Relational term difficulty (comparative, spatial, temporal)

Figurative language and dual definition problems

Conjunction (*and, but, so, because,* etc.) confusion

Naming difficulties may reflect less rich and less elaborate semantic storage or actual retrieval difficulties

Syntax/Morphology

Short, uncomplex utterances

Rule learning difficulties

Run-on, short, or fragmented sentences

Few morphemes, especially verb endings, auxiliary verbs, pronouns, and function words (articles, prepositions)

Overreliance on word order, which takes precedence over word relationships

Difficulty with negative and passive constructions, relative clauses, contractions, and adjectival forms

Article (*a, the*) confusion

Phonology

Limited syllable structure

Fewer consonants in repertoire

Inconsistent sound production, especially as complexity increases

Comprehension

Poor discrimination of units of short duration (bound morphemes)

Impaired comprehension, especially in connected discourse such as conversations

Reliance on context to extract meaning

Wh- question confusion

Overreliance on nonlinguistic cues for meaning

REFERRAL AND SCREENING

Referral may occur at any point in the lifespan. Some children, such as those with identifiable syndromes or those who are at risk for developing a language impairment, might be referred at birth or early infancy; others with LD might go undetected until they begin school; and those with either TBI or childhood aphasia may be of any age.

In a public school, the speech-language pathologist (SLP) may decide to test a child further on the basis of results of screening testing. Screening tests, used to determine only the presence or absence of a speech and language problem, are routinely administered to all kindergarten and first-grade students.

Surveys and parental questionnaires are also effective diagnostic tools. They compare favorably with other language measures (Patterson, 2000; Rescorla & Alley, 2001; Thal, Jackson-Maldonado, & Acosta, 2000).

Referral and subsequent evaluation may occur within an interdisciplinary team of child specialists. The nature of many of the disorders mentioned previously may necessitate input from a pediatrician, neurologist, occupational therapist, physical therapist, developmental psychologist, special education teacher, audiologist, and speech-language pathologist.

CASE HISTORY AND INTERVIEW

The case history questionnaire and interview are the first steps in a formal information-gathering process. In addition to asking the questions presented in Chapter 4, the SLP will want to ask more specific questions relevant to language impairment. Questions would relate to language development, the language environment of the home, and possible causes for language impairment. Table 5.6 presents predictors and risk factors for language change

> Information from referrals, questionnaires, and interviews provides needed background information from which to begin investigating for possible language impairment and determining what that impairment entails.

TABLE 5.6
Predictors and risk factors of language change in toddlers

Predictors

Language

Production:

Small vocabulary with few verbs

Verbs mostly general-purpose, such as *want, go, got,* and *look,*

Comprehension: Six-month delay with large gap between production and comprehension

Phonology:

Few prelinguistic vocalizations and limited variety in babbling

Vowel errors and limited number of consonants

Fewer than 50 percent of consonants correct

Restricted syllable structure

Speech Imitation

Limited spontaneous imitations

Nonspeech

Play: Little combination of play schemes and/or little symbolic play

Gestures: Few gestures or gesture sequences

Social Skills:

Behavioral problems

Few conversational initiations

More interactions with adults than peers and difficulty gaining entrance to activities

Risk Factors

Otitis Media: Prolonged and untreated

Heritability: Family member with persistent language and learning problems

Parents

Low socioeconomic status

Directive style of interaction rather than responsive

Extreme concern

Source: Adapted from Olswang, Rodriguez, & Timler (1998).

in toddlers (Olswang, Rodriguez, & Timler, 1998). Possible questions are presented in Table 5.7

OBSERVATION

Language is heavily influenced by the context in which it occurs. It is helpful, therefore, to observe a child using language in as many contexts as possible. Although it is not always convenient to observe in multiple contexts,

---

TABLE 5.7

Possible questions for questionnaires/interviews when a language impairment is suspected

Language Use

Does the child . . .

Ask for information? How?

Describe things in the environment? How?

Discuss things in the past, future, or outside of the immediate contest?

Make noises when playing alone?

Engage in monologues when playing?

Prefer to play alone or with others?

Express emotions or discuss feelings? How?

Request desired items? How?

Request attention? How?

Direct your attention? How?

Conversational Skills

Does the child . . .

Initiate conversations or interactions with others? What are the child's frequent topics?

Join in when others initiate?

Get your attention before saying something?

Maintain eye contact while talking?

Take turns easily while talking? Interrupt frequently? Are there long gaps between your utterances and the child's responses?

Demonstrate an expectation that you will respond when he or she speaks? What does the child do if you do not respond?

Seem confused or ask for clarification? How? How frequently?

Respond when asked to clarify? How?

Demonstrate frustration when not understood?

Relay sequential information or stories in an organized fashion so that they can be followed? Relay enough information?

Have different ways of talking to different people, such as adults and smaller children?

React more readily to certain people and situations than to others? When does the child communicate best/most?

How does the child respond when you say something? How does the child respond to others?

What emotions does the child express? How?

Are responses meaningful, mismatched, off-top, or irrelevant?

Form and Content

Does the child . . .

Know the names of common events, objects, and people in the environment?

Seem to rely on gestures, sounds, or immediate environment to be understood?

Speak in single words, phrases, or sentences? How long is a typical utterance? Does the child leave out words?

Use words such as *tomorrow, yesterday,* or *last night?*

Use verb tenses?

Put several sentences together to form complex descriptions and explanations?

Follow simple directions?

Source: Adapted from Owens (2004).

a school-based SLP might observe in the classroom, while a clinic-based SLP might observe on a home visit, in the waiting room, or during a freeplay period between the mother and child. In all assessments, testing and sampling periods provide an additional observational period.

THOUGHT QUESTIONS

W hat behaviors might we hope to observe? Might we be interested in the behaviors of others, too? Why or why not?

Behaviors that are observed will vary with the age of the child and the reported disorder. In addition to observing the child's communicative behavior, the SLP is also concerned with the child's interests and the caregiver's style of communicating and method of behavior control. Table 5.8 presents some behaviors that might be observed during an assessment.

Hypotheses about the child's language impairment are formed during observation. These are either confirmed or negated during the remainder of the assessment and during intervention.

It is important for the SLP to remain focused during observation. This requires that she or he define very carefully the behaviors and/or language features that are observed and fully describe the events preceding and following them. For example, one adolescent we knew would scream "Don't hit me" repeatedly. It was observed that this occurred when she was asked a question. The behavior was inconsistent. It was hypothesized that the type of

---

TABLE 5.8

Possible behaviors to observe during an assessment of language impairment

With whom child communicates

Purposes for child's communication

Effectiveness of child's communication

    Obvious patterns of breakdown

Maturity of child's language

    Utterance length

    Verb usage

    Complexity

Relative amounts of initiative versus responsive communication

Relative amounts of nonsocial versus social communication

Responsiveness of caregiver

Turn allocation, relative size of child's and caregiver's turns question influenced the response. The hypothesis was confirmed later in the assessment by careful data collection in which the type of question was modified systematically.

Few formal observational tools exist. Speech-language pathologists, recognizing the importance of observation as a vital portion of assessment, are developing reliable measures (Kaderavek & Sulzby, 1998).

TESTING

After building rapport with a child, the SLP can begin testing. Tasks are varied because of their effect on different children (Fagundes, Haynes, Haak, & Moran, 1998).

Standardized tests are administered to compare a child's performance to others of the same age. Standardized, norm-referenced tests are appropriate for determining if a problem exists, but may be less useful in identifying specific language deficits (Merrell & Plante, 1997). More descriptive test results allow the SLP to explore a child's strengths and weaknesses. In addition, descriptive results can provide useful information for treatment planning.

It is best to use a series of tests to ensure that many features are tested (Gray, Plante, Vance, & Henrichsen, 1999). At the very least, receptive and expressive aspects of language form, content, and use should be tested or sampled in some way. Some widely used tests and their characteristics are presented in Table 5.9.

Test methodology varies widely. Children may be asked to form syntactically similar sentences, to make judgments of correctness, to reconfigure scrambled sentences, or to imitate exactly what they hear. They may have to supply definitions, form sentences, or point to words named. All these tasks require different language skills. Testing is an extraordinary situation being used to measure typical language performance. Unfamiliar tasks may prejudice the results against the child (Peña & Quinn, 1997). Examples of language test tasks are presented in Table 5.10.

The knowledgeable SLP is familiar with many tests and chooses the ones that will yield the information required about the child being assessed. During testing, the SLP will probe the child's performance to try to identify possible effective intervention procedures. Of interest are strategies that either increase production or result in more correct production of a certain language feature (Peña, Iglesias, & Lidz, 2001). Sometimes called **dynamic assessment** (Olswang, Bain, & Johnson, 1990), this probing is invaluable in providing direction for subsequent intervention. Dynamic assessment and techniques that ask children to demonstrate skills that represent realistic learning demands are especially well suited for multicultural populations (Schraeder, Quinn, Stockman, & miller, 1999; Ukrainetz, Harpell, Walsh, & Coyle, 2000).

SAMPLING

If language is influenced by context, then the context of test taking should influence the language a child produces. For some, test structure will de-

> Testing is an extraordinary situation for most children. Typical performance is more likely to be displayed in language sampling.

crease performance. This is especially true for young children, children from minority populations, and those with disabilities.

In addition to testing, the SLP should also engage a child in challenging conversation, so that he or she will attempt to "stretch" language abilities and in the process reveal difficulties (Hadley, 1998). A variety of discourse types, such as conversation, narration, explanation, and interview, should be included in the sample.

Typical performance may be enhanced if parents or teachers interact with the child in familiar settings. The experienced SLP can also be an excellent conversational or play partner for the child. Whenever possible, it is best to collect at least two samples of the child with different partners, locations, and activities or topics.

THOUGHT QUESTIONS

Does sampling ensure that we will get a child's typical performance? Can you think of some contexts in which a child's typical language performance would not occur?

Samples may be either very open ended, in which topics and interactions are not defined, or more closed, in which the SLP tries to elicit specific language features. Responses vary; for example, more restrictive question-answer techniques elicit fewer complex utterances than more conversational strategies (Bradshaw, Hoffman, & Norris, 1998). Narratives are especially helpful for exhibiting deficits in older children or those with TBI because of the demands on a speaker (Chapman, 1997). In addition, narratives tend to elicit a large number and variety of syntactic structures (Gummersall & Strong, 1999). Table 5.11 presents two very different types of language samples.

Language samples are recorded for later transcription and the SLP is careful to transcribe the child's exact words.

The language transcript can be analyzed in several quantitative and qualitative ways to determine the extent and nature of the child's language difficulty. Values such as the average length of the child's utterances in morphemes, referred to as the *mean length of utterance (MLU)*, the average number of clauses per sentence, and the number of different words used within a given period of time can be compared to the values for typical children of the same age or developmental level (Johnston, 2001). Samples might also provide information on the percent correct for a language feature, such as past tense *-ed*. More descriptive measures might be the variety of intentions expressed by the child, the number of conversational styles used, and the types of repair the child uses when the conversation breaks down (Yont, Hewitt, & Miccio, 2000). Being as thorough as possible, the SLP attempts to analyze the sample for all aspects of form, content, and use appropriate for the particular assessment. For example, with bilingual clients, the SLP might consider **code switching** or the movement between two languages, dialect, English proficiency, and contextual effects in addi-

TABLE 5.9
Characteristics of common language tests

Test	Source	Target
Carrow Elicited Language Inventory (CELI) E. Carrow-Woodcock	DLM Teaching Resources	Identification of children with language problems; can be used to determine which specific linguistic structures may contributing to the child's problems
Clinical Evaluation of Language Fundamentals—Preschool (CELF-Preschool) (1992) E. Wiig, W. Secord, E. Semel	Psychological Corp.	Expressive and receptive language skills: basic concept, sentence structure, word structure, naming, recalling sentence in context, linguistic concepts
Clinical Evaluation of Language Fundamentals III (CELF-3) (1995) E. Semel, E. Wiig, W. Secord	Psychological Corp.	Expressive and receptive language skills: semantics, syntax, morphology, and memory
Fullerton Language Test for Adolescents, second edition (FTLA-2) (1986) A. R. Thorum	Consulting Psychologists Press, Inc.	Linguistic processing to identify language-impaired adolescents. Auditory synthesis, oral commands, convergent and divergent productions, syllabication, idioms, and morphological competency.
Peabody Picture Vocabulary Test, third edition (PPVT-III) L. & L. Dunn	American Guidance Service	Receptive vocabulary
Preschool Language Scale, fourth edition (PLS-4) (1992) I. L. Zimmerman, V. Steiner, R. Pond	Psychological Corp.	Auditory comprehension and verbal ability
Test of Adolescent and Adult Language, third edition (TOAL-3) D. Hammill, V. Brown, S. Larsen, J. Wiederholt	Pro-Ed	Expressive and receptive language, semantic and syntactic skills assessed in spoken and written form
Test of Auditory Comprehension of Language—third edition (TACL-3) (1999) E. Carrow-Woodcock	Pro-Ed	Auditory comprehension of word classes and relations, grammatical relations, and elaborated sentences
Test of Early Language Development, 3rd ed. (TELD-3) (1999) W. Hresko, D. Reid, D. Hammill	Pro-Ed	Receptive and expressive language
Test of Language Development—Primary, 3rd ed. (TOLD-P:3) (1997) P. Newcomer, D. Hammill	Pro-Ed	Receptive and expressive language, semantics, syntax, phonology
The Word Test—Adolescent L. Bowers, R. Huisingh, M. Barrett, J. Orman, C. LoGuidice	Lingui-Systems	Expressive vocabulary and semantics

Age	Notes
3–8 years	Administration of the test takes 10 minutes, and scoring takes 1 hour and 30 minutes. Child's responses must be transcribed phonetically.
3–6 years	Meets PL 99-457 and PL 94-142 guidelines.
6–21 years	Provides a guideline for areas of language that are in need of further observation and testing. Takes 45 minutes to score and administer. Provides supplementary oral and written expression sections for additional information.
11–18.5 years	Standardized: provides means and standard deviation for each subset and age group. Three score breakdowns: competence level, instruction level, and frustration level.
2.5–90 years	A standard. Child points to one of four black-and-white pictures named.
0–6 years	Widely used. Wide variety of receptive and expressive tasks using pictures and toys.
12–25 years	Test requires reading and writing for some of the subtests; 1–3 hours to administer; can be administered to a group for 6 of 8 of the subtests; requires several separate booklets to administer.
K to grade 4	Individually administered, no oral response required. Child points to one of three pictures named.
2 to 7–11 years	Individually administered in about 30 minutes; normed on children from 35 states, representing U.S. population.
4 years to 8–11 years	Administered in about one hour; computer scoring is available.
12–17 years	Administration time: 25 minutes. Results: standard scores, percentile ranks, age equivalencies, no basal or ceilings. Is designed to assess a subject's facility with language and word meaning using common as well as unique contexts, surveys 4 semantic and vocabulary tasks reflective of school assignment, as well as language usage in everyday life.

TABLE 5.10
Examples of language test tasks

Test Procedure	Example
Grammatical completion	I'm going to say a sentence with one word missing. Listen carefully, then fill in the missing word. *John has a dish and Fred has a dish. They have two _____.*
Receptive vocabulary	Look at the pictures on this page. I'm going to name one, and I want you to point to it. *Touch (Show me) the officer.*
Defining words	I'm going to say some words. I want you to tell me what each word means or use it in a sentence in a way that makes sense. For example, if I said "coin," you might respond "money made from metal" or "I put my coin in the vending machine."
Pragmatic functions	I'm going to tell you a story and ask you to imagine what the person in the story might say. *Mary lost her money and she must call home for a ride after band practice. She decides to borrow a quarter from her best friend Julie. Before practice begins, she sits down next to Julie and says _____.*
Sentence imitation	I'm going to say some sentences, and I want you to repeat exactly what I say. Let's try one. *We are going to play ball after school tomorrow.*
Parallel sentence production	Here are two pictures. I'll describe the first one, and then you describe the second one using the same type of sentence as I use. For example, for this picture I would say, "The girl is riding her bike," and for this one you would say, "The man is driving his car."
Grammatical correctness	I'm going to say a sentence, and I want you to tell if it is correct or incorrect. If it is incorrect, you must correct it. For example, if I say, "Thems is going to the dance," you would respond, "Incorrect. They are going to the dance."

tion to aspects of both languages (Gutierrez-Clellan, Restrepo, Bedore, Peña, & Anderson, 2000).

For school-aged clients experiencing literacy difficulties, the SLP also will want to collect samples of written language (Greene, 1996). These are discussed in Chapter 6, "Developmental Literacy Impairments."

INTERVENTION

The complexity of language necessitates a multiplicity of intervention methods. Different intervention approaches target specific aspects of language

TABLE 5.11
....
Examples of different types of language samples

Open-Ended	Structured
Clinician: I'll play with this farm set, and you can too or you can pick another toy.	*Clinician:* Well, here's the puppy. What should we say to him?
Child: Want farm.	*Child:* Hi puppy. [GREETING]
Clinician: Oh, you want the farm. We can share. I wonder what should we do first.	*Clinician:* Hi Timmy. I'm hungry. We need to get someone to help us get those cookies.
Child: Open door. Animals come out.	*Child:* You help. Want cookie. [REQUESTING]
Clinician: Okay.	*Clinician:* I wonder how I can reach it.
Child: You be horsie and I man.	*Child:* Get chair. [HYPOTHESIZING]
Clinician: Oh, the farmer.	*Clinician:* Oh, get on the chair. Should I (mumble).
Child: Farmerman chase horsie in barn.	*Child:* Yeah. [DOES NOT REQUEST CLARIFICATION]
Clinician: Oh, he did. I better run fast.	*Clinician:* You want me to (mumble)?
Child: Man go fast in barn.	*Child:* What's that? [REQUESTS CLARIFICATION]
	Clinician: Which do you want, the cookie or the chair?
	Child: Want cookie. No chair. [CHOICE MAKING]

and employ a variety of procedures. Within limits, we shall explore these diverse approaches to remediation of language impairments.

Increasingly, SLPs are including other individuals from the child's environment in the training. For example, without training, day care providers fail to finely tune their language for individual children's needs (Girolametto, Hoaken, Weitzman, & van Lieshout, 2000). With the aid of the SLP, parents may learn how to be better language partners for their young children. Many successful models of the classroom collaborative model mentioned in Chapter 4 have evolved (Prelock, 2000). Even peers can serve as effective tutors or models for children with language impairments (McGregor, 2000).

TARGET SELECTION AND SEQUENCE OF TRAINING

The goal of intervention is the maximally effective use of language to accomplish communication goals within everyday interactions. Although most SLPs would agree on this overall goal, less unanimity exists on the route to achieving it. Decisions on target selection and training vary with each child and each SLP.

Using different criteria, several SLPs might not select the same targets for the same child. A strict developmental model might suggest that a child achieve all behaviors within a given stage of language development before progressing to the next stage. A less strict developmentalist would use language acquisition knowledge as a general guide. A functional model would

The criteria for target selection will vary with the child, the affected aspects of language, the child's disorder, and the needs of the environment.

suggest that training begin at the point of communication breakdown and frustration. Classroom approaches might suggest training for language used within the class. Another approach might be to begin with language features that are emerging, such as those produced correctly 10 to 50 percent of the time.

Decisions must be made as to where to begin once the target is selected. Once again, the SLP must determine the point at which communication breakdown occurs. Some SLPs prefer to begin with receptive language training and progress to expressive. Others will start with expressive training. Expressive training may be bottom-up, in which one begins at the symbol level and works toward conversational goals; top-down, in which training is placed within a conversational framework; or a combination of the two. Obviously, the child's abilities are an important determiner of the method selected. Training should be placed within meaningful communicative contexts.

THOUGHT QUESTIONS

Can you think of reasons why you might begin with receptive training? Expressive? At the individual symbol level? With conversation?

INTERVENTION PRINCIPLES

The needs of children with language impairment suggest several principles that should guide intervention services. These principles, presented in Table 5.12, recognize the need to target a child's language abilities in their entirety rather than to focus exclusively on one deficit area. The interrelatedness of all areas of language and the importance of communication context on the form and content of language necessitate a more holistic approach.

INTERVENTION PROCEDURES

It is important to remember that speech-language pathologists, wherever they may work, are teaching communicative skills. A few basic tenets of good teaching behavior include, but are not limited to, the following:

- *Model the desired behavior for the client.* Modeling may include multiple exposures, called *focused stimulation,* that occur before the child is required to produce the language feature (Cleave & Fey, 1997). The need for modeling decreases as the feature is learned. Older elementary school children and adolescents may also benefit from an explanation of the targeted behavior and a rationale for why its correct use is important.

- *Cue the client to respond.* Carefully selected cues, such as the use of the word *yesterday* to signal a past-tense response, will serve as aids for the client in conversation. Cues may range from very specific, such as *say, imitate,* or *point to,* to more general conversational cues, such as *I wonder what I should say now* to elicit a specific linguistic structure in context or *Maybe Carol can help us if we ask* to elicit a question.

TABLE 5.12
Principles of language intervention

1. The goal of intervention should be greater facility of language use in conversation, narration, exposition, and other textual genres in hearing, speaking, reading, and writing.

2. Deficit areas are rarely, if ever, the only areas of language that should be targeted in an intervention program.

3. Select intermediate goals that stimulate a child's language acquisition processes rather than goals that focus solely on deficit areas.

4. Select specific goals of intervention based on a child's readiness and need for the targeted goals.

5. Manipulate the context to create more opportunities for the language target to occur.

6. Exploit different genres and modalities to develop appropriate contexts for intervention targets.

7. Manipulate clinical discourse so targeted areas are more noticeable and important in various contexts.

8. Systematically contrast a child's language performance with more mature adult usage by recasting a child's utterances.

9. Provide good models of easily comprehended, well-formed phrases and sentences.

10. Use a variety of verbal and nonverbal strategies to elicit and modify a child's language and to give a child practice in using language to accomplish her or his communication needs.

We are deeply indebted to the fine work of Mark Fey, Steven Long, and Lizbeth Finestack (2003) upon which this table is loosely based. See Fey, M.E., Long, S.H., and Finestack, L.H. (2003). Ten principles of grammar facilitation for children with specific language impairment. *American Journal of Speech-Language Pathology, 12,* 3–15.

Cues may be verbal or nonverbal. Verbal cues attempt to elicit the language feature by providing a linguistic framework; nonverbal cues use the context of an event to evoke the feature.

- *Respond to the client in the form of reinforcement and/or corrective feedback.* Reinforcement varies from very direct and obvious forms, such as "Good, that was much better," to more conversational responses. Conversational responses come in many varieties, including imitating the child, imitating but expanding the child's utterance into a more mature version, replying conversationally, and asking for clarification. With some clients, especially those with vocabulary deficits, the relationship of the responsive to the content of the child's utterance has more effect on the child's language than the structural input of the clinician's feedback (Girolametto, Weitzman, Wiigs, & Steig Pearce, 1999).

SLPs are teachers of language. They must plan their behaviors well to teach without overly relying on less natural strategies such as drill and the use of edible reinforcers.

Natural reinforcers flow from the training target. The most obvious example is one in which a child obtains a desired object upon responding to the cue "What do you want?" Conversational responses can be very natural.

Corrective feedback may range from a gentle reminder to instruction. In general, as a language feature is produced more correctly by the client, the SLP relies less on both direct forms. When a client infrequently is using a language feature incorrectly, conversational feedback, such as "What?" or "I don't understand," may be sufficient to cause the client to self-correct.

- *Plan for generalization of the learned feature to the everyday use environment of the client.* SLPs can help generalization by selecting training targets that are highly likely to occur in the client's everyday communication and by including in the training elements of the everyday use environment, such as familiar locations, people, and objects. Parents are often included in the training of young children, while teachers may be involved in the intervention of school-age children and adolescents.

Specific examples of each teaching tenet are presented in Table 5.13.

INTERVENTION THROUGH THE LIFESPAN

Targets of intervention will vary with the age and functioning level of the client. An infant in an early intervention program would have different training targets than an adolescent with LD. However, an infant may be receiving some of the same training as an adolescent who has profound retardation and is functioning below age 1 year. Although reasonable professionals disagree, it seems best to use at least some instruction in two languages with children experiencing difficulties in both (Gutierrez-Clellan, 1999).

Early intervention, especially for children with MR and autism, can have very positive benefit. Initial training may target presymbolic communicative skills and cognitive abilities, such as physical imitation, gestures, and receptive understanding of object names. The SLP may attempt to establish an initial communication system using an augmentative/alternative communication system, such as gesturing, a communication board, or an electronic device. Augmentative/alternative communication will be discussed in more detail in Chapter 15. Parents may be trained to treat their child's behaviors as having some communicative value or to interpret consistent behaviors as attempts to communicate.

Early symbolic training may focus on vocabulary acquisition, semantic categories, word combinations, and an array of early intentions. The beneficial effects of treatment for children with delayed language extend beyond the trained targets into other areas of linguistic and overall development (Brand Robertson & Ellis Weismer, 1999).

Children at the preschool language level usually work on language form in both conversations and narratives. Longer utterances, bound morphemes, and early phonological processes may be intervention goals. Vocabulary will continue to be targeted.

TABLE 5.13

Examples of teaching methods

Method	Example
Modeling	
Focused stimulation	I'll pretend to make a cake first. Watch to see if I make a mistake. I'm *putting* the eggs in the bowl and *taking* them to the table. I'm *cracking* the eggs. Now I'm *beating* the eggs. Next, I'm *sifting* the flour. I'm *adding* the flour to the eggs and *mixing* them. Now I'm *measuring* the sugar and *pouring* it into the mix. . . .
Cuing	
Direct Verbal	
Imitation	Say "I want cookie."
Cloze	This is a _____. She should say _____.
Question	What should I say now? What's this? Which one's this?
Indirect Verbal	
Pass it on	I wonder if Joan knows the answer. How could we find the answer? [TARGET IS FORMATION OF QUESTIONS]
Nonverbal (Inherent in the activity)	Not giving child all the materials needed to complete a task. Not explaining how to accomplish an assigned task. Playing dumb.
Responding	
Direct Reinforcement	Good, I like the way you said that. Much better than the last time.
Indirect Reinforcement	
Imitation	*Child:* I go horsie. *Clinician:* I go horsie.
Expansion	*Child:* I go horsie. *Clinician:* I'm going to go on the horsie.
Extension	*Child:* I go horsie. *Clinician:* Yes, cowboys go on horses too.
Corrective Feedback	Remember, when we use a number like two, three, or more, we say /s/ on the word. Listen. One cat. Two cats.

Intervention with higher functioning children may focus on pragmatic skills in conversations and semantic targets, such as figurative language, multiple meanings, abstract terms, and more advanced relational terms. Academic skills, including summarizing a reading and different types of writing and note taking, may also be targeted. SLPs may use computerized programs to supplement more face-to-face intervention. These must be used with caution and should mesh well with the SLP's overall clinical philosophy and the child's individual needs (Gillam, 1999). Language enhancement—metalinguistics, phonology, and language use—can be infused into the reading curriculum (Fleming & Forester, 1997). Speech-language pathologists may work with the child on both spoken and written language. It is also important for children with language impairment to learn to navigate the curriculum and to understand expectations (Westby, 1997).

Language intervention doesn't end with childhood. Adolescents may continue to exhibit language impairments and be in need of services (Nippold, 2000). Adults with severe ASD or MR will most likely require continued intervention for language and communication deficits and a range of self-care, educational, and vocational needs. Individuals with LD may require additional support in postsecondary education (Downey & Snyder, 2000; Olivier, Hecker, Klucken, & Westby, 2000).

SUMMARY

In this chapter, we have discussed several disorders that are associated with language impairment. It is sometimes difficult for beginning students to remember the differences between children with mental retardation, learning disability, specific language impairment, autism and pervasive developmental disorder, brain injury, neglect and abuse, and fetal alcohol syndrome and drug addiction. Refer to Table 5.4 for the major differences between these disorders.

As the definition and the many associated disorders suggest, language impairments are very complex and many faceted. We have only touched the surface in this chapter. The number of associated disorders, the language features that are affected, and the individual differences among children result in each child's language being very individualistic. It is very important to remember that each child is a unique case. Given this fact, assessment becomes the search to find and describe each child's individual language abilities. This is accomplished through referral, collection of a case history, interviews, observation, testing, and language sampling.

As a result of the assessment process and through repeated assessment during intervention, the speech-language pathologist attempts to find the most efficient and effective method for teaching new skills. The SLP identifies targets for intervention and trains these through a combination of techniques in various settings with the aid of additional language facilitators. Some children may just be learning to communicate and may need to use augmentative and alternative communication methods, while others are working to become more efficient conversationalists, and still others are learning word retrieval strategies.

Obviously, every SLP needs thorough training and extensive experience with a variety of language impairments to serve children with these disabilities. With a firm foundation of speech and language development, speech-language pathologists take several courses in language impairment in both children and adults and complete practica with both populations.

REFLECTIONS

- What are the characteristics of language impairment?
- What disorders are associated with language impairment? Describe each one briefly.
- What are the steps in a typical assessment in language impairment?
- What is the overall design of language intervention?

SUGGESTED READINGS

Nelson, N. W. (1998). *Childhood language disorders in context: Infancy through adolescence* (2nd ed.). Boston: Allyn and Bacon.

Owens, R. E. (2004). *Language disorders: A functional approach to assessment and intervention* (4th ed.). Boston: Allyn and Bacon.

Lloyd, L. L., Fuller, D. R., & Arvidson, H. H. (1997). *Augmentative and alternative communication: A handbook of principles and practices.* Boston: Allyn and Bacon.

Reed, V. A. (2005). *An introduction to children with language disorders* (3rd ed.). Boston: Allyn and Bacon.

Sanders, M. (2001). *Understanding dyslexia and the reading process.* Boston: Allyn and Bacon.

ONLINE RESOURCES

gopher://gopher.sasquatch.com   Traumatic brain injury gopher with lots of information.

http://www.asha.org   American Speech-Language-Hearing Association. Information for members, students, and others who are interested in careers in speech-language pathology or audiology, and anyone with a concern about communicative disorders.

http://www.chadd.org   Children and Adults with Attention Deficit/Hyperactivity Disorders

http://www.autism.org   Center for the Study of Autism

http://www.asel.udel.edu/at-online/   Augmentative/alternative communication. Links and pointers to a variety of AAC topics.

http://www/irsc.org/down.htm   Down syndrome. Index with many web links.

http://www.ldresources.com/   Variety of writing on language learning disability and software to download.

http://www.ninds.nih.gov.healinfo/disorder/autism/autism.htm   Autism fact sheet from NIH.

http://www.autism-society.org   Autism Society of America. Information on education and an online glossary. Good consumer and practitioner information.

http://cnet.shs.arizona.edu/childneuro_list.html   National Center for Neurogenic Communication Disorders Children's language disorders.

Developmental Literacy Impairments

6

CHAPTER
LEARNING
GOALS

When you finish this chapter, you should be able to:

- Describe the aspects of literacy that are of concern to the SLP
- Explain how literacy develops
- Explain the deficits in literacy experienced by children with language impairment
- Describe an assessment of literacy
- Give examples of intervention for literacy

Case Study 6.1

Case Study of a Child with Literacy Impairment: Juan

An athletic 7-year-old, who loves video games and riding his bike, Juan immigrated to the United States from Colombia when he was 4 years old. With three older sisters, he was the baby of the family and received plenty of attention. His mother reported that his Spanish language development was similar to that of his sisters and that she was not concerned, although her son's speech was sometimes difficult for people outside the family to understand. When the family immigrated, the children began to learn English. As the youngest, Juan learned quickly, but experienced some problems with English speech sounds. He received speech and language services in kindergarten, although he was not classified as having a communication disorder.

In first grade, Juan's development of reading was fine initially, but gradually he fell more and more behind his peers. By second grade, he was nearly a year behind his classmates. The speech-language pathologist, reading specialist, and the classroom teacher met with the parents to suggest a thorough reading diagnostic. The evaluation confirmed that

Juan was reading below his age, and the reading specialist pledged to redouble her efforts. The speech-language pathologist noted Juan's especially poor performance on phonological awareness tasks and with the other team members recommended clinical intervention in this area.

Although she was unsure of the actual factors relating to Juan's difficulties, the speech-language pathologist believed that they might be related to his learning of a second language. As if to confirm this estimate, Juan quickly excelled in both phonological awareness and reading. As his phonological awareness skills improved, his speech sound production also became more accurate.

As you read the chapter, think about

- Possible explanations for Juan's reading problems.
- Possible ways in which the evaluative team could explore different aspects of reading.
- Possible explanations for Juan's success.

Democracy is based on the premise that we are an informed people. In the beginning of the American republic, those who were best informed were literate. What does being informed mean today? Is literacy still important, and what level of proficiency is required to be a fully participating citizen? Should we be concerned when one segment of the population has deficits in literacy learning? And who is responsible for aiding these individuals? These questions go to the heart of the issue of developmental literacy impairments.

Let's begin with literacy itself. What is it? **Literacy** is the use of visual modes of communication, specifically reading and writing. The interrelatedness of aspects of literacy is illustrated by the correlation between reading and spelling ability (Bosman & van Orden, 1997; Greenberg, Ehri, & Perin, 1997; Griffith, 1991). Poor readers tend to be poor spellers (Treiman, 1997). But literacy is more than just letters and sounds. Literacy encompasses language; academics; cognitive processes, including thinking, memory, problem solving, planning, and execution; and is related to other forms of communication.

Although spoken and written language have much in common, they differ in very significant ways (Kamhi & Catts, 2005). Reading and writing are not just speech in print. In addition to the obvious physical difference, reading and writing lack the give-and-take of conversation, are more permanent, lack the paralinguistic features (stress, intonation, fluency, etc.) of speech, have their own vocabulary and grammar, and are processed in a different manner.

As in other forms of communication, use of literacy presupposes that the user can encode and decode, but more importantly, that he or she is able to comprehend and compose messages for others. In other words, literacy rests on a language base—and so do literacy impairments.

Many of the disorders mentioned under both childhood and adult language impairments (Chapters 5 and 7) figure prominently in literacy impairments. In fact, as high as 60 percent of children with language impairment may experience difficulties with literacy (Wiig, Zureich, & Chan, 2000). Children with language impairments may be unprepared for literacy learning because they lack preliteracy skills and an oral language base. When compared to children developing typically, preschoolers and kindergarteners with language impairments may be less able to recognize and copy letters and less likely to pretend to read or write, to engage in daily preliteracy activities, or to engage adults in question-answer activities during reading and writing (Marvin & Wright, 1997).

Many literacy impairments do not disappear as children mature (Catts, Fey, Zhang, & Tomblin, 1999). As adults, those who experienced literacy deficits in childhood may continue to struggle with reading and writing. One intelligent man in his 50s — known by one of the authors — has continually worked in manual labor positions because his lack of literacy skills disqualified him from managerial positions. Hopefully, with advances in intervention research, the future will see better and more evidenced-based intervention with increasingly better outcomes.

As adults, some of us may experience a neuropathology such as aphasia or progressive dementia. Whether the loss of language is sudden, as in aphasia, or more gradual, as in progressive dementia such as Alzheimer's, literacy usually is affected in some way. If there is a problem with language, there will be a problem with the methods of transmission.

Literacy deficits vary in complexity and severity. Maybe you are a college student with dyslexia or some other literacy problem who has been able to succeed academically by adjusting to, compensating for, or overcoming deficits in your reading or writing. All of the authors of this text have worked with college students who have had to overcome literacy difficulties.

Although primary responsibility for teaching reading and writing still rests with the teacher and other educational specialists, the SLP is interested in children's language deficits and the ways in which these deficits influence the acquisition of literacy. In recognition of the special skills that SLPs bring to this area, the American Speech-Language-Hearing Association (ASHA) (2001d) recommends that SLPs play a role in literacy intervention.

As a consequence, SLPs are involved in literacy intervention from preschool through adulthood. At both the preschool and early elementary school level, speech-language pathologists focus on preventive intervention. According to ASHA, SLPs have the following responsibilities:

- Educate both teachers and parents in the oral language-literacy relationship.

Of necessity, the concerns of SLPs will differ with the maturational level and preliteracy or literacy abilities of children.

- Identify children at risk.
- Make referrals to good literacy-rich programs.
- Recommend assessment and treatment in preliteracy skills when needed. (Snow, Scarborough, & Burns, 1999)

Because children with language impairments are at a high risk for literacy disabilities (Lewis, O'Donnell, Freebairn, & Taylor, 1998), preliteracy, reading, and writing assessment should be a portion of any thorough language evaluation when appropriate.

With older children and adults, a speech-language pathologist is concerned with improving reading and writing skills. The SLP continues to help children and adolescents develop a strong language base and addresses both reading and writing. Assessment and intervention for literacy are also a vital part of any thorough rehabilitative strategy for adults with neurological impairments (see Chapter 7, "Adult Language Impairments").

As with most communication impairments mentioned in this text, SLPs often work as part of a team, collaborating with teachers to design literacy-based programs on vocabulary, language, and thinking skills (Farber & Klein, 1999; Silliman & Wilkinson, 2004). By working with teachers, SLPs provide opportunities for children with developmental literacy impairments to use skills taught in intervention within meaningful activities in the classroom. Effective collaboration should include curriculum planning, naturalistic language facilitation, and careful teaming of personnel (Hadley, Simmerman, Long, & Luna, 2000).

THOUGHT QUESTIONS

Does literacy seem like a logical extension of the areas of concern for speech-language pathologists? Does the SLP bring a particular expertise to the table? What additional professional training might be needed?

A literacy intervention team may include the classroom teacher, reading specialist, school psychologist, and parent. Other professionals may be included, especially in cases in which specific medical-related problems are present.

In the remainder of the chapter, we'll discuss literacy and associated skills, disorders, assessment, and intervention, first with reading, and then writing. Most language impairments discussed in Chapter 5 will also affect literacy acquisition. As in many disorder areas, the SLP will work with a team that includes educators, literacy specialists, and parents.

READING

Several steps are involved in reading and reading comprehension. Both language and written context play a role in word recognition and in the ability to construct meaning from print (Gillam & Gorman, 2004). A reader's interpretation of print emerges from the interaction of letter, sound, word meaning, grammatical and contextual processes, and a reader's prior knowledge.

The first step is **decoding** the printed word which consists of breaking or segmenting a word into its component sounds and then blending them together to form a word recognizable to the reader. Words are then combined via syntax and interpreted based on grammar, word meanings and context. There is an interaction between the print of the page and linguistic and conceptual information brought to the task be the child (Whitehurst & Lonigan, 2001). Given these processes, it shouldn't surprise us that children with oral language impairments might have reading problems as well. Figure 6.1 is a model of this dynamic process of text interpretation.

Obviously, comprehension requires much more than simply decoding or even interpreting a word. The active reader is concerned with self-monitoring, semantic organization, summarization, interpretation, mental imagery, connection with prior knowledge, and metacognition of knowledge about knowledge, to name some of the skills involved. But let's not get ahead of ourselves; more of this later.

N otice your own reading with a magazine or novel. Does the process seem automatic? Are you conscious of the process? Does this change when reading a text?

THOUGHT QUESTIONS

In summary, reading basically consists of decoding and text comprehension. While phonological skills are essential for decoding, other areas of language—syntax, morphology, semantics, and pragmatics—are needed for comprehension (Nation & Norbury, 2005). The reader uses language and experience to interpret the message conveyed by the author. This may give you some idea why language and literacy go hand in hand. Let's look briefly at two aspects of reading that are of particular interest to SLPs, phonological awareness and comprehension.

PHONOLOGICAL AWARENESS

Necessary for reading, **phonological awareness** is knowledge of the sounds and syllables and of the sound structure of words. Phonological awareness includes **phonemic awareness,** the specific ability to manipulate sounds, such as blending sounds to create new words or segmenting words into sounds. As you might guess, better phonological awareness, specifically phonemic awareness, is related to better reading skills (Cupples & Iacono, 2000; Hogan & Catts, 2004). In addition, phonological awareness skills also are the best predictor of spelling ability in elementary school (Nation & Hulme, 1997).

Phonological awareness consists of many skill areas, including syllabication and phoneme identification, alliteration, rhyming, blending, and seg-

Yes, it does seem easy to confuse terms. Simply put, phonological awareness is an alertness of phonology, so yes, it contains the elements of phonology.

FIGURE 6.1

Reading comprehension.

Beginning with print, a reader uses the letters and speech sounds to decode words that are then recognized based on lexical or vocabulary memory. Words are combined with other words and syntax, semantics, and context are used to interpret and comprehend.

Source: Adapted from Gillam, R.B., & Gorman, B.K. (2004). Language and discourse contributions to word recognition and text interpretation. In E.R. Silliman & L.C. Wilkinson (Eds.), *Language and literacy learning in schools* (pp. 63–97). New York: Guilford.

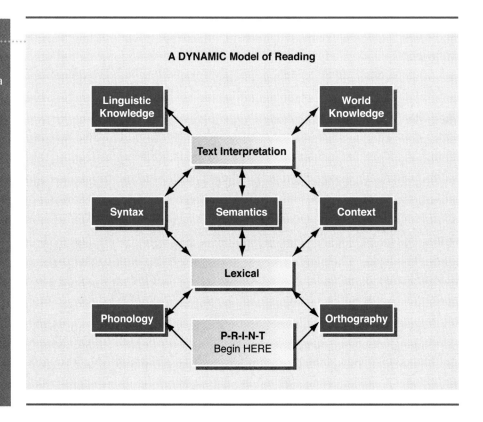

mentation. Not all of these skills are required for reading. The phonemic skills of **segmentation,** or creating a word when a phoneme or syllable is deleted, and **blending,** or creating a word from individual sounds and syllables, plus being able to compare initial phonemes for likeness and difference are areas of phonological awareness that are particularly important for the development of reading (Stanovich, Cunningham, & Crammer, 1984; Yopp, 1988).

COMPREHENSION

Several levels of text comprehension exist. At the basic level, a reader is primarily concerned with decoding. Meaning is actively constructed by blending understanding from the words and sentences with personal meanings and experiences. Above this level is **critical literacy** in which a reader actively interprets *between the lines,* analyzes, and synthesizes information and is able to explain the content. A reader builds meaning by engaging in inferential processes that actively bridge the gaps between what is written and what is meant (Caccamise & Snyder, 2005). At the highest level of **dynamic literacy,** a reader is able to interrelate content to other knowledge through both deductive and inductive reasoning. Dynamic literacy is reading *across and beyond the lines* or across multiple texts, comparing and contrasting, integrating, and using ideas for problem raising and solving (Westby, 2005).

The reader's mental representation of meaning is composed of the text and the model the reader creates through the comprehension process. Comprehension occurs as a reader builds mental models representing a combination of the textual material, text grammar, and the reader's world knowledge and experience—models that are organized into internalized schemes or concepts of the content (Kintsch, 1998; Sanford & Garrod, 1998). The scheme facilitates and is the basis for assimilation, inferencing, summarization, comprehension, and memory of text information.

Reading is a goal-directed activity. For example, the reader may be gathering information to be used in a problem-solving task. Knowing what to do and how to do it is called **metacognition,** knowledge about knowledge and about cognitive processes. Metacogniton has two aspects important for reading. One aspect is self-appraisal or knowledge of one's own cognitive processes.

The other aspect of metacognition is called **executive function.** Executive function is self-regulation and includes the ability to attend; to set reasonable goals; to plan and organize to achieve each goal; to initiate, monitor, and evaluate your performance in relation to the goal; and to revise plans and strategies based on feedback.

During reading, the efficient reader uses self-regulation. Unknown words may be clarified in the dictionary, or the reader may look back to clarify some point in the text. Speed changes with the difficulty of the material. The reader makes hypotheses and predictions and confirms or does not confirm these.

> Each reader must interpret what she or he reads in light of personal experiences and knowledge. In other words, our comprehension will differ based on our own unique self.

READING DEVELOPMENT THROUGH THE LIFESPAN

You may believe that literacy development begins with reading and writing instruction in school. Actually, literacy development begins much earlier and continues throughout our lives.

Emerging Literacy

Reading development begins within social interactions between the child and caregiver(s) at around age 1, as parents or others begin to share books with toddlers. Book sharing is usually conversational in tone with the book serving as the focus of communication. Here's an example:

Adult: This is a book about a . . .

Child: Bear.

Adult: Yeah. And you found him right here. What do bears say?

Child: Grrrrrrrr.

Adult: Um-hm, they growl. Can you find his eye?

Reading the story is secondary to and will be included in the conversation. Notice the importance of language throughout this process.

By age 3, most children in our culture are beginning to develop **print awareness.** Early print awareness consists of knowledge of the meaning and function of print, basic concepts concerning the direction print proceeds across a page and through a book, and recognition of some letters (Snow et al., 1999). Later developing skills include recognizing words as discrete units, being able to identify letters, and using terminology, such as *letter, word,* and *sentence.* At this age, children lack knowledge of the phoneme-grapheme or sound-letter correspondence that they will learn later.

Language forms the basis for the stories children hear and tell. Children with good language skills seem to enjoy reading activities more that children with poor language and will pretend to read at an early age.

By age 4, children begin to notice phonological similarities and syllable structure in words they hear. This is the beginning of phonological awareness, mentioned previously. Four-year-olds also appreciate both sounds and rhymes. At this age, a young child may find rhyming words very funny and may fabricate nonsense words that rhyme. Children who have been exposed to a home literacy environment and to print media have better phoneme awareness, letter knowledge, and vocabulary (Foy & Mann, 2003).

Phonological awareness may arise from a child's need to store words in his or her brain with increasingly more detailed representation. This becomes necessary as a child's vocabulary grows and there are more and more words, some very similar in sound, to store (Metsala & Walley, 1998).

In a "literacy-rich" kindergarten environment, children begin to decode the alphabetic system and to broaden their experience with print (Snow et al., 1999). Five kindergarten variables seem to predict reading success by second grade: letter identification, sentence imitation, phonological awareness, rapid automatized naming (RAN), and maternal education level (Catts, Fey, Zhang, & Tomblin, 2001). RAN is the ability to name a series of items in a category quickly, such as clothes or food.

THOUGHT QUESTIONS

W*hy is maternal education important? How can this influence a child?*

In first grade, children are introduced to reading instruction and learn the sound-letter correspondence called **phonics.** Words read by a child are linked with words and meanings stored in memory. Most of the child's effort goes into decoding the letters, leaving little cognitive energy for either comprehension or interpretation. This is one reason why we don't assign *War and Peace* to first graders.

While phonology (sound) and orthography (letters) are important for early reading, the contribution of grammar and meaning increases as children begin to read multisyllabic words (Ehri & McCormick, 1998). Knowledge of morphology, for example, may aid students to read all portions of a word and to use their knowledge of word parts in interpretation. Children learn to break words apart, recombine them and to create new words (Berninger, Abbott, Billingsley, & Nagy, 2001).

As a child improves, reading becomes more automatic or fluent, especially for familiar words. Fluency is aided by the use of grapheme-phoneme patterns in the child's memory and by analogy, the process of relating unfamiliar words to familiar ones based on similar spelling.

By third grade, there is a shift from *learning to read* to *reading to learn* (Snow et al., 1999). As language continues to improve, so does comprehension with a resultant increase in reading fluency.

Mature Literacy

Although all reading begins with the printed word, mature readers use very little cognitive energy determining word pronunciation. At a higher level of processing, language and world knowledge or experiences are used to derive an understanding of the text, which is monitored automatically to ensure that the information makes sense (Snow et al., 1999). The skilled reader then predicts the next word or phrase and glances at it to confirm the prediction. Printed words are processed quickly, automatically, and below the level of consciousness most of the time. In less than one-quarter of a second, your brain retrieves all the information from a word or phrase that is needed to confirm the prediction and form another prediction of the next word or phrase. Obviously, this entire process, presented in Figure 6.2, is highly dependent on language.

For the beginner, the reading process is less automatic and relatively more energy is used in decoding. This leaves little energy for comprehension and prediction. As a result, reading is more labored and slow. As word recognition and comprehension increase, reading becomes more fluent.

Mature readers don't so much simply read the text as dialogue with it. Reading is an active process in which ideas and concepts are formed and modified, details remembered and recalled, and information checked. Much of this is the unconscious process of the brain partaking of new information, but other activities, such as looking up a definition, are very conscious.

> Establish a habit of reading now. It will serve you well as you mature.

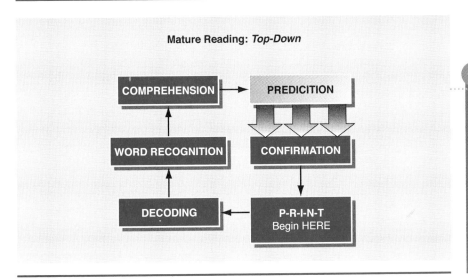

Mature Reading: *Top-Down*

FIGURE 6.2

Model of mature reading.

Mature readers use their language skills to predict what words or phrases will appear next in the text, then momentarily glance at the print to confirm their predictions before predicting anew what will follow.

As we mature, the types and purposes of reading change, but we can continue to enjoy the process throughout our lives. Reading skill continues to be strong through adulthood if we exercise our ability and do not experience any neuropathologies, such as those in Chapter 7. Reading is one of the primary ways by which adults increase their vocabulary and knowledge.

READING PROBLEMS THROUGH THE LIFESPAN

Public Law 107-110, the No Child Left Behind Act (NCLB) passed in 2002, states that all children in third grade, even those with disabilities, will read proficiently by 2013/2014. In short, this law requires annual testing of students in grades 3 through 8 in reading and mathematics. States that fail to meet national standards are held accountable. This law clearly emphasizes the importance of reading and of instructional and intervention methods that are *evidence-based*, meaning they really are effective.

Conceptually, reading impairments can be divided into groups on the basis of both decoding and comprehension (Catts & Kamhi, 2005b; Kamhi & Catts, 2002). This dichotomy suggests that a one-size-fits-all reading intervention model is inappropriate.

Children with dyslexia have poor word recognition or decoding abilities, accompanied by problems with phonological processing, but average comprehension. *Dyslexia,* a type of learning disability, is neurobiological in origin and characterized by difficulties with accurate and/or fluent word recognition and decoding abilities and by poor spelling (Lyon, Shaywitz, & Shaywitz, 2003). Slower letter- and word-naming speeds, reflecting insufficient phonological processing abilities, impede decoding and word-recognition processes (Kamhi, 1998). Many children with dyslexia also exhibit delayed language development, listening comprehension problems, and poor phonological awareness (Catts, 1996). Difficulties are not related to other cognitive abilities or to the efficacy of classroom instruction.

In contrast, other children with LD have poor word recognition and poor comprehension. Although decoding difficulties can seriously hamper reading, children with LD often have difficulty comprehending and learning from text even when they are able to decode adequately (Williams, 1998). In fact, children with LD do better on recall with oral narratives than with written, although both are below that of typical children of the same age. The story of a young man with learning disabilities is presented in Case Study 6.2.

Children with SLI may be similar to those with LD, exhibiting grapheme-phoneme (letter-sound) errors and syntactic, semantic, and pragmatic errors or misinterpretations when reading. Comprehension also may be impaired and may be related to a child's poor vocabulary.

A third group, children with hyperlexia, has poor comprehension but typical or above word recognition abilities. Hyperlexia is a near-obsessive interest in letters and words found in some children with autism spectrum disorder (ASD). Although these children appear very precocious in their reading ability, they often have extremely limited comprehension (Healy, 1982).

Case Study 6.2

Justin, A Young Man with Learning Disabilities

Justin grew up in a midwestern suburb and attended public schools. He's the youngest child of four and the only male. As an adult, he's personable and friendly, works part-time, and is attending the local community college. His sisters, especially the next oldest, help him with his homework when possible.

As a preschooler, Justin cared little for books. His language was slow in developing when compared to his sisters, but his parents assumed that he would be fine and that he didn't talk much because his sisters talked for him. Still, his mom enrolled him in preschool to encourage his development. He scored low on his kindergarten readiness test and, when admitted, was recommended to repeat because of a lack of pre-academic skills needed for first grade. His parents reluctantly agreed.

When he began school, Justin adjusted well, but quickly began to fall behind other children in both reading and writing. An evaluation at the end of first grade resulted in Justin's being labeled as learning disabled. It was recommended that he remain in a regular classroom with additional instruction in literacy. At home, his parents worked closely with him on his reading and written assignments.

Through most of elementary school, Justin saw a reading specialist and a speech-language pathologist several times each week. His SLP focused on Justin's language and listening skills and on his reading comprehension.

When Justin entered junior high school, he stopped seeing both the reading specialist and the speech-language therapist. Instead, it was decided by his team, including both him and his parents, that other measures would be attempted in order to compensate for his deficits. These included use of a word processor, recording of class lessons, and pre-preparation of lecture notes by his teachers. All through junior and senior high school, Justin met with different teachers after school for extra instruction.

When he graduated, Justin had few plans. He drifted from job to job for nearly a year before his sisters convinced him to apply to community college. Going part-time, he was able to do well in his courses and has just been accepted into the physical therapy assistant major. Reading and writing are still difficult, but Justin is determined to do well and his family, especially his sisters, are extremely supportive.

Causal factors for literacy impairment may be extrinsic or intrinsic to an individual (Catts & Kamhi, 2005a). Extrinsic factors may include experience and the manner of instruction. Intrinsic factors may include genetics, vision-based deficits, auditory processing problems, attention deficits, language impairment, and neurology. For example, there appear to be both white and grey matter differences in the brains of children with dyslexia when compared to typical children (Eckert, Leonard, Wilke, Eckert, Richards, Richards, & Berninger, 2005). Differences have been found in the left temporal-parietal region (interior to the left ear), in both the left and right linguistic processing areas, and in the cerebellum (near the brain stem). Neural pathways in the left temporal-parietal area of the brain are important in the development of fluent reading (Deutsch, Dougherty, Bammer, Siok, Gabrieli, & Wandell, 2005). Deficits in cerebellar processing are similar to those in children with fetal alcohol syndrome (FAS) (Coffin, Baroody, Schneider, & O'Neill, 2005).

Although many kindergarteners, both those with language impairments and those without, know some letter names and letter-sound relationships, their knowledge is incomplete (Ehri, 2000). In attempting to read, some children with language impairments, especially those with poor phonological skills but average or above average intelligence, may use memorized word shapes, letter names, or guessing rather than relying on letter-sound correspondence and word-attack skills. As a result, they are unable to decode unfamiliar words. Without word attack or decoding skills, by second grade, when formal decoding instruction ends, these children begin to fail.

Most initial reading problems are related to deficient phonological processing and phonological awareness (Catts & Kamhi, 2005a). In fact, children with reading impairments, even those with dyslexia, make some of the same phonological errors as younger children (Treiman, 1997). For example, consonant clusters are especially difficult for both children with reading impairment and beginning readers. Phonological awareness difficulties seem to be related to failure to analyze words into syllables and these, in turn, into smaller phonological units (Bird, Bishop, & Freeman, 1995).

Language deficits also contribute to literacy problems in other ways, such as impaired comprehension. If a child isn't comprehending, he or she isn't reading. Some children will have difficulty interpreting written narratives because they have poor oral narrative abilities (Naremore, 2001). They may lack the story framework or linguistic skills for telling narratives.

In addition to poor oral language abilities, poor readers often fail to use contextual and visual cues, such as pictures, to aid comprehension. Reading comprehension is, in part, dependent not only upon a person's language abilities and experiences with print but also upon communication, especially social inferencing and interpersonal reasoning (Donahue & Foster, 2004). Given the low social competence of some children with language impairments, it may be easy to see why this aspect of reading might also be difficult (Brinton & Fujiki, 2004).

Good readers guide and control their reading behavior purposefully and flexibly (Anderson, Hiebert, Scott, & Wilkenson, 1985; Baker & Brown, 1984). In contrast, poor readers lack such strategies, reflecting their misconceptions of the task and possible deficits in executive function (Johnston & Winograd, 1985; Torgesen, 1980). They may approach reading as a random, unfathomable process.

Executive function deficit is most evident in children with TBI who seemingly are unable to consider the consequences of their behavior and unrealistic in their self-evaluation (Sohlberg, Mateer, & Stuss, 1993; Ylvisaker & Feeney, 1995). In addition, children with ADHD have been described as inattentive and impulsive, disorganized, unable to inhibit behavior, and ineffective learners, characteristics of those with impaired executive function.

THOUGHT QUESTION

Does it seem logical that impairments such as learning disability, which have a perceptual component, might also be evident in reading and writing?

As children experience repeated reading failure, they may become frustrated or passive. Lacking persistence and with low self-esteem, they may become apathetic and resigned to failure (Butkowsky & Willows, 1980). In contrast, some poor readers may become aggressive or display acting-out behaviors. All of these behaviors interfere with further learning and development (Winograd & Niquette, 1988).

In short, children with language impairments may be at risk for reading impairment for several reasons (Hambly & Riddle, 2002; Miller et al., 2001; Stanovich, 1986). In general, they

- Begin with less language and may have difficulty catching up.
- Have poor comprehension skills because they lack language knowledge that would enable them to integrate what they read.
- Have poor metalinguistic skills.
- Possess linguistic processing difficulties.

When something goes wrong in the reading process, the result is reading that is less automatic and less fluent. Word decoding or text understanding may be impaired. A child who has difficulty interpreting spoken language may have difficulty interpreting written language, especially if classroom instruction focuses primarily on phonetics.

> Competent readers and writers approach the task with a purpose that guides their behavior.

> In case you've forgot, *metalinguistics* includes the ability to consider language out of context, to make judgments about its correctness, and to understand to some extent the process of using language.

ASSESSMENT OF DEVELOPMENTAL READING

SLPs should be alert to potential reading problems among children with phonological problems or those at risk because of other diagnosed disorders such as LD, TBI, or SLI. In this section we'll discuss overall assessment with a more detailed discussion of assessment of phonological awareness, word recognition, comprehension, and executive function.

As mentioned in Chapter 4, assessments begin with an initial data gathering step that may include use of questionnaires, interviews, referrals, and screening testing. Table 6.1 presents a checklist designed to identify kindergarten and first-grade school children at risk for language-based reading difficulties (Catts, 1997). No one item alone will indicate a possible problem.

W*hat might be some clues that a preschool child might have later literacy difficulties?*

THOUGHT QUESTIONS

Children who read poorly may exhibit learned helplessness or have negative attitudes toward the reading process. This information can be gathered from interviews with teachers, parents, and the child and by observation within the classroom. Interview questions should include the child's perceptions of the importance of reading and different types of reading and difficulties, along with self-perceptions (Wixson, Bosky, Yochum, & Alvermann, 1984). Observation can confirm the child, teacher, and parent responses.

Collaborative reading assessment should include standardized reading assessment, oral language samples, oral reading samples including analysis

TABLE 6.1

Checklist for early identification of language-based reading disabilities

The child . . .

_____ Has difficulty remembering words or names

_____ Has problem with verbal sequences (i.e., alphabet, days of the week)

_____ Has difficulty following instructions and directions and may respond to a part rather than the whole

_____ Has difficulty remembering the words to songs and poems

_____ Requests multiple repetitions of instructions/directions with little improvement in comprehension

_____ Relies too much on context to understand what's said

_____ Has difficulty understanding questions

_____ Has difficulty understanding age-appropriate stories and making inferences, predicting outcomes, drawing conclusions

_____ Frequently mispronounces words and names

_____ Has problems saying common words with difficult sound patterns (i.e., *spaghetti, cinnamon*)

_____ Confuses similar-sounding words (i.e., the **Specific** Ocean)

_____ Combines sound patterns of similar words (i.e., **nucular** for *nuclear*)

_____ Has speech that is hesitant, contains fillers (i.e., *you know*), or words lacking specificity (i.e., *that, stuff, thing, one*)

_____ Has expressive language difficulties, such as short sentences and errors in grammar

_____ Lacks variety in vocabulary and overuses words

_____ Has difficulty giving directions or explanations

_____ Relates stories or events in a disorganized or incomplete manner

_____ Provides little specific detail when relating events

_____ Has difficulty with rules of conversation, such as turn taking, staying on topic, requesting clarification

_____ Doesn't seem to understand or enjoy rhymes

_____ Doesn't easily recognize words that begin with the same sound

_____ Has difficulty recognizing syllables

_____ Demonstrates problems learning sound-letter correspondences

_____ Doesn't engage readily in pretend play

_____ Has a history of language comprehension and/or production problems

_____ Has a family history of spoken or written language problems

_____ Has limited exposure to literacy in the home

_____ Seems to lack interest in books and shared reading activities

Source: Adapted from Catts, H.W. (1997) The early identification of language-based reading disabilities. *Language, Speech, and Hearing Services in Schools, 28,* 86–89.

miscues, and written story retelling (Gillam & Gorman, 2004). Formal reading testing might be accomplished by a school's reading specialist, but the SLP may wish to give selected subtests that focus on phonological awareness and ability to derive meaning from print. In a more informal task, a child might be asked to read previously unread curricular materials in an attempt to assess her or his ability to function within the classroom (Nelson & Van Meter, 2002). The child's aloud reading can be recorded for later analysis of the child's miscues. Comprehension can be assessed by using questions, retelling or paraphrasing.

Phonological Awareness

Phonological awareness assessment is multifaceted and should be accomplished within an overall assessment of reading, spelling, phonological awareness, verbal working memory, and rapid automatized naming (RAN). In addition to formal testing, the SLP can use informal methods of assessing rhyming, syllabication, segmentation, phoneme isolation, deletion, substitution, and blending. It is especially important to assess both segmenting and blending with school-age children.

Word Recognition

Decoding skills, especially knowledge of sound-letter correspondence, is the basis for word recognition. Of interest to the SLP will be decoding of consonant blends, long (*day*) and short (*can*) vowels, different syllable structures, and morphological affixes.

Word recognition assessment should adhere to the following guidelines (Roth, 2004):

- Materials should be based on age and developmental appropriateness.
- Tasks should be of various types to assess different level of processing.
- Several measures should be used.
- A student's cultural and linguistic background must be considered.
- Test selection should be based on test quality and appropriateness.
- Unfamiliar test tasks may need to be demonstrated and trained.
- Reading deficits are not limited to children with emergent literacy skills.
- Observation and interpretation of test behaviors is extremely important.

Although traditional assessment procedures stress standardized testing, alternative approaches such as curriculum-based measures and dynamic assessment may be more appropriate for children with language impairment or with cultural and linguistic differences (Roth, 2004). Materials for curriculum-based assessment usually come from the local curricula and use criterion-referenced scoring, which measures a child against himself or herself over time. In this way progress is measured without reference to some abstract norm. Dynamic assessment often takes a test-teach-test format in which a child is assessed for the amount of change she or he can make during the assessment process.

Word recognition is more than just the ability to decode a word in isolation. Readers use a variety of strategies in order to predict words that make sense, fit grammatically and pragmatically, and begin with certain sounds. Sighting the word confirms or does not confirm the prediction. It's important, therefore, that word recognition testing be accomplished with a various clues available to the child and with words both in isolation and within text. More important than test scores is describing a child's strengths and the strategies used.

When analyzing recorded reading data, the SLP notes all discrepancies in the recorded reading samples. All attempts at word decoding, repetitions, corrections, omitted words and morphemes, extended pauses, and dialectal usages should be noted and analyzed for possible strategies used by the child. Miscues can be analyzed at the word level by type, such as word order is changed, word substitutions, additions, and deletions (Nelson, 1994; Nelson & Van Meter, 2002). The percentage of incorrect but linguistically acceptable words indicates the extent of a child's use of linguistic cues to predict the correct word. In addition, the SLP should note the way in which the child sounds out words (Nelson & Van Meter, 2002).

Text Comprehension

Assessing text comprehension abilities of children is complicated by the many cognitive and linguistic processes involved. At the very least, the SLP or other team members should assess a child's

- Oral language with special attention to a child's use of the more elaborate syntactic style used in literature.
- Knowledge of narrative schemes and text grammar schemes.
- Metacognition. (Westby, 2005)

Narrative schemes or the events in a story might be assessed by having a child tell a narrative from pictures or by asking questions about the pictures that relate to the organization of the story. A child's text grammar, consisting of the parts of a story, can be assessed through spontaneous narratives or by retelling previously heard narratives.

The self-appraisal or awareness aspect of metacognition can be assessed through tasks that ask children questions demonstrating their knowledge of *know, remember, forget,* and *guess* (Wellman, 1985). Awareness of cognition is not the same as self-regulation. This aspect of metacognition will be discussed in the following section on executive function.

Although several norm-referenced tests measure reading comprehension, they should be supplemented by other measures of a child's ability to identify grammatical units, interpret and analyze text, make inferences, and construct meaning by combining text with personal knowledge and experience (Kamhi, 2003).

Executive Function

While poor readers act as if reading is simply sounding out words rapidly and fluently, good readers expect text to make sense and to be a source for learning information. As a result, good readers read actively and with purpose, constructing mental models and organizing information as they go.

Self-regulation in reading can be assessed in many ways, including (Westby, 2004):

- Interview questions about different strategies used for different reading tasks.
- Think-Alouds or verbalizing thoughts accompanying reading.
- Error or inconsistency detection while reading.

Errors and inconsistencies can be planted in texts specifically for the assessment.

INTERVENTION FOR DEVELOPMENTAL READING IMPAIRMENT

As in several of the disorders discussed in this text, intervention for developmental literacy impairments should be a team effort. Members should include the classroom teacher, reading specialist, speech-language pathologist, parents, and when appropriate older adolescent clients. It is very tempting to teach reading *per se,* but that is not the primary role of an SLP. Rather, he or she supports the efforts of all team members and the explicit instruction of the classroom teacher and reading specialist.

Team members might cooperate in an embedded/explicit model of intervention in which children participate both in literacy-rich experiences embedded in the daily curriculum and in explicit, focused, therapeutic teaching of reading (Justice & Kaderavek, 2004; Kaderavek & Justice, 2004). The literacy-rich environment might include a message board where children learn to decode an "important" message left daily by the teacher, snack activities in which sounds are embedded in snack names, recipes, music and print, book and speech sound play, rhyming pictures, and book sharing with the teacher and others (Towey, Whitcomb, & Bray, 2004).

Effective intervention for reading should include sound and letter processes used in word identification, grammatical processes, and the integration of these with meaning and contextual processes (Gillam & Gorman, 2004). Training phonological (sound) and orthographic (letter) processing together seems to offer a more effective strategy than working on phonological awareness skills in isolation (Fuchs, Fuchs, Thompson, Otaiba, Yen, Yang, Braun, & O'Connor, 2001; Gillon, 2000).

Beginning in preschool, the SLP can increase children's print awareness with print-focused reading activities (Justice & Ezell, 2002). Print-focused strategies emphasis word concepts and alphabetic knowledge and include cues such as the following:

Show me how to hold the book so I can read.

Do I read this way or this way?

Where is the last word on the page?

How many words do you see?

Find the letter C. Whose name starts with C?

Such print-focused prompts are easy to teach, and parents have been successful at home with only minimal training.

Reading intervention might begin with a two-prong intervention model (van Kleeck, 1995). In one part, called *meaning foundation,* the teacher or SLP *scaffolds* or guides reading for children by placing the text in context and asking questions to guide comprehension. The child learns that print contains the meaning and gains phonological awareness and letter knowledge. In a parallel thrust, called *form foundation,* phonological awareness and alphabetic knowledge are emphasized. This model is illustrated in Figure 6.3. Later reading intervention might target both linguistic and metalinguistic skills, including recognition of key words, use of all parts of the text such as the glossary and the index, and application of general learning strategies, such as graphic organizers containing photos, drawings, and print (Wallach & Butler, 1995). Now let's look at phonological awareness, word recognition, comprehension, and executive function again.

Phonological Awareness

As mentioned, ASHA has recommended that SLPs become active in prevention of literacy impairments as well as in intervention. Phonological awareness is an area of prevention that can be targeted with young children. Evidence-based practice tells us that children who receive phonological awareness training have higher phonemic awareness, word attack, and word identification skills at the end of kindergarten than children who do not receive such training (Ekelman, Fitzpatrick, Vail, Woods, Sloan-Brown, Sopko, Hunter, Warstler, & Minich, 2004). In addition to working with individual students, SLPs can offer phonological awareness instruction to teachers, stressing the importance of phonological awareness and its integration into the reading curriculum (Hambley & Riddle, 2002).

Whenever possible with older children, phonological awareness should be taught within meaningful text experiences, such as systematic and ex-

FIGURE 6.3

Two-stage intervention.

Intervention with young readers should focus on both word meaning and sentence formation.

Two-stage intervention model for pre- and early readers

Word meaning foundation

At Word Level:
　Vocabulary Instruction
　Words that are important,
　　utilitarian, conceptually easy,
　　and frequently used
At Text Level:
　Providing Scaffolding

Sentence form foundation

Understanding underlying
　structure
Relational terms

plicit classroom instruction, so that the emergent nature of both literacy and phonological awareness can support each other (McFadden, 1998). Phonological awareness training alone is insufficient to increase reading comprehension (Pugh & Klecan-Aker, 2004).

Within intervention, the SLP can address both segmentation (*cat → c-a-t*) and blending (*c-a-t → cat*), working at the phoneme and syllable levels. In general, programs focusing on one or two phonological awareness skills yield better results than those that try to teach with a broader focus (National Reading Panel, 2000). It's best if the SLP teaches skills that will directly impact the child's performance of an everyday task.

Intervention can begin with sound recognition and identification and be both receptive and expressive. Next, the SLP can move to syllable segmentation and blending (*stapler → stap-ler*) and, finally, to phoneme segmentation and blending (*c-a-t → cat*). At each level segmentation is easier for most children than blending. Real words are also easier than nonsense ones and will decrease the memory load for children.

Phoneme intervention might progress from recognition of a target sound in isolation, through identification when paired with other sounds, to sounds in syllables, then words (Gerber & Klein, 2004). It is best to work with one or two sounds at a time. Memory can be aided by pairing sounds with the real objects or pictures and finally with printed letters and words. Letters also give additional input, are a potential memory aid, and hopefully will generalize to reading. To aid reading, children can be encouraged to tell a story that is taped by the SLP for later transcription. The SLP and child can then "read" the story together as the child identifies the target phoneme.

Consonant clusters are especially difficult and may require special emphasis. It's advisable to concentrate on one type of cluster at a time rather than mixing all possible ones together. Vowels also offer a particular problem in English because of the many vowel sounds and their inconsistent spellings.

The goal of phonological awareness intervention at the syllable level is to help children segment and blend syllables in order to read and spell multisyllabic words (Hambley & Riddle, 2002). The concept of syllables can be introduced as naturally occurring "beats" in a word. Multisensory approaches are also helpful and can make the training interesting. Clapping hands or drum beats can be used to help children recognize and identify syllables. Other examples include dropping objects into cans, stacking toys, playing hopscotch, or taking turns in any number of child games during auditory recognition training.

Word Recognition

The goals of intervention for word recognition are

- To teach phonemic decoding skills, resulting in accurate and fluent reading of new words.
- To develop a rich vocabulary of sight words.
- To improve reading comprehension. (Torgesen, al Otaiba, & Grek, 2005)

Success in the last two depends on achievement of the first. Although teaching decoding skills can be difficult, explicit, intense, supportive intervention can result in gains, followed by increases in reading accuracy, fluency, and comprehension (Torgesen, 2005). Support for learning can be provided by encouragement and positive feedback and by scaffolding or guiding learning by breaking tasks into smaller steps or by giving a child as much direction as necessary to complete the task successfully.

Context can be used to help children predict words in text. Intervention might begin with obvious words, such as *I took my umbrella because it looked like _____.* Training can then move to more ambiguous choices and the use of other strategies that include morphological and orthographic cues, such as *Let's have _____ for lunch* followed by *Let's have p_____ for lunch* or *Let's have p_____s for lunch.*

Reading fluency is related to word recognition and comprehension. In short, "reading fluency shows the most improvement when students reread a text many times to many different people, using progressively more difficult text with feedback and correction." (Kamhi, 2003).

Text Comprehension

Children who lack internalized story frameworks might begin intervention with telling stories (Naremore, 2001). A child must learn how to go from knowing to telling before he or she can understand the elements of narration and interpret the stories of others, whether oral or written.

Intervention can begin at the oral narrative telling and progress to oral then written narrative interpretation (Boudreau & Larson, 2004). Storybook reading can be divided into before, during, and after reading activities. Postreading might include story mapping and other graphic organizers, retelling, and creating novel narratives. Narratives can be divided into story parts and recombined.

Comprehension may also be enhanced by teaching children the more explicit and precise descriptive language style found in written communication (Westby, 2005). This style can be taught through tasks in which children must follow very explicit oral instructions to be successful or tasks in which contextual cues, such as objects or pictures, are present. Literate vocabularies can be enhanced through prereading activities that focus on the words to be encountered and through use of visual or verbal memory aids. Complex grammar may be taught through books with familiar stories or books in which the grammar becomes increasingly complex through added elements.

Reading comprehension can be improved for children with LD and dyslexia by also focusing on before, during, and after reading strategies (Vaughn & Klingner, 2004). During prereading, teachers can focus on the purpose of reading and on motivation. Vocabulary and concepts in the reading can be *pretaught* and the teacher can help students build a bridge from their current knowledge to the text. During and after reading, the teacher can use questioning, determining the main idea, and summarizing. Graphic organizers, such as word maps, can aid in learning vocabulary and concepts.

As children read, comprehension intervention strategies may include use of summarization, instruction in story grammar or story structure, and mental imagining of the ideas in the text (Pressley & Hilden, 2004). Children can learn to interact with the text through thought questions, such as *Why might you want to be friends with the main character?* Narratives can be connected to personal experience through the use of personal journals.

At another level, comprehension includes a social dialogue with the authors and characters. Comprehension training should also include discussion of the author's goals, and the feelings and motivations of characters (Donahue & Foster, 2004). Knowledge of the text can be used to predict a character's behavior within a narrative.

Executive Function

Specific areas of executive function that might be targeted in intervention include nonverbal working memory, self-directed speech, emotional control, and problem solving (Westby, 2004). Just teaching self-regulating strategies is not enough. The SLP and classroom teacher must help each child achieve independent and appropriate use of these strategies. "Students must understand the purpose of the reading activities, develop a metacognitive ability to reflect on the knowledge they have, and have the motivation to develop goals and procedural knowledge to implement strategies to achieve the goals." (Westby, 2004, p. 413).

Of importance is *distancing* or moving away from dependence on the text and toward independent thinking. This can be accomplished by questions that move from answers explicitly stated in the text to ones in which the question is generated by something in the text but the answer is generated from the student's knowledge.

RITING

As with all modes of communication, writing is a social act. Just like a speaker, the writer must consider the audience, but because the audience is not present when the writing occurs, writing demands more cognitive resources for planning and execution than does speaking (Golder & Coirier, 1994; Graham & Harris, 1996, 1997; Scott, 1999).

In short, writing is using knowledge and new ideas combined with language knowledge to create text (Kintsch, 1998). It's a complex process that includes generating ideas, organizing and planning, acting on that plan, revising, and monitoring based on self-feedback (Scott, 1999). Writing involves motor, cognitive, linguistic, affective, and executive processes.

Writing is more abstract and **decontextualized** than conversation and requires internal knowledge of different writing forms, such as narratives and expository writing. Decontextualized means outside of a conversational context. When you write, the entire context is contained in the writing. You create the context with your language rather than having the context created by your conversational partners.

There are several aspects to the writing process, consisting of (Berninger, 2000):

- handwriting, word-processing, text-messaging
- spelling
- executive function
- text construction or going from ideas to written texts
- memory

As mentioned previously, executive function is self-regulation and includes attending, goal setting, planning, and the like. Memory provides ideas for content and language symbols and rules to guide the formation of that content and is used for word recognition and storage of ideas as they are worked and reworked. As you can see, writing is a very complicated process. Let's look more closely at spelling and then writing development and impairment, followed by assessment and intervention.

SPELLING

Your brain doesn't store words letter-by-letter, rather it stores them by more useful units. For example, *stand* is probably stored as *st-and,* which enables you to spell *land, band, hand, bland, strand,* and so on.

Spelling of most words is self-taught using a trial-and-error approach. It is estimated that only 4,000 words are explicitly taught in elementary school. Rather, classroom teachers focus on strategies and regularities that children can use to determine word spelling.

Many people wrongly assume that spelling is just use of memorized words. Good spellers use a variety of strategies and actively search words for patterns and consistency (Hughes & Searle, 1997). More specifically, mature spellers, like you, rely on memory; on spelling and reading experience; phonological, semantic, and morphological knowledge; orthographic knowledge and mental grapheme representations; and analogy (Apel & Masterson, 2001). Semantic knowledge is concerned with the interrelationship of spelling and meaning, while morphological knowledge is knowing the internal structure of words, affixes (*un-, dis-, -ly, -ment*) and the derivation of words (*happy, unhappily*). Mental grapheme representations are best exhibited when you ask yourself "Does that word look right?" Your representations are formed through repeated exposure to words in print. Finally, through analogy, the speller tries to spell an unfamiliar word using prior knowledge of words that sound the same.

Spelling competes with other aspects of writing for your formidable but limited cognitive energy. Excessive energy expended at the phonological (sound and syllable) processing and orthographic (letter) processing levels comes at the cost to higher language functions. As a result, poor spellers generally produce poorer, shorter texts.

WRITING DEVELOPMENT THROUGH THE LIFESPAN

Writing and speaking development are interdependent and parallel, and many aspects of language overlap both modes. In turn, writing development includes development of several previously mentioned interdependent processes.

Emerging Literacy

Initially, children treat writing and speaking as two separate systems. Three-year-olds, for example, will "write" in their own way but don't yet realize that writing represents sounds. By age 4, some real letters of the parent language may be included (Tolchinsky-Landsmann & Levin, 1985).

As with reading, in early writing, children expend a great deal of cognitive energy on the mechanics, such as sound-letter associations and letter forming. Gradually, spelling, like reading, becomes more accurate and fluent or automatic.

For a few years, the spoken and written systems converge and children write in the same manner as they speak, although speech is more complex. Around age 9 or 10, talking and speaking become differentiated as children become increasingly literate. Writing slowly overtakes speech as written sentences become longer and more complex than speaking. Children display increasing awareness of the audience through their use of syntax, vocabulary, textual themes, and attitude (Kroll, 1981). Some language forms are used almost exclusively in either speech or writing, such as using *and* to begin many sentences in speech but only rarely in writing.

Mature Literacy

In a phase not achieved by all writers, speaking and writing become consciously separate. The syntactic and semantics are consciously recognized as somewhat different and the writer has great flexibility of style. You may or may not have achieved this phase yet. If you find yourself using an enlarged vocabulary when writing or pondering how sentences flow from one to the next, then you are probably there. As with reading, practice results in improvement that should continue throughout the lifespan. In general, the writing of adults as compared to adolescents contains longer, more complex sentences and uses more abstract nouns, such as *longevity* and *kindness,* and more metalinguistic and metacognitive words, such as *reflect* and *disagree* (Nippold, Ward-Lonergan & Fanning, 2005).

When you write, do you consciously think about the way your finished *product will affect a reader? Do you add variety to keep a potential reader's interest?*

THOUGHT QUESTIONS

As you probably suspect, the developmental process is not that easy. You may recall that writing consists of handwriting, word processing, or text messaging; spelling; executive function; text construction or going from ideas to written texts; and memory. Let's discuss, in that order, the ones of particular interest to speech-language pathologists.

Spelling

Spelling development is a long, slow process. Initial *preliterate* attempts at spelling consist of mostly of scribbles and drawing with an occasional letter

For some children, reading and writing seem to be arbitrary, unfathomable processes.

thrown in (Henderson, 1990). Later children use some phoneme-grapheme knowledge along with letter names. Gradually, they become aware of conventional spelling and are able to analyze a word into sounds and letters, although vowels will be difficult for some time. As mentioned earlier, mature spellers are able to call on multiple learning strategies and different types of knowledge (Rittle-Johnson, & Siegler, 1999; Treiman & Cassar, 1997; Varnhagen, McCallum, & Burstow, 1997).

As knowledge of the alphabetic system emerges, the child slowly connects letters and sounds and devises a system called "invented spelling" in which the names of letters may be used in spelling, as in *SKP* for *escape* or *LFT* for *elephant* (Henderson, 1990). One letter may represent a sound grouping, as in **set** for **street**. Because children lack full knowledge of the phoneme-grapheme system, they have difficulty separating words into phonemes (Treiman, 1993).

As spelling becomes more sophisticated, children learn about spacing, sequencing, various ways to represent phonemes, and the morpheme-grapheme relationship (Henderson, 1990). The parallel development of reading aids this process.

Children who possess full knowledge of the alphabetic system can segment words into phonemes and know the conventional phoneme-grapheme correspondences. As children begin to recognize more regularities and consolidate the alphabetic system, they becomes more efficient spellers (Ehri, 2000). Increased memory capacity for these regularities is at the heart of spelling ability.

Many vowel representations, phonological variations, such as *later-latter,* and morphophonemic variations, such as *sign-signal,* will take several years to acquire (Treiman, 1993). Gradually, children learn about consonant doubling, stressed and unstressed syllables (**report-re*port***), and root words and derivations (*add-addition*) (Henderson, 1990).

Most spellers shift from a purely phonological strategy to a mixed one between second and fifth grade (Goswami, 1988; Lennox & Siegel, 1996). As words and strategies are stored in long-term memory and access becomes fluent, the load on cognitive capacity is lessened and can be focused on other writing tasks.

Adults spell in several ways, letter-by-letter, by syllable, and by sub-syllable unit, such as *ck,* used for *back, stick,* and *rock* but never in *ckar* (car). The method used seems to vary with the task.

Next time you're word processing, notice if your spelling is conscious and letter-by-letter. Obviously, sounds are helpful, but the phoneme-grapheme relationship is not one-to-one. Your accumulated knowledge is also important.

Executive Function

It is not until early adulthood — about where most of you are right now — that writers develop the cognitive processes and executive functions needed for mature writing (Berninger, 2000; Ylvisaker & DeBonis, 2000). It takes this long because of the protracted period of anatomical and physiological development of your brain's frontal lobe where executive function is housed.

Until adolescence, young writers need adult scaffolding or guidance in planning and revising their writing. By junior high school, teens are capable of revising all aspects of writing. Improved long-term memory results in improved overall compositional quality (Berninger, Cartwright, Yates, Swanson, & Abbott, 1994).

Text Generation

Once children begin to produce true spelling, even if it is unconventional, they begin to generate text. In first grade, text may consist of only a single sentence, as in *My dog is old.* Early compositions often lack cohesion and use structures repeatedly, as in the following:

> *I like school. I like gym. I like recess. I like art.*

Mature writers use more variety for dramatic effect. The facts and events characteristic of early writing evolve into use of judgments and opinions, parenthetical expressions, qualifications, contrasts, and generalizations (Berninger, 2000).

Initially, compositions lack coherence and organization. Later, ideas may relate to a central idea or consist of a list of sequential events. Written narratives or stories emerge first, followed by expository texts. Expository writing, the writing of the classroom, is of several genres: procedural, descriptive, opinion, cause-and-effect, and compare-and-contrast. Essays include at least a unifying topic sentence, comments referenced to the topic, and elaborations on the comments.

WRITING PROBLEMS THROUGH THE LIFESPAN

Children with language deficits often have writing deficits too. Unfortunately, their writing difficulties may remain through the lifespan, and the gap between their writing abilities and that of children developing typically widens.

Children with LD may have difficulties with all aspects of the writing process (Graham, Harris, MacArthur, & Schwartz, 1991; McFadden & Gillam, 1996; Roth, Spekman, & Fye, 1991; Troia, Graham, & Harris, 1999; Vallecorsa & Garriss, 1990; Wong, 2000). Sometimes called **dysgraphia,** a neurobiological disorder, these writing problems are characterized by spelling errors, word omissions and substitutions, punctuation errors, agrammatical sentences, and a lack of organization. A sample of the writing of a child with LD is presented in Figure 6.4. Because they have little knowledge of the writing process, these children fail to plan and make few substantive revisions. They are easily discouraged and may devote very little time on a given task. Clarity and organization are forsaken for spelling, handwriting, and punctuation, leaving little cognitive capacity for text generation. In the process, meaning suffers.

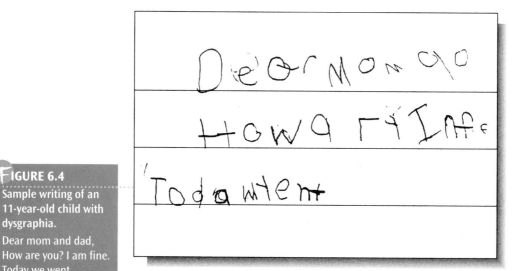

FIGURE 6.4

Sample writing of an 11-year-old child with dysgraphia.

Dear mom and dad, How are you? I am fine. Today we went . . .

Deficits in Spelling

Poor spellers view spelling as arbitrary, random, and seemingly unlearnable (Hughes & Searle, 1997). Misspellings are characterized by omission of syllables, morphological markers such as plural "s," and letters; letter substitutions; and confusion of homonyms such as *to/too/two*. Even adults, especially those with LD, often cite spelling as their primary area of concern (Blalock & Johnson, 1987).

Usually, deficits in spelling represent poor phonological processing and poor knowledge and use of phoneme-grapheme information. While most spellers shift to greater use of analogy between second and fifth grade, poor spellers tend to rely on visual matching skills and phoneme position rules as compensation for their limited knowledge of sound-letter correspondences (Kamhi & Hinton, 2000). Some spellers seem incapable of changing their spelling techniques (Treiman, 1997).

THOUGHT QUESTION

Does an inability in changing spelling habits suggest other cognitive rigidity that might make learning and problem solving difficult?

Deficits in Executive Function

When you write, you begin with ideas. Your ideas are converted into language. In other words, you have something to say. At this point, executive function becomes important.

When executive function or self-regulation is impaired, communication and even problem-solving abilities are diminished, especially in socially demanding or complex linguistic tasks, such as writing. Lacking self-regula-

Literacy-rich environments are critical for children with literacy impairments.

tion, some children with LD follow a "retrieve-write" writing strategy in which they put on paper whatever comes to mind, each sentence stimulating the next, with little thought to planning. They produce and elaborate little, revise ineffectively and with seeming indifference to their intended audience, detect errors poorly, and experience difficulty executing intended changes (Graham & Harris, 1999). Planning is difficult because language formulation difficulties affect what the writer wishes to convey.

One adult professional with LD, known to the authors, uses different templates for his reports in which he fills in the blanks. Otherwise, the task of planning, writing, and revising a report would overwhelm his executive abilities. Until he and his spouse devised the templates, he would call from work each day to be talked through the report writing process.

Deficits in Text Generation

In narrative writing as in storytelling, children with language impairment may lack mature internalized story models or be unable to visualize the words even from their own spoken narratives (Graves, Montague, & Wong, 1990, Montague, Graves, & Leavell, 1991; Roth et al., 1991; Vallecorsa & Garriss, 1990). When compared to the narratives of chronological age-matched peers with typical language, the narratives of children with LD contained shorter, less complex sentences (Scott & Windsor, 2000). As a result, both the oral and written narratives often are shorter with fewer episodes, contain fewer details, and fail to consider the needs of the listener.

Expository writing tasks follow a format, such as statement of a problem, examination of several factors, and a conclusion. Children with lan-

Just as the poor reader expends all his or her energy in decoding, the poor writer becomes bogged down in the mechanics of the writing and spelling process. Both leave the poor reader or writer with little energy for higher cognitive functions such as comprehension or text generation, respectively.

guage impairment have difficulty with these writing tasks and approach them with seemingly little thought or planning. The results are often extremely short, poorly organized, and containing numerous errors of grammar, punctuation, and spelling. There is often little revision. In addition, children with LD have substantial difficulty in written samples with morphological endings, such as regular past tense and regular plurals, even when they demonstrated accuracy with these units in their speech (Windsor, Scott, & Street, 2000).

ASSESSMENT OF DEVELOPMENTAL WRITING

The best writing samples are actual writing from varying contexts. One method of assessing writing in the classroom is through the use of portfolios of children's writing (Paratore, 1995). A portfolio is a collection of meaningful writing collaboratively selected by the child, the SLP, and the teacher that contains samples of the child's writing over time, thus enabling the child to demonstrate progress. The wide variety helps to increase the validity of the sample. Items in a portfolio may include SLP observation notes, work samples, and first drafts of writing samples, such as journal or learning log entries, and projects/papers, final drafts of the same, and peer and teacher evaluations.

Narratives are best for young elementary school children (Nelson, 1998). Older elementary school children or adolescents can provide expository writing samples.

> Executive function is very difficult to assess without some task to accomplish, thus the context is very important.

Executive function is best measured within actual writing tasks as part of an overall writing assessment rather than separate from functional communication tasks (Fey, 1986). Samples should be written in ink to allow for analysis of revisions. It's helpful to allow children to plan and to write drafts. All notes and plans and should be collected along with the finished product and added to the portfolio mentioned previously.

Whenever possible, the SLP, teacher, or an instructional aide can observe the writing process for evidence of planning and organizing, drafting, writing, revising, and editing. Added information can be obtained if children read their paper aloud while being recorded. This procedure aids the SLP or teacher in interpreting garbled or poorly spelled words.

Writing can be analyzed on several levels, including textual, linguistic, and orthographic (spelling). At a textual level, the SLP can note length, any indication of the amount of effort, overall quality, and structure or the way in which comments support the topic (Berninger, 2000). Of interest are the total number of words, clauses, and sentences, as well as the structural complexity as measured in words/clause and clauses/sentence. Writing conventions, such as capitalization and punctuation, plus the use of sentences and paragraphs, should be noted.

Assessment of Spelling

Spelling deficits are very complex and can be difficult to describe. Collection should be of sufficient quantity to allow for a broad-based analysis. Spelling deficits should be assessed through both dictation and connected writing such as that in a child's portfolio (Masterson, & Apel, 2000). Standardized tests should also be included and can be administered by a classroom teacher, writing specialist, or school psychologist. Informal assessments should be developmental in nature and include several phoneme-grapheme variations, such as single consonants in various positions in words, consonant blends (*str-*), morphological inflections (*-est, dis-*), diphthongs, digraphs (two letters for one sound, as in ch" and "sh"), and complex derivations.

Although single-word spelling may be somewhat helpful, it does not measure a child's ability in a real communicative context (Moats, 1995). Connected writing, such as that found in a portfolio, can offer samples closer to actual practice.

*D*oes the necessity of assessing several aspects of writing in an actual writing situation tell you anything about other types of assessment? Does it suggest the importance of context?

Descriptive analysis should focus on patterns evident in the child's spelling (Bear, Invernizzi, Templeton, & Johnston, 2000). Of interest are the most frequent and the lowest level patterns. Table 6.2 presents a possible classification system that suggests several intervention strategies.

Assessment of Text Generation

SLPs and teachers can assess a child's writing using the papers assembled in his or her portfolio. Analysis may include the total number of words and the number of different words. This is an overall measure of a child's vocabulary and flexibility in its use. Other measures might include the maturity of the words used, clause and sentence length, and coherence. Narratives and expository writing can be analyzed for the presence or absence of elements of both. For example, does a narrative include a setting statement of *who, what, when, where?*

INTERVENTION FOR DEVELOPMENTAL WRITING IMPAIRMENT

Intervention for writing may involve both general training and more specific and explicit techniques for both narrative and expository forms. To learn to write, you must write, so intervention needs to focus on the actual writing process.

Spelling

Spelling intervention should be integrated into real writing and reading within the classroom. Words are the vehicles for teaching alphabetic and orthographic principles (Berninger, Vaughan, Abbott, Brooks, Abbott, Reed, Rogan, & Graham, 1998). Ideally, intervention can occur when a child is actually writing and can be reminded of alphabetic and orthographic principles (Scott, 2000). Spelling can be taught within teaching of general

TABLE 6.2

Examples of language-based spelling analysis

Phonological: Segmenting, blending, and phonemic awareness

Omission of internal and unstressed phonemes and cluster reduction

> Stop → SOP   Sand → SAD

Syllable deletion

> Elephant → ELFANT

Letter reversal (most common with liquids and nasals)

> Sing → SIGN

Orthographic: Sound-symbol relationship (/k/ = k, c, ck, cc, ch, q, x), letter combinations, letter and positional patterns, and grapheme representations

Letter sound confusion

> Cash → CAS

Non-allowable letter sequences

> Dry → JRIE   Queen → KWEN

Possible spellings that violate location-pattern rules

> Chip → TCHIP   Corn → CKORN

Different spellings on repeated attempts (no cognitive representation or graphemic representation of word)

Morphological: Inflectional (-ed, -ing, -s) and derivational (un-, dis-, -er, -ist, -ment) morphemes, relationship of root word and inflected or derived form

More difficult if a form has more than one meaning (fast**er**, teach**er**), multiple pronunciations (walk**ed**, jogg**ed**, collid**ed**), and both phonological and orthographic properties are changed when inflected or derived (*ascend* and *ascension*).

Semantic: Effect of spelling on meaning

Homophone confusions

> Won → ONE   They're → THER   Which → WITCH

executive function in which the child is taught to proofread, correct, and edit.

The way children spell is indicative of the way they read (Templeton, 2004). This would suggest that spelling intervention should be integrated with reading to enable a child to learn and to use word knowledge. Spelling is not just sounds and letters but the integration of these with morphemic and semantic knowledge (Venezky, 1999).

Words selected for intervention should be individualized for each child and reflect the curriculum, the child's desires, words attempted but in error, and error patterns (Bear, Invernizzi, Templeton, & Jonhston, 2004; Graham, Harris, & Loynadhan, 1994). Spelling strategies can be discussed with the child using the data from the SLP's analysis. The goal is to learn strategies of spelling and rules rather than specific words. For example, if the child's errors are primarily morphologic, the SLP can target root words and the influence of various morphemes through morpheme finding and word building tasks. In contrast, the child's errors are orthographic in nature, the SLP can teach rules through key words, demonstrating alternative spellings and acceptable sound-letter combinations.

Children with LD benefit from multisensory input such as pictures, objects, or actions (Graham, 1999). Several multisensory techniques using colors or blocks have been proposed in which the child may complete any of several steps, including listening to the SLP say and spell the word, saying the word aloud while looking at it or touching it, writing it while saying it, checking spelling, saying the letters in sequence, tracing the word while saying it, closing his or her eyes and visualizing the word, and rewriting the word and checking or comparing the spelling (Berninger et al., 1998a; Graham & Freeman, 1986; Horn, 1954).

Word analysis and sorting tasks can be used to strengthen the alphabetic principle (Scott, 2000). Sorting tasks will differ based on the targeted error patterns found in the child's misspellings (Scott, 2000). Pairs of words that differ on the bases of these patterns can be used to demonstrate the consequences of misspelling (Masterson & Crede, 1999). For example, word meaning could be used to help the child note the difference between *head* and *hid*. Listening skills would also be targeted. Other contrasting words might include *dead-did, read-rid,* and *lead-lid.* The SLP should begin with known, frequently used words and gradually introduce less frequently used and unknown words to facilitate generalization. Different spelling/meaning patterns might strengthen the conceptual connections among known words and provide clues to the meaning and spelling of unfamiliar ones (Templeton, 2003). For example, a child might be helped to see the relationship between *evaluate* and *evaluation.* Some principles for word study and spelling intervention are included in Table 6.3.

Although use of word processing can encourage editing in children, spell checkers, as you know, are not foolproof, and a child may learn little. In general, spell checkers miss words in which the misspelling has inadvertently produced another word. Suggested spelling may also confuse the child with poor word attack skills. In addition, suggested spellings may be far afield if the original word is seriously misspelled. Spell checkers help only 37 percent of the time for children with LD, a lower percentage than found among children developing typically (MacArthur, Graham, Haynes, & DeLaPaz, 1996).

If children with literacy impairments are taught to spell phonetically when unsure of the correct spelling, spell checkers generate more correct suggestions. Proofing and editing on a hard copy also seems to increase the number of correctly spelled words (McNaughton, Hughes, & Ofiesh, 1997).

> The SLP should not be teaching this week's spelling words from class. SLPs target spelling strategies, not individual words.

TABLE 6.3
Principles for guiding spelling intervention

Focus on what students are "using but confusing" in their spelling rather than beginning with focusing on what a child doesn't know.

Step back and consolidate learning before moving forward.

Use words students know and can read, so that one literacy aspect influences another.

Compare words "that do" with words "that don't" by contrasting what a child knows with what or she does not.

Help a child look at words in many ways through sorting tasks that include sound, sight, and meaning.

Begin with obvious contrasts first; ones that are easy to hear or clearly demonstrate a rule.

Don't hide exceptions, rather deal with them, because they will enhance generalization.

Avoid rules until a child has learned enough examples to see the rule clearly.

Work for sorting and spelling fluency.

Glean words from a child's writing and reading, and then return to meaningful tasks and texts.

Source: Adapted from Bear, D.R., Invernizzi, M., Templeton, S., & Jonhston, F. (2004). *Words their way: Word study with phonics, vocabulary, and spelling instruction* (3rd ed.) Upper Saddle River, NJ: Merrill/Prentice-Hall.

Internet searches can foster spelling learning because correct spelling is needed to complete searches successfully.

On the other hand, word prediction programs reduce spelling errors of children with language impairment by over half, although the user must get the initial letters correct for the program to work effectively (Newell, Booth, Arnott, & Beattie, 1992). Word prediction programs such as *Co:Writer* (D. Johnston, 1998), *Write Away 2000* (Information Services, 1989), and *Clicker Plus* (Crick Software, 1997) are helpful for spelling (MacArthur, 2000; Ylvisaker & DeBonis, 2000). It's important that a word prediction program's vocabulary match the writing task, and several programs can incorporate word frequency or various topics (MacArthur, 1999; Zhang, Brooks, Fields, & Redelfs, 1995).

Executive Function

Executive function can be targeted within the writing process using a goal-plan-do-review format (Ylvisaker & Feeney, 1996; Ylvisaker & Szekeres, 1989; Ylvisaker, Szekeres, & Feeney, 1998). The SLP can provide external support to enable children to experience some level of success (Ylvisaker & DeBonis, 2000).

Intervention can begin by allowing children to select their own topics. This increases motivation and shifts the focus to ideas. In the planning phase, the SLP and child can brainstorm ideas for inclusion in the writing (Troia et al., 1999). Drawings and ideational maps or "spider diagrams" can help. It is also helpful for the child to focus on the potential audience. The SLP can ask questions such as the following (Graham & Harris, 1999):

Who will read this paper?

What do the readers know?

What do the readers need to know?

Why are you writing?

The SLP and child may prefer to use computers as an assistive technology for writing (MacArthur, 2000). Software, such as *Inspiration* (Inspiration Software, 1997), can aid text generation, and the result is easily modifiable by the child or teacher. Children with LD who receive training in executive function along with word processing make greater gains in the quality of their writing than children instructed only in executive function or word processing alone (MacArthur, & Graham, 1987; MacArthur, Graham, Schwartz, & Schafer, 1995; Vace, 1987). Grammar checkers miss many errors, especially if there are multiple spelling errors, and can easily confuse the writer who is left to figure out just what the error is. Although speech recognition software allows a child to compose by dictation, the software can not overcome oral language difficulties although these can be moderated with the additional use of grammar checkers.

*E*ver find your grammar or spell checker baffling? Imagine what it might be like if you didn't have the excellent language base that you possess.

THOUGHT QUESTION

Narrative Text Generation

For some children, narrative writing intervention may need to begin at the oral narrative level (Naremore, 2001). They may need to learn to tell common event sequences and the elements of a narrative, called a **story grammar.**

Children with language and writing impairments may not realize that they know a narrative or how to get it started. Story swapping with peers, spin-offs from reading or real life, draw-tell-write methods, or topic selection from a prepared list can all be used to facilitate this process (Tattershall, 2004). Once a topic is selected, a child can be encouraged to write one statement, then another and another. A child can be guided by narrative-enhancing questions from the classroom teacher or SLP and by graphic organizers.

During the writing process, the SLP or classroom teacher can guide a child's writing through the use of brainstorming of ideas, story guides, prompts, and acronyms to aid a child. Story guides are questions that help the student construct the narrative, while prompts are story beginning and ending phrases (Graves et al., 1990; Montague et al., 1991; Thomas, Englert, & Morsink, 1984). Acronyms, such as SPACE for **s**etting, **p**roblem, **a**ction, and **c**onsequent **e**vents, can also act as prompts for guiding writing (Harris & Graham, 1996). Children can be encouraged to write more with verbal prompts such as "Tell me more" or "What happened next?" Feelings and motivations can be encouraged with pictures and questions such as "How do you think she felt?" (Roth, 2000).

Written narration may require explicit instruction in story grammar or structure. Story maps using pictures or story frames may be necessary initially. Story maps may be pictures that highlight a narrative's main events. Story frames (Fowler, 1982) are written starters for each main story grammar element. The child completes the sentence and continues with that portion of the narrative. Cards or checklists can also be used to remind the child of story grammar elements (Graves et al., 1990; Montague et al., 1991).

TABLE 6.4

Strategies for teaching expository writing

Include other students in a supportive environment.

Place training within a literacy-rich environement.

Provide extensive modeling.

Teach

Writing explicitly and systematically.
Various types of writing.
Planning and organizing strategies

Use

Verbal prompts to support self-regulation.
A variety of strategies to address different needs.
Graphics for display and as a means of storing test-relevant information, such as words, grammar, and ideas.

Move from oral to written forms by integrating the two.

Provide ample opportunity for for communication and language to develop.

Collaborate with teachers in mentoring students to write.

Ensure the seamless integration of language intervention and classroom instruction and learning.

Source: Adapted from Singer, B.D., & Bashir, A.S. (2004). EmPOWER, A strategy of teaching students with language learning disabilities how to write expository text. In E.R. Silliman & L.C. Wilkinson (Eds.), *Language and literacy learning in schools* (pp. 239–272). New York: Guilford.

TABLE 6.5

Sample prompts for opinion writing

Section of Paper	Examples
Introduction	In my opinion. . .
	I believe. . .
	From my point of view,. . . .
	I agree with. . .
	I disagree with. . .
	Supporting words: first, second, finally, for example, most important is. . ., consider, think about, remember
Counter Opinion	Although. . .
	However,. . . .
	On the other hand,. . .
	To the contrary,. . .
	Even though. . .
Conclusion	In conclusion,. . .
	After considering both sides,. . .
	To summarize,. . .

Sources: Adapted from Wong (2000); Wong et al. (1996).

Expository Text Generation

Procedures for intervention with expository writing may include collaborative planning and scaffolding with SLP/teacher and peer input; individual, independent writing; conferencing with the SLP/teacher and peers; individual, independent revising; and final editing (Van Meter, Nelson, & Ansell, 2004; Wong, 2000). Collaborative planning is important. Children should think aloud and solicit opinions. Such brainstorming often provides a child with alternative views.

One promising method of teaching expository text writing is called Em-POWER, which treats writing as a problem-solving task involving six steps: **E**valuate, **M**ake a **P**lan, **O**rganize, **W**ork, **E**valuate, and **R**ework (Englert, Raphael, Anderson, Anthony, Fear, & Greg, 1988). In addition, research has indicated that certain strategies are effective with children with LLD (Singer & Bashir, 2004). These are presented in Table 6.4.

Once a topic is selected and discussed in small groups, with a peer, and/or with the SLP, the SLP can give the child a planning sheet to help organize her or his thoughts. After the child has completed the sheet, the SLP can help the child organize the information. This is a great time to challenge and help a child clarify views and prepare for independent writing.

Writing, even independent writing, can be fostered through the use of a prompt card containing key words for each major section of the paper (Wong, Butler, Ficzere, & Kuperis, 1996). Table 6.5 presents some sample prompts.

After a child has completed the paper, he or she can conference with peers for feedback while the SLP mediates. The child then revises the paper based on this feedback.

At each stage in the process, a child can record progress on a checklist that provides a model for the writing process. The checklist can also motivate a child as she or he notes progress.

SUMMARY

Although many aspects of literacy impairment clearly are the domain of the classroom teacher and reading specialist, some justifiably belong in the speech-language pathologist's realm. Working with a team, the SLP helps the child obtain language-based skills upon which literacy is based. This is a natural extension of the SLP's concern for language in all modes of communication, something you will note in Chapter 7, "Adult Language Impairments."

REFLECTIONS

- How do reading and writing differ?
- Briefly explain the development of both reading and writing.
- How are language and literacy impairments related?
- How would you assess for literacy impairment?
- Suggest some intervention methods for literacy impairments.

SUGGESTED READINGS

Catts, H. W., & Kamhi, A. G. (2005). *Language and reading disabilities* (2nd ed.). Boston: Allyn and Bacon.

McGee, L. M., & Richgels, D. J. (2004). *Literacy's beginnings: Supporting young readers and writers* (4th ed.). Boston: Allyn and Bacon.

ONLINE RESOURCES

http://members.tripod.com/~Caroline_Bowen/pre-literacy.html
Caroline Bowen offers a wealth of ideas for encouraging preliteracy skills in children with speech and language disorders.

http://www.maccs.mq.edu.au/ddoll/r_tests.htm

Macquarie University site offers reviews of materials and helpful information for parents, teachers, and researchers.

http://www.ld.org/

National Center for Learning Disabilities site offers links to new and research on literacy impairments.

www.asha.org/about/publications/literacy

Facts on literacy, information for SLP's role, grant opportunities, and links from ASHA.

7

Adult Language Impairments

CHAPTER
LEARNING
GOALS

When you have finished this chapter, you should be able to:

- Differentiate between aphasia, right hemisphere injury, traumatic brain injury, and dementia

- List the concomitant or accompanying deficits found with aphasia

- Explain the different types of aphasia and stroke

Many language impairments found in childhood continue into the adult years. Mental retardation, autism, and learning disability do not disappear, although they may change or their effect on language may alter. Other language impairments may lessen or disappear, such as specific language impairment.

This chapter is not about those impairments. Rather, this chapter focuses on language disorders that occur or develop during adulthood. Specifically, we discuss aphasia, right hemisphere syndrome, traumatic brain injury, and degenerative neurological conditions. We will be describing language problems related to interruption of blood supply to the brain, direct destruction of neural tissue, or a pathological process. This will be your introduction, and, of necessity, it will only scratch the surface. Although the speech-language pathologist is concerned primarily with communication, the disorders described in this chapter necessitate an understanding of the medical conditions from which they originate.

THOUGHT QUESTION

If children are still learning language and adults have completed most of that learning, might we expect language impairments, even those with similar causes, to be manifested in different ways? How?

Case Study 7.1

Case Study of an Adult with Language Impairment: Marsha

A single mom, Marsha has been the sole breadwinner in her family for several years. Two of her three children are grown and her youngest is in high school. With no high school diploma, Marsha has had to work in sales or housekeeping jobs to make ends meet. Most recently, she has been a sales associate in the women's fashions section of a large department store.

Nearly a year ago, Marsha awoke one morning with a very strong headache. Although she felt somewhat unsteady on her feet, she determined that she should go to work anyway. Her right leg became weak as she walked to the bus stop and she collapsed before she had reached her destination.

She awoke in the hospital several hours later, confused and disoriented. She tried to talk with the staff and with her family but seemed unable to comprehend their speech and to form replies. Her medical team, consisting of her physician, a neurologist, the speech-language pathologist, a physical therapist, and an occupational therapist, recom-

mended that Marsha be released from the hospital after one week and that she receive services in a rehabilitation center. Both of her older children were eager to help.

The speech-language pathologist worked with Marsha and her family on strengthening Marsha's comprehension and production of language and on her speech. Her intervention services were comprehensive and involved both physical and occupational therapy as well. To date Marsha has recovered much of her speech and language. Some speech sounds are slightly slurred and she still has some lingering word retrieval difficulties. She was able to return to her job and is able to communicate well.

As you read the chapter, think about

- Possible causes of Marsha's stroke.
- Possible ways in which the team could coordinate services and work together.
- Possible problems Marsha might still experience at work.

In this chapter, we will explore adult language development and four neurological impairments that affect adult language. Within each impairment we'll discuss characteristics, causes, lifespan issues, and assessment and intervention for language deficits.

Space precludes examining all possible neurological disorders. For example, we will not be discussing impairments such as chronic schizophrenia, which typically affects pragmatic aspects of language, such as turn-taking, topic selection, and intentions (Meilijson, Kasher, & Elizur, 2004).

LANGUAGE DEVELOPMENT THROUGH THE LIFESPAN

By adulthood, speech and language have matured and adults are able to communicate in a variety of modes, using not only speech and language, but paralinguistic and nonlinguistic signals effectively. A subtle pause or shift in word emphasis can signal vast differences of meaning in speech. Reading and writing are also essential communication tools.

Unless debilitated in some way through accident, disease, or disorder, adults continue to refine their communication abilities throughout their lives. Writing and speaking abilities continue to improve with use, new words are added to vocabularies, and new styles of talking are acquired.

> Language and communication should continue to develop throughout one's life.

Language development proceeds slowly throughout adulthood. Even people with delayed development, such as individuals with MR, experience continued but slowed language growth.

USE

Through the use of various communication techniques, competent adults can influence others, impart information, and make their needs known. Some adults are even capable of oratory on a par with that of a Winston Churchill or a Martin Luther King, which can call up the heroic and the unselfish in others.

> Adult language use is extremely flexible because of the variety of language forms, the large size of the vocabulary, and the breadth of language uses.

Compared to children, adults are very effective communicators and skilled conversationalists who have a variety of styles of talking from formal to casual. Styles require modification not only in the manner of talking, but also in the topics introduced and the vocabulary used. As the Little Prince noted when talking with adults (Saint-Exupéry, 1968):

> I would talk . . . about bridge, and golf, and politics, and neckties. And the grown-up would be greatly pleased to have met such a sensible man.

Competent adult communicators quickly sense their role in an interaction and adjust their language and speech accordingly. For example, some people are addressed as *sir* and some as *honey,* and adults do well not to confuse the two. Communication may vary from direct, as in *Turn up the heat,* to indirect, as in *Do you feel a chill?* The goal is the same, but the linguistic methodology is very different.

The number of communicative intentions increases gradually so that adults are able to hypothesize, to cajole, to inspire, to entice, to pun, and so on. The skilled speaker knows how to fulfill these intentions and when to use them.

CONTENT

Adults continue to add to their personal vocabularies and most use between 30,000 and 60,000 words expressively. Receptive vocabularies are even larger. Specialized vocabularies develop for work, religion, hobbies, and social and interest groups. Some words fade from the language and are used less frequently while new words are added. For example, you no longer *dial* a telephone number. Multiple definitions and figurative meanings are also expanded.

FORM

Within language form, adults continue to acquire prefixes, morphophonemic contrasts, and infrequently used irregular verbs. Conversations become more cohesive through more effective use of linguistic devices, such as pronouns, articles, verb tenses, and aspect (which, for example, allows us to talk about the past from the vantage point of the future, as in *Tomorrow, I'll look back and say "That was a great picnic"*). In general, written language is more complex than spoken language.

THOUGHT QUESTIONS

Are there more things to learn about language form as an adult? Try some of these. Can you state the past tense of the verbs "lay" and "lie"? What is the difference between "effect" and "affect"? Do "uninterested" and "disinterested" mean the same thing?

APHASIA

Aphasia means literally "without language," a feature that describes the most severe varieties of this impairment. The aphasic population is extremely diverse. Although aphasia results from localized brain damage, the exact locations and the resultant severity and type of aphasia are not a perfect match. Nor does all brain damage result in aphasia. Damage to the brain may result in loss of motor or sensory function, impaired memory, and poor judgment, while leaving language intact. Although mildly aphasic individuals may have language that is similar to that of typical elderly persons, individuals with aphasia usually exhibit greater deficits in expressive language and overall efficiency of communication (Ross & Wertz, 2003).

It is estimated that over one million Americans have aphasia (http://www.ninds.nih.gov/disorders/aphasia/aphasia.htm, 2005). Over 200 individuals—primarily adults—become aphasic in the United States each day. For these people, language has suddenly become a jumble of strange and seemingly unfamiliar words that they are unable to comprehend and/or produce. Most of you, regardless of whether your chosen profession is speech-language pathology, are likely to have some experience with aphasia through a relative, friend, neighbor, or possibly firsthand.

Many severities and varieties of aphasia exist. Problems in two areas, auditory comprehension and word retrieval, seem to be common to varying degrees in all. Word retrieval difficulties suggest that memory may also be impaired in some way. Aphasia is not the result of a motor speech impairment, dementia, or the deterioration of intelligence.

> *C*an you imagine the horror and confusion of going to bed with a headache and awakening in a hospital unable to speak or comprehend the speech around you?

THOUGHT QUESTION

Aphasia may affect listening, speaking, reading, and/or writing as well as specific language functions such as naming. Related language functions such as arithmetic, gesturing, telling time, counting money, or interpreting environmental noises such as a dog's bark may also be difficult. Given the great variation possible, it may be better to think of aphasia as a general term that represents several syndromes.

Expressive deficits may include reduced vocabulary, either omission or addition of words, stereotypic utterances, either delayed and reduced output of speech or hyperfluent speech, and word substitutions. Each of these characteristics is an example of a deeper language-processing problem. **Hyperfluent speech,** very rapid speech with few pauses, may be incoherent, inefficient, and pragmatically inappropriate.

Language comprehension deficits, whether spoken or written, involve the impaired interpretation of incoming linguistic information. Although individuals with aphasia may have normal hearing and vision, difficulty comes in the interpretation or the ability to make sense of the incoming signal.

Severity may range from individuals with a few intelligible words and little comprehension to those with very high-level subtle linguistic deficits that are barely discernible in normal conversation. Severity is related to several variables, including the cause of the disorder, the location and extent of the brain injury, the age of the injury, and the age and general health of the client. Differences in individual brains may account for different aphasic characteristics and for the lack of similar characteristics when similar areas of the brain are injured.

Although individuals with aphasia differ greatly, several patterns of behavior exist that enable us to categorize the disorder into numerous types or *syndromes*. While categories of the disorder describe certain similarities among individuals with aphasia, they do not adequately characterize any one individual. Speech-language pathologists and other professionals, such as neurologists and psychiatrists, must thoroughly assess each individual and describe individual strengths and weaknesses.

It is rare that brain injury is so precise as to affect only language. Other related areas of cognitive function and motor behaviors may also suffer damage.

Other neurogenic disorders—those that affect the central nervous system—such as apraxia or dysarthria often exist along with aphasia, and these complicate classification. Apraxia and dysarthria will be discussed in Chapter 12. Individuals with aphasia may also experience seizures and depression. Depression is also a common condition in neurological disorders.

CONCOMITANT OR ACCOMPANYING DEFICITS

Hemi means "half," as in "hemisphere."

Physical and psychosocial problems may accompany aphasia and be traced to the same cause. Physical impairments may include hemiparesis, hemiplegia, and hemisensory impairment. **Hemiparesis** is a weakness on one side of the body in which strength and control are greatly reduced. In contrast, **hemiplegia** is paralysis on one side. Finally, **hemisensory impairment** may accompany either and is a loss of the ability to perceive sensory information. The client may complain of cold, numbness, or tingling on the affected side and may be unable to sense pain or touch.

Vision is one aspect of sensory impairment that may affect communication. Individuals with deep lesions in the left hemisphere interior to the ear and across the top of the brain may experience blindness in the right visual field of each eye. Called **hemianopsia,** this condition will affect the individual's ability to read.

When paresis, or paralysis, and/or sensory impairment involve the neck and face, the client may have difficulty chewing or swallowing. There may be accompanying drooling or gagging. This condition, known as **dysphagia,** is also the concern of speech-language pathologists and will be addressed in Chapter 13.

In addition, brain damage may result in seizure disorder or epilepsy seen in approximately 20 percent of aphasic adults. Seizures may be of the tonic-clonic type, which result in periods of unconsciousness, or the *petit mal* and psychomotor type, in which the client may lose motor control but remain conscious. The discussion of aphasia is complicated and uses terminology that might be unfamiliar to you. As we discuss each, try to think of it as an extreme form of some behaviors that you already manifest. For example, occasionally, we all have difficulty recalling a name or remembering a word. In its extreme form, we call this *anomia.* Some of the more common terms are listed below with a brief description. Examples of these expressive deficits of adults with aphasia are presented in Table 7.1 and Figure 7.1.

Agnosia: A sensory deficit accompanying some aphasias that makes it difficult for the client to understand incoming sensory information. The disorder may be specific to auditory or visual information.

Agrammatism: Omission of grammatical elements. Individuals with aphasia may omit short, unstressed words, such as articles or prepositions. They may also omit morphological endings, such as the plural *-s* or past-tense *-ed.*

Agraphia: Difficulty writing. Writing may be full of mistakes and poorly formed. Clients may be unable to write what they are able to say.

TABLE 7.1
Examples of the expressive language deficits in the speech of adults with aphasia

Deficit	Characteristic	Example
Agrammatism	Omission of unstressed words; telegraphic speech	Take dog walk. Go home. Make instant coffee, watch T.V.
Anomia	Difficulty naming entities	It's a . . . a . . . thing . . . that thing that you do that with . . . you know, that thing for doing stuff with.
Jargon	Meaningless or irrelevant speech with typical intonational patterns	We went for the cookies to laugh in the elephants, didn't we?
Neologism	Novel word	Cow juice and cookies; that's what I like, especially mixed up chocolate (*chocolate milkshake*).
Paraphasia	Word and phoneme substitutions	I need the pen . . . pen . . . pencil and the sheet . . . peeper . . . peeper sheet to color on.
Verbal stereotype	An expression repeated over and over	I see, I see, I see, I see.

Agrammatism, jargon, and neologisms may be present in written language as well as in spoken.

Alexia: Reading problems. Clients may be unable to recognize even common words they use in their speech. Paraphasia and neologisms may be present.

Anomia: Difficulty naming entities. Clients may struggle greatly. Individuals who have recovered from aphasia report that they knew what they wanted to say but could not locate the appropriate word. An incorrect response may continue to be produced even when the client recognizes that it is incorrect.

Jargon: Meaningless or irrelevant speech with typical intonational patterns. Responses are often long and syntactically correct although containing nonsense. Jargon may contain neologisms.

Neologism: A novel word. Some individuals with aphasia may create novel words that do not exist in their language, using these words quite confidently.

Comb hair

knif the butter

Quarter money

Broca's aphasia

I have a comb in my pocket.
I put the knife in my drawer.
I bought the quarter in my pocket.

Wernicke's aphasia

FIGURE 7.1

Examples of the expressive language deficits in the writing of adults with aphasia.

Paraphasia: Word substitutions found in clients who may talk fluently and grammatically. Associations to the intended word may be based on meaning, such as saying *truck* for *car;* on similar sound, such as *tar* for *car;* or on some other relationship.

Verbal stereotype: An expression repeated over and over. One young man responded to every question with "I know," occasionally stringing it together to form "I know I know I know." Sometimes the expression is an obscene word or expletive or a neologism. One Mother Superior, seen in the clinic, continually uttered the same obscene word with great gusto, to her total embarrassment but seeming inability to stop.

THOUGHT QUESTIONS

How does the term "jargon" as used here relate to the same term used to refer to the speech of a developing child of approximately 10 months? What are the similarities in meaning?

TYPES OF APHASIA

Aphasias can be classified into two large categories based on the ease of producing speech: **fluent aphasia** and **nonfluent aphasia.** In turn, these can be subdivided into *syndromes.* The most common syndromes and their characteristics are presented in Table 7.2.

TABLE 7.2

Characteristics of fluent and nonfluent aphasias

Aphasia Type	Speech Production	Speech Comprehension	Speech Characteristics	Reading Comprehension	Naming	Speech Repetition
Wernicke's	Fluent or hyperfluent	Impaired to poor	Verbal paraphasia, jargon	Impaired	Impaired to poor	Impaired to poor
Anomic	Fluent	Mild to moderately impaired	Word retrieval and misnaming, good syntax and articulation	Good	Severely impaired in both speech and writing	Good
Conduction	Fluent	Mildly impaired to good	Paraphasia and incorrect ordering with frequent self-correction attempts, good articulation and syntax	Good	Usually impaired	Poor
Transcortical Sensory	Fluent	Poor	Paraphasia, possible perseveration	Impaired to poor	Severely impaired	Unimpaired
Broca's	Nonfluent	Relatively good	Short sentences, agrammatism; slow, labored, with articulation and phonological errors	Unimpaired to poor	Poor	Poor
Transcortical	Nonfluent	Mildly impaired	Impaired, labored, difficulty initiating, syntactic errors	Unimpaired to poor	Impaired	Good
Global	Nonfluent	Poor, limited to single words or short phrases	Limited spontaneous ability of a few words or stereotypes	Poor	Poor	Poor, limited to single words or short phrases

> Adults with fluent aphasia have typical rate, intonation, pauses, and stress patterns.

Fluent Aphasias

The fluent aphasias are characterized by word substitutions, neologisms, and often verbose verbal output. Lesions in fluent aphasia tend to be found in the posterior portions of the left hemisphere.

Wernicke's Aphasia

As a fluent aphasia, **Wernicke's aphasia** is characterized by rapid-fire strings of sentences with little pause for acknowledgment or turn taking. Content may seem a jumble and may be incoherent or incomprehensible although fluent and well articulated. Characteristics include the following:

1. Fluent or hyperfluent speech
2. Poor auditory and visual comprehension
3. Verbal paraphasia or unintended words and neologisms
4. Sentences formed by strings of unrelated words, called jargon
5. Mild to severe impairment in naming and imitative speech

Intonational patterns and sound-combination patterns are maintained.

Poor comprehension extends to reading as well as listening. In addition, poor auditory comprehension affects verbal repetition. The client might not be able to repeat back what was said to him or her. Further, clients may demonstrate reduced ability to comprehend their own speech as well as that of others.

Damage in Wernicke's aphasia is near Wernicke's area in the posterior portions of the left temporal lobe (interior to the left ear). The following is an example of the speech of a client with Wernicke's aphasia:

> I love to go for rides in the car. Cars are expensive these days. Everything's expensive. Even groceries. When I was a child you could spend five dollars and get a whole wagon full. I had a little red wagon. My brother and I would ride down the hill by our house. My brother served in World War II. He moved away after the war. There was so little housing available. My house is a split-level.

An audio sample of a person with Wernicke's aphasia is presented on the accompanying CD-ROM.

Anomic Aphasia

As the name suggests, **anomic aphasia** is characterized by naming difficulties. Most aspects of speech are normal with the exception of word retrieval. Other characteristics include the following:

1. Severe anomia in both speech and writing
2. Fluent spontaneous speech marred by word retrieval difficulties
3. Mild to moderate auditory comprehension problems

Names may be unavailable, or entities may be misnamed with both related and nonrelated words. Imitated or repetitive language is less affected.

Brain damage seems to be at the convergence of the parietal-temporal-occipital cortex (above and posterior to the left ear). Memory difficulties are evident. The following is an example of the speech of a client with anomic aphasia:

> It was very good. We had a bird . . . a big thing with feathers and . . . a bird . . . a turkey stuffed . . . turkey with stuffing and that stuff . . . you know . . . and that stuff, that berry stuff . . . that stuff . . . berries, berries . . . cranberry stuffing . . . stuffing and cranberries . . . and gravy on things . . . smashed things . . . Oh, darn, smashed potatoes.

Conduction Aphasia   Like the other fluent aphasias, **conduction aphasia** is characterized by conversation that is abundant and quick, though filled with paraphasia. Characteristics include the following:

1. Anomia
2. Only mild impairment of auditory comprehension, if any
3. Extremely poor repetitive or imitative speech
4. Paraphasia or the inappropriate use of words formed by the addition of sounds and incorrect ordering of sounds or by substituting related words

Paraphasia may be severe enough to make the individual's speech incomprehensible. Given the good comprehension skills of many individuals with conduction aphasia, self-correction attempts are frequent, although the client may be unable to benefit from the verbal cues of others.

Damage may be deep below the brain surface between areas where language is formulated and speech programmed. The following is an example of the speech of a client with conduction aphasia:

> We went to me girl, my girl . . . oh, a little girl's palace . . . no, daughter's palace, not a castle, but a pal . . . place . . . home for a sivit . . . and he . . . visit and she made a cook, cook a made . . . a cake.

Transcortical Sensory Aphasia   The rarest of the fluent aphasias, **transcortical sensory aphasia** is characterized by conversation and spontaneous speech as fluent as in Wernicke's aphasia, but filled with word errors. Characteristics include the following:

1. Unimpaired ability to repeat or imitate words
2. Verbal paraphasia or word substitutions
3. Lack of nouns and severe anomia
4. Poor auditory comprehension
5. Ability to repeat or imitate words, phrases, and sentences

The unimpaired imitative ability may be perseverative or may become so persistent as to seem echolalic. Echolalic speech is characterized by an immediate or delayed whole or partial repetition of the speech of another speaker. Brain damage seems to isolate language areas from other areas of cortical control.

Subcortical Aphasia   Although its existence had been hypothesized, **subcortical aphasia** could not be confirmed until the advent of neuroimaging techniques. Lesions occur deep in the brain without involvement of the cerebral cortex. Characteristics include the following:

1. Fluent expressive speech
2. Paraphasia and neologisms
3. Repetition unaffected
4. Auditory and reading comprehension relatively unaffected

Additional language characteristics may include word-finding difficulties, perseveration, and spontaneous speech. Other characteristics, including dysarthria, have been related to specific sites in the basal ganglia (Kirshner, 1995).

Nonfluent Aphasias

Nonfluent aphasia is characterized by slow, labored speech and struggle to retrieve words and form sentences. In general, the site of lesion is in or near the frontal lobe.

Broca's Aphasia   **Broca's aphasia** is associated with damage to the anterior or forward parts of the frontal lobe of the left cerebral hemisphere, centered in Broca's area. The most common traits are the following:

1. Short sentences with agrammatism in which auxiliary or helping verbs, the verb *to be,* prepositions, articles, and morphological endings are omitted
2. Anomia
3. Problems with imitation of speech because of overall speech problems
4. Slow, labored speech and writing
5. Articulation and phonological errors

Auditory comprehension seems unimpaired, although careful testing may reveal subtle deficits in understanding.

The following is an example of the speech of a client with Broca's aphasia:

Foam, foam, phone, damn, phone . . . not ude . . . phone not ude . . . ude . . . ude . . . use . . . can't ude . . . no foam can ude.

Transcortical Motor Aphasia   This is the nonfluent counterpart of transcortical sensory aphasia. Characteristics of this syndrome include the following:

1. Impaired speech, especially in conversation
2. Good verbal imitative abilities
3. Mildly impaired auditory comprehension

Individuals with **transcortical motor aphasia** may have difficulty initiating speech or writing.

Severely impaired speech is characteristic of damage to the motor cortex. Actually, the areas that are affected may go well below the surface of the brain.

> Adults with nonfluent aphasia have slow rate, less intonation, inappropriately placed and abnormally long pauses, and less varied stress patterns than typical speakers.

Global or Mixed Aphasia   As the name implies, **global or mixed aphasia** is characterized by profound language impairment in all modalities. It is considered the most severely debilitating form of aphasia. Mixed aphasia is a milder form. Other characteristics include the following:

1. Limited spontaneous expressive ability of a few words or stereotypes, such as overlearned utterances or emotional responses

2. Imitative speech and naming affected

3. Auditory and visual comprehension limited to single words or short phrases

Global aphasia has both the auditory comprehension problems found in some fluent aphasias and the labored speech of nonfluent aphasias.

These symptoms are associated with a large, deep lesion in a subcortical area well below the brain's surface. Often, both the anterior speech and posterior language areas of the left hemisphere are involved.

Can you imagine how your life might change if you had global aphasia? What would happen to your social life? Family life? Career plans?

THOUGHT QUESTIONS

Additional Types of Aphasia

Not all aphasias can be neatly classified within the fluent-nonfluent system. Other aphasias may affect primarily one communication modality, such as writing. Examples of these specific aphasias include the following:

Alexia with agraphia: Reading and writing impairment

Alexia without agraphia: Reading impairment with no accompanying writing difficulty

Pure agraphia: Severe writing disorder

Pure word deafness: Lack of auditory comprehension with error-free spontaneous speech

Crossed aphasia: Aphasia accompanying right hemisphere damage

Aphasia classification and its relation to the location of lesions are controversial issues and areas of continued study.

CAUSES OF APHASIA

The onset of aphasia is rapid. Usually, it occurs in people who have no former history of speech and language difficulties. The lesion or injury leaves an area of the brain unable to function as it had just moments before.

The most common cause of aphasia is a **stroke** or **cerebrovascular accident,** the third leading cause of death in the United States. Strokes affect half a million Americans annually. Seventy percent of these are over 65 years of age (http://www.strokecenter.org/pat/stats.htm, 2005). Although some

Stroke is caused by an interruption of the blood supply to the brain.

children suffer strokes, this is rare. In 1990, the National Institute on Neurological Disorders and Stroke estimated that as a result of strokes, approximately 80,000 people become aphasic each year.

THOUGHT QUESTION

*A*re you leading a healthy life that could reduce your chances of stroke?

Strokes are of two basic types: ischemic and hemorrhagic. **Ischemic strokes** result from a complete or partial blockage or occlusion of the arteries transporting blood to the brain as in cerebral arteriosclerosis, embolism, and thrombosis. **Cerebral arteriosclerosis** is a thickening of the walls of cerebral arteries in which elasticity is lost or reduced, the walls become weakened, and blood flow is restricted. The resulting ischemia, or reduction of oxygen, may be temporary or may cause permanent damage through the death of brain tissue. An **embolism** is an obstruction to blood flow caused by a blood clot, fatty materials, or an air bubble. The obstruction may travel through the circulatory system until it blocks the flow of blood in a small artery. For example, a clot may form in the heart or the large arteries of the chest, break off, and become an embolus. As in cerebral arteriosclerosis, blockage results in a lack of oxygen-carrying blood, depriving brain cells of needed oxygen. Similarly, a **thrombosis** also blocks blood flow. In this case, plaque buildup or a blood clot is formed on site and does not travel. The result is the same.

A **hemorrhagic stroke** is one in which the weakened arterial walls burst under pressure, as occurs with an aneurysm or arteriovenous malformation. An **aneurysm** is a saclike bulging in a weakened artery wall. The thin wall may rupture, causing a cerebral hemorrhage. Most aneurysms occur in the meninges, the layered membranes surrounding the brain, and blood flowing into this space can damage the brain or cause death.

Arteriovenous malformation is rare and consists of a poorly formed tangle of arteries and veins that may occur in a highly viscous organ such as the brain. Malformed arterial walls may be weak and give way under pressure.

Patterns of recovery differ with the type of stroke. Often, with ischemic stroke, there is a noticeable improvement within the first weeks after the injury. Recovery slows after three months. In contrast, the results of hemorrhagic strokes are usually more severe after injury. The period of most rapid recovery is at the end of the first month and into the second as swelling lessens and injured neurons regain functioning.

The results of a stroke are further complicated by the prestroke storage patterns for language.

Damage from stroke may occur in any part of the brain. In all right-handed individuals and in some left-handed ones, injury to left hemisphere language areas produces aphasia. Injury to the right hemisphere results in aphasia in only 3 percent of the cases, usually left-handed individuals whose right hemisphere is more important for language (Calvin & Ojemann, 1980).

Aphasia-like symptoms may be noted with head injury, neural infections, degenerative neurological disorders, and tumors. In most of these cases, however, other cortical areas are also affected, resulting in clinically different disorders.

The human brain is extremely complex. Categorizing the types of aphasias that we have discussed helps to bring some understanding to the subject of brain disorders but may have little practical clinical value. Most clients will present mixed aphasia. It is all the more important, therefore, that speech-language pathologists describe each client's abilities and disabilities carefully and clearly.

LIFESPAN ISSUES

Most individuals with aphasia previously lived healthy productive lives. The risk of stroke is increased if the individual has a history of smoking, alcohol use, poor diet, lack of exercise, high blood pressure, high cholesterol, diabetes, obesity, and previous strokes. Although children and adolescents can experience aphasia, especially accompanying brain tumors, most victims are adults in middle age and beyond. Usually, the onset of symptoms is rapid when the cause is vascular, but it can take months or years to become evident with tumor or degenerative disease. These patterns are presented in Figure 7.2.

In the most common situation, the individual suffers an ischemic stroke, depriving the brain of a needed supply of oxygenated blood. First indications may be loss of consciousness, headache, weak or immobile limbs, and/or slurred speech. This condition may be temporary in which function returns quickly or more permanent in nature. Some individuals may experience a series of "ministrokes" spaced over a period of years before they become alarmed. Some ministrokes go undetected by the individual.

Usually, the individual is rushed to the hospital. Approximately one-third of individuals will die from the stroke or shortly thereafter. For those who survive, there may be a period of unconsciousness, followed by confusion. Deep long-lasting periods of unconsciousness or coma are associated with poorer eventual recovery (Carlsson, Svardsudd, & Welin, 1987).

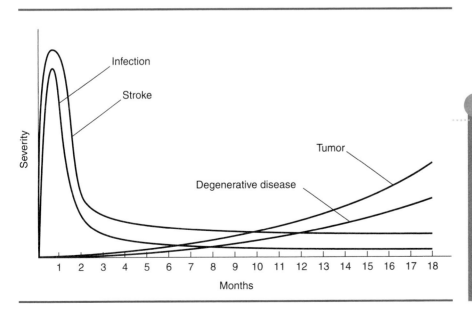

FIGURE 7.2

Severity of symptoms by neurological condition. Individuals will differ in severity and path of the disorder. *Source:* Adapted from Brookshire, R. H. (1997). *Introduction to neurogenic communication disorders* (5th ed.). St. Louis, MO: Mosby-Year Book.

Most individuals remain in acute care for only a few days until their condition stabilizes. Following this, an individual may receive a variety of care depending on the severity of the stroke. These include rehabilitative hospitalization, outpatient rehabilitation, or nursing home care. Most return home but with some impairment.

Although intervention services may occur for years, most individuals receive services for at least the first several months. In addition to neuromuscular deficits, seizures, and dementia, the individual with aphasia may exhibit behavior changes, including perseveration, disinhibition, and emotional problems. *Perseveration* is the repetition of inappropriate responses in which the client may become fixed on a single task or behavior and repeat it. *Disinhibition* is a seeming inability to inhibit certain asocial or inappropriate behaviors, such as touching others. Finally, brain damage may contribute to exaggerated swings in emotion in which the emotion is appropriate but the magnitude and the suddenness of the emotional shift are not. Emotional behavior must be considered in light of the extreme frustration experienced by some individuals with aphasia.

Given the variety of possible symptoms following a stroke, the individual will most likely receive services from a team of professionals. Team members may include a neurologist, physical therapist, occupational therapist, nutritionist, speech-language pathologist, and audiologist. Life changes and family concerns may necessitate the services of a counseling social worker, psychologist, psychiatrist, and/or pastoral counselor.

Immediately after the incident, neurological functioning is most severely affected. Within days, the body's natural recovery process begins. As swelling is reduced, injured cells may recover and begin to function normally. Adjacent areas of the brain that shared brain functions with the injured area may begin to play a larger role. The course and extent of this recovery process are difficult to predict, but the rate is fastest during the first few weeks and months after the stroke, then slows, and usually ceases after six months. During this process, the entire syndrome that the client presents may change and most certainly will lessen in severity. The most frequent linguistic gains are in auditory comprehension (Kertesz & McCabe, 1997). In general, less severely affected individuals, those who are younger, in general good health, and left-handed, recover from aphasia better and faster than those who are more severe, older, in poor health, and right-handed.

With or without spontaneous recovery, assessment and intervention begin as soon as the client's individual condition permits. Clients who are most responsive are probably the best candidates for intervention services. A general rule is that the earlier the treatment, the better the rate of recovery, but clients do not all recover similarly (Robey, 1994, 1998). The SLP's first goal is to determine the feasibility of clinical intervention. Although it is not possible to accurately predict how much gain will be the result of spontaneous recovery and how much the outcome of intervention, the SLP attempts to determine which clients will benefit most from clinical intervention (Marshall, 1997).

Loss of the ability to use language efficiently changes the social role of each individual with aphasia and can result in social isolation. This situation is complicated by the often incorrect assumption that cognitive abilities are

Communication is so entwined in our social interactions and in our very definition of who we are that the effects of aphasia reach well beyond speech and language.

also damaged. In addition, inability to communicate may cause the affected individual to become dependent on others for the simplest of daily tasks. Family roles and responsibilities may also change. Wives, husbands, and children may have to take on new responsibilities. If the individual supported the family prior to the incident, there may be economic problems in addition to medical ones. Case Study 7.2 presents the story of one individual with aphasia.

Case Study 7.2

Personal Story of an Adult with Aphasia

When Mr. W. was 55 years of age, he looked fitter than most men ten years his junior. Having earned a master's degree in labor relations from Cornell University, Mr. W. was employed for many years as a labor mediator by the small city in which he lived. Mr. W. was viewed as cheerful by his circle of friends, primarily fellow hikers with whom he explored mountain trails almost every Saturday.

Although Mr. W. had been rugged and capable of vigorous outdoor activity, he knew that he had high blood pressure, and he was taking medication under a doctor's care. Mr. W. was rarely ill, and he had been hospitalized only once, for acute appendicitis, before his stroke.

One Sunday afternoon, Mr. W. decided to lie down after a four-hour cross-country ski outing. He had a bad headache, and he hoped that a short rest would relieve it before a dinner date with skiing buddies. When he awoke from his nap, he got up to go to the bathroom but collapsed. His friends were concerned when he failed to meet them. They phoned and got no answer, so someone went to his home. Mr. W. was found on the floor, breathing but unconscious. He had suffered a cerebrovascular accident (CVA), or stroke.

Mr. W. was taken to the emergency room of the local hospital. When he became conscious, he was confused, did not seem to understand what was said to him, and was unable to speak. The right side of his body was partially paralyzed. The medical report stated that he had "sustained a left CVA that resulted in right hemiplegia and aphasia." He remained hospitalized for six weeks. In addition to the attending neurologist and family physician, Mr. W. was seen by a speech-language pathologist and a physical therapist. The SLP performed an initial bedside assessment and counseled family members and friends. The SLP's initial report stated that "Mr. W. presented with severe expressive/receptive aphasia characterized by severe oral motor apraxia and a severe auditory comprehension deficit with moderate to severe reading comprehension deficits for single words."

When Mr. W. was discharged from the hospital, he moved in with his sister and her family. He was cared for largely by family and friends, and he was taken for medical appointments and twice-weekly physical and speech-language therapy. Early goals were simple auditory comprehension requiring yes/no head nods as responses, and the expression of needs such as "eat."

Two years after the stroke, Mr. W. was able to walk with a walker. Family members reported that they could understand approximately 85 percent of his intentional speech. Strangers could understand only about 20 percent. He used gestures and largely unintelligible sounds to express himself. Mr. W.'s ability to comprehend language had improved dramatically, and he was now able to follow directions that contained three critical elements ("put the pencil on top of the card and then put it back"). Friends reported that he often seemed agitated, but he apparently liked their visits. Since Mr. W. had always enjoyed being outdoors, his friends frequently took him for short walks. Family members said that they tried to sing together on a regular basis and that Mr. W. joined in to the extent that he was able.

Recently, Mr. W. was evaluated for augmentative/alternative communication. He has received an electronic voice output system and is being taught how to use it. He will never be able to speak normally, but this device should greatly facilitate his ability to communicate.

ASSESSMENT FOR APHASIA

Assessment and intervention may begin in the hospital and continue as outpatient service. Successful intervention is a team effort. The relative importance of each specialist will change as the client recovers. In addition, a spouse, other family member, or close friend may be a critical participant in the recuperative process.

Before beginning any intervention, it is necessary to complete a thorough assessment of each client's abilities and deficits. This process may continue in several stages as the client stabilizes and experiences **spontaneous recovery,** a natural recovery process that proceeds with or without professional intervention.

The assessment procedures outlined in Chapter 4 provide a model. Especially important are the client's medical history, the interview with the client and family, the oral peripheral examination, the hearing testing, and direct speech and language testing. The medical history can reveal information about general health and previous cerebrovascular incidents. In addition, current neurological reports and progress notes provide valuable information on present and changing status.

During the interview, it will be necessary for the SLP to provide as much information as he or she receives from the client and family. The client may be confused and need reassurance. Family members will have many questions regarding recovery. Unspoken questions may center on family dynamics, income, medical expenses, and the like. It is important for families to know the extent of the injuries and to have a realistic appraisal of recovery with and without professional assistance. Although it is unethical to promise a "cure" (see Appendix 1.1, "Code of Ethics"), the SLP should give the family an honest estimate of expected progress.

THOUGHT QUESTIONS

*W*hy is it unethical to promise to cure aphasia? Is there real danger, especially with this disorder, that the client and family may be vulnerable to such promises?

Counseling with the family will be ongoing. The family and client may need professional counseling to cope with the enormous changes that have occurred in their lives.

The oral peripheral examination is important because of the potential for either neuromuscular paralysis or weakness. Speech disorders such as apraxia and dysarthria frequently are associated with aphasia and should be described or ruled out. See Chapter 12, "Neurogenic Speech Disorders," for a fuller discussion.

Possible hearing loss must be ascertained, especially given the older age of most individuals with aphasia. It is important to separate hearing loss from comprehension deficits.

Finally, careful observation is essential, especially shortly after the incident, when more formal testing is not possible. It is important to observe the client's general speech and language behavior and to listen and observe what is communicated and how. Observing spontaneous language use can give the SLP important information on the nature and extent of the disorder (Davis, 1993; Helm-Estabrooks & Albert, 1991).

Initial testing, often at the bedside, may be very informal with probes of the client's knowledge of her or his name, date and year, personal history, and the ability to produce automatic language, such as counting or reciting the days of the week. Table 7.3 presents an outline of an informal bedside evaluation. More formal testing and sampling phases should assess overall communication skills as well as receptive and expressive language within all modalities—reading, writing, auditory comprehension, expressive language, and gestures and nonlinguistic communication—and across all five aspects of language: pragmatics, semantics, syntax, morphology, and phonology. With higher functioning clients, the SLP will want to assess higher language skills such as verbal reasoning and analogies, figurative language, categorization, and explanations of complex tasks. Table 7.4 is an overview of the areas that ASHA recommends be evaluated in a functional assessment of communication abilities.

Several standardized tests are available for assessing specific language skills. Table 7.5 presents some frequently used aphasia batteries. Formal tests must be selected carefully, given the varying range and scope of different instruments. Overall test construction varies from those that view aphasia as a multimodality disorder, such as the *Minnesota Test of Differential Diagnosis of Aphasia* (Schuell, 1972) and the *Porch Index of Communicative Abilities* (Porch, 1981), to those that consider performance in each modality to be somewhat distinct and help in describing different syndromes, such as the *Boston Diagnostic Aphasia Examination* (Goodglass & Kaplan, 1983a). Some measures, such as the *Functional Communication Profile* (Sarno, 1969) and *Communication Abilities in Daily Living* (Holland, 1980), follow neither model and attempt to describe the client's communicative abilities in daily

> Comprehensive testing of clients with aphasia should include at least the two input modalities of vision and audition and the three output modalities of speech, writing, and gestures.

TABLE 7.3

Components of an informal bedside evaluation

What is your name?

How old are you?

Where do you live?

Count to 20 (*or* Tell me the days of the week *or* Tell me the months of the year).

Can you tell me the names of these objects? (Use common household objects.)

Point to the objects (or pictures) named.

Repeat the following sentences.

Read the following sentences.

TABLE 7.4

ASHA recommendations for a functional assessment of communicative abilities with adults with aphasia

Assessment Domains	Behaviors
Social communication	Use names of familar people
	Express agreement and disagreement
	Request information
	Exchange information on the telephone
	Answer yes/no questions
	Follow directions
	Understand facial expressions and tone of voice
	Understand nonliteral meaning and intent
	Understand conversations in noisy surroundings
	Understand TV and radio
	Participate in conversations
	Recognize and correct communication errors
Communication of basic needs	Recognize familiar faces and voices
	Make strong likes and dislikes known
	Express feelings
	Request help
	Make needs and wants known
	Respond in an emergency
Reading, writing, number concepts	Understand simple signs
	Use reference materials
	Follow written directions
	Understand printed material
	Print, write, and type name
	Complete forms
	Write messages
	Understand signs with numbers
	Make money transactions
	Understand units of measure
Daily planning	Tell time
	Dial telephone numbers
	Keep scheduled appointments
	Use a calendar
	Follow a map

Source: Adapted from American Speech-Language-Hearing Association. (1994). *Functional assessment of communicative skills for adults (FACS)*. Washington, DC: Author.

TABLE 7.5
Frequently used aphasia batteries

Aphasia Assessment Battery

Boston Diagnostic Aphasia Exam (Goodglass & Kaplan, 1983a)

Boston Naming Test (Goodglass & Kaplan, 1983b)

Communication Abilities in Daily Living (Holland, 1980)

Minnesota Test of Differential Diagnosis of Aphasia (Schuell, 1972)

Porch Index of Communicative Abilities (Porch, 1981)

Western Aphasia Battery (Kertesz & McCabe, 1982)

living tasks. Most tests include picture or object naming, pointing to pictures named, automatic language, repeating sentences, describing pictures and answering questions, reading and answering questions and/or drawing conclusions, and writing. It is important for the SLP to remain flexible and to continue to probe the client's behavior for the duration of intervention, especially as behaviors change.

Interpretation of client behavior during testing is extremely important. It is critical, for example, whether the client failed to respond because she or he could not retrieve the answer or because she or he did not comprehend the verbal cue.

Most test tasks involve decision making or problem solving, the endpoints of several cognitive and linguistic processes. Subcomponents of the process are not assessed individually. *Online* assessment, which measures effects at various points within the process, may be more sensitive to individual client strengths and weaknesses (Shapiro, Swinney, & Borsky, 1998). To date, most online analysis is limited to research, but such procedures are slowly being adapted for clinical use.

Because most individuals with aphasia have some residual communication impairment, the goal of intervention is to maximize communication effectiveness in the face of this impairment.

INTERVENTION

The overall goal of intervention is to aid in the recovery of language and to provide strategies to compensate for persistent language deficits (Rosenbek, LaPointe, & Wertz, 1989). Individual intervention goals are determined by the results of the assessment and by the desires of both the client and family. Goals will be individualized according to the type and severity of the aphasia and upon the individual needs of each client. Ideally, the goals are mutually acceptable to the client, family, and SLP. All members of the team coordinate their efforts to strengthen treatment received from others. Some guidelines for working with individuals with aphasia are presented in Table 7.6.

Intervention approaches reflect the SLP's theoretical position on aphasia plus a strong dose of practical knowledge regarding the most effective

---

TABLE 7.6
Guidelines for intervention with individuals with aphasia

Treat the client in an age-appropriate manner.

Keep your own language simple, clear, and unambiguous and control for length and complexity.

Adjust your language and the speed of production for the processing capabilities of the client.

Use everyday items and tasks and involve the family.

Use repetition and familiar routines, situations, and responses to facilitate learning.

Structure tasks to improve performance and adjust the amount of structure just enough to support the client's efforts but not foster dependency.

Provide a context to supportive the client's language processing.

Increase the demands made on the client gradually based on the client's abilities.

Teach the client to use his or her strengths to compensate for weaknesses.

---

techniques. Each clinician must decide whether to work on underlying skills, such as memory and auditory comprehension, or to begin with specific skill deficits, such as naming. If the SLP decides that the client's brain needs help to reorganize, he or she may choose cross-modality training, such as reading aloud while tracing the letters with one's finger.

The SLP can also take advantage of cross-modality generalization in which skills trained in one modality generalize to another. For example, some individuals with agrammatism benefit from comprehension training more than production training (Jacobs & Thompson, 2000). Comprehension training seems to generalize to comprehension and production. Similarly, generalization occurs across linguistically related structures and from more complex structures to less complex ones (Thompson, Shapiro, Kiran, & Sobecks, 2003).

Conversational techniques can provide language therapy and therapeutic support (Holland & Fridriksson, 2001). Within a therapeutic conversation, the client carries as much of the "communication burden" as possible. Mindful of small improvements by the client, the SLP revises the demands made of the client. In short sessions using conversation, the SLP reassures, explains what's happening to the client, and points out positive changes. As clients progress, the SLP provides less support and provides a variety of communication contexts and experiences.

Another method of intervention is to have the client attempt to access the language in the left hemisphere by bridging from the right. This might be attempted by teaching the client to gesture or sign and simultaneously attempt to say the names of familiar objects. It is reasoned that gestures or signs, being visuospatial in nature, are stored in part in the right hemisphere. Another method, called *melodic intonational therapy* (Sparks, Helm, & Albert, 1974; Sparks & Holland, 1976), uses the client's usually intact right hemisphere ability to sing or produce intonational patterns. Words and phrases are taught by using different patterns of rhythm and melody. In either example, the signs or the intonational patterns are gradually faded as the client begins spontaneously to produce the targeted words and phrases without their aid.

As in many areas of language intervention, unanimity on cross-hemispheric treatment methods does not exist. Many SLPs prefer to remediate language deficits by more direct multimodality stimulation of the affected cognitive processes (Heiss, Kessler, Thiel, Ghaemi, & Karbe, 1999; Peach, 2001; Warburton, Price, Swinburn, & Wise, 1999). The goal is reactivation of speech areas in the dominant hemisphere.

Sign, gesture, or some other form of augmentative/alternative communication may become the primary communicative modality for clients who possess profoundly impaired language and/or speech disorders. Communication boards or electronic forms of communication may be appropriate for those who also have neuromuscular impairments. Amerind, or American Indian signs, may also be useful because many require only one hand and are easily guessable by others. See Chapter 15. "Augmentative and Alternative Communication."

Speech and language services are part of a team approach to intervention.

Intervention might also focus on cognitive abilities, such as memory and attention, in addition to more linguistic targets (Murray, Holland, & Beson, 1997, 1998). Clinician-assisted training may also be supplemented by more minimally assisted training, such as computer-provided reading tasks including visual matching and reading comprehension (Katz & Wertz, 1997).

Might some forms of augmentative/alternative communication be utilizing the intact right hemisphere as in melodic intonational therapy?

THOUGHT QUESTION

Assuming that the family is amenable, it is best to involve them in an intense, around-the-clock communication training program. The familiar atmosphere of the home and the objects, actions, and people in it can provide

Augmentative/ alternative communication may become the primary mode of communication or may be used as a facilitative tool to access verbal language.

a context that can facilitate a client's recovery and strengthen his or her re-learned communicative behaviors. It is important for professionals to remember that the beneficial involvement of the family must not be at their emotional expense. Family members must not be made to feel guilt if the client progresses little.

Volunteers can also be trained to support the conversational attempts of individuals with aphasia (Kagan, Black, Duchan, Simmons-Mackie, & Square, 2001). These individuals need to acknowledge and respond to a client's interactive behaviors. This feedback can affect motivation and performance and is an essential part of intervention (Simmons-Mackie, Damico, & Damico, 1999).

CONCLUSION

Aphasia is a complex impairment varying in scope and extent across individuals. In addition, clients may have other impairments, such as paralysis, as a result of their injury. Only a careful description of individual abilities and deficits in each specific modality of communication will enable the SLP to plan and carry out effective intervention. The individual variation in symptoms and severity, the team approach to intervention, and the possibility of spontaneous recovery complicate our efforts to measure intervention effectiveness and offer opportunities for those of you interested in research.

RIGHT HEMISPHERE INJURY

The term **right hemisphere injury or syndrome (RHI)** refers to a group of deficits that result from damage to the right hemisphere of the brain, the nondominant hemisphere for nearly all language functions. Deficits may be neuromuscular, perceptual, and linguistic. In addition, individuals may exhibit unusual behaviors. One client would regularly take a shower with his clothes on and try to go outside nude. Families report personality and mood changes including indifference and apathy. Even less-involved clients can have unrealistic estimates of their own condition and prognosis. An apparent lack of concern may actually mask a client's confusion.

Less information exists on RHI than on damage to the left hemisphere, although approximately half the individuals who have suffered stroke have right hemisphere involvement. The communication disorders that clients with RHI experience are not language based. Rather, a combination of cognitive deficits results in the communication problem. As a result, the efficiency, effectiveness, and accuracy of communication are affected.

Approximately 4 percent of the population are either right-hemisphere dominant for language or have bilateral language processing. If these individuals become aphasic as a result of left-hemisphere damage, they usually experience milder impairment and quicker recovery than those who are left-hemisphere dominant. The role of the right hemisphere is unclear in the recovery of left-dominant individuals with aphasia.

CHARACTERISTICS

Deficits in RHI are not as obvious as those that result from left-hemisphere damage. The most common include the following (Meyers, 1999):

1. Neglect of all information from the left side
2. Unrealistic denial of illness or limb involvement
3. Impaired judgment and selfmonitoring
4. Lack of motivation
5. Inattention

Deficits may be very subtle but can have a great effect on everyday life. Although these deficits may seem nonlinguistic in nature, they can have a great effect on communication (Meyers, 1999; Tompkins, 1995).

Disturbances can be grouped into attentional, visuospatial, and communicative. Attentional disturbances are characterized by client's lack of response to information coming from the left side of the body. This phenomenon is exhibited in the drawings of individuals with mild RHI who may omit all or provide few left-side details. Figure 7.3 shows an example of left-side neglect in a drawing. More severely impaired individuals may even refuse to look to the left side.

> About half of individuals with RHI have communication impairments.

*D*oes it seem odd that the damaged right hemisphere would ignore information from the left side? What can you recall about contralateral neural pathways and sensory information?

THOUGHT QUESTIONS

FIGURE 7.3

Drawings of an individual with mild RHI that demonstrate left side neglect.

Visuospatial deficits may include poor visual discrimination and poor scanning and tracking. The client may have difficulty recognizing familiar faces, remembering familiar routes, and reading maps. Some clients not only fail to recognize family members, but may be convinced that they are actually impostors (Bienemann, 1989).

Communication impairments can be divided into linguistic and paralinguistic deficits. Linguistic difficulties occur in both reception and expression. Of the various aspects of language, pragmatics seems to be the most impaired. For example, topic maintenance, appreciation of the communication situation, and determination of listener needs are impaired. Clients with RHI may exhibit poor auditory and visual comprehension of complex information and limited word discrimination and visual word recognition. They may also incorrectly interpret complex information, possibly because of a tendency to respond to superficial qualities of stimuli and not to observe relationships among them. In general, individuals with RHI fail to suppress irrelevant or inappropriate information, which in turn affects comprehension (Tompkins, Baumgaertner, Lehman, & Fassbinder, 2000). In addition, clients may fail to make use of other contextual, paralinguistic, and nonlinguistic cues (Meyers, 1999). Contextual information may be misinterpreted and the client may fail to integrate sensory information.

Understanding may be very concrete with literal interpretation of humor, indirect requests, and common figurative expressions, such as *hit the roof*. In indirect requests, the speaker does not state his or her request or demand directly. For example, a speaker might say, *I think I'll get my sweater* when meaning *Please turn up the heat*. Clients with RHI also exhibit poor judgment in determining which incoming information is important and which is not.

A similar pattern of difficulty with selectivity is noted in expressive use of language. Clients may include unnecessary, irrelevant, repetitious, and unrelated information, seemingly unable to organize their language in meaningful ways or to present it efficiently. Other problem areas include naming, repetition, and writing, especially letter substitutions and omissions.

Paralinguistic deficits include difficulty comprehending and producing emotional language. The speech of individuals with RHI lacks normal rhythm or prosody and the emphasis used to express joy or sadness, anger or delight.

ASSESSMENT

As with aphasia, the assessment of individuals with RHI is a team effort involving many of the same professionals and diagnostic tasks. The SLP is interested in visual scanning and tracking, auditory and visual comprehension of words and sentences, direction following, response to emotion, naming and describing pictures, and writing. For example, the client may be asked to re-create patterns with blocks or to find two objects or pictures that are the same; to recall words or sentences heard, seen in print, or both; and to describe a picture accurately enough for the SLP to re-create it. Sampling and observational data are essential in assessing the client's pragmatic abilities in conversational contexts.

Portions of aphasia batteries, standardized tests for RHI, and nonstandardized procedures may be used in the assessment. Standardized batteries include the *Right Hemisphere Language Battery* (Bryan, 1989) and the *Mini Inventory of Right Brain Injury* (Pimental & Kingsbury, 1989). Tasks include reading and writing, affective language, and figurative language. The *Rehabilitation Institute of Chicago Evaluation* (RICE) *of Communicative Problems in Right-Hemisphere Dysfunction* (Burns, Halper, & Mogil, 1985) is a nonstandard testing procedure that includes interviewing, observation, and ratings of the client's behavior along with testing of communication.

INTERVENTION

Intervention often begins with visual and auditory recognition. These skills are essential before progressing to more complex tasks, such as naming, describing, reading, and writing. Self-monitoring and paralinguistics are introduced, and the complexity of the content is gradually increased.

> Because of the diffuse effects on behavior seen in RHI, we know less about the treatment of these patients.

Clients are helped to respond appropriately to common communicative initiations and to track increasingly complex information in conversations. Beginning with questions from the SLP that require precise information, the client learns to make responses that come to the point. These questions become more open-ended as the client learns to make off-topic responses less frequently. Similarly, time restraints may limit conversational turns to keep the client from rambling.

Sequencing tasks and explanations of common multistep actions, such as making coffee, will be introduced to help the client organize linguistic content and make relevant contributions. Cues such as objects or pictures may be used initially to aid organization.

Finally, within conversations, the SLP will help the client to synthesize these many skills. Visual and verbal cues may aid in turn taking. Important nonlinguistic markers such as eye contact, body language, and gestures may be targeted. Topic maintenance and relevant conversational contributions are stressed.

TRAUMATIC BRAIN INJURY (TBI)

Adolescents and young adults (15–24 years of age) are the age groups most at risk for head injury. The increase in motor vehicles, motorcycles, and off-road vehicles is also directly related to the increase in TBI. Another disturbing increase is the rise in attempted homicides and gun-related injuries, especially in urban areas. The authors have seen adult clients with TBI as the result of automobile, motorcycle, and bicycle collisions; falls; violent crime; and failed suicide attempts involving firearms.

Every minute, nearly two people in the United States suffer serious head injury. Annually approximately 260,000 individuals sustain TBI of a serious enough nature to require hospitalization (http://www.cdc.gov/doc.do/id/

0900f3ec800101eB, 2003). Of these, approximately 200,000 die. Most others are treated for concussion and recover. Approximately 80,000–90,000 have significant impairment requiring further care and have altered their lives for the foreseeable future (http://www.cdc.gov/doc.do/id/0900f3 ec800101eB, 2003). Approximately 70 percent of these are males. The statistics tell a chilling story but do not begin to explain the pain and suffering or the long struggle to recover. Case Study 7.3 presents the personal story of one young man with TBI.

You will recall from our discussion of children that, unlike stroke, which injures a specific area of the brain, TBI is a diffuse injury to the entire brain; it is nonfocused. Damage may result from bruising and laceration of the brain caused by forceful contact with the relatively rough inner surfaces of the skull and from secondary **edema** or swelling due to increased fluid, which can lead to increased pressure; infection; hypoxia (oxygen deprivation); intracranial pressure from tissue swelling; **infarction,** or death of tissue deprived of blood supply; and **hematoma,** or focal bleeding (Sohlberg & Mateer, 1989). Aphasia-like symptoms are rare, but linguistic impairments related to cognitive damage are not. In addition, the individual with TBI may have sensory, motor, behavioral, and affective disabilities. Neuromuscular impairments may include epilepsy, hemisensory impairment, and hemiparesis or hemiplegia. The symptoms and the life changes that result can be profound.

CHARACTERISTICS

The behavioral characteristics of adults with TBI are similar to those of children who are similarly injured. Adults with TBI are a heterogeneous group with a diverse collection of physical, cognitive, communicative, and psychosocial deficits. Usually, the most devastating aspect is an inability to resume interests and daily living tasks to the level that existed before the injury. Some clients exhibit near total dependence on others. Cognitive difficulties may be evident in orientation, memory, attention, reasoning and problem solving, and executive function, or the planning, execution, and self-monitoring of goal-directed behavior (Sohlberg & Mateer, 1989).

Language may be affected in three out of four individuals with TBI (McKinlay, Brooks, Bond, Martinage, & Marshall, 1981). The two most commonly reported symptoms for TBI are anomia and impaired comprehension (Coelho, 1997).

As with children, the most disturbed language area and that with the most pervasive problems is pragmatics (Sohlberg & Mateer, 1989). Most published tests target language form and content and may miss pragmatic deficits that are evident in conversation. Pragmatic impairments result from the inability to inhibit behavior and from errors of judgment. The result may be rambling speech and incoherence, as manifested by off-topic and irrelevant comments and inability to maintain a topic, and poor turn-taking skills, such as frequent interruption of others. In addition, communication may be marked by poor affective or emotional language abilities and inappropriate laughter and swearing.

Case Study 7.3

Personal Story of a Young Man with TBI

His family called him Felipe, but he preferred to use the more Americanized nickname "Chip" that his friends had given him. He was excited to be leaving home for college. Thoughts of being on his own thrilled him with endless possibilities. Even though he was only a freshman, he planned to live with some older friends in their off-campus apartment.

A few weeks after school began, Felipe decided to hitchhike home to surprise his mother, who missed him a great deal. He stuck out his thumb early on Friday afternoon but never made it home. After his first ride, he bought a soda and began to thumb anew. Shortly afterward, he was struck in the head by the mirror on a pickup truck. Luckily, Felipe was carrying identification in his backpack, and his family was alerted shortly after he was admitted to the hospital.

When he regained consciousness, a few hours after the accident, Felipe was extremely disoriented. He made no attempt to speak and was very lethargic. Although he seemed to recognize his family, he made no attempt to communicate with them. Over the next few weeks, his condition slowly stabilized. Physicians were initially concerned about swelling in the area of the injury. There was evidence of some internal bleeding, but it was not a major problem.

Once the swelling began to recede, Felipe's abilities slowly returned. He began to recall the names of family members and common objects. Walking was extremely difficult because of paralysis on the right side of his body. He dropped out of college and remained at home, where he received intervention services. As an outpatient, he was seen by the speech-language pathologist, physical therapist, and occupational therapist.

After a year's absence from school, Felipe returned and was able to be successful with some adaptations, such as the use of a tape recorder and extra time for completing written tests. He retains a slight limp in his right leg and some minimal weakness in his right arm. His language and speech skills have returned, although he has some mild word-finding difficulties. His cognitive abilities are more concrete than those he had before the accident, and problem-solving tasks require a greater effort. All indications are that he will be successful in his academic pursuits, although his physical and cognitive limitations will continue to affect him.

Deficits are not limited to language and may include speech, voice, and swallowing difficulties. Approximately one-third of all individuals with TBI exhibit dysarthria, a disorder resulting from weakness or incoordination of the muscles that control speech production (Sarno, Buonaguro, & Levita, 1986) (see Chapter 12). Language deficits reflect underlying disruptions in information-processing, problem-solving, and reasoning abilities. In addition, psychosocial and personality changes may include disinhibition or impulsivity, poor organization and social judgment, and withdrawal or aggressiveness. Physical signs may include difficulty walking, poor coordination, and vision problems. A more complete list of the possible outcomes of TBI is presented in Table 7.7.

Severity seems to be related to initial levels of consciousness and post-traumatic amnesia. Consciousness levels can be classified along a continuum from extended states of unconsciousness or coma, in which the body responds only minimally to external stimuli, to consciousness with disorientation, stupor, and lethargy. Amnesia, or memory loss, is a frequent result of TBI. The duration of both coma and amnesia has been used successfully, but not infallibly, as a predictor of severity and prognosis. In general, the

TABLE 7.7

Possible outcomes of TBI

Cognition	*Emotion/Personality*
Inattentive	Aggression/withdrawal
Disoriented	Apathy and indifference
Poor memory	Denial
Poor problem-solving abilities	Depression
	Disinhibition and impulsivity
Language, Speech, and Oral Mechanism	Impatience
Dysphagia	Phobias
Dysarthria	Socially inappropriate behavior and comments
Possible mutism	Suspiciousness and anxiety
Pragmatic difficulties (talks better than can communicate)	
Confused language—irrelevant, confabulatory, circumlocutionary, tangential to the topic, lacks logical sequencing, misnaming	

shorter both are, the less severe the resultant deficits of TBI and the better the potential outcome.

LIFESPAN ISSUES

Most adults with TBI are young and have experienced an auto or motorcycle accident. Imagine that you, a college student, are riding in a friend's car. The next thing that you remember is waking in the hospital, dazed, confused, and unaware of your surroundings. You may have language or other impairments that will change your life forever or at least for the immediate future.

Several stages of recovery have been described and clinical intervention varies with each (Hagan & Malkamus, 1979). Most individuals will not reach full recovery and some residual deficits will most likely remain. Initially, the individual may be nonresponsive to stimuli and need total assistance in a hospital setting.

When the individual does begin to respond, his or her responses may be undifferentiated, whole body responses that do not reflect the varying nature of the stimuli. Responses may be delayed. Vocalizations seem purposeless.

Gradually, the individual begins to respond differently to different stimuli and to recognize some familiar individuals. Response to commands is often inconsistent.

As the individual becomes more alert, he or she may be confused or agitated. Short-term memory and goal-directed behaviors may be poor. Although able to sit and walk, these behaviors are performed without purpose. Subject to violent mood swings, the individual may have incoherent, inappropriate, or emotional language. The individual may still need rehabilitative hospital care but has recovered enough to move from intensive care.

As agitation fades and language continues to return, the individual can remain alert for short periods of time and hold brief conversations if strong external cues are used. There are still periods of nonpurposeful behavior. Short-term memory is still severely impaired. With structure, the individual can perform learned tasks but is unable to learn new behaviors.

As the individual continues to improve, he or she needs less assistance. Able to attend for up to 30 minutes with redirection, the individual is aware of the appropriate responses to self, family, and basic needs, which become more goal-directed. Relearned tasks exhibit some carryover, although new learning exhibits none. Language is used appropriately in highly familiar contexts.

Gradually, the individual becomes oriented to persons and place. Time is still confusing and the individual demonstrates only superficial understanding of his or her condition. Usually in outpatient status, the individual is able to learn and carry over this learning to other tasks and to monitor his or her own behavior with minimal assistance. Still unable to recognize inappropriate social behavior, the individual is often uncooperative, unrealistic in his or her expectations, and unaware of the needs and feelings of others.

As the individual gains more of an understanding of his or her condition and is able to plan and initiate routine tasks, frustration may build, and the individual become depressed, argumentative, irritable, or overly dependent or independent. Living at home and possibly having returned to work, the individual may be able to concentrate for an hour even with distractions, to recall past and present events, and to learn new tasks with only minimal assistance.

Increasing abilities may not reduce the individual's low tolerance for frustration, although behavioral responses may be less. In the later stages of recovery, the individual can shift between tasks for up to two hours and initiate and carry out familiar tasks. Able to acknowledge his or her impairment, the individual is able to consider the consequences of his or her actions and to recognize the needs and feeling of others.

Finally, the individual may be able to consistently act in a socially appropriate manner, to respond appropriately to others, and to plan, initiate, and complete both familiar and unfamiliar tasks. Periodic depression may occur and irritability may reappear with illness, inability to perform a task, and in emotional situations.

The individual with TBI may face a long period of rehabilitation. Even those who have made a near-full recovery will have some lingering deficits. The authors have worked with college students who were able to gain their degrees with only minimal adaptations.

ASSESSMENT

The SLP is a member of an interdisciplinary team of rehabilitation specialists who collaborate in assessment of and intervention with persons with TBI (Ylvisaker, 1994). As such, the SLP is responsible for assessing all aspects of communication, cognitive-communicative functioning, and swallowing.

Unlike individuals with aphasia, those with TBI progress through recognizable stages of recovery. Assessment must be ongoing and varies with each stage. Neurological, psychiatric, and psychological reports will aid in the planning of both assessment and intervention. Observation can aid the SLP in deciding which areas to probe, especially in determining pragmatic deficits that may be missed in formal testing.

To date, few comprehensive tools exist for assessment of language skills in individuals with TBI. Many SLPs working with this population have compiled a series of individual tests for aspects of both language and cognition. These tests are often portions of larger test batteries. Language testing must be comprehensive. Tests that emphasize language form and content may fail to adequately assess pragmatics, thus underestimating the extent of the language impairment.

Sampling is essential because pragmatic behavior that varies across communicative contexts cannot be adequately assessed in a testing context alone (Starch & Falltrick, 1990). Sampling contexts should include functional activities, such as talking on the phone or grocery shopping, in natural environments, such as the home. Sampling should occur within a discourse unit, a series of related linguistic units that convey a message (Coelho, Liles, & Duffy, 1995).

INTERVENTION

With or without intervention, the pattern of recovery for individuals with TBI is predictable. Unlike those with focal damage such as a stroke, who progress smoothly, those with TBI recover in a stepwise or plateau fashion characterized by periods of little or no change interspersed with periods of rapid improvement. After a period of unconsciousness, the person often responds indiscriminately and seemingly without purpose. Attention may be fleeting, and overall level of arousal may fluctuate. The client is often hyperresponsive to stimuli and easily irritated and agitated. Clients may become very emotional and exhibit shouting, biting, and repetitive, stereotypic movements such as rocking. With recovery, clients become more clear thinking, and their behavior becomes more purposeful, although restlessness and irritability may persist.

As the client becomes more oriented in place and time, he or she is better able to respond to simple requests, although attention span is short and distractibility high. Memory and abstract reasoning may continue to be a problem even as the client becomes better able to manage daily living and to begin to function independently.

Intervention for cognitive-communicative deficits with individuals with TBI is called **cognitive rehabilitation,** a treatment regimen designed to in-

Cognitive rehabilitation promotes independent functioning in daily life by focusing on specific cognitive processes such as memory and language processing.

crease functional abilities for everyday life by improving the capacity to process incoming information. The two primary approaches are restorative and compensatory (Ben-Yishay & Diller, 1993). The restorative approach attempts to rebuild neural circuitry and function through repetitive activities, while the compensatory approach concedes that some functions will not be recovered and develops alternatives. Restorative techniques might include classification tasks and word associations. In contrast, compensatory strategies to improve memory might include focused attending and rehearsal of new information. Traditionally, restorative strategies are attempted first and may include rehearsal and encoding strategies and the use of memory aids (Hutchinson & Marquardt, 1997). Compensatory methods are used when the restorative attempts have failed. Slowly, professionals are recognizing that compensatory strategies aid in restorative development, and both methods are being used simultaneously (Coelho, 1997).

The SLP is responsible for designing and implementing treatment programs to decrease the effects of impairment. In addition to providing direct intervention, the SLP helps to identify functional supports, such as memory logs, and work adjustments that aid in successful independent living.

Intervention programs vary depending on the stage of recovery. During the early stages, intervention focuses on orientation, sensorimotor stimulation, and recognition of familiar people and common objects and events. Early intervention results in shorter rehabilitation and higher levels of cognitive functioning (Mackay, Bernstein, Chapman, Morgan, & Milazzo, 1992).

In the middle stages, training becomes more structured and formal. The goals are to reduce confusion and improve memory and goal-directed behavior. Much of the training involves increasing the client's orientation to the everyday world. Consistency and routines are important in orientation training. The SLP may target active listening and auditory comprehension and following directions with increasingly more complex information. Word definitions, descriptions of entities and events, and classification of objects and words are also targeted. Conversational speech training is also attempted. One SLP, recognizing that the act of taking a conversational turn is too difficult for some clients, begins by using a beanbag or other object, which is passed back and forth to signal turn changes.

During the late stages of recovery, the goal is client independence. Targets include comprehension of complex information and directions and conversational and social skills. The SLP helps the client to explore alternative strategies for word recall, memory, and problem solving. Conversational problem-solving tasks are also targeted, along with self-inhibition and self-monitoring. Real-world contexts are emphasized, especially those that are potentially confusing or emotional.

DEMENTIA

We live in a youth-oriented culture. Commercial images lead to the stereotype of older people with deteriorated bodies and minds. While physical decline with age is inevitable, intellectual capacity is frequently unimpaired.

Dementia is an impairment of intellect and cognition.

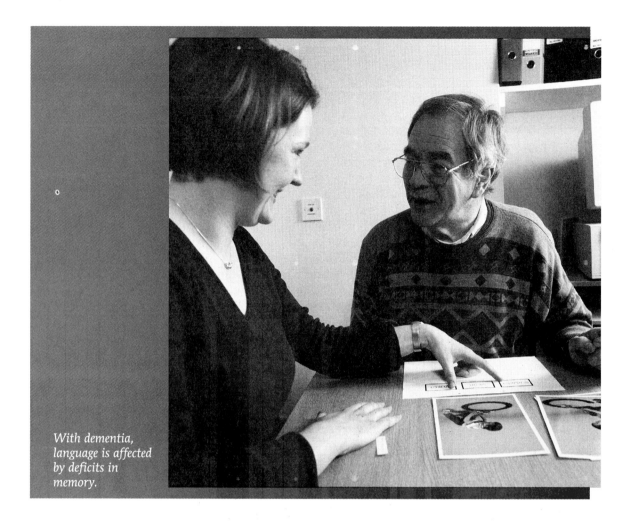

With dementia, language is affected by deficits in memory.

Fewer than 15 percent of the elderly experience dementia, and as many as 20 percent of these positively respond to treatment (Shekim, 1990). The incidence of dementia is increasing rapidly as the percentage of the U.S. population over age 65 increases. It is estimated that as high as 48 percent of new admissions to long-tern care facilities have a diagnosis of dementia (Magaziner, German, Itkin Zimmerman, Hebel, Burton, Bruber-Baldini, May, & Kittner, 2000).

THOUGHT QUESTIONS

Do you ever assume that seniors have lost some of their cognitive abilities? Is occasional confusion always a sign of deteriorating cognitive abilities? Do you equate physical frailty with mental frailty?

Dementia is an umbrella term for a group of both pathological conditions and syndromes. It is acquired and is characterized by intellectual decline due to neurogenic causes. Memory is the most obvious function affected (American Psychiatric Association, 1994). Additional deficits include poor reasoning or judgment, impaired abstract thinking, inability to attend to relevant information, impaired communication, and personality changes.

Dementia can be divided into cortical and subcortical types based on patterns of neurophysiological impairment (Cummings & Benson, 1992). The characteristics of cortical dementias, such as Alzheimer's and Pick's diseases, resemble those of focal impairments such as aphasia and RHI. These include visuospatial deficits, memory problems, judgment and abstract thinking disturbances, and language deficits in naming, reading and writing, and auditory comprehension. Alzheimer's disease accounts for over 50 percent of the dementia cases and may affect 20 million people worldwide.

Subcortical dementias may accompany multiple sclerosis, AIDS-related encephalopathy, and Parkinson's and Huntington's diseases. A slow, progressive deterioration of cognitive functioning occurs with deficits in memory, problem solving, language, and neuromuscular control. Those disorders that involve neuromuscular functioning will be discussed in Chapter 9, "The Voice and Voice Disorders," and Chapter 12, "Neurogenic Speech Disorders."

The language functions that are most dependent on memory seem to be primarily affected. A significant decline is noted in naming and word retrieval. Language form—phonology, morphology, and syntax—is generally less disordered, although syntax may be less coherent than before as the client struggles with anomia. As a consequence, conversations may lack coherence and may be filled with repetitions, stereotypic utterances, false starts, verbal repairs, jargon, neologisms, and the use of phrases such as *that one* and *you know* (Shekim & LaPointe, 1984). One client would repeat "I know" several times.

ALZHEIMER'S DISEASE

Alzheimer's disease is a cortical pathology that affects approximately 10 percent of individuals over age 65 and possibly as high as 50 percent of those over age 85 (http://www.alz.org/AboutAD/Statistics.asp, 2005). Given the aging U.S. population, the prevalence of Alzheimer's disease will increase 27 percent by 2020, 70 percent by 2030, and almost 300 percent by 2050, unless science finds a way to slow the progression of the disease or prevent it (http://www.alzheimersupport.com/library/showarticle.cfm/id/1959/searchtext/prevalence/, 2003). A heterogeneous population, individuals with Alzheimer's may be primarily impaired in memory, language, or visuospatial skills (DeSanti, 1997). Alzheimer's is two or three times as common in women as in men.

The cause of Alzheimer's disease is unknown but may be a combination of genetic and environmental factors. The neuropathology is characterized by the presence of twisted neurofilaments in the cytoplasm of neurons that deteriorate cell functioning. These tangles are most pronounced in the temporal lobe and in associational areas of the brain. Nerve fibers degenerate, resulting in brain atrophy that may decrease brain weight as much as 20 per-

Alzheimer's is characterized by microscopic changes in the neurons of the cerebral cortex.

cent, especially in the temporal, frontal, and parietal lobes (Kemper, 1984; Koo & Price, 1993). Other physical changes include extensive damage to the hippocampus, located on the interior portion of the temporal lobes (interior to the ears) and formation of senile plaques within the cortex that affect nerve cell interactive functioning.

Mild dementia may be characterized by name recall difficulties, occasional disorientation, and memory loss. Memory problems are the most obvious changes. Retention of newly learned information is most impaired (Convit, deLeon, Tarshish, DeSanti, Tsui, Rusinek, & George, 1995). Long-term memory is unimpaired initially but deteriorates as the disease progresses.

Language is not affected in all individuals initially. Early problems involve word finding, off-topic comments, and comprehension. At these early stages, deficits are mostly pragmatic and semantic-conceptual in nature, while syntax is relatively unaffected compared to that of elderly individuals not affected by Alzheimer's disease (Kavé & Levy, 2003).

Later characteristics include paraphasia (word substitution) and delayed responding. In more severe stages, expressive and receptive vocabulary and complex sentence production become reduced; pronoun confusion, topic digression, and inability to return to and to shift topic are more pronounced; and writing and reading errors occur (Mentis, Briggs-Whittaker, & Gramigna, 1995). In its most severe form, the language of individuals with Alzheimer's is characterized by naming errors and the use of generic words (*this, that*), syntactic errors, minimal comprehension, jargon, echolalia, or mutism (DeSanti, 1997). As might be expected, increased severity results in more conversational breakdowns (Orange, Lubinsky, & Higginbotham, 1996).

Lifespan Issues

Alzheimer's disease is a genetic disorder that lies in hiding, although early screening is possible in some cases. Genetic and environmental factors seem to be important. Often the person who will be afflicted with the disease is unaware and/or ignores early signs. At present there are no cures, but some early drug therapies seem to lessen the effects.

In the early stages, the individual experiences memory loss, especially of new information. The individual experiences word retrieval problems and some difficulty with higher language functions, such as humor and analogies. The individual may seem indifferent and initiate little communication. Able to live at home, the individual can become an increasing burden on an elderly spouse or on adult children with families of their own.

As the disease progresses, memory loss increases with the effect that vocabulary decreases. Comprehension is reduced. Language production may be reduced to ritualistic or high-usage phrases accompanied by poor topic maintenance and repair of errors, frequent repetition and word retrieval problems, and insensitivity to conversational partners. Irritability and restlessness may increase. The individual may be able to live at home with visiting nurse care to help with daily living routines.

In the most advanced stages of the disease, all intellectual functions including memory are severely impaired and almost all individuals reside in nursing homes. Language may be meaningless or the individual may be mute or echolalic. Most clients cannot recall the names of loved ones and may undergo radical personality changes. Motor function is also severely impaired and the individual will need total care.

Assessment

Definitive diagnosis of Alzheimer's is difficult in the early stages of the disease. Use of magnetic resonance imaging (MRI) may help in early identification. Pupil dilation tests may also indicate the presence of the disease in the early stages.

Working as a member of a diagnostic team, SLPs usually help identify changes in language performance that may signal intellectual deterioration and aspects of behavior amenable to change (Hopper, 2005). The results of this assessment may help differentiate Alzheimer's disease from other neuropathologies.

Genetic history and general and neurological health data are important elements in the assessment process. Observation of the individual in different communication environments is also important. In the early stages, dementia may be confused with other disorders, such as depression. The progressive nature of the disorder makes it imperative that the SLP remain current on the changing condition and learning ability of a client.

Although few language tests for this population exist, the *Arizona Battery for Communicative Disorders of Dementia* (Bayles & Kazniak, 1987) has been specifically designed to assess the retrieval, perceptual, and linguistic deficits common to dementia. Cognitive-communicative strengths may be measured using the *Functional Linguistic Communication Inventory* (Bayles & Tomoeda, 1994), assessment of the client's ability to participate in the give-and-take of daily communication in a number of areas.

Several scales exist for rating the severity of a client's loss. Of particular importance are the memory deficits that are common (Azuma & Bayles, 1997). In addition, many assessment batteries that are used with individuals with aphasia can be helpful in evaluating the communication skills of persons with dementia. Detailed understanding of a client's strengths and weaknesses is essential for helping family members choose the most effective communicative strategies (Causino Lamar, Obler, Knoeful, & Albert, 1994).

Intervention

Intervention with those with progressive disorders can sometimes feel like trying to hold back the tide. Decline is inevitable, given the present state of our knowledge. That does not mean that we do nothing. Quite the contrary, clinical intervention by an SLP can help to maintain the client at her or his highest level of performance and help others to maximize the client's participation in conversational interactions. It is imperative, therefore, that the SLP emphasize the use of intact cognitive abilities to compensate for deficient ones (Hooper, 2005).

Intervention is not undertaken in isolation. As in the other disorders discussed in this chapter, the SLP is a member of a team. Professionals consult with one another and with the client and family on the best course of action.

The SLP may target memory or word retrieval by working on word associations and categories, auditory attending and comprehension in conversa-

Appropriate and effective intervention requires that the SLP understand what the family of the client is experiencing.

tional contexts, coherent verbal responses, and formation of longer, more complex utterances with the help of memory aids. Family members can be helped to keep conversations focused on the present, to validate the client's comments, to reduce distractions and limit the number of participants, and to foster comprehension and participation by slowing the rate and decreasing the complexity of their utterances, using nonlinguistic cues and yes/no response questions (Shekim, 1990; Small & Perry, 2005). Interactive strategies that result in the least communication breakdown include eliminating distractions, speaking in simple sentences, and employing yes/no questions (Small, Gutman, Makela, & Hillhouse, 2003). Relatively intact reading and visual memory can be used to facilitate verbal memory (Hopper, 2005).

New drug and gene therapies and bioengineering techniques hold the promise that many of the diseases that cause dementia may one day be controllable. At present, intervention that stimulates cognitive processes combined with pharmacological approaches that increase certain neural chemicals important for memory is best. Embryonic stem cells may also be used to someday regenerate brain tissue.

SUMMARY

Aphasia, right hemisphere injury, traumatic brain injury, and dementia result in very different types of language impairment. Aphasia, the result of a focal brain injury, most likely a stroke, may result in a wide variety of impairments that may affect one or more modalities of communication, although comprehension, speech, and naming are usually impaired. Stroke is also the primary cause of right hemisphere injury. Comprehension and production of paralinguistics and complex linguistic structures are affected. Pragmatics is the most affected aspect of language. This is also true for traumatic brain injury, which, in contrast to the previous two, is a nonfocused rather than a focal injury. Finally, dementia, particularly that caused by Alzheimer's disease, is a degenerative disease. Word-finding difficulties, off-topic comments, and comprehension deficits are the most common characteristics.

In the adult language impairments discussed, the SLP functions as a member of a multidisciplinary collaborative team. The role of the SLP includes assessment of communicative abilities and their implication of other cognitive deficits, swallowing, and associated neurological disorders. Other responsibilities include treatment planning and programming, direct intervention services, interdisciplinary consultation, and family training and counseling. Intervention usually focuses on retrieval of language skills and on compensatory strategies.

REFLECTIONS

• What are the major differences between aphasia, right hemisphere injury, traumatic brain injury, and dementia?

- What are the concomitant or accompanying deficits found with aphasia?
- What are the two main types of aphasia and the characteristics of each?
- Describe the different types of stroke or CVA.

SUGGESTED READINGS

Brookshire, R. H. (1997). *Introduction to neurogenic communication disorders* (5th ed.). St. Louis, MO: Mosby.

ONLINE RESOURCES

alzheimer@wubios.wustl.edu
   Alzhemer's discussion group.
cnet_strode_dem_head_injury@listserv.arizona.edu Stroke discussion group.
   TBI gopher points to other sites.
http://www.asha.org/fact_14.htm
   #14 Neurological/Fluency/Voice Disorders in Multicultural Populations
http://www.nyneurosurgery.org/
   Head injury tutorial with information on classification and treatment for head injury.
http://www.ninds.nih.gov/healinfo/disorder/alzheimr/alzheimers.htm
   NIDCD publication on Alzheimer's disease including information and a current bibliography.
http://www.stroke.org/
   Information on causes and treatment of stroke with available low-cost materials.
tbi-sprt@maelstrom.stjohns.edu
   TBI discussion group.

Fluency Disorders

8

CHAPTER LEARNING GOALS

When you have finished this chapter, you should be able to:

- Describe differences between fluent and stuttered speech

- Describe the onset and development of stuttering

- Describe some stuttering treatment techniques that are used with children

- Describe some stuttering treatment techniques that are used with adults

Fluent speech is the consistent ability to move the speech production apparatus in an effortless, smooth, and rapid manner resulting in a continuous, uninterrupted forward flow of speech. Several conditions that adversely influence speech and language production can have a disruptive effect on the fluency of speech. Dysarthria, apraxia, cerebral palsy, and some forms of aphasia affect the fluency of speech. These disorders and their effects on speech and language production are discussed in Chapters 7 and 12 of this book. Another condition called *cluttering* also adversely affects speech fluency. Cluttering is characterized by rapid bursts of unintelligible speech. The primary focus of this chapter is on a disorder of speech called "developmental stuttering." Developmental stuttering, or simply "stuttering," primarily influences the speaker's ability to produce fluent speech. Stuttered speech is characterized by involuntary repetitions of sounds and syllables (i.e., b-b-b-ball), sound prolongations (i.e., mmmmm-mommy), and broken words (i.e., b—oy). All three of these interruptions are considered to be stuttering behaviors, and they have a negative impact on the speaker's ability to produce fluent speech.

Case Study 8.1

Case Study of a Child with Stuttering: Tamara

Mrs. Fisher brought her 4-year-old daughter, Tamara, to the speech and hearing clinic at a nearby university. In an interview with the clinic's director, Mrs. Fisher explained that when Tamara was about 3½ years old she had trouble starting to speak because she repeated the first sounds and syllables at the beginning of each utterance like "C-c-c-can I have some ice cream?" or "Ba-ba-ba-ba-baseball is boring." This difficulty lasted about two weeks, and then it went away as abruptly as it began. Tamara's speech was free of such disruptions for the next six months. Mrs. Fisher further explained that about two weeks prior to her visit to the clinic, Tamara's speech interruptions reappeared. And, she showed great concern when she told the clinic director that in addition to repeating sounds and syllables at the beginning of utterances she was holding or prolonging sounds at numerous places in her utterances like "I-I-I-I want to sssssssssssit over there."

The clinic director observed Mrs. Fisher and her daughter interacting with one another in an adjoining room via a one-way mirror. The clinic director observed that Mrs. Fisher spoke at a very rapid rate and that she tended to use complex sentence structures when she spoke to her daughter. A formal evaluation of Tamara's speech revealed that she produced an average of 15 instances of stuttering per 100 words spoken, she would frequently lose eye contact with the examiner, and she scored 30 points on the *Stuttering Prediction Instrument*. Based on these findings, it was recommended that Tamara be seen in direct therapy two times per week and that Mrs. Fisher be given instruction regarding reducing her speaking rate and sentence complexity.

Following four months of the start of direct intervention with Tamara and parental counseling, Tamar's disfluent behaviors were markedly reduced, falling well within normal limits. And Tamara's mother had dramatically slowed her speaking rate and she spoke in relatively simple sentence structure when she conversed with her daughter.

As you read this chapter, think about

- The nature of the speech interruptions Tamara had developed.
- The developmental course of Tamara's disfluent behaviors.
- Why the clinic director recommended direct therapy for Tamara and parental counseling for her mother.

In this chapter, we define stuttering and discuss how stuttering begins and develops as a disorder, paying particular attention to how stuttered speech differs from fluent speech. Consideration will be given to some of the major theories regarding stuttering, the clinical diagnosis of stuttering, stuttering treatment, and, finally, treatment efficacy. As you begin reading this chapter, consider carefully the thoughts of the late Charles Van Riper, a pioneer in the treatment of stuttering. His words set the tone for this chapter. In the dedication to his 1992 book entitled *The Nature of Stuttering,* Van Riper wrote:

> To the ancient birch tree to whom, when I was a youth and it was a sapling, I swore an oath to find the cause and cure of the stuttering that afflicted me and so many others. Though I have failed and we have both grown old I did my utmost and am content. Others will take up my quest. (dedication page)

Dr. Charles Van Riper was a distinguished professor of speech-language pathology for many years at Western Michigan University. Dr. Van Riper learned to control his stuttering and spent most of his life searching for the cause and cure of stuttering. Therapy techniques that he developed are still in use today.

Many people have indeed taken up Van Riper's quest to find the cause of stuttering and a cure for it, but neither has been discovered. The cause of stuttering is elusive, and our understanding of stuttering is incomplete, despite its long and diverse history. Stuttering has been part of the human condition for all recorded time. Clay tablets found in Mesopotamia dating from centuries before the birth of Christ record the disorder, hieroglyphics from the twentieth century B.C. depict stuttering, and poems written in China more than 2,500 years ago allude to stuttering (cf. Van Riper, 1992). Stuttering affects people worldwide. Physicist Sir Isaac Newton, author W. Somerset Maugham (*Of Human Bondage*), and statesman Winston Churchill stuttered. Performers James Earl Jones, Carly Simon, Marilyn Monroe, and Bruce Willis stuttered. Stuttering is insensitive to race, creed, color, intellect, and virtually any other attribute that could be used to distinguish one human being from another.

The number of adults who report that they had stuttered at some time in their life is 5 percent (Andrews et al., 1983; Conture & Guitar, 1993). However, this 5 percent incidence rate includes the high percentage of children who spontaneously recover from the disorder before the age of 6 (Conture, 1996). Relatively new information indicates that 65 to 75 percent of children will recover from stuttering within the first two years after its onset and 85 percent will recover within the next few years. Given a recovery rate of about 85 percent (i.e., more than four out of five children), the 5 percent lifetime incidence percentage reduces down to about a 1 percent incidence (Conture, 1996; Yairi & Ambrose, 1992a; Yairi & Ambrose, 2004; Yairi, Ambrose, & Nierman, 1993). It is not well understood why some children spontaneously recover from stuttering and others do not. For example, females appear to recover from stuttering more frequently than males.

The prevalence of stuttering is determined by ascertaining the number of cases in a given population (usually school-age children) during a given period of time. Research findings of many studies conducted in various regions around the United States suggest an average prevalence rate of 0.97 percent for school-age children (Bloodstein, 1995). This figure is consistent with the 1 percent incidence estimate and with prevalence estimates from European and Near East countries. The prevalence of stuttering is stable from the first to the ninth grade with a precipitous decline in stuttering during grades 10, 11, and 12.

THOUGHT QUESTION

What might be some of the reasons for the decline in stuttering during grades 10, 11, and 12?

Stuttering affects more males than females, the reported sex ratio differences ranging from 2.3 to 1 to 3.0 to 1. This difference has been attributed to differences in the physical maturation rates of boys and girls and to differences in speech and language development, but genetic factors may also be involved.

Stuttering has a high degree of familial incidence. Fifty percent of people who stutter report that they have a relative who stuttered at some time in his or her life. Fifteen percent of first-degree relatives (parents, sisters, and brothers) of people who stutter are current or recovered stutterers. This threefold increase over the reported 5 percent lifetime incidence for the general population is genetically significant (Felsenfeld, 1997; Felsenfeld, Kirk, Zhu, Statham, Neale, & Martin, 2000; Kidd, 1984). Additionally, if one twin stutters, there is a high probability that the other twin will stutter, and the rate of concordance (both twins exhibiting the disorder) is higher for monozygotic twins (genetically identical) than for dizygotic (fraternal) twins.

Recent genetic research has indicated that stuttering may be linked to a specific single gene, although the location and nature of such a gene is unknown (Ambrose, Yairi, & Cox, 1993; Shugart, Mundorff, Kilshaw, Doheny, Doan, Wanyee, Green, & Drayna, 2004). Continued genetic research will ultimately play a role in our understanding of stuttering, but the actual contributions of such research "remain over the horizon" (Felsenfeld, 1997, p. 20).

FLUENT SPEECH VERSUS STUTTERING

Anyone who has listened carefully to a young child speak can attest to the fact that the flow of most children's speech is not continuously forward and uninterrupted. Children exhibit many hesitations, revisions, and interruptions in their utterances. Children are not born as fluent speakers. Fluency requires some degree of physical maturation and language experience, but it does not develop linearly as the child matures. Longitudinal research indicates that children around 25 months of age are more fluent than they will be at 29 months and at 37 months of age (Yairi, 1981, 1982). There is a gradual increasing in disfluent behaviors beginning around 2 years of age that peaks around the third birthday. Fluency then improves after the third birthday, and the types of disfluency change.

NORMAL DISFLUENCIES

The type of disfluency exhibited by the normally developing child changes between the ages of 25 and 37 months. At approximately 2 years of age, typical disfluencies are whole-word repetitions (I-I-I want a cookie), interjections (Can we-uhm-go now?), and syllable repetitions (I like ba-baseball). Revisions such as "He can't—he won't play baseball" are the dominant disfluency type when the child is approximately 3 years old (Yairi, 1982). Normal disfluencies persist throughout the course of one's life, but they do not tend to adversely affect the continuous forward flow of speech. Normally fluent speakers frequently interrupt the forward flow of speech by repeating whole multisyllablic words (I really-really like hockey), interjecting a word or phrase (He will, uhhhhh, you know, not like that idea), repeating a phrase (Will you, will you please stop that), or revising a sentence (She can't—She didn't do that).

Some parenthetical interjections or asides that are common interruptions in adult speech are devices that help to maintain listener interest. An example of a parenthetical interjection is "When John slipped on the stairs—like Mary slipped in the same spot last week—he broke his ankle."

What are some normal speech disfluencies that you might exhibit under conditions such as speaking in front of a large audience or to a professor whom you find intimidating?

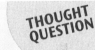
THOUGHT QUESTION

STUTTERED DISFLUENCIES

What is stuttering and how is it different from normally fluent and normally disfluent speech? These are not simple questions, and there are no simple answers. Consider the words of English literary genius Samuel Johnson (1709–1784) when he mused about poetry: "Sir, what is poetry? Why, sir, it is much easier to say what it is not" (Gregory, 1981, p. 416). We might say the same about stuttering.

The chances are that you know what stuttering is, but could you explain what it is? For example, if you viewed a cartoon featuring Porky Pig and were then asked to classify Porky's speech, it is highly likely that you would classify it as stuttering. But what exactly are you reacting to? What aspects of Porky's speech led you to such a conclusion? Your best friend might also classify Porky's speech as stuttering, but is your friend reacting to the same aspects of speech as you are? Clinical and research evidence suggests that even though both of you classify Porky as a stutterer, you might be using different aspects of his speech to lead you to that classification.

The issue of what stuttering is and how to define it lies at the center of some unresolved issues (Ingham & Cordes, 1997). Can clinicians determine reliably if and when stuttering has occurred? Do normal disfluencies and stuttered disfluencies lie along the same continuum or are they categorically different behavioral events? There are no absolute answers to these questions. At present, no universally accepted definition of stuttering exists. However, a reasonable framework from which one can begin to distinguish between normal disfluencies and those that are likely to be regarded as stuttered disfluencies has been proposed:[1]

> Speech, like many other human behaviors, is occasionally produced by speakers with hesitations, interruptions, prolongations and repetitions. These disruptions in . . . ongoing speech behavior are termed *disfluency* and the frequency, duration, type, severity and so forth of these speech disfluencies vary greatly from person to person and from speaking situation to speaking situation. Some speech disfluencies, particularly those which involve within-word disruptions (such as sound or syllable repetitions), are most apt to be classified or judged by listeners as *stuttering*. (Conture, 1990a, p. 2)

Specifically, stuttering or stuttered speech involves part-word repetitions, sound prolongations, monosyllabic whole-word repetitions, and/or within-word pauses (Conture, 1990b). Tense pauses and hesitations between words may also be regarded as stuttering. In other words, stuttering is "any cessation in the forward flow of speech marked by audible or inaudible repetitions or prolongations of word/syllable fragments, including periods of silence between words/syllables" (Prins, Hubbard & Krause, 1991, p. 1012). Examples of stuttered speech can be heard and seen on the book's CD-ROM.

Disfluencies that occur within a word unit that are likely to be regarded as stuttering include monosyllabic whole-word repetitions (he-he-he-he-hit me), sound repetitions (p-p-p-p-pail), syllable repetitions (ba-ba-ba-ba-baseball), audible prolongations (sssssss-snow), and inaudible prolongations, (g——irl). Table 8.1 lists some between-word and within-word disfluency types. More than one type of within-word disfluency may be present in a given disruption that interferes with the forward flow of speech. Consider the following disfluent production of the word "mommy" that contains elements of both a sound repetition and an audible prolongation: "m-m-m-mmmommy" (Yaruss, 1997). Such productions, called "clustered disfluencies," are quite common in the speech of children who stutter. Some researchers have suggested that the presence of clustered disfluencies may indicate incipient (just beginning, in an early stage) stuttering and that they may help to differentiate children who stutter from children who do not stutter.

Within-word disfluencies and some between-word disfluencies are considered to be the cardinal, universal features of stuttering, but there are other behaviors that may accompany instances of disfluency. Behaviors that occur concomitantly with stuttered disfluencies are called secondary symptoms, or accessory behaviors, and are widely varied and idiosyncratic. Some common secondary symptoms include blinking of the eyes; facial grimacing; facial tension; and exaggerated movements of the head, shoulders, and arms. Interjected speech fragments that are superfluous to the utterance are also considered to be secondary symptoms, particularly when they are in connection with a disfluency. An example of an interjected speech fragment is the superfluous phrase "that is to say" in the utterance "I met her in T-T-T-

---

[1]See also Guitar's (1998) definition of stuttering.

TABLE 8.1

Types of within-word (stuttered) and between-word (normal) speech disfluencies

Disfluency Type	Within-Word	Between-Word	Examples
Sound/syllable repetitions	X		He's a b-b-b-boy. G-g-g-g-go away. Yes, puh-puh-please.
Sound prolongation	X		Sssssee me swing! T——oronto is cool.
Broken word	X		Base-(pause)-ball.
Monosyllablic whole-word repetitions	X	X	I-I-I-hit the ball. It's my-my-my-turn.
Multisyllabic whole-word repetitions		X	I'm going-going home.
Phrase repetition/ interjection		X	She hit—she hit me. I like, uh, ya know, big boats.
Revisions		X	He went, he came back.

Source: Adapted from Conture (1990b).

T, that is to say, I met her in Toronto." An example of secondary symptoms can be seen on the book's CD-ROM.

The speaker may have adopted these behaviors in an effort to minimize stuttering (Bloodstein, 1995). The person who stutters discovers through trial and error that some action (e.g., bodily movements) momentarily distracts from the act of speaking and that action appears to help terminate or avoid an instance of stuttering. Behaviors such as eye blinking, however, soon lose their apparent power to reduce stuttering, and the individual is forced to replace the ineffective behavior with a new behavior, such as shrugging the shoulders, to reduce stuttering. Unfortunately, the eye blinking behavior may have become so strongly habituated that it will remain permanently associated with a person's stuttering. How do these cardinal stuttering behaviors and secondary symptoms develop and how do they change over the course of an individual's life?

Do you have a friend who stutters? Can you describe his or her speech behaviors and secondary symptoms?

THOUGHT QUESTIONS

THE ONSET AND DEVELOPMENT OF STUTTERING THROUGH THE LIFESPAN

Although stuttering can develop at any age, the most common form of stuttering begins in the preschool years and is called **developmental stuttering.** Developmental stuttering is contrasted with the second form of stuttering, called **neurogenic stuttering,** which is typically associated with neurological disease or trauma. Neurogenic stuttering differs from the more common developmental stuttering in several ways.

Disfluencies associated with developmental stuttering usually occur on content words (e.g., nouns, verbs), whereas disfluencies associated with neurogenic stuttering tend to occur on function words (e.g., conjunctions, prepositions) and content words. People who have developmental stuttering frequently exhibit secondary symptoms and anxiety about speaking, whereas neurogenic stutterers do not. Finally, developmental stuttering tends to occur on the initial syllables of words, whereas neurogenic stuttering is more widely dispersed throughout the utterance (Ringo & Dietrich, 1995). We will focus primarily on developmental stuttering in this chapter.

It is generally accepted that the onset of developmental stuttering occurs between the ages of 2 and 5 and that the risk of developing stuttering is mostly over by the time the child is 3½ years old (Yairi, 1983, 2004; Yairi & Ambrose, 1992a, b, 2004). The onset of stuttering is gradual for the majority of children who develop the condition, with stuttering severity increasing as the child grows older. When stuttering develops in a gradual manner, some general trends regarding stuttering behaviors, reactions to stuttering, and conditions that seem to promote stuttering can be observed. We will outline some of these developmental trends (Bloodstein, 1995). Not all children will exactly follow this developmental framework of stuttering, but it generally does capture the onset and progression of the disorder. This developmental framework is divided into four phases that have a sequential relationship to each other.

Phase One corresponds to the preschool years, roughly between the ages of 2 and 6. During Phase One, periods of stuttering are followed by periods of relative fluency. The episodic nature of stuttering is an indication that stuttering is in its most rudimentary form. The child may stutter for weeks at a time between long interludes of normally fluent speech. The child will tend to stutter most when he or she is upset or excited, and in conditions of communicative pressure, such as when a parent forces a child to recite in front of friends or relatives. Sound and syllable repetitions are the dominant feature, but there is also a tendency to repeat whole words. Stuttering tends to occur at the beginnings of sentences, clauses, and phrases on both content words (e.g., nouns, verbs) and function words (e.g., articles, prepositions, etc.) unlike more advanced forms of stuttering, in which disfluencies are generally confined to content words. Finally, during Phase One, most children are unaware of the interruptions in their speech.

Phase Two represents a progression of the disorder and is associated with children of elementary school age. In Phase Two, stuttering is essen-

TABLE 8.2

Summary of Bloodstein's four phases of the onset and development of stuttering

Phase	Age	Highlights
One	2–6 years	Stuttering is episodic.
		Most stuttering occurs when the child is upset or excited.
		Sound/syllable repetitions are the dominant speech feature.
		Child seems unaware of the stuttering.
Two	Elementary school age	Stuttering is chronic.
		Stuttering occurs on content words (nouns, verbs).
		Child regards himself or herself as a stutterer.
Three	8 years to adulthood	Stuttering is situational (speaking on the telephone, speaking to large groups).
		Certain words are regarded as more difficult than others.
		Circumlocutions and word substitutions are frequent.
Four	8 years to adulthood	Stuttering is at its apex of development.
		There is fearful anticipation of stuttering.
		Certain sounds, words, and speaking situations are avoided.
		Increased circumlocutions and word substitutions are present.

tially chronic, or habitual, with few intervals of fluent speech. The child has developed a self-concept as a person who stutters and will refer to himself or herself in that way. Stuttering in Phase Two occurs primarily on content words with much less tendency to stutter only on the initial words of sentences and phrases. Stuttering is more widely dispersed throughout the child's utterances. Although the child has a self-concept as a person who stutters, he or she exhibits little or no concern about the stuttering. Stuttering in Phase Two also increases under conditions of excitement.

Phase Three is associated with individuals who can range in age from about 8 years to young adulthood. Stuttering in Phase Three seems to be in response to specific situations such as speaking to strangers, speaking in front of groups, or talking on the telephone. Certain words are regarded as more difficult than others, and the person who stutters will attempt to avoid such words by using word substitutions and circumlocutions. An example of a word substitution is "I want a ni-ni-ni—five cents"; the child substitutes

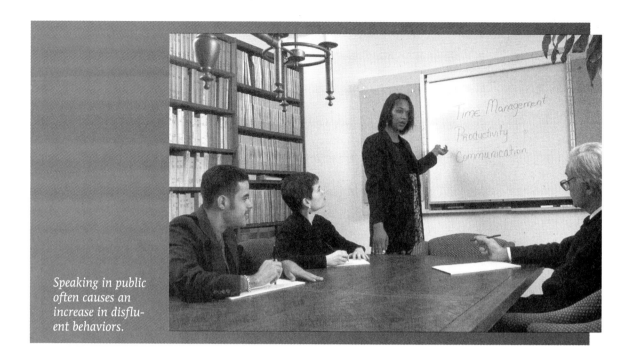

Speaking in public often causes an increase in disfluent behaviors.

"five cents" for the originally intended word "nickel." Circumlocutions are roundabout or indirect ways of speaking. A circumlocution used to avoid the term "fire truck" in a child's request for a toy might take on the following form "I want a—ya know—red thing—sirens and ladders—truck for my birthday." Despite the individual's awareness of stuttering, he or she will present little evidence of fear or embarrassment and will not avoid specific speaking situations.

In Phase Four, the apex of development, stuttering is in its most advanced form. A primary characteristic of Phase Four is vivid and fearful anticipation of stuttering. Certain sounds, words, and speaking situations are feared and avoided, word substitutions and circumlocutions are frequent, and there is evidence of embarrassment. Stuttered words may have associated audible vocal tension and rising pitch, which can be seen on the book's CD-ROM. These phases are summarized in Table 8.2. See Case Study 8.2 for the personal story of a young man whose fear of speaking prevented him from eating his favorite food.

THOUGHT QUESTIONS

What factors might contribute to the changes in a person's reactions to his or her stuttering? What speaking situations do you have that are fearful or very difficult?

Stuttering does not always develop gradually. For some individuals, when stuttering is first diagnosed in young children, the symptoms appear to be very advanced and secondary symptoms may be present (Van Riper, 1982;

Yairi, 2004; Yairi & Ambrose, 1992a, b, 2004; Yairi, Ambrose, & Nierman, 1993). The onset may be a distinct and sudden event for as high as 36 percent of children, and the stuttering behaviors may be considered to be moderate to severe (Yairi & Ambrose, 1992a). More research is needed on the onset and development of stuttering.

Case Study 8.2

Personal Story of a Young Man with Stuttering

Geoff was a teenage boy who was first seen at the speech and hearing clinic on his thirteenth birthday. His parents explained, during an initial interview, that Geoff had begun stuttering when he was around 4 years old. They further explained that the stuttering would come and go, and he would sometimes have fluent periods that lasted two months. Although the parents were concerned about Geoff's stuttering behaviors, they thought that he would outgrow the stuttering. This belief was reinforced by his long periods of fluency.

Geoff was evaluated by an SLP. Formal tests of stuttering placed him as a severe stutterer, most of his stuttering behaviors taking the form of long sound prolongations. Geoff told the SLP that his grades in school were falling because he would not speak in class and that he didn't like to interact with his classmates because they "always make fun of the way I talk." He also reported that there were certain words that he could not say without stuttering severely.

The SLP recommended that Geoff enroll in therapy twice a week for a trial period of six months. The parents and Geoff agreed. He made good progress during this trial period and stayed in therapy for an additional four months. At the end of ten months of therapy, he was dismissed, exhibiting good control over his stuttering.

Two months later, he and his mother came back to the clinic for a reevaluation of his fluency skills. During the reevaluation, Geoff told the SLP that he was happy with his new speech because he could say any word he wanted without stuttering. He told the SLP that he loved to go to McDonald's or Burger King to eat cheeseburgers and French fries. But before therapy, if he had to place his own order, he wouldn't order the French fries because he knew he would stutter on the word "French." He went without the fries more times than he cared to recall. Nowadays, Geoff is enjoying his cheeseburgers *with* the French fries that he orders himself. According to Geoff, that makes him the "happiest kid on the planet."

THE EFFECTS OF STUTTERING THROUGH THE LIFESPAN

Stuttering almost always has its onset in early childhood. Research conducted at the University of Illinois indicates that in 68 percent of the children studied, stuttering onset occurred by 36 months of age and in 95 percent of the children studied by 48 months of age (Yairi, 2004; Yairi & Ambrose, 2004). Although the prevalence of stuttering (the number of persons in the population who stutter) is 1 percent, research indicates that "the magnitude of the problem is much larger among young children" (Yairi & Ambrose, 2004, p. 5). To put the effects of stuttering throughout the lifespan in perspective, however, we will briefly discuss the model developed by the World Health Organization.

From within the context of this model, stuttering is considered to be a *handicap* or a *handicapping condition*. Specifically, a handicap comprises "the disadvantages that result from reactions to the audible and visible events of a person's stuttering, including those of the person who stutters" (Conture, 1996, p. S20). Both informal and formal observations suggest that stuttering has a negative effect on a wide variety of daily life activities, especially in three main venues of life, school, work, and social interactions. Children may withdraw and refuse to communicate orally in school, adults may select professions that require little or no oral communication, and both children and adults may avoid social contact because of a fear of speaking.

Let us first consider the negative impact stuttering can have on a child's school performance. Stutterers, on the whole, are poorer in educational adjustment than normal speakers. This conclusion is based on the amount of retention in grade at school. On average, children who stutter are delayed about half a year or half a grade level. Schoolchildren who stutter are older than their classmates who do not stutter, a finding suggesting that children who stutter are more likely to be held back in school. If so, timely and appropriate treatment should be expected to improve the academic performance of children who stutter (Bloodstein, 1995; Conture, 1996). An additional concern is children's vulnerability to being bullied. School-age children who stutter were significantly more likely to be bullied and/or teased than their peers who do not stutter (Blood & Blood, 2004).

The educational and personal disadvantages stuttering may pose on a young person do not end when the child leaves school. Stuttering can also have a negative impact in the workplace and is a vocationally handicapping condition because employers view it as a disorder that decreases employability and opportunities for promotion (Hurst & Cooper, 1983). Despite this view, when an employee who stutters seeks treatment, there is an attendant improvement in the employer's perception of the employee (Craig & Calvert, 1991). This enhanced perception is reflected by increased numbers of job promotions among employees who sought treatment and were successful in maintaining fluency following treatment.

Stuttering's potential effects on an individual's social interactions and quality of life are not well understood. Clinical observations suggest that successfully treated individuals, particularly adults, experience an improvement in their social interactions, but the nature and significance of these changes in social behavior are not well documented (Conture, 1996). However, considerable research has indicated that people who stutter do not as a group exhibit consistent, recognized patterns of psychoneurotic disturbance, but mild forms of social maladjustment are frequently reported (Bloodstein, 1995). Further research is needed to determine whether and to what extent stuttering treatment influences psychosocial adjustment (Conture, 1996).

THOUGHT QUESTIONS

What kinds of jobs require a great deal of speaking? What kinds of jobs do not require a great deal of speaking? Do you think it likely that people who stutter might choose to avoid jobs that require a great deal of speaking? Explain.

*T*HEORIES AND CONCEPTUALIZATIONS OF STUTTERING

An examination of some of the more prominent etiological theories of stuttering will provide you with an appreciation of the various models that have influenced stuttering research and treatment for over eighty years in this country. Additionally, various aspects of some of the theories we will consider are implicitly present in contemporary stuttering research and treatment. Etiological theories of stuttering can be classified into three categories: organic, behavioral, and psychological.

ORGANIC THEORY

Organic theories propose an actual physical cause for stuttering. Speculations about a physical cause for stuttering date back to the writings of Aristotle, who suggested that stuttering was a disconnection between the mind and the body and that the muscles of the tongue could not follow the commands of the brain (Rieber & Wollock, 1977). Many organic theories have been proposed since Aristotle's writings, but they have all failed in one manner or another to explain stuttering satisfactorily. For example, the *theory of cerebral dominance* or the "handedness theory" proposed by Samuel Orton and Lee Travis in the 1930s (Bloodstein, 1995) assumed that when neither cerebral hemisphere was dominant, both would send competing neural impulses to their respective muscles of speech, resulting in a discoordination between the right and left halves of the speech musculature. This discoordination was believed to result in stuttering. Subsequent research and clinical observation ultimately led to the demise of this theory.

Speculations about potential organic origins of stuttering reemerged in the 1970s, based largely on the observations of Marcel Wingate. Wingate (1969, 1970) developed the modified vocalization hypothesis, which asserted that stuttering was reduced greatly in conditions in which voicing was absent (whispering) or modified in some way through singing or speaking with delayed auditory feedback. (Delayed auditory feedback is discussed later this chapter.) A great deal of research conducted in the 1970s indicated that the amount of stuttering was reduced proportionally as the rapid shift between voiced and unvoiced sounds associated with spontaneous speech was reduced. Such research findings led Wingate and other investigators to suggest that stuttering was a discoordination between the muscles used for phonation and other muscles that are used during speech production.

The continued search for a specific organic cause of stuttering has been enhanced recently by developments in medical technology. Researchers are currently studying the central nervous system of people who stutter using techniques such as computerized tomography, magnetic resonance imaging, and the measurement of regional cerebral blood flow. The findings of this research, although preliminary, indicate that stuttering may be linked to the failure of a neurophysiological system that integrates motoric, linguistic, and cognitive processes (Watson & Freeman, 1997). Future brain imaging research may facilitate the development of a comprehensive neurophysio-

Many stuttering treatment programs include specific behavioral modification techniques such as rewarding fluent speech and punishing stuttered speech. Clinical research investigating the behavioral technique of contingent time-out from speaking following a stuttered utterance is showing great promise.

logical model for both fluent and stuttered speech that could lead to new stuttering prevention and treatment methods (c.f., Ingham, Ingham, Finn, & Fox, 2003).

BEHAVIORAL THEORY

Behavioral theories assert that stuttering is a learned response to conditions external to the individual. A prominent behavioral theory, the *diagnosogenic* theory, was developed by Wendell Johnson during the 1940s and 1950s. Johnson contended that the speech hesitations of children whose parents believed their children to be stuttering did not differ from the speech hesitations of children whose parents did not consider them to be stuttering. The differences between these two groups of children lay in the parental reactions to these hesitations. Johnson's conclusions stand as a formal statement of his theory:

1. Practically every case of stuttering was originally diagnosed, not by a speech expert, but by a layperson—usually one, or both, of the child's parents.

2. What these laypersons had diagnosed as stuttering was, by and large, indistinguishable from the hesitations and repetitions known to be characteristic of the normal speech of young children.

3. Stuttering . . . as a definite disorder was found to occur, not before being diagnosed, but after being diagnosed (Bloodstein, 1995, p. 77).

For Johnson, stuttering began in the parent's ear, not in the child's mouth. Overly concerned parents would react to the child's normal speech hesitations and repetitions with negative statements admonishing the child to speak more slowly and not to stutter. Such parental behaviors made the child anxious about speaking, and the child's anxiety fostered further hesitations and repetitions. The parents would react with increased criticism and punishment, which in turn raised the child's anxiety level about speaking and increased disfluent speech behaviors. The child's disfluent behaviors soon became a habitual manner of speaking. Although the basic premises of the theory have been seriously questioned, parent-child communicative interactions play a pivotal role in certain contemporary therapeutic regimes to be discussed later in this chapter.

THOUGHT QUESTIONS

In what ways could a parent's speech pattern influence the speech pattern of his or her child? For example, could the rate of a parent's speech affect the child's speech?

PSYCHOLOGICAL THEORY

Psychological theory contends that stuttering is a neurotic symptom with ties to unconscious needs and internal conflicts, treated most appropriately by psychotherapy. Some psychological theories regard people who stutter as individuals with neuroses; other theories regard stuttering as a phobic manifestation. However, research indicates that psychotherapy is not an effective method for the treatment of stuttering. Some people who stutter may indeed have neuroses, but psychological theory has yet to provide a cogent explanation for the underlying cause of stuttering or its onset and development.

CURRENT CONCEPTUAL MODELS OF STUTTERING

The *covert repair hypothesis,* based on a language production model, assumes that stuttering is a reaction to some flaw in the phonetic plan of speech (Postma & Kolk, 1993). Speakers have the capability of monitoring their speech as it is being formulated and detecting errors in the speech plan. People who stutter have poorly developed phonological encoding skills that cause them to introduce errors into their speech plan. If there are more errors in the speech plan, there will be more occasions for error correction. Stuttering is not the error. Rather, stuttering is a "normal" repair reaction to an abnormal phonetic plan.

Another relatively new conceptualization of stuttering is the *demands and capacities model* (DCM) (Starkweather, 1987, 1997). This model asserts that stuttering develops when the environmental demands placed on a child to produce fluent speech exceed the child's physical and learned capacities. The child's capacity for fluent speech depends on a balance of motor skills, language production skills, emotional maturity, and cognitive development. Children who stutter presumably lack one or more of these capacities for fluent speech. Parents of a child who lacks the required motor skills for fluency might talk rapidly; rapid rates of speech may put a time pressure on the child that exceeds his or her motoric ability to respond. Other parents might insist on the use of advanced language structures that are in excess of the child's language development. In every case of stuttering within the DCM, there is an imbalance between the environmental demands that are placed on the child and the child's capacity for fluent speech.

The DCM is not a theory of stuttering, and it does not suggest a cause for stuttering. Rather, the DCM is a useful tool that helps clinicians to understand the dynamics of forces that contribute to the development of stuttering. Therapeutically, the DCM provides useful guidelines for understanding what capacities a child may lack for fluent speech production and the elements of the child's environment that may be challenging those capacities.

One more theoretical construct regarding stuttering is worthy of mention. The EXPLAN model (Howell, 2004) is an account of the production of spontaneous speech that applies to both fluent speakers and speakers who stutter. In this model, speech planning (PLAN) is the linguistic process of language formulation, and execution (EX) is the motor activity related to production of the language formulation. Although some theoretical accounts of stuttering have placed the primary site of disruption in the language formulation phase and other accounts have placed the primary site at the instructions sent to the motor system, the EXPLAN model posits that stuttering results from a failure in normal interactions between the PLAN and EX processes (Howell, 2004). Fluency failures occur when linguistic plans are sent too slowly to the motor system. This detailed, scientifically sophisticated model may further our understanding of the basic nature of stuttering and also the basic nature of stuttering treatment.

THOUGHT QUESTION

Your professor has called on you in class to explain a problem that was part of the homework assignment that you didn't complete. What happens to your speech patterns?

THERAPEUTIC TECHNIQUES USED WITH YOUNG CHILDREN

When parents are concerned that a child is stuttering, it is the speech-language pathologist's (SLP) responsibility to determine whether there should be concern and, if so, to plan an appropriate course of action. Two important components of the evaluation of a child suspected of stuttering are observations of the child and parents interacting with one another and a detailed parental interview (see Table 8.3 for some common questions for parents with a disfluent child).

THE EVALUATION OF STUTTERING

A number of aspects of parent-child interactions have been identified as contributing to stuttering in children, including excessive parental speech rates exceeding 200 words per minute, the use of complex linguistic structures that are too sophisticated for the child, and frequent parental interruptions. Although these parental behaviors do not cause stuttering, they are quite likely to exacerbate or perpetuate the stuttering (Conture, 1990b). Careful observation of parent-child interactions will provide vital information that will be used later in parent counseling.

A second important component of the stuttering evaluation is a detailed analysis of the child's speech behaviors. The SLP determines the average number of each type of disfluency the child produces (e.g., within-word repetitions, sound prolongations). Three or more within-word disfluencies per 100 words spoken may indicate that the child has a fluency problem (Conture, 1990b). The percentage of the total disfluency that each type of disfluency contributes is another important evaluative measure. For example, if the child produces 10 disfluencies per 100 words spoken and 6 of them are sound prolongations, then 60 percent of all the disfluencies are sound prolongations. A high percentage of sound prolongations may indicate a

TABLE 8.3
Common questions for parents of a disfluent child

Introduction

Why are you here today?

Tell us (me) about your child's problem.

General Development

Tell us (me) about your child's development from birth to present.

How does this compare with his or her siblings?

Family History

Do any other family members have speech, hearing, or language problems?

Did they receive speech therapy?

Speech/Language Development

When did your child say his or her first words?

When did your child say his or her first phrases and sentences?

History/Description of the Problem

Describe your child's speaking problems.

When did the problem start?

What was your reaction? Did you bring the

problem to your child's attention?

Can you describe your child's stuttering when it first began?

Has it changed over time?

Does your child lose eye contact when talking to you?

Does your child have excessive body movements when talking?

Does he or she avoid speaking situations?

Have you done anything to help your child stop stuttering?

Family Interactions

What do you and your child do when you spend time together?

What kind of things do you do as a family?

How do you handle sibling hostilities?

Wrap Up

If you could wish for three things for your child, what would you wish for?

Source: Adapted from Conture (1990b).

chronic fluency problem. The SLP will also measure the duration of several disfluencies. Longer durations and/or multiple sound or syllable repetitions may represent an increase in the severity of the stuttering problem.

Standardized tests such as the *Stuttering Prediction Instrument* (SPI; Riley & Riley, 1981) may also be used in the fluency evaluation. The SPI yields a numerical score based on a number of stuttering-related behaviors such as the duration of disfluencies and stuttering frequency. The numerical score is converted to a verbal stuttering severity rating. Finally, the SLP will record the types of secondary symptoms that the child presents. A wide assortment of secondary symptoms may indicate a progression of the disorder.

The SLP's decision to recommend therapy is not based on any single behavior or test result. Therapy may be recommended if two or more of the following behaviors are observed:

1. Sound prolongations constitute more than 25 percent of the total disfluencies produced by the child.

2. Instances of sound or syllable repetitions or sound prolongations on the first syllables of words during iterative speech tasks (e.g., iterative productions of pa-ta-ka, pa-ta-ka, pa-ta-ka).

3. Loss of eye contact on more than 50 percent of the child's utterances.

4. A score of 18 or more on the SPI (Conture, 1990b).

INDIRECT AND DIRECT STUTTERING INTERVENTION

If the SLP determines that the child has a stuttering problem or a high probability of developing stuttering, therapeutic intervention is indicated. In general, two broad intervention strategies can be used with young children who stutter: indirect therapy and direct therapy. Indirect approaches are considered viable for children who are just beginning to stutter and whose stuttering is fairly mild. Direct approaches are typically reserved for children who have been stuttering for at least a year and whose stuttering is moderate to severe.

An indirect approach does not explicitly try to modify or change the child's speech fluency, focusing instead on the child, the child's parents, and the child's environment. Important aspects of indirect therapy are information sharing and counseling in which the parent is encouraged to reduce communicative pressure on the child and provide a slow, relaxed speech model for the child. Play-oriented activities that encourage slow and relaxed speech are the central component of such intervention. There is no explicit discussion about the child's fluent or stuttering speaking behaviors. The goal of indirect therapy is to facilitate fluency through environmental manipulation.

THOUGHT QUESTION   :   *What kinds of activities might be used to encourage slow, relaxed speech?*

Direct approaches involve explicit and direct attempts to modify the child's speech and speech-related behaviors. In direct therapy, concepts such as "hard" and "easy" speech are introduced. Hard speech is rapid and relatively tense (such as a tense sound prolongation of /s/ in sssssssss-snake), whereas easy speech is slow and relaxed. The terms "hard" and "easy" are simple and carry little negative connotation for the child. Children are taught to identify both types of speech by first monitoring their tape-recorded utterances and later by identifying these types of speech in their ongoing productions. Once the child is able to accurately and reliably identify hard and easy speech segments, the SLP teaches the child strategies that will help him or her increase easy speech and change from hard speech to easy speech when required. The therapeutic sequence of identification followed by identification/modification forms the core elements of many strategies for children and adults.

PARENTAL COUNSELING

Whether or not a young child is recommended for therapy, parental counseling is almost always indicated. In addition to providing the parents with information about normal speech and language development, the SLP needs to suggest ways that will help their child to speak in an easy, effortless manner. There are some important issues that need to be stressed in a parental counseling session (Perkins 1992). First, parents and other family members should provide relaxed and slow speech models for the child. Relaxed and slow speech can be accomplished by prolonging vowels, delaying response times, and pausing frequently during conversational speech. Simply telling the child to "slow down" or "relax" might cause the child to feel self-conscious or anxious about speaking, which in turn might increase stuttering behaviors. Slow and relaxed communicative situations facilitate fluency by reducing pressure on the child to compete for time on the floor. Another way to reduce communicative pressure is to have one parent spend time with the child in a one-to-one context. One-to-one speaking situations provide an opportunity for the child to communicate without interruptions from other children or adults. Parents should also be counseled to reduce the general level of excitement in the home and to avoid negative verbal interactions between the child and other family members. Finally, parents should not pressure the child to talk or perform verbally.

What are some other ways a parent could reduce communicative pressure on his or her child?

THOUGHT QUESTION

THERAPEUTIC TECHNIQUES USED WITH OLDER CHILDREN AND ADULTS WHO STUTTER

Individuals who continue to stutter into their teenage years and beyond will likely have many negative reactions to speaking situations that may affect their social lives and vocational goals. Many of these individuals will have had previous unsuccessful speech therapy and perhaps other forms of remediation to combat the fluency problem. The adult who stutters "brings a complexity of attitudes, experiences, and coping attempts to the therapeutic process, and these must be dealt with directly or indirectly" (Gelfer, 1996, p. 160).

The primary focus of this section is on therapeutic techniques that are used to manage adulthood stuttering. In particular, we will explore direct techniques that are used to establish fluency. Changing certain aspects of one's speaking behavior is of fundamental importance in stuttering intervention and is often a source of confusion among clinicians who treat the adults who stutter (Sommers & Caruso, 1995).

Delayed auditory feedback systems use a microphone and earphones. A person wearing the earphones speaks into the microphone, which transmits the speech to a device that electronically delays sending the speech to the earphones. If the delay were set at 250 milliseconds (or ¼ second) the speaker would hear his or her utterance ¼ of a second after it was uttered. Delaying the auditory feedback causes the speaker to reduce the rate of speaking.

Therapeutic techniques designed to modify stuttering behaviors are classified generally into two broad categories: *fluency-shaping techniques* and *stuttering modification techniques.* When used properly, both techniques have a powerful effect in reducing stuttering. Fluency-shaping techniques involve changing the overall speech timing patterns of the individual. This is typically accomplished by lengthening the duration of sounds and words and greatly slowing down the overall rate of speech. Stuttering modification techniques involve changing only the stuttering behaviors. This is typically accomplished by lengthening the duration of or in some way modifying only the speech segment on which the stuttering is occurring.

A different and perhaps more useful way of classifying therapeutic techniques considers those that modify the "timing of speech movements" and those that modify the "physical tension of speech movements" (Max & Caruso, 1997). Although we will be discussing various techniques that modify speech timing and physical tension as individual entities, combinations of these various individual techniques can be used therapeutically. That is, many of these techniques are not mutually exclusive, and elements of several techniques can be used simultaneously in the treatment of stuttering. It is not well understood exactly how these various techniques reduce stuttering, and their genesis has come largely from the clinical trenches of trial and error. Techniques that modify the timing of speech movements will be discussed first.

MODIFYING THE TIMING OF SPEECH MOVEMENTS

Reducing the rate of speech, known as *prolonged speech,* is one of the most frequently used techniques to reduce stuttering. Prolonged speech may be a specific therapeutic goal, or it may be used as strategy to control the occurrence of stuttering (Max & Caruso, 1997). The term "prolonged speech" arose from research conducted in the 1960s regarding the effects of delayed auditory feedback (DAF) on speech production. DAF is a condition in which a speaker hears his or her own speech after an instrumental delay of some finite period of time, such as 250 or 500 milliseconds. When a person speaks under DAF, his or her speech is slowed down involuntarily because the duration of syllables is prolonged. For example, when people who stutter speak under conditions of DAF, speaking rates decrease dramatically, and the longer the delay, the slower the speech. The slowed speaking rate associated with DAF is accompanied by a substantial decrease in stuttering.

When DAF is used clinically to prolong speech, the feedback delay is set to promote speaking rates of approximately 30 to 60 syllables per minute. During this initial phase, the person who stutters is taught to prolong the duration of each syllable but not to increase the duration of pauses between syllables (Boburg & Kully, 1995; Max & Caruso, 1997). This prolonged speech pattern is systematically altered over the course of intervention by adjusting the DAF times to reduce the magnitude of syllable prolongation while maintaining fluent speech. Speech rates ranging from 120 to 200 syllables per minute are typical targets for the termination of therapy. An example of DAF-facilitated prolonged speech can be seen on the book's CD-ROM.

Another clinical rate reduction technique, called *pausing/phrasing,* is designed to lengthen naturally occurring pauses (clause and sentence boundaries) and to add pauses between other words or phrases. Additionally, pausing/phrasing techniques may attempt to limit utterance length to 2 to 5 syllables. Both this strategy and DAF have an ameliorative or lessening effect on the frequency of stuttering. A formal stuttering treatment known as the *Gradual Increase in Length and Complexity of Utterance* (Ryan, 1974) capitalizes on the underlying principles of pausing/phrasing techniques.

Three techniques developed by Charles Van Riper can be placed under the general rubric of modifying the timing of speech movements. Van Riper conceptualized stuttering as a disorder of speech timing, and he later proposed that his techniques were designed to improve the sequential ordering and timing of speech motor acts (Van Riper, 1982). As such, three of these widely used techniques, known as *cancellations, pull-outs,* and *preparatory sets,* are considered under modifying speech timing movements.

These three techniques are introduced therapeutically in sequential order, beginning with stuttering cancellation. During the cancellation phase of therapy, an individual is required to complete the word that was stuttered and pause deliberately following the production of that stuttered word. The individual pauses for a minimum of three seconds and then reproduces the stuttered word in slow motion. This ostensibly provides practice with the motoric integration and speech timing movements that are required for a fluent production of that word. When the individual reaches a criterion level of cancellation proficiency, he or she will move to the second technique, known as pull-outs.

During the pull-out phase of therapy, the individual does not wait until after the stuttered word is completed to correct the inappropriate behavior. Rather, the individual modifies the stuttered word during the actual occurrence of the stuttering. This modification involves slowing down the sequential movements of the syllable or word when stuttering occurs in a fashion similar to the slowed and exaggerated movements that were learned in the cancellation phase of therapy. In essence, the individual is modifying the stuttering online, "pulling out" of the stuttering behavior and completing it with a more fluent production of the intended word. Once again, when the individual reaches a criterion level of proficiency, he or she will move to the last stage, known as preparatory sets.

Preparatory sets involve using the slow-motion speech strategies that were learned during the first two phases of therapy, not as a response to an occurrence of stuttering, but in anticipation of stuttering. A person who stutters typically knows when and on what word a stuttering will occur. When an individual anticipates a stuttering, he or she will start preparing to use the newly learned fluency producing strategies before the word is attempted. The goal of this phase of therapy is to initiate the word in a more fluent manner even though the individual is producing consecutive speech movements and transitions in a slowed manner.

MODIFYING THE PHYSICAL TENSION OF SPEECH MOVEMENTS

Techniques designed to modify the physical tension of speech movements reduce the amount of physical tension in the speech musculature before and

People who stutter frequently use excessive articulator pressure when producing sounds. They may, for example, press the tongue very hard on the roof of the mouth during the production of /t/ and /d/ sounds. Teaching the individual to reduce such pressure, or make light articulatory contacts, promotes fluency.

during occurrences of stuttering. Some of the common forms of these techniques are discussed below.

Light articulatory contacts are particularly germane to the production of stop consonants (/b/, /p/, /t/, /d/, /k/, and /g/) because production of this class of speech sounds requires a complete constriction somewhere in the vocal tract (Max & Caruso, 1997). The therapeutic use of light articulatory contacts involves instructing an individual to use less tension in the articulators used for the constriction. It is believed that reducing articulatory tension will prevent the occurrence of prolonged articulatory postures that interfere with smooth articulatory transitions from sound to sound. Light touches promote continuity and ease of articulation by preventing excessive pressure and tension in the articulators (Boburg & Kully, 1995).

There are two related intervention techniques that are used to modify the manner in which a person who stutters initiates his or her voice; both are powerful fluency enhancers. These two techniques are called *gentle voicing onsets* (GVOs) and *speaking after exhalation has begun* (Max & Caruso, 1997). Gentle voicing onsets are a cardinal feature of many therapy programs, and they are known by many different names, such as Fluency Initiation Gestures (FIGS) (Cooper, 1984). The basic characteristic of GVOs is a tension-free onset of voicing that gradually builds in intensity. One can appreciate the dynamics of this technique by initiating production of the vowel /a/ in a whisper, gradually engaging the vocal folds such that the vowel is produced with a breathy voice quality, and finally increasing the vowel's intensity. The apparent fluency enhancing effects of GVOs are presumably related to reduced vocal fold tension, which reduces tense adduction of the vocal folds. In most therapeutic programs, GVOs are learned in a hierarchical fashion beginning with vowel production, followed by syllable productions, and then word productions.

THOUGHT QUESTION

*C*an you initiate a vocalization using GVO? Try producing the /a/ or any vowel as described above.

A technique related to GVOs is speaking after exhalation has begun. This technique delays initiation of speech until after exhalation has begun rather than initiating voicing at the onset of exhalation (Max & Caruso, 1997; Neilson & Andrews, 1993). In clinical application, an individual is taught to inhale, begin to exhale, and then initiate speech shortly after the exhalation has begun. This technique is first taught in single syllables with gradual increases in utterance length up to the conversational level (Culatta & Goldberg, 1995; Max & Caruso, 1997).

SELECTING INTERVENTION TECHNIQUES

The SLP's selection of a specific fluency-establishing technique will depend on many factors, including the severity of the stuttering problem, the motivation and specific needs of the person who stutters, and the SLP's knowledge of the specific techniques available. Careful and detailed observation of an individual's stuttering behaviors before initiating treatment and during the treatment process is an essential component of successful clinical management. Such observation will assist the SLP in "selecting, combining, and modifying available techniques in order to teach the client how to alter timing and tension aspects of his or her speech movements" (Max & Caruso, 1997, p. 50). In short, a one-size-fits-all clinical program does not and should not exist. Inherent differences among individuals within the stuttering population prohibit the use of inflexible clinical protocols that cannot be modified to meet the individual's needs.

THE EFFECTIVENESS OF STUTTERING INTERVENTION THROUGH THE LIFESPAN

Determining how effective stuttering treatment is depends largely on how "effectiveness" is defined. This is a complex issue. However, a "treatment for stuttering might be considered *effective* if it resulted in the individual's being able to speak with disfluencies within normal limits whenever and to whomever he or she chose, without undue concern or worry about speaking" (Conture, 1996, p. S20). The treatment of stuttering differs across an individual's lifespan in terms of frequency and nature of therapy, and rates of recovery. Therefore, the review of treatment efficacy is probably best considered relative to four age groups: preschoolers, school-age children, teenagers, and adults.

EFFICACY OF INTERVENTION WITH PRESCHOOL-AGE CHILDREN

In general, the findings of most recent studies are quite encouraging and indicate the potential benefits of early diagnosis and treatment of stuttering. As many as 91 percent of preschool children who had been in a stuttering treatment program maintained their fluent speech five years subsequent to their initial evaluation (Fosnot, 1993). Among preschool-age children enrolled in a parent-conducted therapy program, all maintained their fluent speech four years after dismissal from treatment (Lincoln & Onslow, 1997). In another study, 100 percent of 45 preschool-age children who stuttered had maintained fluent speech two years following dismissal from treatment (Gottwald & Starkweather, 1995).

EFFICACY OF INTERVENTION WITH SCHOOL-AGE CHILDREN

One noteworthy study of stuttering treatment effectiveness utilized four different treatment approaches with school-age children and reported an average 60 percent posttreatment improvement (Ryan & Van Kirk Ryan, 1983). Even better results were found in another study in which 96 percent of the school-age children enrolled in two treatment programs maintained fluent speech fourteen months after treatment (Ryan & Van Kirk Ryan, 1995).

The findings of nine investigations of the effectiveness of stuttering treatment involving 160 school-age children are mildly encouraging. The findings of these studies indicated a 61 percent average (range of 33 percent to over 90 percent) decrease in stuttering frequency and/or stuttering severity across the nine studies. As with the stuttering treatment efficacy findings among preschool-age children, these studies suggest cautious optimism (Conture, 1996).

EFFICACY OF INTERVENTION WITH ADOLESCENTS AND ADULTS

Teenagers who stutter can be difficult to manage clinically, and very little information is available regarding specific therapy programs for this age group (Daly, Simon, & Burnett-Stolnack, 1995; Schwartz, 1993). In sharp contrast, many reports of treatment outcomes for the adult who stutters are available. A wide variety of adult stuttering treatment techniques have been investigated, ranging from operant conditioning techniques to drug therapies. Collectively, these studies suggest a 60 to 80 percent improvement rate regardless of the therapeutic technique that was used. However, two specific treatment techniques seem to yield superior benefits for the adult stutterer. These two treatments use the techniques of prolonged speech and/or gentle voicing onsets (Andrews, Guitar, & Howie, 1980; Conture, 1996; Ingham, 1990). Both of these techniques seem to result in both short- and long-term reductions in stuttering frequency and severity. These two stuttering therapies, as well as many other stuttering therapies, will soon be under serious scientific scrutiny in conjunction with ASHA's recent initiative to have speech-language pathology become an evidence-based discipline. For a general discussion of evidence-based practice with regard to stuttering, see Kully and Langevin (2005).

In summary, stuttering intervention across all age groups results in an average improvement for about 70 percent of all cases, with preschool-age children improving more quickly and easily than people who have a longer history with stuttering. The clinical research that we have considered indicates that effective treatment of stuttering is increasingly able to improve the daily life of people who stutter by increasing their ability to communicate whenever and with whomever they choose without undue concern about speaking.

SUMMARY

Stuttering is a handicapping condition primarily characterized by sound and syllable repetitions and sound prolongations that interrupt the smooth forward flow of speech. Stuttering is a universal problem that affects males more than females. In most cases, stuttering appears between the ages of 2 to 4 years, and as the disorder progresses, it increases in severity. Stuttering can adversely affect an individual's school performance, employment, and social interactions. The treatment of stuttering is most effective when it is initiated in early childhood, although treatment at any age can reduce stuttering.

A number of theories—organic, behavioral, and psychological—attempt to account for the onset and development of stuttering, but its cause is unknown. Solving the riddle of stuttering will undoubtedly require expertise from many specialists including SLPs, neurolinguists, geneticists, and medical specialists. Perhaps one of you reading this text will find your own birch tree and take up Van Riper's quest to find the cause and a cure for stuttering.

REFLECTIONS

- What is the difference between the incidence and the prevalence of stuttering? What are the incidence and prevalence of stuttering?
- How can stuttering affect one's life in school, at work, and in one's social interactions?
- What are normal disfluencies and how do they differ from stuttering?
- Briefly describe the onset and development of stuttering using Bloodstein's phases.
- What are the general stuttering treatment procedures that are used with children who stutter?
- What are rate reduction techniques and what are cancellations, pull-outs, and preparatory sets?
- How effective is stuttering treatment for preschool-age children, school-age children, and adults?

SUGGESTED READINGS

Bloodstein, O. (1995). *A handbook on stuttering.* San Diego: Singular Publishing Group.

Conture, E. G. (1990). *Stuttering* (2nd ed.). Englewood Cliffs, NJ: Prentice-Hall.

Curlee, R. F., & Siegel, G. M. (1997). *Nature and treatment of stuttering: New directions.* Boston: Allyn and Bacon.

Guitar, B. (1998). *Stuttering: An integrated approach to its nature and treatment* (2nd ed.). Baltimore, MD: Williams and Wilkins.

Onslow, M. (2004). Advice to students of stuttering treatment. *Contemporary Issues in Communication Science and Disorders, 31,* 5–24.

Yaruss, J. S. (1997). Clinical measurement of stuttering behaviors. *Contemporary Issues in Communication Science and Disorders, 24,* 33–44.

Yaruss, J. S. (2004). Documenting individual treatment outcomes in stuttering therapy. *Contemporary Issues in Communication Sciences and Disorders, 31,* 49–57.

ONLINE RESOURCES

http://www.stuttersfa.org Website of the Stuttering Foundation of America. Available catalogs, referral lists, videotapes, and excellent information about stuttering.

The Voice and Voice Disorders

9

CHAPTER LEARNING GOALS

When you have finished this chapter, you should be able to:

- Explain the normal phonation process
- Describe the perceptual signs of a voice disorder
- Describe voice disorders that are associated with vocal misuse or abuse, medical or physical conditions, and psychological or stress conditions
- Describe the major goals of voice therapy

Voice is our primary means of expression and is an essential feature of the uniquely human attribute known as speech (Boone & McFarlane, 2000; Colton & Casper, 1996; Titze, 1994). Your voice reflects gender, personality, personal habits, age, and the general condition of health. Research has shown that certain characteristics of the voice reflect various personality dimensions, and these vocal characteristics correlate well with standardized tests of personality (Colton & Casper, 1990; Markel, Meisels, & Houck, 1964). Your voice is an emotional outlet that mirrors your moods, attitudes, and general feelings. Expressions of anger can be achieved by shouting, and expressions of affection can be achieved by speaking softly; these types of vocal expression have great potential to evoke emotional responses from a listener. Evoking emotional responses from listeners through controlled vocal expression is key to a successful operatic performance. Dramatic actors achieve pathos through deliberate and controlled vocal expression. The evocative nature of vocal expressions, however, is hardly limited to stage performances. We constantly vary the tone of our voices to achieve some specific meaning or intention. Your voice is a powerful tool that delivers a message and simultaneously adds to the meaning of that message (Colton & Casper, 1990).

THOUGHT QUESTIONS

Has anyone ever told you "I don't like the tone of your voice"? What does that expression mean?

Case Study 9.1

Case Study of a Young Man with a Voice Impairment: Lamar

Lamar, a 20-year-old college student, was seen at the university medical center's communicative disorders unit on a Monday late in October. Lamar, an avid college football fan, attended all his school's home games. He had attended the home football game that was held the Saturday before he reported to the communicative disorders unit. Lamar reported that he was yelling loudly during much of Saturday's game until his voice became weak. He further reported that when he woke on Sunday morning it felt like there was something stuck in his throat. As he spoke, the SLP noted that his voice quality was very hoarse and excessively breathy.

The SLP referred Lamar to the otolaryngology department of the medical center. There, an otolaryngologist examined Lamar's vocal folds using a flexible fiberoptic endoscope. The otolaryngologist reported that Lamar had a large unilateral sessile polyp on his right vocal fold, and she recommended that the polyp be removed surgically. It was further recommended that following the removal of the polyp Lamar should be scheduled for voice therapy.

One month following surgery, Lamar began attending voice therapy. The principal focus of therapeutic intervention was to educate Lamar regarding conditions that are detrimental to vocal fold tissue and to educate him regarding proper vocal hygiene. Lamar remains an avid football fan, but he uses his voice in a healthy fashion when he attends games.

As you read this chapter, think about

- Why the SLP referred Lamar to the otolaryngologist.
- Why Lamar required voice therapy following the polyp's removal.
- What possible strategies Lamar was taught to promote vocal hygiene.

CHANGES IN VOICE PRODUCTION THROUGH THE LIFESPAN

The manner in which you use your voice changes with each major stage of life: infancy and childhood, adulthood, and advanced age. Changes in the voice are related to biological, cognitive, social, and emotional maturation Sapienza et al., (2004).

INFANCY AND CHILDHOOD

Crying is how an infant uses the voice to express pain, hunger, or displeasure and is the major avenue for infant communication. Cooing is how the infant uses the voice to express pleasure, happiness, and contentment. Both crying and cooing reflect the beginning of the infant's ability to control his or her voice and, in turn, his or her environment.

As children mature, they begin to use voice for the production of speech sounds and to express ideas and moods. Mature intentional patterns are mimicked before children learn words to fit these patterns. Later, pitch and intensity changes are used to denote differences of meaning and intention.

ADULTHOOD

The adult voice is achieved by about the age of 18 years (Kahane, 1982; Titze, 1994). At this age, the individual has full control over the voice and is capable of using many variations of pitch, loudness, and vocal expression. Under normal circumstances, the average speaking pitch or frequency of your voice should remain constant for the next several decades, and the way your voice is used will be determined by specific situational demands.

Adults frequently abuse their voice through excessive misuse. Some jobs, for example, require speaking in the presence of loud machinery or background noise. Such conditions might require the use of very loud vocal production, which can affect the voice negatively. Smoke and alcohol adversely affect the voice. Even if a person recognizes that he or she is engaging in abusive vocal habits, making the necessary changes to eliminate the aggravating condition is frequently difficult. In addition to vocal abuse, certain disease processes such as cancer or neurological dysfunctions can adversely affect the adult voice (Colton & Casper, 1990).

Do you like the music of Elton John? He had trouble with his voice during a tour of the United States in 1986 and was forced to cancel engagements. Fortunately, his voice problem was associated with a nonmalignant lesion that was corrected surgically. Do you think that vocal performing might injure vocal fold tissue?

THOUGHT QUESTIONS

ADVANCED AGE

The voice begins to decline in much the same way that other body functions begin to decline after the age of 60 or so. Typical voice changes include increases or decreases in vocal pitch, a decreased capacity to control the vocal loudness, and diminished vocal quality (Colton & Casper, 1990; Kahane, 1982; Titze, 1994). For example, with advanced age, the pitch of the voice tends to decrease in females and to increase in males. Such unidirectional gender-linked voice pitch changes have been associated with decreased estrogen levels in females and decreased testosterone levels in males (Hollien, 1987; Kent, 1997; Titze, 1994).

By simply listening to someone's voice, even untrained listeners can make reasonable estimates of that person's chronological age. Additionally, physiological age, which is determined by standard measures of blood pressure, heart rate, vital capacity, and the like, more closely determines the quality of one's voice than chronological age (Ramig & Ringel, 1983; Shipp, Qi, Huntley, & Hollien, 1992; Titze, 1994). Staying in shape pays many dividends.

Demands on the voice are different for the adult of advanced age than for younger adults. For example, the retired college professor no longer needs to deliver lengthy lectures that can strain the voice in large classrooms.

Despite the general physiological decline in aged individuals, the voice retains its central importance for communication. Verbal communication may be the only manner in which a person of advanced age can "maintain human contact and control the environment" (Colton & Casper, 1990, p. 5).

From this brief introduction, it should be clear that the human voice is a dynamic multidimensional tool that is central to verbal communication.[1] In Chapter 3, we discussed the basic concepts related to normal voice production. We will extend some of these basic concepts in this chapter with a discussion of how one changes the pitch and loudness of the voice. Next, we will discuss voice disorders in children and adults associated with vocal misuse and hyperfunction, abnormal medical and physical conditions, and psychological and stress conditions. Finally, assessment, treatment, and treatment efficacy issues will be discussed.

> During one complete vibratory cycle of vocal fold vibration, the vocal folds move from a closed or adducted position to an open or abducted position and back to the closed position.

PITCH AND THE PITCH-CHANGING MECHANISM

You are probably aware that the relative pitch of your voice is somewhat dependent on your sex and age. *Pitch* of the voice is the perceptual counterpart to fundamental frequency associated with the speed of vocal fold vibration. As the speed of vocal fold vibration increases, the perceived pitch of the voice increases. As we discussed in Chapter 3, the speed at which the vocal folds vibrate is called the fundamental frequency of the voice. Frequency is measured in **hertz (Hz),** or the number of complete vibrations per second.

---

[1]It should be noted that the primary biological functions of laryngeal structures, including the vocal folds, are to prevent foreign objects from entering the trachea and to impound air for forceful expulsion (coughing) of such objects.

The fundamental frequency of the voice varies considerably during speaking, but each individual speaker has an average fundamental frequency, or *habitual pitch*. Each individual also has a particularly suitable pitch level known as the **optimal pitch level,** which is largely determined by vocal fold structure. For example, on average, adult men have fundamental frequencies of around 130 Hz (the vocal folds open and close 130 times per second), whereas adult women have fundamental frequencies around 250 Hz. Therefore, the perceived pitch of male voices is, on average, lower than the perceived pitch of female voices. The fundamental frequency of young children's voices can be as high as 500 Hz, resulting in a very high-pitched voice. The difference in vocal fundamental frequency (and resulting vocal pitch) among men, women, and children is due largely to the structure of the vocal folds themselves.

At birth, the infant larynx is positioned relatively high in the neck, at about the level of the third cervical vertebra. The epiglottis is in contact with the soft palate. The elevated laryngeal position allows the infant to breathe while nursing and reduces the risk of choking (Kent, 1997; Zemlin, 1998). The infant larynx begins to descend in the neck shortly after birth, reaching the level of the sixth cervical vertebra by about 5 years of age. Laryngeal descent continues until the larynx reaches the level of the seventh cervical vertebra between 15 and 20 years of age.

At birth, the vocal folds are approximately 3 mm long for both sexes. The growth rate of the vocal folds is approximately 0.4 mm/year in females and 0.7 mm/year in males, but this difference in growth rate does not result in appreciable average pitch differences between boys and girls (Titze, 1994). Males and females have similar fundamental frequencies until about 12 years of age. During puberty, however, male vocal folds rapidly increase in length by about 10 mm and, importantly, they also thicken. The increase in vocal fold length and thickness during the pubertal period results in a large drop in the male's vocal fundamental frequency. In comparison, female vocal folds lengthen by approximately 4 mm during puberty with no significant thickening of the folds. Female fundamental frequency drops only about three musical tones during puberty. Postpubertal vocal fold length ranges from 17 mm to 20 mm in males and from 12.5 mm to 17 mm in females (Zemlin, 1998). In general, because of their larger structure, male vocal folds vibrate with a lower fundamental frequency than female vocal folds, resulting in a lower-pitched male voice. The structural changes of the vocal folds and the relationship to vocal fundamental frequency are summarized in Table 9.1.

T hink about the strings on a piano or a guitar. What is the relationship between the thickness of the string and the sound it produces when it vibrates?

THOUGHT QUESTION

Although individuals have a habitual speaking frequency (average pitch), the frequency of the voice constantly varies during speech produc-

TABLE 9.1

Summary of laryngeal development and fundamental frequency characteristics through the lifespan

Time	Structural Development	Fundamental Frequency
Birth	Larynx positioned high in the neck; vocal fold length is 3 mm	Average is about 400 Hz; unstable
4 years	Little sex difference in vocal fold length until about 10 years	Stable from 4 to 10 years with little sex influence
Puberty	10 mm increase in vocal fold length for males; 4 mm increase for females	One octave decrease for males; decreases 3 musical tones for females
Adulthood	Vocal fold length is 20 mm in men; vocal fold length is 17 mm in women	Males' average is 130 Hz; females' average is 250 Hz

Source: Adapted from Kent (1997).

tion. A monotonous or **monotone** voice is the result of not varying the habitual speaking frequency during speech production. People who use a monotone voice are not terribly interesting to listen to, and listeners will quickly lose interest in what is being said. Varying the pitch of the voice also has linguistic significance. Consider these two sentences:

Tom has a dog.

Tom has a dog?

The words in these two sentences are identical, but the sentences' meanings are quite different. "Tom has a dog" is a statement of fact (a declarative), whereas "Tom has a dog?" is a question (an interrogative). Say those two sentences out loud, paying particular attention to what happens to your pitch at the end of each sentence. For the declarative, the pitch of your voice will decrease or fall off as you are saying the word "dog." In contrast, for the interrogative, the pitch of your voice will increase when you are saying the word "dog."

How does one change the pitch of the voice? Modifications in the length and tension of the vocal folds are necessary to produce pitch change. Lengthening and tensing the vocal folds via intrinsic muscle contraction will increase the pitch of the voice, whereas relaxing these muscles will decrease pitch.

VOCAL INTENSITY AND THE INTENSITY-CHANGING MECHANISM

Like changing the pitch of the voice, changing vocal intensity is also necessary for adequate communication. Vocal intensity is measured in **decibels**

(dB), and in general, as vocal intensity increases, the perceived loudness of the voice increases. The loudness of normal conversational speech, such as conversations at the dinner table, averages around 60 dB. Changes in vocal intensity require the vocal folds to stay together longer during the closed phase of vibration, but subglottic pressure is the major determinant of vocal intensity (Kent, 1997; Zemlin, 1998). As discussed in Chapter 3, subglottic pressure is the pressure placed on the inferior aspects of the vocal folds by the lungs. Every time subglottic pressure doubles, there is an 8 to 12 dB increase in vocal intensity. The *Guinness Book of World Records* reports that the loudest scream ever recorded was produced at 123.2 dB, and a man named Anthony Fieldhouse won the World Shouting contest with a yell that was registered at 112.4 dB (Kent, 1997). Unless you are a record seeker, this kind of behavior is not recommended, as we will see later in the chapter.

DISORDERS OF VOICE

Normal voice production requires that voice quality, pitch, loudness, and flexibility be relatively pleasing and audible to a listener. Disordered voice production involves deviations of voice quality, pitch, loudness, and flexibility that may signify illness and interfere with communication (Aronson, 1990). Voice disorders can affect people of any age. For example, it is estimated that approximately 3 to 6 percent of school-age children have voice disorders (Ramig & Verdolini, 1998) and that school teachers have a higher prevalence of voice disorders than non-teaching (11.0% vs 6.2%) adults (Roy, Merrill, Thibeault, Parsa, Gray, & Smith, 2004). Children's voice disorders are characterized by abnormal pitch, loudness, quality, or combinations thereof (Aronson, 1990). Such voice disorders are related generally to vocal misuse or abuse and in most cases are temporary. The primary focus of the remainder of this chapter will be concerned with voice disorders that develop in adulthood.

It is estimated that 3 to 9 percent of the adult population of the United States have a voice disorder and that males are more commonly affected than females. Data from the National Center for Voice and Speech (Ramig & Verdolini, 1998) suggest that approximately 3 percent of the working population in the United States have occupations (e.g., police, air traffic controllers, pilots) in which use of their voice is necessary for public safety. More recently, reported that "approximately 10 percent of the workforce in the United States would be classified as 'heavy occupational voice users (Roy, 2005, p. 8)." Given these statistics, it is clear that the occurrence of voice disorders in adults is "potentially one of great magnitude from a health, as well as an economic standpoint" (Laguaite, 1972, p. 151). In contrast to children, adult voice disorders are quite varied; we will discuss some of the specific disorders later in the chapter.

Perceptual signs of a voice disorder are related to specific characteristics of a person's voice, which can be evaluated by a clinician. Clinically, perceptual signs in conjunction with a person's case history serve as the initial benchmarks in the differential diagnosis of a voice disorder. Perceptual signs of the voice can be divided into five broad categories: pitch, loudness, quality, nonphonatory behaviors, and aphonia, or the absence of phonation (Colton & Casper, 1996).

DISORDERS OF VOCAL PITCH

As we stated earlier in this chapter, pitch is the perceptual correlate of fundamental frequency. Three aspects of pitch may suggest a voice disorder. The first is **monopitch.** A monopitch voice lacks normal inflectional variation and, in some instances, the ability to change pitch voluntarily. Monopitch may be a sign of a neurological impairment or a psychiatric disability, or it may simply reflect the person's personality. **Inappropriate pitch** refers to the voice that is judged to be outside the normal range of pitch for age and/or sex. A vocal pitch that is too high may indicate underdevelopment of the larynx, whereas a vocal pitch that is excessively low may be related to endocrinological problems such as hypothyroidism. It is also possible that a vocal pitch that is excessively high or low may be related to personal preference or habit.

Pitch breaks are sudden uncontrolled upward or downward changes in pitch. Pitch breaks are common among males who are going through puberty, but this condition usually resolves itself over time. Certain types of laryngeal pathologies and/or abnormal neurological conditions can be related to pitch breaks.

DISORDERS OF VOCAL LOUDNESS

Loudness is the perceptual correlate of vocal intensity. Two aspects related to vocal loudness may indicate a voice disorder. The first is **monoloudness.** A monoloud voice lacks normal variations of intensity that occur during speech, and there may be an inability to change vocal loudness voluntarily. Monoloudness may be a reflection of neurological impairment or psychiatric disability or merely a habit associated with the person's personality. **Loudness variations** are extreme variations in vocal intensity in which the voice is either too soft or too loud for the particular speaking situation. The inability to control vocal loudness may reflect a loss of neural control of the respiratory or laryngeal mechanism. Psychological problems may also contribute to abnormal variations in vocal loudness.

DISORDERS OF VOCAL QUALITY

Several perceptual characteristics of the voice are related to vocal quality. *Hoarseness/roughness* is the first. A hoarse/rough voice lacks clarity, and the voice is noisy. Pathologies that affect vocal fold vibration can result in a hoarse/rough vocal quality. Some of these pathologies are discussed later in this chapter. A hoarse/rough voice can also be a temporary condition that results from minor forms of vocal misuse or abuse that produce vocal fold swelling called edema.

Have you ever attended a sporting event or rock concert at which you shouted or yelled excessively to root for your team or to overcome the loud background noise and music? How did your voice sound the following day? What do you think happened to make your voice sound that way?

Breathiness is the perception of audible air escaping through the glottis during phonation. Excessive airflow through the glottis usually indicates inadequate glottal closure during vocal fold vibration. The inability to close the glottis during vocal fold vibration may be related to the presence of a lesion on the vocal folds that prevents closure or some form of neurological impairment.

Tremor involves variations in the pitch and loudness of the voice that are not under voluntary control. **Vocal tremor** is usually an indication of a loss of central nervous system control over the laryngeal mechanism. **Strain and struggle** behaviors are related to difficulties initiating and maintaining voice. During speech production, the voice fades in and out, and actual voice stoppages may occur. Strain and struggle behaviors are usually related to neurological impairment, but psychological problems may also cause them.

Some research suggests that normal female voices are perceived to be more breathy than normal male voices. Research also suggests that young women use more air than young men to produce a syllable.

NONPHONATORY VOCAL DISORDERS

Stridor is noisy breathing or involuntary sound that accompanies inspiration and expiration. Stridor is indicative of a narrowing somewhere in the airway. Stridor is always abnormal and serious because its presence represents a blockage of the airway.

Excessive throat clearing, a frequent accompaniment to many voice disorders, is an attempt to clear mucus from the vocal folds. Although throat clearing is a normal behavior, it is considered abnormal when it occurs with excessive frequency.

Consistent aphonia is the persistent absence of voice and is perceived as whispering. Aphonia may be related to vocal fold paralysis, disorders of the central nervous system, or psychological problems. **Episodic aphonia** is uncontrolled, unpredictable aphonic breaks in voice that can last for a fraction of a second or longer. Central nervous system disorders and psychological problems can contribute to episodic aphonia. The perceptual signs of voice disorders are summarized in Table 9.2.

Before we turn our attention to specific voice disorders, it should be noted that many of the perceptual signs of voice disorders can be objectively quantified with clinical instruments that are readily available to the SLP (Behrman & Orlikoff, 1997). Briefly, quantitative assessments of the voice are easily made by using specially designed computer hardware and software. Kay Elemetrics, for example, manufactures a computer-based instrument called the VisiPitch® (see Figure 9.1). It is a user-friendly instrument that permits numerous objective assessments of the physical correlates of pitch,

TABLE 9.2

Perceptual signs of voice disorders

I. Pitch	B. Breathiness
A. Monopitch	C. Tremor
B. Inappropriate pitch	D. Strain/struggle
C. Pitch breaks	IV. Nonphonatory Behaviors
II. Loudness	A. Stridor
A. Monoloudness	B. Excessive throat clearing
B. Inappropriate loudness	V. Aphonia
(soft, loud, uncontrolled)	A. Consistent
III. Quality	B. Episodic
A. Hoarseness/roughness	

Source: Adapted from Colton & Casper (1990).

loudness, and hoarseness/roughness. Objective assessments are valuable for diagnostic purposes as well as monitoring improvements during voice therapy. VisiPitch operations can be seen on the book's CD-ROM.

Instruments are also available that measure airflow and air volume exchanges during phonation that can be used to objectively assess vocal breathiness. These instruments can be interfaced with specially designed computer hardware and software for vocal assessment. Normative data exist for many objective correlates that are related to the perceptual signs of voice disorders (see, e.g., Baken & Orlikoff, 2000).

FIGURE 9.1

Kay Elemetrics VisiPitch®.

Three general etiologies of voice disorders are vocal misuse or abuse (functional) conditions, medical or physical (organic) conditions, and psychological or stress conditions (Ramig, 1994). The exact etiology of a specific voice disorder is not always easy to determine, and some voice disorders may have multiple causes. With this caution in mind, we use these three general etiologies to examine some of the more common disorders of voice.

VOICE DISORDERS ASSOCIATED WITH VOCAL MISUSE OR ABUSE

Vocal misuse and abuse are frequently claimed to contribute to structural damage of vocal fold tissue, which in turn affects vocal fold vibratory behavior. Although there is a fine distinction between vocal misuse and abuse, vocal abuse is considered to be the harsher of the two with a greater risk of injuring vocal fold tissue (Colton & Casper, 1996). Conditions and behaviors that are considered to be vocal misuse and abuse are listed in Table 9.3 and discussed below.

Vocal nodules are a common vocal fold pathology that is secondary to vocal misuse/abuse. Nodules are localized growths on the vocal folds resulting from frequent, hard vocal fold collisions that occur, for example, during yelling or shouting (Colton & Casper, 1996; Gray, Titze, & Lusk, 1987). They are generally bilateral (appearing on both vocal folds), although they can appear on only one vocal fold (see Figure 9.2). Nodules are soft and pliable early in their formation. Over time, however, they become hard and fibrous, interfering greatly with vocal fold vibration. Nodules usually appear at the juncture of the anterior one-third and posterior two-thirds of the vocal folds where contact is greatest. Nodules occur more frequently in adult women, particularly those between 20 and 50 years of age. However, children who are prone to excessive loud talking or screaming may also develop vocal nodules; in this age group, they are more likely to develop in boys (Colton & Casper, 1996).

The primary perceptual voice symptoms of vocal nodules are hoarseness and breathiness. People who have vocal nodules may complain of soreness in the throat and an inability to use the upper third of their pitch range. Newly formed nodules are treated effectively with vocal rest (no talking). To prevent their return, however, people with vocal nodules need to alter the

TABLE 9.3

Common conditions and behaviors that are considered to be misuse or abuse of the voice

Misuse	Abuse
Abrupt voicing onsets	Screaming or yelling
High laryngeal position	Excessive use of alcohol
Lack of pitch variability	Excessive throat clearing and coughing

Source: Adapted from Colton and Casper (1990).

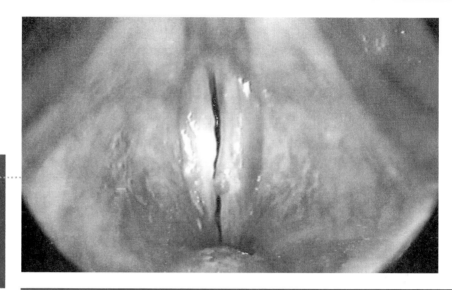

FIGURE 9.2
Unilateral vocal fold nodule. (Photograph courtesy of Robert Orlikoff, Ph.D., Memorial Sloan-Kettering Cancer Center, New York, NY)

vocal behaviors that produced the nodules. Consulting a SLP for voice therapy and education is usually recommended. Longstanding nodules may require surgical removal followed by voice therapy designed to eliminate vocally abusive behaviors. See Case Study 9.2 for the personal story of a college music student with nodules that were effectively treated with therapy and vocal rest. A voice sample of a woman with bilateral vocal nodules can be heard on the book's CD-ROM.

Contact ulcers are reddened ulcerations that develop on the posterior surface of the vocal folds in the region of the arytenoid cartilages. Contact ulcers, like vocal nodules, are usually bilateral, but unlike nodules, they can be painful. Pain is usually unilateral, and it may radiate into the ear. It was once believed that contact ulcers, which occur predominantly in males over the age of 40, resulted from forceful and aggressive speaking behaviors (Colton & Casper, 1996; Titze, 1994). Contemporary thought, however, suggests that the regurgitation of stomach acids into the esophagus and throat (gastric reflux) during sleep may be an important predisposing condition for the development of contact ulcers. Stomach acids irritate vocal fold tissue, promoting excessive throat clearing, which is abusive to the tissue and causes the ulcerations (Colton & Casper, 1996).

The primary voice symptoms of contact ulcers are vocal hoarseness and breathiness. Throat clearing and vocal fatigue accompany the disorder. Although some individuals claim that contact ulcers can be treated effectively with voice therapy (e.g., Boone & McFarlane, 2000), others suggest that successful treatment is questionable and not well documented. Quite frequently, contact ulcers reappear after surgical removal. A voice sample of a man with contact ulcers can be heard on the book's CD-ROM.

Case Study 9.2

Personal Story of a College Woman with Vocal Nodules

Jessica, a music major, decided to pledge a sorority in the fall semester of her sophomore year. A talented vocal performer, Jessica had aspirations to teach singing and to perform professionally. During the fall semester, her course work was demanding, requiring several vocal performances and long hours of rehearsal. Pledging turned out to be demanding vocally also. Jessica was talking excessively all day long and well into the night, in addition to shouting loudly at sorority events.

During the fifth week of the semester, Jessica noted that her voice fatigued easily, she sounded hoarse, and she could not reach some of the high notes required in her singing. Her vocal teacher suggested that she be evaluated at the university's speech and hearing clinic in an effort to determine the cause of her diminished vocal capacity. A perceptual and instrumental evaluation of Jessica's voice was performed by two graduate students enrolled in the university's communication disorders program. The findings of this evaluation suggested the possibility of vocal nodules. During the consultation after the evaluation, the supervising professor and the two graduate students explained their findings to Jessica

and told her that she needed to be examined by an otolaryngologist before they could proceed further. Otolaryngologic examination is required to confirm or disconfirm the presence of nodules, and speech-language pathologists are required ethically to ensure that such an examination has been performed before they initiate therapy.

The otolaryngologic examination confirmed the presence of newly formed bilateral vocal nodules. Her physician prescribed complete vocal rest for a week followed by voice therapy. Jessica enrolled in voice therapy at the university for six weeks. Vocal hygiene was stressed during therapy sessions. Jessica was examined by her otolaryngologist at the end of the sixth week of therapy. Her vocal nodules were significantly reduced in size and were no longer adversely affecting her voice.

Jessica completed her academic semester and sorority pledging successfully, graduated two years later, and went on to graduate school at the Julliard School of Music in New York City. She maintains contact with the university's speech clinic and reports that she continues to practice good vocal hygiene. Jessica and her voice are doing very well.

Vocal polyps, like vocal nodules, are caused by trauma to the vocal folds associated with vocal misuse or abuse. Polyps develop when blood vessels in the vocal folds rupture and swell, developing fluid-filled lesions. Polyps tend to be unilateral, larger than nodules, vascular, and prone to hemorrhage (Colton & Casper, 1996). Unlike vocal nodules, polyps can result from a single traumatic incident such as yelling at a sporting event.

Two general types of polyps have been identified: sessile and pedunculated (Colton & Casper, 1996; Titze, 1994). A **sessile** (closely adhering or attached to vocal fold tissue) **polyp** (see Figure 9.3) can cover up to two-thirds of the vocal fold. A **pedunculated polyp** appears to be attached to the vocal fold by means of a stalk and can be found on the free margins of the vocal folds as well as on the upper and lower surfaces of the folds.

Hoarseness, breathiness, and roughness are the typical vocal symptoms, and individuals who have a vocal polyp may report the sensation of something in the throat. The combination of surgical removal of the polyp and voice therapy to eliminate vocal misuse or abuse is effective in treating this condition (Ramig, 1994).

Have you or anyone you know had a voice disorder? What were the symptoms and how was it treated?

THOUGHT QUESTIONS

Acute and **chronic laryngitis** are inflammation of the vocal folds that can result from exposure to noxious agents (tobacco smoke, alcohol, etc.), allergies, or vocal abuse (Colton & Casper, 1996). Acute laryngitis is a temporary swelling of the vocal folds that can result in vocal hoarseness.

Chronic laryngitis is the result of vocal abuse during periods of acute laryngitis, and it can lead to serious deterioration of vocal fold tissue. The vocal folds appear thickened, swollen, and reddened because of excessive fluid retention and dilated blood vessels in the vocal folds. If chronic laryngitis persists, a marked atrophy (wasting away of tissue) of the vocal folds will occur. The vocal folds become dry and sticky, resulting in a persistent cough, and the individual reports frequent throat aches (Boone & McFarlane, 2000). The voice symptoms of chronic laryngitis range from mild hoarseness to near aphonia. Surgery and subsequent voice therapy are usually both necessary to treat chronic laryngitis effectively.

VOICE DISORDERS ASSOCIATED WITH MEDICAL OR PHYSICAL CONDITIONS

The second major group of voice disorders is those caused by central nervous system (CNS) disorders, organic disease, or laryngeal trauma. A number of the conditions discussed in this section of the chapter have a general deleterious impact on bodily functions. We will focus primarily on how these conditions affect voice production.

Disorders of the CNS can result in speech and voice disorders that are characterized by muscle weakness, discoordination, tremor, or paralysis. Generally called *dysarthrias,* most involve generalized neurological damage resulting in complex patterns of speech and voice symptoms. It is useful to broadly separate CNS disorders that affect the voice into two categories: those that result in **hypoadduction,** or reduced vocal adduction, and those that result in **hyperadduction,** or increased adduction (Ramig, 1994).[2] These categories are related generally to the anatomical location of CNS lesions or disease. CNS disorders will be discussed in more detail in Chapter 12, "Neurogenic Speech Disorders."

VOICE DISORDERS ASSOCIATED WITH HYPOADDUCTION

Parkinson's disease is a CNS disease that results in vocal fold hypoadduction. Muscle rigidity, tremor, and an overall slowness of movement, or hypokinesia, are characteristics of Parkinson's disease (Aronson, 1990; Colton & Casper, 1996). Facial appearance is unemotional and sometimes referred to as masklike. The voice symptoms associated with Parkinson's disease include monopitch, monoloudness, harshness, and breathiness (Aronson, 1990).

Parkinson's disease is a serious medical condition that is treated aggressively with a variety of drugs. Although such neuropharmacological treatments have a positive effect on limb movement, speech and voice symptoms are not consistently improved. Intensive voice therapy aimed at improving vocal fold adduction has been successful in improving vocal loudness and speech intelligibility (Ramig, 1994). A voice sample of a man with Parkinson's disease can be heard on the book's CD-ROM.

Unilateral and bilateral **vocal fold paralysis** is another common hypoadductory disorder that can result from CNS damage. The **recurrent branch** of the tenth cranial nerve (vagus) is the nerve supply for most of the laryngeal muscles associated with voice production. This nerve leaves the brain stem and travels down into the chest cavity, loops around the heart's aorta, and then courses upward, inserting into the larynx from below. Damage to this nerve can occur through injuries to the head, neck, or chest; from viral infections; and sometimes during neck or chest surgery. If the recurrent laryngeal nerve is damaged on one side, unilateral vocal fold paralysis results. If it is damaged on both sides, bilateral vocal fold paralysis results.

The voice symptoms of unilateral vocal fold paralysis include a hoarse, weak, and breathy voice quality. The paralyzed vocal fold is flaccid (limp or weak) in comparison to the nonparalyzed vocal fold. Therefore, the two vocal folds vibrate at different speeds, resulting in **diplophonia,** the perception of two vocal frequencies. The voice is very weak or totally absent in cases of bilateral vocal fold paralysis. If nerve regeneration and improved function are not observed within six months after the injury, surgical treatment may be required to facilitate vocal fold closure. Collagen or Teflon can sometimes be injected surgically into a paralyzed vocal fold to build up its mass. Vocal fold implantation helps to promote vocal fold contact. Voice therapy after surgery will be aimed at increasing vocal fold closure and vocal loudness. Three examples of vocal fold paralysis can be heard on the book's CD-ROM.

The recurrent branch of the vagus nerve was severed frequently in the early days of open heart surgery, resulting in postoperative aphonia. Improved surgical procedures have minimized this problem, although the risk still exists.

[2]Ramig (1994) also proposes a third category, called phonatory instability, which is characterized by involuntary variations of pitch and loudness.

VOICE DISORDERS ASSOCIATED WITH HYPERADDUCTION

Pseudobulbar palsy is a neurological condition that results in vocal fold hyperadduction. This condition can be caused by strokes, brain injuries, and multiple sclerosis (Colton & Casper, 1996). People who suffer from pseudobulbar palsy have great difficulty swallowing and producing speech. These individuals also exhibit emotional lability, breaking into fits of crying or laughing for no apparent reason. Such behaviors appear to be uncontrolled (Colton & Casper, 1996). The prominent voice symptoms include hoarseness, pitch breaks, and a strained or strangled vocal quality; these are characteristic of vocal fold hyperadduction.

Huntington's chorea (a hyperkinetic disorder characterized by abrupt, jerky movements of the head, neck, and limbs), a genetically transmitted disease of the basal ganglia, is also a disorder that results in vocal fold hyperadduction during phonation. The voice symptoms associated with this vocal fold hyperadduction are harshness, monopitch, and a strained or strangled voice quality. People who suffer from this disease also exhibit sudden phonatory arrests that are probably associated with uncontrolled adductory or abductory vocal fold gestures (Ramig, 1986).

The last disorder that we will consider in the hyperadductory category is **spastic dysphonia.** Spastic dysphonia occurs with equal incidence in men and women. This disorder is typically associated with middle age, but it has been observed in people as young as 20 years of age. There is some controversy about the etiology of spastic dysphonia. Some authors claim that the etiology of the disorder is psychological; others believe that the etiology is neurological (Colton & Casper, 1996).

Spastic dysphonia is typically characterized by hyperadduction of the vocal folds, resulting in a strained or strangled voice production with intermittent stoppages of the voice that resemble stuttering (Titze, 1994). Associated symptoms include hoarseness, harshness, and vocal tremor. Surgical resecting (cutting) of the recurrent laryngeal nerve and drug therapy have been used to treat spastic dysphonia. Voice therapy has also been a treatment option for spastic dysphonia to provide relief from the hyperadductory behaviors. A voice sample of a woman with spastic dysphonia can be heard on the book's CD-ROM.

OTHER CONDITIONS THAT AFFECT VOICE PRODUCTION

A number of other conditions unrelated to CNS disorders can affect the larynx and, in turn, voice production. **Laryngeal papillomas** are small wart-like growths that cover the vocal folds and the interior aspects of the larynx. These lesions are caused by a papovavirus and are common in children under the age of 6 years (Boone & McFarlane, 2000; Colton & Casper, 1996). Papillomas are noncancerous, but they can obstruct the airway, hindering breathing. Children with the disorder exhibit stridor during inhalation and may be aphonic (Wilson, 1987). Papillomas must be surgically removed, but they have a strong tendency to reappear, requiring multiple operations that may damage vocal fold tissue.

Congenital laryngeal webbing is present at birth. Congenital webs typically form on the anterior aspects of the vocal folds and can interfere with breathing. Laryngeal webbing must be removed surgically. Webs may produce a high-pitched, hoarse voice quality.

Laryngeal cancer is the most serious organic disorder of the voice; it has been linked to cigarette smoking and the excessive use of alcohol. One of the early signs of laryngeal cancer is persistent hoarseness in the absence of colds or allergies (Ramig, 1994). Once cancer is diagnosed, it is frequently necessary to remove the entire larynx to prevent the spread of the cancer to other parts of the body. When the larynx is removed surgically, the trachea is repositioned to form a stoma (mouthlike opening) on the anterior aspect of the throat for breathing purposes. Two voice samples of a man and a woman with laryngeal cancer can be heard on the book's CD-ROM.

> Over 75 percent of people who are diagnosed with cancer of the larynx are or were heavy cigarette smokers. Particles in tobacco smoke are a major irritant to vocal fold tissue.

Removal of the larynx requires alternate methods of producing voice. Some alaryngeal (without larynx) speakers use a technique called **esophageal speech,** which uses the esophagus as a vibratory source. Essentially, these individuals learn to speak using "burps" as a substitute for actual voice production. Some individuals are incapable of producing esophageal speech. Several prosthetic devices are available to produce an alternative form of voicing for these alaryngeal speakers. One such device is a battery-powered **electrolarynx.** The electrolarynx has a vibrating diaphragm that is placed on the lateral aspects of the neck. This vibration excites the air in the vocal tract and thus serves as an alternate form of voicing. Some alaryngeal speakers may be candidates for devices that are inserted through a surgical opening in the throat. A device called a **tracheo-esophageal shunt (TEP)** directs air from the trachea into the esophagus, allowing the speaker to use respiratory air and a muscle of the esophagus, the cricopharyngeous muscle, for voice production (Ramig, 1994). This device enhances esophageal speech. Voice samples of a man and a woman using a TEP can be heard on the book's CD-ROM. Other augmentative and alternative communication systems are available (see Chapter 15).

Trauma can damage the nerve supply to the larynx or cause structural damage to laryngeal cartilages and vocal folds. For example, a condition associated with surgical intubation of the larynx (respiratory tube placed between the vocal folds) is called **granuloma** (see Figure 9.4).

The severity of this condition is directly related to the size of the tube and the length of time it is in place between the vocal folds (Titze, 1994). Granulomas are ruptured capillaries covered with epithelial tissue (Colton & Casper, 1996). The preferred treatment for granuloma is surgical removal followed by voice therapy.

VOICE DISORDERS ASSOCIATED WITH PSYCHOLOGICAL OR STRESS CONDITIONS

Your voice involuntarily responds to emotional changes. Strong emotional reactions such as extreme sadness, fear, anger, or happiness are reflected by your voice. When experiencing strong emotions, your might not be able to control your voice.

THOUGHT QUESTIONS

Have you ever given a presentation to a large group of people? When you first started speaking, did your voice tremble and quaver? What might cause such vocal behaviors?

Strong emotions, when they are suppressed, can cause *psychogenic* voice disorders. Psychogenic voice disorders that are the result of psychological suppression of emotion are called **conversion disorders** because the person is converting emotional conflicts into physical symptoms (Aronson, 1990). In these cases, the vocal folds are structurally normal, and they function normally for nonspeech behaviors. One type of vocal conversion disorder is called **conversion aphonia.** People who suffer from conversion aphonia whisper to produce voice. Although these individuals are capable of coughing and clearing the throat, indicating the capability of glottal closure, they do not approximate the vocal folds for speech production. In many cases, people with conversion aphonia believe that they have a physical condition that prevents them from using their voice.

It is believed that conversion aphonias develop out of a desire to avoid some type of personal conflict or unpleasant situation in the person's life (Aronson, 1990). Conversion aphonia is not a common condition, and it will likely persist until the person is willing to resolve the emotional conflict. People with deep-rooted psychological problems may require psychotherapy or psychiatric treatment.

FIGURE 9.4
Granuloma. (Photograph courtesy of Robert Orlikoff, Ph.D., Memorial Sloan-Kettering Cancer Center, New York, NY)

THE VOICE EVALUATION AND INTERVENTION

Evaluation and treatment of voice disorders requires a multidisciplinary team approach. The specific nature of the disorder will determine the precise composition of the team. At the very least, however, the team needs to comprise an otolaryngologist and a SLP.

THE VOICE EVALUATION

The first step in the evaluation of any suspected voice disorder is an examination performed by an otolaryngologist. The otolaryngologic examination will provide information about vocal fold tissue damage, presence of nodules, polyps, or other abnormal growths. A direct examination of the vocal folds and other laryngeal structures is essential to determine whether the voice disorder has an organic basis. The otolaryngologist makes direct observation of the laryngeal structures using laryngeal mirrors (similar to the mirror used by a dentist) or with an **endoscope.** An endoscope (see Figure 9.5) is basically a lens coupled with a light source. The light source[3] illuminates the larynx, and laryngeal structures are viewed through the lens. Biopsies of vocal fold tissue may be taken if laryngeal cancer is suspected.

The SLP's role in the voice evaluation typically begins by obtaining a case history. Information regarding the nature of the voice disorder, how it affects daily life activities, the developmental history and duration of the disorder, the person's social and vocational use of the voice, and his or her overall physical and psychological condition are important areas of interest in taking a case history (Colton & Casper, 1996).

A perceptual evaluation will also be conducted to describe the pitch, loudness, and vocal quality characteristics of the voice. In some clinical situations, detailed acoustic and physiological data regarding vocal function will be collected and compared to normative data. The data obtained by the otolaryngologist and the SLP will be considered collectively, and a therapeutic plan will be recommended.

> Fiber optics are specially constructed flexible, tubular-shaped rods of glass that conduct light in only one direction. In an endoscope, small fiber optics transmit light from a source to illuminate an object, and a larger fiber optic transmits light from the illuminated object to a camera lens or viewing instrument.

INTERVENTION FOR VOICE DISORDERS ASSOCIATED WITH VOCAL MISUSE OR ABUSE

Treatment of any voice disorder may involve behavioral voice therapy, surgical intervention, psychological or psychiatric counseling, drug treatments, or various combinations of these. Treatment protocol decisions are based on the specific needs of the individual and the established clinical efficacy of the treatment (Ramig, 1994). Voice therapy is frequently the clinical method of choice for voice disorders that have resulted from vocal misuse or abuse.

---

[3]The light source can be a stroboscopic light that flashes light rapidly in synchrony with vocal fold vibration.

FIGURE 9.5

Van endoscope system.

When voice therapy is the primary treatment method, the SLP will work toward several goals: (1) restore the vocal fold tissue to a healthy condition, (2) regain clear and full vocal function, (3) identify and eliminate behaviors that are abusive to the voice, and (4) establish improved vocal habits (Colton & Casper, 1996). Table 9.4 lists some suggestions for good **vocal hygiene** that the SLP might recommend during a counseling session. When voice therapy is a secondary treatment method, as after the surgical removal of vocal nodules or polyps, the SLP will work toward these goals: restore healthy vocal function, help the individual discover the "best" voice of which he or she is capable, and make environmental changes as necessary (Colton & Casper, 1996).

The SLP will use a number of therapeutic techniques in an effort to reach the goals outlined above: breathing and relaxation exercises, soft glottal attacks (initiation of voice with a whisper), reducing vocal loudness, and a variety of other techniques that facilitate healthy use of the voice. The therapeutic process may also involve discussions regarding personal concerns and it is important that the SLP listen in nonjudgmental fashion. It is also essential that the SLP provide support and encouragement that will help an individual accept a changed or restored voice (Colton & Casper, 1996).

THOUGHT QUESTION

Complete vocal rest for a given period of time is often a therapeutic goal. Consider your own life and think how hard it would be not to talk for a week or two.

INTERVENTION FOR VOICE DISORDERS ASSOCIATED WITH MEDICAL OR PHYSICAL CONDITIONS

Treatment of voice disorders associated with disease processes does not focus on elimination of the disorder (such as reducing the size of a nodule) or on precipitating conditions (frequent yelling at sporting events), but rather on assisting the individual to achieve the best voice possible or on establishing alternative manners to produce voice. For example, voice disorders associated with neurological problems are usually not the primary disability. Therefore, direct treatment of voice disorders associated with certain types of neurolog-

TABLE 9.4
Behaviors that promote good vocal hygiene

Drink plenty of fluids, especially water.	Avoid loud, dry, or smoky environments.
Limit the intake of caffeine.	Do not use "unnatural" voices, such as imitating cartoon characters.
Limit the intake of alcoholic beverages.	Practice vocal rest.
Avoid tobacco products.	Avoid excessive throat clearing and coughing.
Avoid yelling and screaming.	
Speak at a comfortable loudness level; don't "push" your voice.	

ical disease may be a secondary concern to the SLP's treatment of related disabilities such as apraxia, aphasia, or dysphagia (Colton & Casper, 1996).

If voice therapy is indicated, the overriding therapeutic goal is to assist the individual to produce the best voice possible to remain communicatively functional in vocational and social settings. Additionally, the SLP can be helpful in assessing the effects of medications or surgery on voice production. Some of the specific techniques that the SLP uses to establish the best voice possible include increasing breath support, changing the rate of speaking, and changing the overall prosody of speech. It is essential that the SLP recognize the limitations of voice therapy for certain medical or physical conditions and help the individual to achieve the best possible means of communication (Colton & Casper, 1996).

INTERVENTION FOR VOICE DISORDERS ASSOCIATED WITH PSYCHOLOGICAL OR STRESS CONDITIONS

Treatment of voice disorders associated with psychological or stress conditions can be effective if the SLP succeeds in convincing the individual that there is nothing wrong physically with his or her voice. Individuals who have recognized conditions of stress or emotional conflict in their life and the relationship of this stress to their voice problem are the best candidates for voice therapy (Boone & McFarlane, 2000). These individuals want the ability to use their voice again.

A recommended therapeutic technique for voice disorders associated with psychological or stress conditions (conversion aphonia) begins by having the individual initiate voice from a prolonged throat clearing. This strategy is followed by having the individual initiate voice from the production of an "uh-huh." Such techniques provide solid evidence to the individual that he or she is capable physically of normal voice production (Boone & McFarlane, 2000).

Unfortunately, many individuals with conversion aphonia are highly resistant to changing their vocal patterns and habits. For these individuals, psychological counseling is imperative, and the SLP and psychologist should work as a team in an effort to restore the voice.

EFFICACY OF VOICE THERAPY

Assessing the efficacy of the treatment of voice disorders is complex because of the variety of conditions that produce voice disorders; varying severity levels of specific types of voice disorders; the variety and combinations of behavioral, pharmacological, and surgical treatments available; and the manner in which treatment efficacy is defined. Despite these complexities and the fact that not all voice disorders respond well to voice therapy, an impressive amount of clinical and experimental data compiled by Ramig and Verdolini (1998) suggest a general clinical effectiveness. In particular, voice disorders associated with vocal misuse or abuse, including those with structural tissue damage, some voice disorders associated with medical or physical conditions like Parkinson's disease, and voice disorders associated with psychological or stress conditions, respond reasonably well to treatment. Ramig and Verdolini stress the need for continued research regarding voice therapy efficacy.

SUMMARY

The human larynx is a versatile instrument that, in addition to its primary biological function of protecting the lower airways from invasion of foreign substances, serves as the primary sound generator for spoken communication. The human voice reflects one's personality, general state of health and age, and emotional condition. Vocal function changes in predictable ways as one matures. The infant's crying to satisfy some particular need soon gives way to more purposeful communication designed to control his or her environment. Most adults have full control over their voices and are capable of a wide assortment of differentiated vocalizations that convey meaning, attitude, and emotion.

Disorders of the voice affect a substantial number of people in the United States. These disorders can range from relatively uncomplicated abnormalities such as vocal hoarseness resulting from yelling excessively at a sporting event to life-threatening cancer of the larynx. Voice disorders vary in both etiology and severity, and the specific method of treatment will in large measure be dictated the etiology and severity of the disorder.

SLPs play a pivotal role in the treatment of voice disorders, but effective and ethical intervention demands a team approach. In many instances, surgical intervention followed by voice therapy is the treatment protocol of choice; in other instances, voice therapy may precede surgery, perhaps rendering surgery unnecessary. Dealing effectively with individuals with voice disorders requires detailed and specific knowledge about normal and abnormal laryngeal functioning. Because many voice disorders respond well to techniques used by SLPs, it can be a rewarding and exciting clinical endeavor.

REFLECTIONS

- Explain the normal phonation process.
- Describe how the pitch of one's voice changes with age.
- Explain how one changes the pitch of the voice.
- Explain how one changes the loudness of the voice.
- Describe the perceptual signs of a voice disorder.
- Describe voice disorders that are associated with vocal misuse or abuse.
- Describe voice disorders associated with certain medical or physical conditions.
- Describe voice disorders associated with certain psychological conditions.
- Describe the major goals of therapy for voice disorders associated with misuse or abuse.
- Discuss the efficacy of voice therapy.

SUGGESTED READINGS

Colton, R. H., & Casper, J. K. (1996). *Understanding voice problems: A physiological perspective for diagnosis and treatment* (2nd ed.). Baltimore: Williams & Wilkins.

Hollien, H. (1987). Old voices: What do we really know about them? *Journal of Voice, 1,* 2–17.

Titze, I. R. (1994). *Principles of voice production.* Englewood Cliffs, NJ: Prentice-Hall.

The entire issue of the *Language, Speech, and Hearing Services in Schools, 35* (4) (2004) is devoted to the assessment and treatment of children with voice disorders.

ONLINE RESOURCES

http://www.bgsm.edu/voice/index.html Center for Voice Disorders of Wake Forest University.
    One of the first multidisciplinary voice centers in the United States, the Center is housed in the Department of Otolaryngology of the Bowman Gray School of Medicine. The site features extensive links to information about a variety of voice disorders.

http://www.nyee.edu/otolaryn/voicefaq.htm New York Eye and Ear Infirmary, Department of Otolaryngology: FAQs about Voice Disorders.
    Voice disorders are discussed in terms of conditions that influence vocal quality, loudness, pitch, or serviceablility of the voice.

http://www.asha.org/ Voice disorders.
    Click on the "search site" button and type "voice." Many different voice disorders and therapeutic techniques are discussed.

Disorders of Articulation and Phonology

10

CHAPTER LEARNING GOALS

When you have finished this chapter, you should be able to:

- Describe the nature of speech sounds and the relationship between phonology and articulation

- Describe the correlates and causes of disorders of articulation and phonology

- Explain the procedures for assessing speech sound disorders

- Describe the major techniques for treatment of articulatory and phonological disorders

While the written alphabet that we use contains twenty-six letters, spoken English has forty-one to forty-three different speech sounds. In this chapter, we are concerned primarily with speech sounds, or phonemes, which are combined to form spoken words, phrases, and sentences. For example, the word "cat" contains three phonemes [kæt]. Be careful; phonemes and letters are not the same. The word "that" also has three phonemes [ðæt]. Phonemes are generally written between two slashes, as in /p/, while transcribed phonemic combinations such as words are often transcribed between brackets as in [ðæt]. Some phonemes are universal and are found in all languages; other phonemes are used in only a few languages. For example, the tongue clicks that are used in some African languages are not used as phonemes in English. In general, the more phonemes two languages have in common, the more similar the languages sound. The phonemic symbols for standard American English speech sounds are shown in Table 10.1.

In addition to phonemes, which are the building blocks of speech, *phonotactic* rules exist that specify acceptable sequences and locations. For example, the "ks" combination is never used at the beginning of an English word, but it is fine at the end in words such as "books" [bʊks]. Many Polish and Russian names are difficult for English speakers to pronounce because these Slavic languages permit consonant combinations that are not found in English.

Each phoneme is really a family of related sounds and may be said with some variation but still be considered to be that particular phoneme. These

> Allophonic variations contribute to regional and foreign dialects. The examples given in the text do not apply to all English speakers.

Case Study 10.1

Case Study of a Child with an Articulation Disorder: Kee

Although his grandparents are somewhat recent immigrants, Kee was born in the United States and speaks only English. Thoroughly acculturated, he loves baseball and pizza. Now in fifth grade, Kee has no remnants of the articulation problem he experienced as a younger child.

Kee's parents became concerned about his speech when he was a preschooler. Unsure who to ask, they inquired of the family physician, who told them that it was normal for children to have speech sound problems, and they shouldn't worry. Reassured, they made no further inquiries.

In kindergarten, Kee was identified as a child with a possible speech problem and his parents agreed to further testing by the speech-language pathologist. He determined that Kee had difficulty with both the "s" and "sh" sounds and to a lesser extent with the "z," demonstrating a frontal lisp on all three. Prognosis was good because Kee produced the "s" and "sh" correctly 12 and 19 percent of the time, respectively, and the "z" 42 percent of the time.

Kee received speech-language pathology services in school twice per week beginning in kindergarten. In the middle of second grade he was dismissed from therapy because of satisfactory progress.

As you read the chapter, think about

- Possible explanations for Kee's difficulties.
- Possible ways in Kee's speech-language pathologist may have gathered diagnostic data.
- Possible intervention methods that may have contributed to Kee's progress.

TABLE 10.1

Phonemic symbols for standard American English speech sounds

	Consonants				Vowels		
Phoneme	*Example*	*Phoneme*	*Example*	*Phoneme*	*Example*	*Phoneme*	*Example*
/p/	put	/ʃ/	shoe	/i/	eat	/ɔ/	all
/b/	book	/ʒ/	treasure	/ɪ/	it	/ɑ/	hot
/t/	talk	/h/	hello	/e/	ate		
/d/	door	/tʃ/	chair	/ɛ/	elbow		*Diphthongs*
/k/	kiss	/dʒ/	gym	/æ/	apple	*Phoneme*	*Example*
/g/	get	/m/	me	/ʌ/	up	/aɪ/	eye
/f/	fun	/n/	no	/ə/	ahead	/aʊ/	out
/v/	very	/ŋ/	sing	/ɝ/	her	/ɔɪ/	boy
/θ/	thumb	/l/	lime	/ɚ/	mother		
/ð/	the	/w/	wick	/u/	who		
/s/	see	/j/	yes	/ʊ/	could		
/z/	zoo	/r/	red	/o/	go		

Source: Adapted from Edwards (1997).

variations are called **allophones.** Compare the "p" in the words "pot" and "spot." When "p" is at the beginning of a word and followed by a vowel it is pronounced with a little puff of air (**aspiration**), but in most regions of the United States, when "p" is immediately preceded by "s," it is not aspirated. Still, we recognize both as /p/. If the wrong allophone is used, the spoken words do not sound right.

We begin our discussion of articulation and phonology with information about how sounds are produced and classified. We examine the distinction between articulation and phonology, then we go on to describe development of speech and impairments that may be related to articulatory and phonological disorders. The second half of the chapter is devoted to assessment and treatment.

Can you think of any English phonotactic rules in addition to the one mentioned above? Are there consonant sounds that are never blended together? Do you know any phonemes that are used in English but not in some other language?

THOUGHT QUESTIONS

UNDERSTANDING SPEECH SOUNDS

The command center for speech is in the human brain, which stimulates neural impulses to the muscles involved in breathing, phonating, and articulating speech. Figure 10.1 is a simplified model of speech production. You'll notice that the processes of respiration, phonation, and articulation/resonation, which were described in Chapter 3, work together in response to neural impulses and are monitored by auditory and kinesthetic feedback. Phonemes are often categorized as either **vowel** or **consonant.** Very generally, vowels are produced with a relatively open or unobstructed vocal tract, and consonants are made with some degree of constriction.

Consonant phonemes may be classified according to which articulators are used (place of articulation), how the sound is made (manner of production), and whether they occur with laryngeal vibration (voicing). Vowels are normally described according to tongue and lip position and relative degree of tension in these articulators. In addition, the concept of **distinctive features** is sometimes used to describe both vowels and consonants. These methods of characterizing phonemes are described in the next few pages.

All spoken languages have vowels and consonants. The intelligibility of the utterance is determined largely by the consonants, while the sound energy comes primarily from the vowels.

CLASSIFICATION OF CONSONANTS BY PLACE AND MANNER

As was mentioned, consonants are characterized by constriction somewhere along the vocal tract. This point of contact or constriction is used to classify

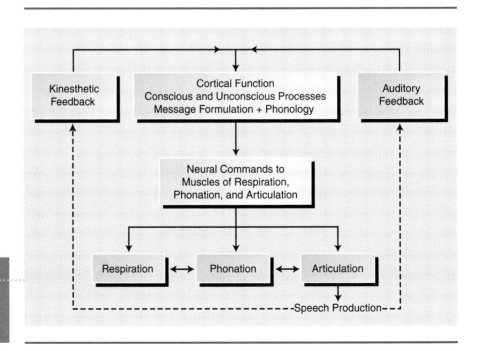

FIGURE 10.1

A simplified view of speech production.
Source: Adapted from Zemlin (1998).

consonants. Consonants in which constriction is made with both lips are called **bilabial,** meaning "two lips." **Labiodental** consonants are made with the bottom lip and upper teeth in contact. **Interdental** consonants are produced with the tongue between the teeth and are sometimes called **lingua-dental. Alveolar** sounds are made when the tongue tip is touching the alveolar or upper gum ridge. In **palatal** consonants, the center of the tongue is near the hard palate. The rear of the tongue approaches the velum or soft palate in the production of **velar** consonants. When the constriction occurs at the level of the vocal folds, the phonemes that are produced are called **glottal.**

Consonants may be *voiced* or *voiceless,* that is, produced with or without laryngeal vibration. **Obstruents,** in which airflow is blocked or obstructed, include stops, fricatives, and affricates. In the production of **stops,** air pressure is built up behind the point of constriction, momentarily stopped, and then released, as in the /p/ sound. **Fricatives** are nonresonants that are made with a narrow passageway for the air to pass through, creating a frictionlike sound. **Affricates** begin as stops, and then are released as fricatives. **Resonants** are the **nasals** and **approximants.** The special characteristic of nasals is that they are produced with resonance in the nasal cavity. Approximants include **glides** and **liquids.** Glides occur when the articulatory posture changes gradually from consonant to vowel. Liquids include /l/ and /ɹ/.

*B*efore looking at Table 10.2, say the phonemes /p/ and /m/. Which one is a stop? How do you know? Which one is nasal? How did you tell? Now place two fingers on the side of your throat and say the following speech sounds: /s/, /z/, /t/, /d/, /f/, /v/. Can you tell which are voiced and which are not voiced?

Table 10.2 depicts the classification of consonants by manner and place of production.

CLASSIFICATION OF VOWELS BY TONGUE AND LIP POSITION AND TENSION

Vowels are produced by resonating the exhaled air within the oral cavity. The exact sound that is made is dependent upon which part of the tongue is elevated (front, center, or back), its relative height (high, mid, or low), and the amount of tension (tense or lax) in the articulators. Whether the lips are rounded (pursed) or retracted (pulled back into a sort of smile) also influences the sound that is produced. Figure 10.2 is a diagram of American English vowels. In the figure, the higher vowel of the front and back paired vowels and /ɝ/ are relatively tense; all other vowels are lax. High and mid back vowels and the back central vowels are produced with the lips somewhat rounded. All other English vowels are unrounded. All English vowels are normally voiced and not nasal. Exceptions occur when you whisper and

TABLE 10.2

Classification of American English consonants by manner and place of production

Manner	Place													
	Bilabial		Labio-dental		Inter-dental		Alveolar		Palatal		Velar		Glottal	
	VL	V*	VL	V*	VL	V*	VL	V*	VL	V*	VL	V*	VL	V*
Nonresonants														
Stops	p	b					t	d			k	g		
Fricatives			f	v	θ	ð	s	z	ʃ	ʒ			h	
Affricates									tʃ	dʒ				
Resonants														
Nasal		m						n				ŋ		
Approximants														
Glides		w								j		w		
Liquids								l		ɹ				

*VL = voiceless; V = voiced.

Note: Affricates are not listed in the 1996 update of the International Phonetic Alphabet; however, the term is still widely used.

Source: Adapted from Small (1999). Used with permission.

when nasal resonance occurs for any number of reasons including proximity to a nasal phoneme, such as /m/ or /n/.

When two vowels are said in close proximity, they produce a special type of phoneme called a **diphthong.** In English, the vowels in the words "sigh," "now," and "boy" are diphthongs. "Sigh" contains /aɪ/, "now" has /aʊ/, and "boy" contains /ɔɪ/.

FIGURE 10.2

Classification of American English vowels by height and frontness/backness of tongue.

Source: Adapted from Shriberg & Kent (1995) and Yavas (1998).

Can you think of additional words containing the phonemic diphthongs /aɪ/, /aʊ/, and /ɔɪ/?

DISTINCTIVE FEATURE ANALYSIS

In an attempt to provide a system for describing phonemes found in all languages, linguists identified the components of individual sounds and called these distinctive features. Each phoneme can then be theoretically identified by the presence or absence of each of these features (Chomsky & Halle, 1968). For example, three English phonemes (/m/, /n/, and /ŋ/) are produced with nasal resonance. They are considered + nasal. All other English phonemes are – nasal. To further distinguish among the nasal phonemes, we might note that /m/ and /n/ are produced with obstruction in the front portion of the mouth; they are + anterior, while /ŋ/ is – anterior. The phonemes /m/ and /n/ can be differentiated on the basis of the distinctive feature "distributed." If the constriction extends for some distance along the direction of the airflow, it is + distributed. In the example we are using, /m/ is considered + distributed, while /n/ is – distributed.

The concept of distinctive feature analysis has been helpful in finding patterns of speech sound errors and thereby facilitating their correction. Table 10.3 contains brief definitions and examples of some of the more commonly used distinctive features.

Contrast the use of distinctive features with classification by place and manner of production. How are the systems similar? How are they different?

SPEECH SOUND DEVELOPMENT THROUGH THE LIFESPAN

Although you gained early control of most of the muscles needed for speech, it took you longer to perfect their movement and to learn to produce all the sounds of American English. Even so, most children can produce English speech sounds by early elementary school.

PRE-SPEECH

Although newborns produce predominantly reflexive sounds, such as fussing and crying, and vegetative sounds, such as burping and swallowing, both decrease with maturation. This disappearance is related to the rapid rate of brain growth and to myelination. **Myelination** is the development of a protective myelin sheath or sleeve around the cranial nerves. Myelination is not completed until adulthood.

TABLE 10.3

Definitions and examples of some common distinctive features

Anterior:	Sounds that are produced with an obstruction in the front portion of the mouth—specifically, labials, dentals, and alveolars
	Examples of + anterior: /m, p, b, f, v, θ, ð, n, t, d/
Consonantal:	Sounds that are produced with obstruction in the oral cavity—specifically, obstruents and nasals
	Examples of + consonantal: /s, z, t, d, m, n, r, l/
	Examples of – consonantal: /æ, i, e, o, u/
Continuant:	Sounds in which the air may flow without interruption—specifically, fricatives, glides, liquids, vowels.
	Examples of + continuant: /f, v, s, z, h, j, r, l, i, e, o, u/
	Examples of – continuant: /p, t, k, b, d, g/
Distributed:	Consonants that are produced with a constriction that extends a relatively long distance along the direction of airflow
	Examples of + distributed: /m, p, b, ʃ,ʒ, tʃ, ʤ/
Nasal:	Phonemes that are produced with a lowered soft palate
	Examples of + nasal: /m, n, ŋ/
Sonorant:	Sounds that are produced with a relatively open vocal tract, such that spontaneous voicing is possible—specifically, vowels, nasals, liquids, glides
	Examples of + sonorant: /æ, o, m, n, l, r, w, j/
	Examples of – sonorant: /p, b, t, d, k, g, ʃ, tʃ
Strident:	Sounds in which the airstream is constricted in such a way as to produce a high-intensity noise
	Examples of + strident: /s, z, f, v/
	Examples of – strident /p, b, i, e, o/
Syllabic:	Sounds that serve as the nucleus of a syllable—specifically vowels, syllabic liquids, syllabic nasals
	Examples of + syllabic: [bʌ tn̩] as in "button"
	Examples of – syllabic: the /b/ and /t/ in "button."
Voiced:	Sounds that are produced with vocal fold vibration—specifically all vowels, nasals, glides, voiced consonants
	Examples of + voice: /i, e, o, m, n, j, w, b, d, g, z, v/
	Examples of – voice: /p, t, k, s, f/

Source: Based on Chomsky & Halle (1968).

Initially, newborns cry on both inhalation and exhalation. The expiration phase—a more efficient sound production source—gradually increases. Crying helps children to become accustomed to air flow across the vocal folds and to modifying their breathing patterns. Since speech sounds originate at the level of the larynx, this early stimulation is necessary. However, noncrying vocalizations are far more important in the development of speech.

T ry saying "Ah-h-h" on inhalation and on exhalation. Inhalation vocalization is very inefficient and may even hurt a little. Although some languages have a few sounds that are produced on inhalation, excessive vocalization in this way may harm the vocal folds.

THOUGHT QUESTION

Noncrying sounds usually accompany feeding or are produced in response to smiling or talking by the caregivers. These noncrying vowellike sounds contain some *phonation* or vibration at the larynx, but the child has insufficient ability to produce full speech sounds.

By 2 months of age, infants develop nondistress sounds called either "gooing" or "cooing." During gooing, infants produce back consonant sounds similar to /g/ and /k/ and middle and back vowel sounds, such as /ʌ/ and /u/, with incomplete resonance.

By 3 months of age, infants vocalize in response to the speech of others. Infants are most responsive if their caregivers respond to them.

At 5 months, infants are able to imitate the tone and pitch signals of their caregivers. Most infant imitative and nonimitative vocalizations are single-syllable units of consonant-vowel (CV) or vowel-consonant (VC) construction. These sound units that begin around 4 months are called **babbling.**

With maturity, longer sequences and prolonged individual sounds evolve. Children produce increasingly more complex combinations. Sounds are now more like adult speech sounds. As muscle control moves to the front of the oral cavity, we see strong tongue projection in 4- to 6-month-olds. Initially, back consonants predominate in babbling, but by 6 months, labial or lip sounds, such as /m/ and /p/, are produced more frequently.

Babbling is random sound play, and even deaf infants babble. During babbling, infants experiment with sound production. With age, children's babbling increasingly reflects the syllable structure and intonation of the caregivers' speech.

At about 6 or 7 months, infants' babbling begins to change to **reduplicated babbling,** which contains strings of consonant-vowel syllable repetitions or self-imitations (CV-CV-CV), such as "ma-ma-ma." Hearing ability appears to be very important. Children with deafness continue to babble, but the range of consonants decreases, and few reduplicated strings are produced.

In contrast to babbling, reduplicated babbling more closely approximates mature speech in its resonant quality and timing. The child is beginning to

The consonant-vowel (CV) syllable becomes one of the predominant building blocks in first words.

adapt the speech patterns of the environment. Regardless of the language, infants' vocalizations and later first words have similar phonological patterns. For example, stops (/p, b, t, d, k, g/), nasals (/m, n, ŋ/), and approximants (/w, j/) constitute approximately 80 percent of the consonants in infant vocalizations and in the first fifty words of Spanish-, Korean-, and English-speaking children.

The period from 8 to 12 months has been called the *echolalic* stage. **Echolalia** is speech that is an imitation of some other speaker. At first, children imitate only those sounds that they have produced spontaneously on their own.

Gradually, infants begin to use imitation to expand and modify their repertoire of speech sounds. At about the same time, they begin using gestures, with or without vocalizations, to communicate. Speech during this period is characterized by **variegated babbling,** in which adjacent and successive syllables in the string are purposely not identical.

In the second half of the first year, children begin to recognize recurring patterns of sounds within specific situations. The child may even produce sounds in these situations. For example, the child might begin to say "M-m-m" during feeding if this sound is modeled for him or her. In response to caregiver conversations, infants may begin to experiment with *jargon,* long strings of unintelligible sounds with adultlike intonation.

THOUGHT QUESTION

T ry to produce jargon yourself. Say the sentence "How are you today?" with exaggerated intonation as if talking to an infant. Now do it again but substitute "la" for each syllable. Congratulations, you're jargonning with the best of 'em!

PCFs are the child's first attempt at consistent use of a sound to represent or "stand for" something else.

Many speech sounds will develop sound-meaning relationships. Called phonetically consistent forms (PCFs), these sound patterns function as "words" for the infant (Dore, Franklin, Miller, & Ramer, 1976). The infant has noticed that adults consistently use certain sound patterns to refer to the same things in the environment.

Word production depends upon sound grouping and sound variation. Children adopt a problem-solving or trial-and-error approach to word production. The resultant speech is a complex interaction of the ease of production and perception of the target syllable and its member sounds.

TODDLER SPEECH

At around 12 months of age, you probably produced your first recognizable word. Sometimes a child's word is easily recognizable to others, but some words may be modified by the child for ease of speaking.

When faced with a difficult word, children adopt similar strategies. Armed with the consonant-vowel (CV) structures of babbling and the CV-

CV-CV strings of reduplicated babbling, children attempt to pronounce the adult words they encounter. It is not surprising, therefore, that many words are reduced to variations of a CV structure or other simplification. These adaptations, called phonological processes, are presented in Table 10.4.

Toddlers often omit final consonants, resulting in a CVC word being produced as CV, as in *cake* pronounced as *ca*. It is also possible that children will add an additional vowel to form the CV-CV *cake-a*. Multisyllable words may be reduced to one or two syllables, or the syllables may be repeated. For example, *telephone* might become *tephone*, and *baby* might be modified to *bebe*. If the syllables are not duplicated, only the consonants may be, as in *doggie* becoming *goggie*. Consonant blends might be shortened to single consonants, as in *stop* becoming *top*. Finally, one type of sound might be substituted for another. For example, all initial consonants in words might be pronounced as the same consonant, as in, *Go bye-bye* becoming *Bo bye-bye*.

TABLE 10.4
Phonological processes of young children

Process	Explanation	Example
Deletion of final consonant	Reduces CVC structure to more familiar CV	*Cat* becomes *ca* (/ka/) *Carrot* becomes *cara* (/kara/) CVCVC → CVCV
Deletion of unstressed syllable	Reduces number of syllables to conform to the child's ability to produce multisyllable words	*Telephone* becomes *tephone* (/tefon/) *Vacation* becomes *cation* (/kaʃən/)
Reduplication	Syllables in multisyllable words repeat	*Baby* becomes *bebe* (/bibi/) *Mommy* becomes *mama*
Reduction of consonant clusters	Reduces CCV+ structures to the more familiar CV	*Tree* becomes *te* *Stay* becomes *tay*
Assimilation	One consonant becomes like another, although the vowel is usually not affected	*Doggie* becomes *goggie* /gɔgi/
Substitution	One group of difficult sounds, such as fricatives (/f/, /v/, /s/, /z/, and others) are replaced by easier sounds, such as stops (/b/, /p/, /d/, /t/, /g/, /k/)	*Face* becomes *pace* *This* becomes *dis*

THOUGHT
QUESTION

*T*ake a three- or four-syllable word and apply several phonological patterns. Note how the word may be altered beyond recognition. Is it any wonder that you might have some difficulty understanding some young speakers?

PRESCHOOL SPEECH

Most of the phonological processes described for toddlers have disappeared by age 4. Consonant blends consisting of two or more adjacent consonants, as in *strong,* continue to be difficult for some children, and simplification strategies, resulting in *tong,* may continue into early elementary school. Children who experience continuing phonological difficulties may persist in the use of more immature phonological processes.

Children continue to master new speech sounds throughout the preschool period. The acquisition process is a gradual one and depends on the individual sound, its location in words, its frequency of use, and its proximity to other speech sounds. A sound may be produced correctly in single words but not in connected speech.

We can make a few generalizations about the speech sound acquisition by young children:

1. Phoneme acquisition is a gradual process.
2. Vowels are easier to master than consonants. Usually, English vowels are acquired by age 3, while some consonants may not be mastered until age 7 or 8.
3. Many sounds are first acquired in the initial position in words.
4. Consonant clusters (*cons*ider) and blends (*str*eet) are not mastered until age 7 or 8, although some clusters appear as early as age 4.
5. Some sounds are easier than others and are acquired first by most children. As a group, stops (/p, b, t, d, g, k/) and nasals (/m, n, ŋ/) are acquired first.
6. Much individual difference exists.

> Development of individual sounds is dependent on the location in words, frequency of use, and the influence of other speech sounds.

This information is presented visually in Table 10.5. Children with neuromuscular problems, sensory deficits, perceptual problems, or poor learning skills are going to have difficulty acquiring all the sounds of the language.

SCHOOL-AGE SPEECH

By early elementary school, your phonological system probably resembled that of adults. A few children will still have difficulty with multiple consonant blends, such as *str* and *sts,* as in *street* and *beasts,* respectively.

Other developments such as **morphophonemic contrasts**—changes in pronunciation as a result of morphological changes—will take several years

TABLE 10.5

Mastery of English speech sounds

Ages by which most children have acquired speech sounds in all positions. Vowels are not included because they are usually mastered by age 2–3 years.

Age 2	p, h, n, b, k
Age 3	m, w, g, f, d
Age 4	t, ʃ ("sh"), j ("y")
Age 5	s, v, ŋ("ng"), r, l, tʃ ("ch"), z, ʤ ("j")
Age 6	θ ("th" in "<u>th</u>in"), ð ("th" in "<u>th</u>e"), ʒ ("zh" in "mea<u>s</u>ure")
Age 8	Consonant blends and clusters

Sources: Compiled from Olmsted (1971); Prather, Hedrick, & Kern (1975); and Sanders (1972).

to master, some extending into adulthood. For example, in the verb *derive,* the second vowel is a long "i," transcribed phonetically as /aɪ/. When we change *derive* to the noun *derivative,* the second vowel is changed to sound like the "i" in *give,* transcribed as /ɪ/. Other contrasts were mentioned in Chapter 2.

Five-year-olds still have difficulty with a few consonant sounds and with consonant blends. Six-year-olds have acquired most English speech sounds. By age 8, children have acquired consonant blends, such as *str, sl,* and *dr.*

PHONOLOGY AND ARTICULATION

The correct use of speech sounds within a language requires knowledge of the sounds of the language and the rules that govern their production and combination, called *phonology.* Speech also requires neuromotor coordination to actually say sounds, words, and sentences; termed *articulation.* To help you understand this distinction, visualize learning a new language such as French. You will be exposed to new words and sound combinations and begin to grasp the nature of that language's sound system or phonology. But you must also be able to form the words with your lips, tongue, and so on. You might find this very difficult because your neuromotor pathways have been trained to make English words; the inability to coordinate your muscles to correctly produce the words is a problem of articulation.

Phonological impairments are disorders of conceptualization or language rules. Remember that phonology is concerned with classes of sounds and sound patterns within words. For example, English has both open and closed syllables at the ends of words. An **open syllable** is one that ends in a vowel—for example, "ba-na-n<u>a</u>"; a **closed syllable** ends in a consonant ("kum-qua<u>t</u>"). A child who uses only open syllables and deletes all final consonants would be exhibiting a disorder of phonology. In this example, the child would say "banana" correctly but produce "kumquat" as "kuqua."

The distinction between phonology and articulation is often difficult to understand. Articulation refers to the actual production of speech sounds; phonology is knowledge of speech sounds within a language and the ways in which they are combined.

Articulation impairments are disorders of production. A child whose only speech error is incorrect production of the /s/ phoneme has a disorder of articulation. Disorders of articulation are typically characterized as

- Substitutions
- Omissions
- Distortions
- Additions

Substitutions occur when one phoneme is replaced with another. For example, a person who says "shair" for "chair" would be substituting "sh" for "ch." An omission is the deletion of a phoneme, as in "chai" for "chair." Distortions occur when a nonstandard form of the phoneme is used. An example of an addition would be "ch<u>uh</u>-air" for "chair." Some individuals have disorders of both phonology and articulation. We will talk more about specific patterns and types of errors later in this chapter.

Associated Disorders and Related Causes

The majority of children with disordered articulation and phonology do not exhibit an identifiable physical reason for the problem.

The causes of phonological and articulatory disorders in most children are not readily identifiable. In these cases, when no cause is known, it may be termed a *functional disorder.* Recognizing the limited usefulness of this concept, researchers have directed their attention to **correlates,** or related factors. Correlation means that two or more things occur together but one does not necessarily cause the other(s). Nevertheless, correlates may offer some clues to causality that should prompt further research. Table 10.6 lists some correlates of phonological impairment. In the next few sections, we describe the characteristics associated with a few well-established correlates of phonological and articulatory impairment. Data from long-term studies suggest that more persistent problems may be related to motor-speech deficits (Flipsen, 2003).

THOUGHT QUESTIONS

*C*an you think of any two things that are correlated but not causally related? What may account for the correlation? Why is it important to distinguish between causality and correlation?

DEVELOPMENTAL IMPAIRMENT IN CHILDREN

Language and speech learning is not easy. Words are composed of phonemes that are typically acquired gradually by 8 years of age. Many children with articulation and phonological difficulties exhibit a developmental impairment in speech sound production with no readily identifiable corollary factors.

Characteristics of Articulation

Table 10.5 lists the consonants that are typically mastered at various ages. When a child's articulation is delayed, you would expect that he or she is not

TABLE 10.6
Possible correlates of phonological and articulatory impairments

Hearing loss

History of otitis media during the first few years of life

Diminished speech sound perception and discrimination ability

Atypical tooth alignment and missing teeth

Impaired oral-motor skills

Eating problems

Tongue thrust swallow after 6 years of age

Neuromotor disabilities

Mental retardation

Language problems

Reading disorders

Family history

producing the phonemes expected that age. Other children may be idiosyncratic in their phoneme use. Some researchers identify these children as "disordered" in their development. This dichotomy is a difficult one, however, because of the wide range of behaviors in young children (Howell & Dean, 1994; Stoel-Gammon & Dunn, 1985).

Phonological Processes

As we discussed, children simplify adult speech in many ways. Children's phonological and phonotactic simplifications are called **phonological processes.** Table 10.4 provides explanations and examples of phonological processes of young children.

Case Study 10.2 describes a young girl who exhibited the phonological process of backing.

Lifespan Issues

The average age of diagnosis of a phonological disorder is 4 years, 2 months (Shriberg & Kwiatkowski, 1994), although the roots of these problems may be seen in infancy and toddlerhood. With maturation and therapy, immature patterns of articulation tend to diminish (Gierut, 1998). If they do not, they may have a negative impact on the individual's academic and professional accomplishments as well as on personal relationships. What was considered "cute" in childhood may be viewed negatively in adulthood.

Children who were unsuccessful in correcting immature speech patterns through therapy may become rebellious and feel punished by continued intervention efforts. These youngsters sometimes benefit from a break from treatment. When they return for therapy, SLPs must be careful to use

Phonological processes involve more than individual phonemes. Final consonant deletion can involve any consonant, as when the target "Give him the book" is produced as "Gi- hi- the boo." Many children exhibit multiple processes.

age-appropriate materials and activities. Although speech sound production can be modified at any stage in life, as we age, old habits become more firmly entrenched, and so change is more difficult.

Case Study 10.2

Personal Story of a Child with a Phonological Disorder

Brandi was just over 3 years of age when she was first brought to the University Speech and Hearing Center by her mother, Mrs. A. Brandi had been identified in a preschool screening program as needing further evaluation. Mrs. A. noted that Brandi mispronounced many words and could not be understood by people outside of the family, and "people say her mouth looks stiff." Brandi's 5-year-old brother frequently interpreted Brandi's speech so that others could understand her. Examination at the center revealed that Brandi had normal hearing and physical structure for speech. Her receptive and expressive language skills were above average in all areas but phonology. Brandi was diagnosed with a moderate-to-severe phonological disorder of unknown cause.

A cycles approach was used in therapy that first targeted the phonological processes cluster simplification, stopping of fricatives, and backing to velars.

An example of Brandi's speech at the beginning of therapy is as follows:

Target: Stop playing with my toy.
Brandi: Kop payin' wid my koy.

Because of her young age and her high spirits, therapy was presented through structured play activities. Brandi enjoyed beanbag tosses and musical chairs. She also demonstrated that she understood the purpose of the speech sessions and attempted to do as the SLP requested of her. By the end of three months, Brandi frequently self-corrected in the clinical setting. At the end of a year of therapy, Brandi's mother reported that Brandi was self-correcting at home. Although Brandi had made good progress, she would receive speech therapy for two more years. She entered first grade with easily intelligible speech and only a few articulation errors.

LANGUAGE IMPAIRMENTS

Children who have language impairments, as described in Chapter 5, may also be impaired in their production of the sounds of the language. It has been estimated that a general impairment in expressive language is present in about 60 percent of children who are hard to understand and who have multiple speech sound errors (Shriberg & Kwiatkowsi, 1994; Tyler & Watterson, 1991). These children have more complicated problems than those of youngsters with isolated phonological or articulatory deficiencies. Some children with learning disabilities (LD) have difficulties not only with listening and speaking, but also with reading, writing, reasoning, and mathematics (National Joint Committee on Learning Disabilities, 1991).

Articulation and Phonological Process Characteristics

The speech sound productions of children with learning disabilities are similar to those with developmental impairments, although complex syllable structures may be especially challenging for those with LD (Orsolini, Sechi, et al., 2001). Children with LD may also have difficulty understanding language and will use simpler and less grammatically correct speech. They are also more likely to exhibit phonological errors that also affect morpheme production (Owen, Dromi, & Leonard, 2001).

*W*hat bound morphemes are affected by omission of the final /s/ in words in the sentence "Tom likes to read Pete's books"?

Lifespan Issues

Although most individuals with learning disabilities are of normal intelligence, phonological impairments may have a deleterious effect on the acquisition of reading and writing skills. Learning to read requires an awareness of phonemes and phoneme combinations. Children with specific language impairments are also more likely than their peers to struggle with academic subjects through the grades and even into college and beyond. They may require support and the use of various strategies to achieve to their full potential (Owens, 2004).

HEARING IMPAIRMENTS

Because hearing is the primary way in which we acquire the speech sounds of a language, it is no surprise that individuals with hearing impairments may have disordered articulation and phonology. Not only are those with hearing loss limited in their ability to hear others, but their ability to monitor their own speech production may be inadequate. It must be recognized that phonology will not be impaired alone, but all parameters of speech, including voice quality, pitch, rate, and rhythm, will similarly be affected.

Articulation and Phonological Process Characteristics

Although the specifics vary, in general, the more severe a person's hearing loss, the less intelligible his or her speech is likely to be (Wolk & Schildroth, 1986). Although an exact relationship between type and degree of hearing impairment and speech cannot be made, certain patterns are frequently observed (Bankson & Bernthal, 1998a).

Articulation errors that tend to occur in the speech of children who are deaf include voicing confusion, as when "toy" is said as "doy," and vowel substitutions, as when "ill" is pronounced as "eel" (Calvert, 1982). More examples are provided in Table 10.7.

Although it is not always the case, children who have a history of frequent bouts of **otitis media** (middle ear infections), resulting in transient conductive hearing loss, are more likely than youngsters who have not had these infections to exhibit phonological and articulatory errors (Bankson & Bernthal, 1998a). Common errors are presented in Table 10.8.

Lifespan Issues

The age at onset and the degree and type of hearing impairment influence the nature of the articulation and phonological disability. Individuals who

TABLE 10.7

Typical speech sound errors in children who are deaf

Sound Substitution Pattern	Examples
Voiced for voiceless sounds	"see" → "zee" [zi]
	"can" → "gan" [gæn]
Nasal for oral consonants	"dog" → "nong" [nɔŋ]
Sounds with easy tactile perception for those difficult to perceive	"run" → "wun" [wʌn]
Tense vowels for lax vowels	"sick" → "seek" [sik]
Diphthongs for vowels	"miss" → "mice" [maɪs]
Vowels for diphthongs	"child" → "chilled" [tʃɪld]

Sources: Adapted from Bankson & Bernthal (1998a) and Calvert (1982).

are born deaf or with severe hearing impairment typically have poorer speech than those who lose hearing later in life. Speech deteriorates over time, however, for those who are initially hearing and become hard-of-hearing or deaf after they have learned to talk. Accuracy of speech sound production can be enhanced by the use of hearing aids (for individuals with some hearing) and appropriate training. (See Chapter 14, "Audiology and Disorders of Hearing.") Even the best speech of many adults with deafness is nearly unintelligible to others.

THOUGHT QUESTIONS

*W*hy do people who lose hearing later in life have less impaired speech than those who were born deaf? Which phonemes do you think a deaf or severely hard-of-hearing person would find most difficult to learn? Why?

NEUROMUSCULAR DISORDERS

People with dysarthric speech have a neuromuscular impairment resulting in muscle weakness and poor coordination that interferes with accurate production of speech sounds.

Dysarthrias are speech problems that are due to neuromuscular impairment that results in poor coordination, weakness, or paralysis of the speech mechanism, described in more detail in Chapter 12, "Neurogenic Speech Disorders." Dysarthrias commonly affect respiration, phonation, resonance, and the rate and rhythm of speech. Clients with dysarthria may also have chewing, sucking, and swallowing problems. (See Chapter 13, "Disorders of Swallowing.")

Cerebral palsy (CP) is a term for several types of congenital neuromotor disorders. About two-thirds of people with cerebral palsy have impaired speech or language. Because it is not a unitary problem, no single pattern of articulation or phonology can be identified. Disorders in articulation are

TABLE 10.8

Phonological processes often observed in children with history of otitis media

Phonological Process	Phonemes Involved	Examples
Stopping of fricatives	/s/, /z/, /ʃ/, /ʒ/, /tʃ/, /dʒ/	"see" → [ti]
	/f/, /v/, /θ/, /ð/	"John" → [dɑn]
		"thumb" → [tʌm]
Initial consonant deletion	Any consonant	"see" → [i]
		"John" → [ɑn]
Glottal fricative replacement	/h/ used for initial consonant	"see" → [hi]
		"John" → [hɑn]
Glottal stop replacement	Any consonant	"see" → [ʔi]
		"John" → [ʔɑn]
Nasal replacement	/m/, /n/, /ŋ/	"my" → [naɪ] or [baɪ]

Source: Bankson, J. E., & Bernthal, N. W. (1998). Factors related to phonologic disorders. In Bernthal, J. E., & Bankson, N. W., *Articulation and phonological disorders.* Fourth Edition. Boston: Allyn and Bacon. Copyright © 1998 by Allyn and Bacon. Reprinted by permission.

often related to some form of CP or *dysarthria* (Air, Wood, & Neils, 1989). The precise symptoms depend largely on the type and extent of the brain lesion.

Characteristics of Articulation

Most people with dysarthric or cerebral palsied speech are imprecise in their articulation of consonants. The errors that an individual exhibits tend to be similar whether she or he is reading aloud, speaking to a group, or in an intimate conversation. In general, the location of the motor neuron impairment in a particular speaker determines which phonemes are involved. For example, a person with loss of lip strength and coordination would likely misarticulate such phonemes as /p/, /b/, and /m/. Someone with primarily tongue tip **paresis,** that is, muscle weakness or partial paralysis, might incorrectly produce /t/, /d/, /l/, and /n/ (Crary, 1993).

Lifespan Issues

In cerebral palsy, the symptoms are present from earliest childhood onward. Speech training or the use of augmentative or alternative communication may be required. Dysarthrias that are the result of a stroke, tumor, or disorders such as Parkinson's disease most often occur in adulthood. At any age, dysarthria or speech difficulties are but one aspect of an individual's diminished physical condition.

APRAXIA OF SPEECH

Individuals with speech apraxia may have adequate muscle strength and often have satisfactory articulation when engaging in automatic speech such as counting, but they exhibit errors in volitional speech that requires motor planning.

Some individuals have no difficulty in conceptualizing speech sounds and have adequate muscle strength and coordination, but their speech is characterized by multiple speech sound errors. These errors may be attributable to an impairment in programming the speech musculature to select, plan, organize, and initiate a motor pattern (Nijland, Maassen, & van der Menlen, 2003). This deficiency is termed *apraxia of speech*. The causes of apraxia are neurological. Apraxia is not due to hearing loss, muscle weakness, low intelligence, impaired receptive language, or an apparent organic condition, although it may coexist with these deficits (Hall, Jordan, & Robin, 1993). Apraxin will be discussed in more detail in Chapter 12, "Neurogenic Speech Disorders."

Characteristics of Articulation

A person with apraxia of speech does not have a typical pattern of misarticulated phonemes; in fact, an individual's errors tend to be inconsistent. However, a commonality of speech production activity can be described. These behaviors include the following:

- Poor speech sound imitation
- Difficulty initiating speech movements characterized by initial consonant deletion
- Vowel misarticulations
- Groping and struggle behavior in producing speech sounds on command
- Rate and rhythm abnormalities
- Poor diadochokinetic performance (ability to rapidly repeat syllables)
- Inconsistent vowel and consonant errors (Bankson & Bernthal, 1998a; Strand & McCauley, 1997)

In addition, clients with apraxia often do not respond readily to speech therapy; their rate of improvement may seem frustratingly slow (Hall et al., 1993).

Lifespan Issues

Brain damage at any age can result in apraxia of speech. When the behaviors described above are observed in a child, it may be called **developmental apraxia of speech (DAS)** or **developmental verbal dyspraxia (DVD).** Apraxia in adults is caused by damage to the left side of the brain, which may be due to a degenerative neurological disease, tumor, stroke, or other trauma.

The articulatory patterns noted above may be seen in adults or children with apraxia; however, older individuals are more likely to exhibit automatic speech—such as counting or naming the days of the week—that is free of error, while words and sentences that are linguistically and intellectually complex show more deterioration. Younger children may not have had the opportunity to develop this automaticity. Many writers suggest that developmental apraxia of speech and adult onset apraxia are clearly distinct disorders because of the differences in etiology (Bankson & Bernthal, 1998a; Bloom & Ferrand, 1997).

CLEFT PALATE

Children who are born with a cleft palate frequently exhibit articulatory errors in their speech. These errors may be due not only to the nature of the cleft, an inadequate or too short palate, and inability to sufficiently close the oral/pharyngeal passageway to the nose, but also to frequently related factors such as misaligned teeth, hearing loss, and delayed development. The type of cleft, the age of the client, and the age at the time of surgical repair(s) also influence the precise nature of the articulatory impairment. For this reason, the SLP must not assume a particular pattern of errors but must take care to assess the child's articulation and phonology fully (Air et al., 1989; Grunwell, 1993). In addition, as we'll see in Chapter 11, "Cleft Lip and Cleft Palate," aspects of voice and resonance are typically also impaired.

Characteristics of Articulation

Despite the variability noted above, certain speech sound errors are particularly common among those with a history of cleft palate. Phonemes that require the buildup of intra-oral pressure are typically affected. These include stops, fricatives, and affricates. Vowels may sound especially nasal. Minor variations of the dimensions of the hard palate and velum do not appear to affect speech articulation; however, surgical removal of any portion of the roof of the mouth and congenital clefts seriously compromise speech intelligibility. Surgery and/or the use of prosthetic devices, called **obturators,** have been found to be effective intervention and, along with speech therapy, permit significant gains in speech articulation.

Lifespan Issues

Although a person may be born with a cleft palate, simple clefts are usually surgically repaired between the ages of 12 and 18 months. More involved clefts may require a number of surgical, orthodontic, and other procedures. In these cases, and if surgery is delayed past the age of 2 years, the child's articulation becomes more disordered and harder to correct. This is because the individual is likely to develop *compensatory* movements to produce sounds that are intended to resemble target phonemes. These maladaptive errors are sometimes labeled "cleft palate speech." Beyond 10 years of age, surgery without speech therapy is insufficient to alter disordered articulation. Although therapy is never a guarantee, it results in positive changes for many speakers. Although some individuals with early surgery develop unimpaired speech without formal training, therapy tends to enhance progress. (Grunwell, 1993). Some compensatory articulations are included in Table 10.9.

Cleft palate is a congenital condition—something you are born with. Occasionally, however, similar inability to achieve velopharyngeal closure occurs later in life. These disruptions may be due to removal of tumors, adenoidectomy, or neurological disorders such as muscular dystrophy. In these cases, speakers probably will not develop compensatory movements, but their speech will contain some misarticulations.

TABLE 10.9

Compensatory articulations often present among individuals born with a cleft palate

Target	Phonemes Involved	Compensatory Articulation
Stop	/p/, /b/, /t/, /d/, /k/, /g/	Glottal stop /ʔ/, stop produced at the glottis
		Pharyngeal stop, stop produced near pharynx
		Middorsum stop, stop produced in middle of tongue
Fricative	/s/, /z/, /ʃ/, /ʒ/	Pharyngeal fricative, closure occurs near pharynx
		Velar fricative, posterior nasal fricative
Affricate	/tʃ/, /dʒ/	Pharyngeal fricative, velar fricative, posterior nasal fricative

The overall effect is speech that is hypernasal and contains nasal emission and weak and distorted consonants.

Source: Adapted from text material in Air, Wood, & Neils (1989).

OTHER ORGANIC ABNORMALITIES

In this section, we review the impact of structural and functional variations on articulation.

Lips

If you were to systematically examine the lip structure of every student in your class, you would observe considerable variation in appearance. Although these structural differences usually do not affect speech sound production, neuromotor problems that impair the ability to purse and retract the lips might slightly affect the way vowels and labial consonants are said. Remember, in English, front vowels usually are said with the lips pulled back, and back vowels typically require lip rounding.

> Although speech articulation requires rapid and accurate movements involving the tongue, teeth, and lips, some individuals with organic problems can compensate and produce acceptable speech in atypical ways.

THOUGHT QUESTION

Look in the mirror as you say the words "eat," "oat," "he," and "who." Do your lips change shape?

Teeth

Both occlusion (tooth alignment) and missing teeth may affect articulation. Most individuals with malocclusions or rotated or absent teeth are able to compensate for these deficiencies. Although an open bite, in which the front teeth do not meet, occurs more often in speakers with articulatory errors, many people with open bite speak normally. Similarly, more children with missing front incisors misarticulate /s/ and other phonemes than children with a full set of teeth. On the other hand, most children whose front incisors are missing do not make articulatory errors (Bankson & Bernthal, 1998a).

Adults with dentures may exhibit misarticulations, particularly of the /s/ phoneme. Readjustment of these prostheses, with particular attention to the upper incisors, is generally effective (Runte, Lawerino, Dirksen, et al., 2001). If this is insufficient, the SLP may work with the client to compensate for any misalignment.

Tongue

Technically, a person who is "tongue-tied" has **ankyloglossia,** or a relatively short lingual frenum (the tissue that connects the underportion of the tongue to the floor of the mouth), which restricts tongue movement. Several decades ago, frenums were frequently clipped soon after birth if there was apparent ankyloglossia. Physicians have become more conservative with this procedure. In fact, although the tip of the tongue must be free to move to produce tongue tip sounds such as /l/, /t/, /d/, it is quite rare for misarticulation to be caused by ankyloglossia (Bankson & Bernthal, 1998a).

Complete or partial **glossectomy,** surgical removal of the tongue, usually as a result of cancer, is likely to impair speech sound production, but again, humans are remarkably adaptable and can often compensate. As might be expected, the greater the amount of tongue that is removed, the more impaired speech intelligibility will be. Fricatives such as /s/, /z/, /f/, /v/, /ʃ/, /ʒ/, /θ/, and /ð/ and stops such as /p/, /b/, /t/, /d/, /k/, and /g/ are most affected (Leonard, 1994). Speech therapy typically is helpful in assisting clients improve their speech intelligibility (Furia, Kowalski, Latorre, et al., 2001).

During the first few years of life, because of the size of the tongue relative to the oral cavity, all youngsters have tongue placement somewhat forward in the mouth with the tongue tip resting against the back of the front teeth. Swallowing during this time also involves a forward movement of the tongue. This pattern has been termed **tongue thrust, myofunctional disorder,** or **reverse swallow.** By age 5, tongue thrust should no longer be apparent; its perpetuation has been associated with dental malocclusion and speech misarticulation. The phonemes that are most likely to be affected by tongue thrust are /s/, /z/, /ʃ/, /ʒ/, /tʃ/, /dʒ/, /t/, /d/, /l/, and /n/ (Hanson, 1994).

LANGUAGE AND DIALECTAL VARIATIONS

If you are a native speaker of American English and went to another country, such as Greece, to live, you would learn Greek to communicate with those around you. When you spoke in Greek, your speech would reveal your American background. You would speak Greek with an "American accent." This is not a speech disorder.

Similarly, if you are from Georgia and moved to Massachusetts, you would bring your Georgia regionalism with you. Again, this is not a disorder

A person whose speech reflects a regional or foreign language influence may also have a speech disorder. However, the regionalism or foreign dialect in itself is not a disorder.

but a dialectal difference to those in your new environment. Many Americans take pride in their regional and linguistic backgrounds and cherish the cultural diversity that characterizes this country.

THOUGHT QUESTIONS

*W*hat do you think the role of speech-language pathologists should be for individuals from diverse linguistic, regional, and cultural backgrounds? Have you ever wanted your speech to sound more "mainstream"? Why or why not?

In assessing phonological skills, an SLP must guard against over- and underdiagnosis, especially with bilingual and minority dialect speakers (Yavas & Goldstein, 1998). The SLP must differentiate between disordered phonology and that which is simply different due to foreign language or dialect influences. This can be accomplished by doing the following:

1. Recognize cultural differences
2. Evaluate phonological competence in all relevant languages whenever possible
3. Select appropriate assessment tools
4. Use nonstandard assessments often with the help of bilingual assistants
5. Describe phonological patterns
6. Diagnose any phonological disorders that exist (Yavas & Goldstein, 1998)

The SLP then plans and engages in intervention as appropriate. If dialect differences are targeted, the SLP must assess the client's attitude toward his or her dialect and the individual's motivation for accent reduction. Some generalizations can be made regarding the speech of individuals from various linguistic and regional backgrounds. Table 10.10 highlights just a few of these.

CHARACTERISTICS OF ARTICULATION AND PHONOLOGY

It is impossible to describe all the variations in articulation and phonology that reflect non-English or dialectal influences. The first language may interfere with languages that are learned later. For example, in Spanish, /d/, and /ð/ are allophones or variations of the same phoneme, whereas in English, these are two separate phonemes, as can be seen in the words "dough" [do] and "though" [ðo]. Native Spanish speakers, however, may confuse the /d/ and /ð/ and pronounce both words the same way (Yavas, 1998). Some first language interferences are neutral or positive.

THOUGHT QUESTION

*H*ow does your articulation differ from that of someone from another part of the country or a different linguistic or dialectal background?

TABLE 10.10
....
Sample phonological characteristics of American English dialects and non-English language influences on spoken English

Rule	Example
African American Vernacular	
Final cluster reduction	"presents" → "presen"
Stopping of interdental initial and medial fricatives	"they" → "dey"
	"nothing" → "noting"
Deletion of "r"	"professor" → "puhfessuh"
Appalachian English	
Addition of "t"	"once" → "oncet"
Addition of initial "h"	"it" → "hit"
Addition of vowel within clusters	"black" → "buhlack"
Portugese, Italian, Spanish	
Final consonant deletion	"but" → "buh"; "house" → "hou"
Cantonese	
Confusion of /i/ and /ɪ/	"heat" → "hit"; "leave" → "live";
	"hit" → "heat"; "live" → "leave"
Spanish	
Confusion of /d/ and /ð/	"they" → "day"
Devoicing of "z"	"lies" → "lice"
Affrication of /ʃ/	"shoe" → "chew"

Sources: Adapted from Iglesias & Goldstein (1998) and Yavas & Goldstein (1998).

LIFESPAN ISSUES

Some adults for whom English is a second (or third or fourth) language choose to modify their foreign accent. Often this desire is based on professional considerations. Teachers of English as a second language and speech-language pathologists may contribute to the improvement of English expression and comprehension. However, once a person is teenaged and beyond, the articulatory patterns of a first language are often firmly established and are difficult to entirely eliminate. The goal, then, is not to make a nonnative speaker sound like a native, but rather to improve intelligibility and thereby the person's communicative effectiveness.

What regional or foreign dialect patterns have you heard in the media? Do you think certain variations occur more often than others? If so, why might this be?

THOUGHT QUESTIONS

ASSESSMENT

No matter what the cause of the speech sound disorder, assessment should be comprehensive. The standard procedures described in Chapter 4, "Assessment and Intervention," are important. Specific formal and informal measures are essential in obtaining a complete picture of the speech of an individual with articulatory and phonological deficits.

The goals of phonological assessment parallel those for any communication disorder and have been described as follows:

- To describe an individual's phonological status
- To identify the differences between the client's articulatory patterns and nondisordered speech
- To determine the communicative implications of the client's phonology
- To assess the client's pronunciation patterns from a developmental viewpoint
- To identify factors that may relate to the etiology and maintenance of the phonological disability
- To plan treatment when appropriate
- To make a prognosis without and with treatment
- To monitor change over time (Bankson & Bernthal, 1998b; Grunwell, 1985)

These objectives may be achieved by assessment that results in a description of phonological status including the following:

- A speech sound inventory
- Characterization of syllable and word structure
- Listing of phonemic errors
- Phonological process analysis when warranted
- An evaluation of intelligibility

The SLP identifies differences in the client's speech that warrant attention based on interference with communication, developmental information, and other factors and collects baseline data from which to measure change over time with or without intervention. The case history, interview, hearing screening, and oral peripheral examination may provide insight into the etiology of the disorder. Predictions for improvement or prognoses are based on the foregoing and on measures of consistency, stimulability, and error sound discrimination. Error consistency appears to be the biggest factor in overall phonological change following intervention (Tyler, Lewis, & Welch, 2003).

Typical assessment procedures are briefly described and explained in the following sections.

DESCRIPTION OF PHONOLOGICAL STATUS

The speech-language pathologist should obtain data on several aspects of speech that relate to articulatory performance. Samples of three children with phonological impairments are presented on the accompanying CD-ROM.

Speech Sound Inventory

A speech sound inventory and description of word and syllable shapes are highly appropriate for children who are at a very early stage of development and for others whose speech is markedly unintelligible. A recommended system for listing phonemes is by manner of production and syllable and word position (Grunwell, 1987; Klein, 1997). Table 10.11 shows a speech sound inventory for Pablo, a 4-year-old boy who is receiving speech and language therapy.

If a client has only one or two speech sound errors and all other phonemes are correctly produced, a statement to that effect is sufficient. A listing of all the correct phonemes is not needed.

Syllable and Word Structure

A listing of the consonant-vowel (CV) patterns that have been produced in words suggests their complexity. The SLP might list the word and syllable shapes that are most characteristic of the client's speech as well as the reductions or simplifications that have occurred. Table 10.12 on provides a list of the words in Pablo's language sample in both standard orthography and phonetic transcription.

Phonemic Error Inventory

In all cases, the SLP needs to identify phonemes that the client misarticulates. This list is typically compiled on the basis of formal testing of sounds in words. The *Goldman-Fristoe Test of Articulation-2* (GFTA-2) (Goldman & Fristoe, 2000) and the *Photo Articulation Test-3* (Lippke, Dickey, Selmar, & Soder, 1997) are two commonly used published tests. Phoneme errors are re-

---

TABLE 10.11

Phonemes produced in various word positions by Pablo, age 4 years

Manner of Production	Syllable Initial Word Initial	Syllable Initial Word Within	Syllable Final Word Within	Syllable Final Word Final
Nasals	/m/ /n/ "more," "no"	/n/ "nana"	/m/ "Sam-uel"	/m/ "drum"
Stops	/p/ /b/ /t/ /d/ "put," "ball," "top," "drum"	/p/ /b/ /d/ "happy," "Toby," "lady"		
Fricatives	/h/ /f/ /s/ "house," "face," "see"	/f/ "coffee"		
Glides	/w/ /j/ "wet," "you"	/j/ "yo-yo"		

Note: Words were taken from spontaneous language sample. Words in quotes are exemplars of produced phoneme in given word position. Accuracy of articulation of the entire word is not suggested.

TABLE 10.12

Words in Pablo's language sample in standard orthography and phonetic transcription

"more" → [mɔə]	"happy" → [hæpi]	"baseball" → [bebɔ]
"no" → [no]	"Toby" → [tobi]	"ice cream" → [aɪtim]
"banana" → [nænə]	"lady" → [ledi]	"face" → [fe]
"Samuel" → [sæmu]	"house" → [hau]	"wet" → [wɛ]
"put" → [pʊ]	"face" → [fe]	"you" → [ju]
"ball" → [bɔ]	"see" → [si]	"yoyo" → [jojo]
"top" → [tɑ]	"shoe" → [su]	"light" → [jaɪ]
"drum" → [dʌm]	"coffee" → [tɔfi]	"balloon" → [bʌju]

The word shapes produced include CV ([no]), CVCV ([jojo]), CVC ([dʌm]), and VCVC ([aɪtim])

The word shapes that were reduced are

CVC → CV	("put" → [pʊ])
CVCVCV → CVCV	("banana" → [nænə])
CVCCVC → CVCV	("baseball" → [bebɔ])
VCCCVC → VCVC	("ice cream" → [aɪtim])

---

ported as **substitutions, omissions, distortions,** and **additions** in syllable/word positions. For example, if 8-year-old Amanda pronounced "lemon" as "wemon," the SLP might record

> w/l (I) [meaning "w" was substituted for "l" in the initial position; i.e., at the beginning of a word]

Errors are compared with norms for the individual's age. A sample of an administration of the GFTA-2 is presented on the accompanying CD-ROM.

THOUGHT QUESTIONS

Can you determine whether Amanda's substitution is typical for her age? At what age do most children correctly produce the /l/ phoneme in all positions of words? Check Table 10.5.

Phonological Process Analysis

Many research studies have shown that targeting a process rather than an individual phoneme has the advantage of encouraging generalization of learning to similar phonemes and phonological contexts (Gierut, 1998). Therefore, if an individual has numerous errors, it is helpful to identify which phonological processes are apparent. The most common processes are shown in Table 10.4 and may include assimilation, fronting, final consonant deletion, weak syllable deletion, stopping, gliding, cluster simplification, deaffrication, and vocalization. Phonological process information may be analyzed by the SLP on the basis of transcriptions of the child's conversational or single word utterances. Often SLPs will use a published test such as the *Khan-Lewis Phonological Analysis-2* (Khan & Lewis, 2002), which analyzes phonological processes on the basis of the findings of the *Goldman-Fristoe Test of Articulation-2* (Goldman & Fristoe, 2000). Other published tests for determining phonological processes include the *Assessment of Phonological Processes—Revised* (Hodson, 1986) and the *Bankson-Bernthal Test of Phonology* (Bankson & Bernthal, 1990). One version of the *Comprehensive Test of Phonological Processing* addresses the needs of older individuals ages 7 through 24 years (Wagner, Torgesen, & Rashotte, 1999).

> While computer analysis of phonological processes might save time, once the program is learned, the SLP must still understand the nature of the processes to effectively work with the client.

Phonological processes also may be analyzed by using a computerized program. These systems often save time and provide more detailed information than hand-scored procedures. Examples of computerized phonological analysis programs include *Diagnostic Report Writer 2000* (Weiner, 2000) and *Macintosh Interactive System for Phonological Analysis* (Mac-ISPA; Masterson & Pagan, 1993). The *Assessment of Phonological Processes* noted in the previous paragraph is also available in a computerized version called *Computerized Analysis of Phonological Processes* (Hodson, 1985).

In the case of Amanda above, if her only phoneme error was /l/ → /w/ (I), this would not be indicative of a phonological process; it is a *single* phonemic substitution, an error of articulation. If, on the other hand, Amanda produced /l/ → /w/ (I,M) and /r/ → /w/ (I,M), this *pattern* could be described as the phonological process gliding of liquids, since /l/ and /r/ are liquids and they were said as the glide /w/.

*W*hy was final position not included in the examples of Amanda's use of /w/ for /l/ and /r/? Are these sounds produced differently in this position?

THOUGHT QUESTIONS

Intelligibility

Speech **intelligibility** refers to how easy it is to understand the individual. Poor intelligibility has a negative impact on communicative effectiveness. Intelligibility depends on such factors as the number, type, and consistency of speech sound errors. The person's voice, fluency, rate, rhythm, language, and use of gesture also contribute to ease of comprehension, and these should be noted. Other factors beyond the speaker include the listener's hearing acuity, familiarity with the speaker, and experience listening to disordered speech, plus, environmental noise, message complexity, and environmental cues. Table 10.13 illustrates a commonly used subjective way of reporting intelligibility.

TABLE 10.13

Subjective descriptors of intelligibility

1. Readily intelligible even when the context is not known

2. Intelligible with careful listening when the context is not known

3. Intelligible with careful listening when the context is known

4. Unintelligible with careful listening even when the context is known

A more objective measure of intelligibility is percentage of intelligible words. If speech is exceedingly poor, intelligibility may be measured in terms of syllables or consonants (Strand & McCauley, 1997). A recorded sample of continuous speech is transcribed, and the percentage of intelligible words is computed as follows:

$$\text{Percentage of Intelligible Words} = \frac{\text{Number of Intelligible Words}}{\text{Total Number of Words}} \times 100$$

The percentage of intelligible syllables or consonants is computed in a similar fashion. Intelligibility measures are becoming increasingly common in research and clinical use (Shriberg, Austin, Lewis, McSweeney, & Wilson, 1997; Wilcox & Morris, 1999).

In general, highly unintelligible speech signals a severe disorder, while readily intelligible speech suggests that the disorder may be mild. Severity is also based on expectations for a child's age and the presence of additional communication impairments.

PROGNOSTIC INDICATORS

The detailed description of the client's speech will provide some insights into the likelihood of improvement without and with therapy. Background information on family models and support, illnesses, ear infections, and the like may help the SLP to predict the client's improvement. Prognosis may also be determined by the consistency of the phoneme errors, the stimulability of the client, and possibly the individual's ability to discriminate error sounds from target phonemes.

Consistency

Think about your own speech. If you are reading aloud in front of a class, you are likely to be very careful in how you produce all the sounds of the words. On the other hand, when you are speaking casually to a friend, your articulation is probably far less precise. Inconsistency is normal, and it may be a clue to the exact nature of an articulation or phonological error. Let's go back to Amanda. If her misarticulation of /l/ occurs only when she is in conversational speech and then only at the beginning of words, her speech sound error may be more amenable to change. Lack of consistency is considered a positive prognostic indicator. Ironically, an individual with consistent errors may be easier to understand than someone whose error pattern is inconsistent. Consistency of phoneme errors is achieved by evaluating the client's speech during more than one task and in more than one word position and phonemic context (Bernhardt & Holdgrafer, 2001).

Stimulability

Assessment should always include trial therapy. **Stimulability** is the ability of an individual to produce the target phoneme when given focused auditory and visual cues. Typically, the SLP will say, "Look at me. Listen to me. Now say exactly what I say: _____." The SLP will first prompt correct production of the error phoneme or pattern within the word in which it had been misarticulated. If the client does not correctly imitate the SLP, the prompt is moved to the syllable or phoneme level.

Although stimulability is often a positive prognostic indicator, research studies suggest a more complex relationship. Children who are stimulable may respond more quickly to correction of the target phoneme and may also be more likely to self-correct without therapy than those who are not stimulable. Those sounds for which a child is not stimulable are highly unlikely to change without treatment. On the other hand, among children in therapy, those with low stimulability scores often make more progress, especially with untreated sounds, than do those who are more stimulable.

Error Sound Discrimination

It is possible that a child does not perceive the difference in his or her speech. This would be a weakness in **external error sound discrimination.** A fairly common exchange between a parent and young child goes something like this:

Child: Oh, I see a wabbit

Parent (exaggerating the /r/): You see a rabbit!

Child: Yeah, I see a wabbit!

Parent: Say "er."

Child: "er."

Parent: say "er abbit."

Child: "er wabbit."

While the above dialogue is an example of a parent trying to stimulate the child to correctly produce a word, it may also probe whether a child hears the difference between the parent's and the child's utterances.

> Intuition suggests that the easier it is for a person to produce a target phoneme, the more likely it is that the individual will make rapid progress.

> Improvement in nontargeted phonemes, in addition to those that are taught, is often made when the targets are relatively difficult.

Do you think the child can discriminate between his or her production of the word "rabbit" and the parental model? Why? What other explanations could account for the differences?

THOUGHT QUESTIONS

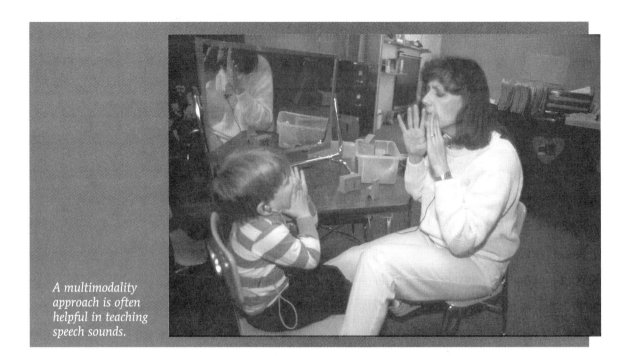

A multimodality approach is often helpful in teaching speech sounds.

Error sound discrimination is often assessed both externally and internally. External discrimination, or **interpersonal error sound discrimination,** refers to the ability to perceive differences in another person's speech. For example, in external discrimination, the SLP might ask the client, "Are these the same or different: 'wemon'—'lemon'?" Sometimes two words are contrasted, and the client is asked to point to pictures that can be labeled using either the targeted phoneme or the one that was substituted; for example, shown two pictures, the client is told "Point to awake. Now point to a lake." **Internal error sound discrimination,** sometimes termed **intrapersonal error sound discrimination,** is the ability to judge one's own ongoing speech. The client may be asked to judge the accuracy of her or his phoneme productions.

The relationship of speech sound discrimination to articulation and phonology remains unclear. Perception of a contrast such as /r/ or /l/ and /w/ usually precedes production in children who are developing typically (Strange & Broen, 1980). In addition, children who are better at internal discrimination have been reported to have more correct articulations (Lapko & Bankson, 1975). From this, we might conclude that error sound discrimination ability signals a more favorable prognosis than the absence of this ability. Two warnings about phoneme discrimination testing are warranted: (1) Only the error phonemes appear to relate to therapeutic prognosis, so only these should be routinely assessed. (2) Many young children do not understand the concept of same versus different; therefore, their error sound discrimination is difficult to judge.

INTERVENTION

If the results of the assessment suggest that treatment is appropriate, the SLP must determine how to proceed. Initial questions to be answered include the following:

- Where will therapy occur? (Clinic, center, school, or home setting?)
- How frequently will the client be seen? (Once or twice a week or three, four, or five times weekly?)
- How long will the sessions be? (Twenty to sixty minutes is the typical range.)
- Will therapy be individual, group, or within a classroom?

Answers to these questions will be related to the facilities that are available as well as to the needs of the child. In addition to such administrative type decisions, the SLP must determine the following:

- What should be the therapy targets?
- What treatment approach appears most suitable?

Parents may be enlisted to reinforce therapy under the guidance of a speech-language pathologist. Carefully structured home-work assignments can provide a client with additional beneficial practice.

*W*hat might be some relative advantages and disadvantages of different therapy settings and schedules?

THOUGHT
QUESTION

TARGET SELECTION

The major goal of therapy should be to make the client easier to understand, that is, to improve his or her intelligibility in a way that will have a positive impact on the person's life. One factor is the frequency of a particular misarticulated phoneme within the language: For example, /ʒ/, as in "treasure" ([trɛʒɚ]), does not occur in many American English words, so it would not normally warrant early attention. On the other hand, targets that may generalize to correction of phonological processes would be extremely helpful in improving intelligibility. If a child exhibits the process stopping of fricatives, as in saying "see" as [ti] and "five" as [paɪb], intervention for correct production of /s/ may generalize to other fricatives, including /f/ and /v/.

A second factor in target selection is likelihood of success. The SLP might initially choose targets that the client will probably master relatively quickly. The best predictors of ease of mastery are stimulability and inconsistency. If the client can produce the target phonemes when prompted to imitate with increased visual and auditory stimulation, this is a favorable sign. In addition, if the client does not misarticulate a particular target in all words or situations, this demonstrates that successful intervention is likely (Edwards, 1983).

Some current research studies have demonstrated that greater generalization to nontarget phonemes occurs when the targets are more difficult for the child—that is, not stimulable, consistent, later developing, and more phonetically complex (Gierut, 1998). It is up to the SLP to determine whether early success on a few targets or more long-term progress on multiple phonemes is best for the individual client.

INTERVENTION APPROACHES

A variety of therapy approaches and techniques exist. The SLP might target one phoneme at a time, work with phonological processes, emphasize motor movements, or focus on the nonsegmental aspects of speech such as rate, rhythm, and melody. Most SLPs will adjust their approach to suit each client and combine procedures to provide individually tailored therapy. In the next few sections, we provide highlights of just a few of the well-known therapy approaches.

Single-Phoneme Targets

A single-phoneme target approach may be valuable for individuals who have a limited number of phoneme errors and who do not have significant neuromotor impairment. This approach consists of four stages, each one following the previous or overlapping (Van Riper & Erickson, 1996).

Perceptual or **ear training** is normally the first stage. It in turn contains four steps:

1. Identification of a target sound
2. Location of target sound
3. Stimulation
4. Discrimination

First, the client is made aware of the target phoneme. If the target is /s/, it might be called the "snake sound," and a picture might be used to highlight this association. Second, the client might signal every time she or he hears the target. Soon the client might specify whether the target phoneme occurred at the beginning, middle, or end of a presented word. Third, the SLP stimulates the client to recognize the sound in sentences that contain multiple examples of the target. For example, if the target is /f/, the SLP might say "Find the funny fox." Naturally, for children, these utterances would be accompanied by appropriate activities. Fourth, ear training culminates with the client learning to discriminate correct from incorrect productions.

Production training refers to teaching the client to say the target phoneme first in isolation, then in syllables, words, phrases, and finally, sentences. Exercises, drills, and games are used to provide opportunities for learning and practice in progressively more difficult utterances. At the sentence level, carrier phrases are often used. For example, if the target is /f/, the client may be instructed to say "I found X," X being a variety of items beginning with /f/, such as "five," "fork," "foot," and "finger." Phonemic contexts are also varied so that the client practices the target in all positions of words and in all combinations.

Stabilization involves activities that will reinforce and review the learned target. Many different activities will be used to ensure stabilization.

Structured conversations will give way to more spontaneous situations always with the goal of correct production of the previously misproduced phonemes. The client will be expected to engage in self-monitoring and self-correction of errors.

Finally, the client needs to transfer or **carry over** correct production into everyday conversation. Most SLPs encourage their clients to use what they have learned in conversation outside of the clinical setting as early as feasible. Homework assignments and activities that are naturalistic are used to ensure that what was accomplished clinically becomes automatic and habitual. In doing this, it is important that adequate guidance is provided to parents, teachers, or others who are to assist in carryover.

What should parents, caregivers, teachers, and others know to effectively assist in carryover? Can you think of a situation in which an untrained person might do more harm than good?

Stimulability Training

Since the ability to imitate sounds is an important predictor of success in producing these sounds spontaneously, some SLPs work to enhance stimulability. This is particularly useful for children who have few phonemes in their repertoire and are not stimulable for many sounds. In working with preschoolers, one method uses stimulus characters and associated gestures in playlike activities. For example, to teach the child to imitate /s/, the clinician would present a picture of a "silly snake" and slinkily move a finger up his or her arm, while modeling the sound and encouraging the child to repeat it. Since the clinician wants to avoid frustrating the child by only presenting sounds that the child is unable to produce, stimulable sounds are also included in the sessions (Miccio & Elbert, 1996).

When a youngster has multiple phonemic errors, these generally can be described as phonological processes. It is more efficient to target a process than to attempt to correct one phoneme at a time.

Phonological Process Targets

Children who have multiple phonemic errors and are highly unintelligible may benefit from phonologically based treatment that focuses on phonological processes, rather than individual phonemes as the primary targets. In the **cycles approach,** the basis for choosing targets is the ease with which the client is likely to master them (Hodson & Paden, 1991). The first target would be the pattern for which the child is most *stimulable.*

Each session in the cycles approach follows a particular structure. First, the previous session's target words are reviewed. Then the child listens to about twelve words containing the target pattern, which are presented with slight amplification (**auditory bombardment**). The child is asked to say three to five production practice words that contain the target in a carefully selected phonemic context. These words are then used in carefully planned play activities. Some conversation is introduced each session so that the SLP can observe whether targets are being generalized to spontaneous speech.

Possible targets for the next session are probed, and the most stimulable target is selected for the next session. Auditory bombardment is repeated, and the list of words is given to the parent or caregiver to read aloud to the child for about two minutes each day.

The **metaphon** approach incorporates of the child's active cognitive participation in remediation of the disorder. For therapy to be effective, metaphon theorists state that the client must be aware that his or her articulatory production is inappropriate, want to modify it, know the relevant articulatory targets, and have the neuromotor capability of accurately producing the targets with adequate speed in a variety of phonetic contexts (Hewlett, 1990).

Metaphon therapy is divided into two basic phases. In Phase One, the client develops phonological awareness. The goal is to make the client interested in the sound system of the language and prepared to learn about how sounds are produced and how they differ from one another. During Phase Two, the client transfers the knowledge acquired in Phase One to communicative situations and learns to self-monitor and modify output to improve message transmission. The concept of minimal pairs (described later in this chapter) is a useful tool in metaphon and other therapy (Howell & Dean, 1994).

Articulatory Training

Both single-phoneme and phonological process approaches depend heavily on auditory stimulation and the ability to hear and then reproduce target speech sounds. Some individuals for various reasons are unable to imitate what they've heard even when they understand the objective. Consider, for example, that you are learning to speak Mandarin Chinese, a language that uses melodic patterns or tones to communicate word meaning. Although you "hear" what is said to you and you understand what is required, you may have difficulty correctly imitating and differentiating between two words differing only by melodic pattern. You simply cannot get your vocal mechanism to act the way it must to say the Chinese words.

Articulatory techniques focus on the neuromotor processes needed in phoneme production. We will briefly describe two approaches that are sometimes used particularly with children who do not respond easily to auditory stimulation. These approaches are sensory-motor and oral-motor.

In **sensorimotor training** the client is made aware of the tactile and proprioceptive sensations associated with the production of sounds in syllables and words. The client is asked to imitate targets and then describe, for example, where the tongue is placed, where air can be felt, and so on. The focus is not on the individual phoneme but on overlapping movements that occur in connected speech (McDonald, 1964).

Oral-motor training goes beyond the mouth and provides suggestions for appropriate body posture and breathing for speech. Six principles of oral-motor dynamics have been suggested (Boshart, 1998):

1. Motor development is continuous, sequential, and cumulative. We move from generalized movements and reflexes to more precise voluntary oral gestures.

2. Correct speech sound production depends on the correct oral-facial resting posture from which movement is possible. The lips are closed, the tongue is up, and the jaw is gently relaxed.

3. Speech requires adequate muscle strength, tone, and endurance. Tone refers to the muscle's state of readiness to act, and endurance means that the movement can be held and/or repeated many times.

4. Tactile and proprioceptive feedback permit the speaker to self-monitor. Remember the last time you were at the dentist and received novocaine? Your sense of touch (tactile) and position (proprioception) within your mouth were impaired. You probably had difficulty speaking normally. Speakers constantly make tiny adjustments based on how things feel as well as how they sound (auditory feedback).

5. Stability is critical to movement. Try to say the word "temperature" while moving your jaw from side to side. You will find it difficult. Speakers learn to isolate one part of the oral mechanism while holding everything else stable.

6. Speech requires well-coordinated, subtle movements. The lips must be able to move independently of the jaw. Movement of the tongue tip must be isolated from that of the back of the tongue.

Specific exercises are recommended for accomplishing each of these principles. In essence, the SLP prepares the client motorically before actually teaching speech sounds. The oral-motor principles identified above relate broadly to speech production. Diminishment of oral apraxia without relating this to speech motor control may do nothing to improve speech movements (Hall et al., 1993).

Minimal Pairs

Minimal pair contrasts are used in many types of articulation and phonological therapy. Two words are presented that are the same with the exception of a single phoneme, for example, boy/toy, chip/ship, or fine/pine. At least three types of contrasts are possible: error phoneme/target phoneme, **minimal contrast,** and **maximal contrast** or **maximal opposition.**

In error phoneme/target phoneme minimal pairs, the SLP usually chooses one phoneme at a time. The SLP attempts to reproduce the target as normally said by the client and contrast this with a correct production. For example, if the client typically pronounced "chair" as "share," the SLP might begin by presenting both utterances and asking the client whether they are the same or different. From there, the SLP may have the client point to pictures representing each member of the pair. Additional exercises include using both words in sentences and asking the client whether the sentences make sense or not—for example, "He sat on the share." Production exercises follow, in which the client is expected to produce the minimal pair in designated contexts.

In minimal contrasts, several phoneme pairs that differ in a single distinctive feature may be targeted. Actually, the example above of error phoneme contrast is also a minimal contrast. An additional example of a

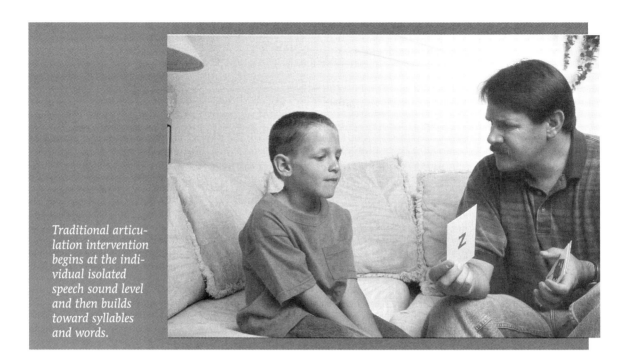

Traditional articulation intervention begins at the individual isolated speech sound level and then builds toward syllables and words.

minimal contrast would be "Sue" and "zoo." The "s" and "z" differ only in that the "s" is voiceless and the "z" is voiced.

Maximal contrasts, sometimes called maximal opposition, pair phonemes that differ in more than one distinctive feature. For example, in the words "man" and "fan," "m" and "f" differ in manner of production, voicing, and nasality. Maximal contrasts are sometimes used earlier in therapy, since they might be easier for a client to differentiate. In addition, maximal contrast training may lead to modification of error phonemes beyond that which is immediately targeted (Gierut, 1989).

When minimal pair contrasts are used in the metaphon approach, the client is asked how he or she knows whether the utterance and picture match (or whether the sentence makes sense). Focus of discussion is always on the communicative success of the transaction rather than on the "correctness" of the articulation. When the client is asked to name pictures, the clinician responds on the basis of what is said, regardless of whether it is what the client intended (Howell & Dean, 1994).

However minimal pairs are used, they are a valuable tool in the remediation of articulation and phonology (Bauman-Waengler, 2000).

Computer Applications

Computer programs are available that can be used as an adjunct to intervention by the SLP. These programs provide exercises in both perception of phonemic targets and production. They are helpful in providing immediate

TABLE 10.14

A basic progression in phonemic therapy

1. Prepare the client for correct phoneme production.

   a. Auditory, visual, and oral-motor training are applied as necessary.

   b. Listening exercises and oral-motor drills may be used.

2. Facilitate target production in a minimally complex context.

   a. Auditory, visual, and oral-motor training provide techniques for correct productions.

   b. Isolated phonemes and processes may be targeted.

3. Increase the level of complexity as the client is ready.

   a. Target words become longer and more phonologically challenging.

   b. Target words are embedded in phrases and sentences.

4. Encourage self-monitoring, self-correction, and generalization.

   a. The client is challenged to take responsibility for correct productions.

   b. Situations for using targeted phonemes are extended to conversations and different communicative partners and settings.

feedback on the client's performance. School-age children with few phonemic errors often respond especially well to drills that are presented in computer game format. Computer exercises provide an opportunity for independent practice as well as for variety within a therapy session. It is up to the SLP to ensure that mastery goes beyond simple exercises and that improvement is reflected in conversational speech (Gierut, 1998).

Combination

Most speech-language pathologists use a combination of approaches and select features of each that are appropriate to the needs of the particular client. Table 10.14 outlines the basic steps of intervention.

GENERALIZATION AND MAINTENANCE

Once the client has achieved an acceptable level of correct phoneme production, the SLP must ensure that slippage does not occur and that the new speech pattern becomes habitual. Many SLPs introduce self-monitoring exercises from the very beginning of therapy. In this way, clients understand that they are ultimately responsible for their own success. Once the SLP believes that the client is ready for dismissal from therapy, follow-up sessions may be scheduled at progressively longer intervals. If the progress has been maintained over time, the remediation has been effective.

Success of therapy is determined by the application of what has been learned in a clinical setting to everyday life.

SUMMARY

Producing the sounds of a language during speech is a complex process. It involves an inner conceptualization of phonemes and phonotactic rules so that in our "mind's ear" we know how the language we are speaking should sound. Speech production also requires the neuromotor ability to move our articulators to form the desired sounds in a smooth, rapid, and automatic fashion. As children develop spoken language, they typically employ phonological processes that simplify adult forms. If these persist beyond the expected ages, they may present difficulties. Hearing disorders, neurological impairments, and organic abnormalities may contribute to phonological and articulatory disorders. Foreign language background and regional dialects contribute to variations in speech. Assessment of articulation and phonology includes a detailed description of the individual's phonological output, as well as investigation of etiology and determination of prognosis. Intervention strategies may include ear training, oral-motor facilitation, and production enhancement techniques. The general goal is improved intelligibility in spontaneous speech.

REFLECTIONS

- What systems are used for classifying speech sounds? Why is it important to do this?
- What disorders are associated with articulatory and phonological impairments?
- Identify the steps in the assessment of articulation and phonology.
- What factors are considered in selecting targets for articulatory and phonological improvement?
- How do speech-language pathologists modify articulatory and phonological production?
- What is the major goal of articulatory and phonological intervention?

SUGGESTED READINGS

Ball, M. J., & Kent, R. D. (1997). *The new phonologies: Developments in clinical linguistics.* San Diego, CA: Singular.

Baumann-Waengler, J. (2000). *Articulatory and phonological impairments: A clinical focus.* Boston: Allyn and Bacon.

Bernthal, J. E., & Bankson, N. W. (1998). *Articulation and phonological disorders* (4th ed.). Boston: Allyn and Bacon.

Crary, M. A. (1993). *Developmental motor speech disorders.* San Diego, CA: Singular.

Grunwell, P. (1985). *PACS: Phonological assessment of child speech.* San Diego, CA: College-Hill.

Hodson, B., & Paden, E. (1991) *Targeting intelligible speech: A phonological approach to remediation* (2nd ed.). Austin, TX: Pro-Ed.

⊙NLINE RESOURCES

http://www.americandialect.org/   Home page of the American Dialect Society. Dedicated to the study of the English language in North America and its relationship to other languages. Highlights related news such as recent books and conferences on language.

http://www.tandf.co.uk/journals/ft/02699206.html Clinical Linguistics & Phonetics.
The tables of contents of recent issues are available online. Articles are featured on such topics as phonetic disorders of speech, clinical dialectology, phonetics of hearing impairment, and disordered communication in multicultural settings. If you sign up, you also can view a free sample issue.

http://www.arts.gla.ac.uk/IPA/   The International Phonetic Association. Website contains the latest version of IPA, phonetic fonts for word processing, and information about the International Congress of Phonetic Sciences and the *Journal of the International Phonetic Association.*

http://www.ling.upenn.edu/phono_atlas/NationalMap/NationalMap.html   A national map of the regional dialects of American English.
A phonological atlas showing the major dialect regions of the United States and linguistic features that characterize the areas.

Cleft Lip and Cleft Palate

11

CHAPTER LEARNING GOALS

When you have finished this chapter, you should be able to:

- Describe the embryological development of the face and palate

- Describe how clefts of the lip and palate form

- Describe the clinical features and possible causes of a cleft of the lip

- Describe the clinical features of bilateral and unilateral clefts of the lip and palate

- Describe the team approach and general management procedures used for treating people with clefts

The roof of your mouth is called the palate. The anterior two-thirds of the palate is the hard palate, which is composed of bony plates that are fused along their midline. If you run the tip of your tongue along the roof of your mouth in a front-to-back direction, you will trace roughly the fusion line of your hard palate. The hard palate is stationary and serves to separate the anterior aspects of the oral and nasal cavities. **Mucosal tissue,** pinkish-colored tissue lining the inside of the mouth, covers the hard palate.

The soft palate, called the *velum,* constitutes the posterior one-third of the palate and is composed of muscle and mucosal tissue. The velum and muscles in the back of the throat, or **pharynx,** constitute the **velopharyngeal mechanism.** This mechanism acts like a valve; it can be open, allowing a coupling between the oral and nasal cavities, or it can be closed, partitioning the oral and nasal cavities. For example, when you breathe

Case Study 11.1

Case Study of a Child with Cleft Palate: Colin

Colin is a 6-year-old boy with a repaired bilateral complete cleft of the lip and palate. When Colin was born presenting with the bilateral complete cleft, he was taken to the major medical center in his home town for surgical repair of his lip and palate. In the years following his surgery, Colin was followed carefully by the craniofacial team at the medical center. This team of different specialists ensured that Colin received appropriate dental and orthodontic care, otologic and audiologic management, and speech-language therapy. During his preschool years, Colin had received speech therapy at the medical center. He was dismissed from therapy when he was 4½ years old because his speech and language production was within normal limits.

When Colin enrolled in kindergarten at his local school, he received a standard speech-language screening that was administered to all new students. The SLP who screened Colin noted that he had a mild nasal resonance, particularly on vowels adjacent to nasal consonants, and a small degree of nasal emission noted primarily during production of stop consonants. When the school SLP informed Colin's parents about the problem, they asked her to add Colin to her caseload. The SLP declined their request explaining that Colin should be thoroughly evaluated by the craniofacial team. The SLP explained that such

an evaluation would ensure that Colin's velopharyngeal mechanism was physically capable of closure during speech production. If it was determined that the velopharyngeal mechanism was physically incapable of closure, speech therapy may be contraindicated.

Colin was evaluated by the medical center's craniofacial team. Multidimensional videofluoroscopy revealed that Colin's velopharyngeal mechanism was capable of closure. The hypernasal resonance and nasal emission in his speech was determined to be the result of faulty learning subsequent to Colin's dismissal from speech therapy. The team recommended that Colin resume speech therapy in school. The school SLP agreed to keep the craniofacial team apprised of Colin's progress.

As you read this chapter, think about

- The types of speech problems that result from structural abnormalities of the upper lip, and of the hard and soft palate.
- Why Colin demonstrated nasal emission on stop consonants.
- Why Colin demonstrated hypernasal resonance on vowels that were adjacent to nasal consonants.

through your nose, the soft palate hangs like a curtain coupling the nasal and oral cavities. Air passes through the nose into the pharynx, trachea, and lungs.

Put your index finger under your nose and say the /p/ sound several times. You will observe that no air escapes from your nose. During production of the /p/ sound, your velopharyngeal mechanism closed, separating the oral and nasal cavities. Separation of the oral and nasal cavities is required during swallowing and for the production of most speech sounds. This separation is accomplished through muscle contraction that moves the velum in a superior (upper) and posterior direction. The **velopharyngeal portal,** or conduit connecting the oral and nasal cavities, is closed, and separation of the oral and nasal cavities is complete when the velum makes contact with the posterior and lateral aspects of the pharynx. In addition to elevation of the velum, closure of the velopharyngeal portal is assisted by active movement of the lateral walls of the pharynx.

Velopharyngeal incompetence (VPI) is a term that we will be using frequently in this chapter. It means that the velopharyngal mechanism is incapable of separating the oral and nasal cavities during swallowing and speech production (Pannabacker, 2004). VPI is a frequent result of palatal clefts and is associated with velar soft tissue and muscle tissue deficiencies. We will have more to say about VPI later in the chapter.

You can see a portion of your soft palate by looking into a well-illuminated bathroom mirror. You will also see a structure projecting inferiorly (downward) called the **uvula;** the uvula is the termination of your soft palate.

When you swallow, your velum elevates, separating the oral and nasal cavities. What would happen if your velum didn't close the velopharyngeal portal during swallowing?

THOUGHT QUESTION

In this chapter, we will explore **craniofacial anomalies** or congenital malformations involving the head and face and affecting speech. There are hundreds of different craniofacial anomalies, many of which are accompanied by malformations of the upper lip, hard palate, and soft palate. Malformations of the upper lip and hard and soft palate are called **clefts.** A cleft is an abnormal opening in an anatomical structure (Shprintzen, 1995), representing a failure of structures to fuse or to merge early in embryonic development. This fusion process will be discussed later in this chapter.

Clefts may involve an entire anatomical structure, such as the entire hard palate, or only a part of it. Clefts of the lip that may involve the dental arch (**alveolus**) and the anterior aspect of the hard palate (**premaxilla**) develop between the fifth and eighth weeks of gestation. Isolated clefts of the hard and/or soft palate develop between the eight and twelfth weeks of gestation.

Clefts of the lip and palate create a condition that interferes with basic biological functions such as breathing and swallowing, and they can inhibit severely a child's development of speech and language. We will discuss some of the unique communicative problems associated with palatal clefts and the wide range of medical, dental, and behavioral treatments that children with clefts require. We will also discuss the necessity of an interdisciplinary treatment approach for people with clefts.

Clefts of the lip and palate may present challenges well beyond infancy, and these challenges will change across the individual's lifespan. We will briefly consider some of the major challenges that present themselves across the lifespan of persons with clefts.

*P*HYSICAL CHALLENGES OF CLEFTS THROUGH THE LIFESPAN

At birth, the person with a cleft may have obstructive breathing problems and need immediate medical attention. Depending on the severity of the cleft, the child may also have problems with food intake. Typical feeding problems include poor oral suction, lengthy feeding times, nasal regurgitation, gagging, and excessive air intake. Unfortunately, there is no single feeding method that will be successful for infants with different types of clefts. The infant's performance during the initial feedings will dictate the feeding method and individual modifications will need to be made to ensure adequate nutrition. SLPs, occupational therapists, nutritionists, and nurse practitioners will be involved in assisting the mother and infant (Kummer, 2001).

During the first year of life, clefts of the lip will be surgically closed and the infant will be carefully monitored for possible middle ear infection. Approximately a year following closure of the lip, surgeons will close the clefts of the hard and soft palate, and subsequent to this surgery, the SLP will begin evaluating the individual for VPI. Frequently, very successful cosmetic surgery does not result in adequate velopharyngeal function.

When the child is around 2 years of age, dental specialists will begin reconstruction of abnormal dentition and dental occlusion. SLPs will work closely with dental specialists to ensure normal speech and language development. The adolescent child may require extensive orthodontic treatment in addition to secondary surgeries for VPI and/or cosmetic improvements. Psychological counseling and speech-language therapy may also be required.

From the teenage years through adulthood, a number of potential issues may require attention. These include middle ear disease, potential hearing loss, psychological status, and genetic counseling regarding the risk of having an infant with a cleft. Generally, however, adequate and appropriate health care and specialized services throughout the lifespan will result in an individual who is capable of leading a fulfilling life. We will now turn our attention to a more detailed discussion of the information presented above.

DEVELOPMENT OF THE FACE AND PALATE

To begin our discussion of cleft lip and palate, we will focus on the normal development of the face and the palate. A brief examination of how the face and palate are formed will shed light on the underlying nature of clefts and how they form. The third through the twelfth week of gestation are when the face and the palate are formed. The formation of cleft lip with or without cleft palate and of isolated cleft palate are well understood.

FACIAL DEVELOPMENT

The face and anterior aspects of the mouth are formed between the fifth and eighth weeks after conception. Normal development of the face and mouth is a result of a complex fusion among five embryonic processes: the right and left **mandibular processes,** the **frontonasal process,** and two **maxillary processes.** These processes are illustrated in Figure 11.1a.

Fusion of the right and left mandibular processes, which forms the mandible and the lower lip, occurs early in the development of the face, during the fourth and fifth weeks of gestation. The right and left mandibular processes grow toward one another and fuse in the midline of the face. This fusion process has been completed in the 6-week-old embryo shown in Figure 11.1a. Mandibular fusion is relatively simple when considered in light of fusion processes that occur above the mandible.

During the fifth week of gestation, the frontonasal processes grow in a downward direction, separating into two distinct tissue masses on both sides of the face called the **nasomedian processes** and the **lateral nasal processes.** Depressions between the nasomedian and lateral nasal processes called the **olfactory pits** will ultimately become the right and left nasal cavities. The lateral nasal processes fuse with the maxillary processes to form the **nasal alae** (the flared portion of the nostrils) and the anterior aspects of the face just beneath the eyes as shown in Figure 11.1b.

The nasomedian processes also fuse with the paired maxillary processes. Primitive tissue contained in the nasomedian processes will become the anterior portion of the upper lip, the anterior aspect of the alveolus (the portion of the maxilla or upper jaw that holds teeth) containing the upper frontal incisor teeth, and the anterior aspect of the hard palate, called the premaxilla. Facial development is completed during the eighth week of gestation, as shown in Figure 11.1b. Clefts of the lip that may include a cleft alveolus and premaxilla occur when the fusion process between the nasomedian and maxillary processes has been interrupted by some abnormal genetic condition or by environmental agents (e.g., certain drugs, chemicals, nicotine, irradiation) called **teratogens** that adversely affect the developing child.

G̶iven that development of the face begins around the fourth week of pregnancy, why is it important for couples planning on having a child to be as drug-free as possible?

THOUGHT QUESTION

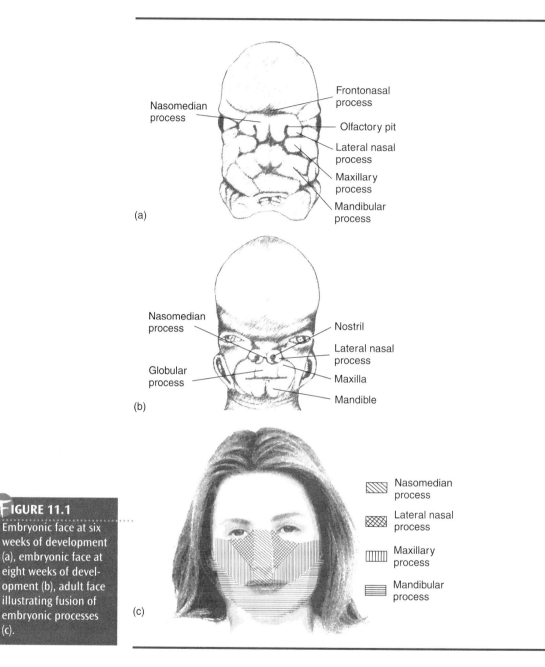

FIGURE 11.1

Embryonic face at six weeks of development (a), embryonic face at eight weeks of development (b), adult face illustrating fusion of embryonic processes (c).

DEVELOPMENT OF THE SECONDARY PALATE

The secondary palate includes the bony hard palate and the soft palate. Although development of the anterior aspects of the face is complete by the end of the eighth week of gestation, complete separation of the oral and nasal cavities has not yet been achieved. Between the eighth and twelfth weeks of gestation, embryonic processes that give rise to the hard and soft palate will fuse, separating the oral and nasal cavities.

Two **palatal shelves,** which are wedge-shaped tissue masses, grow downward from the inner aspects of the maxillary processes. Up to the ninth week of gestation, the tongue projects into the nasal cavity. A rapid growth spurt during the eighth and ninth weeks of gestation increases the length and width of the mandible, pulling the tongue downward and away from its position between the palatal shelves, which then begin fusing with one another in an anterior to posterior fashion. Figure 11.2 shows the general aspects of this anterior to posterior fusion process. As the palatal shelves are fusing, the nasal septum grows downward to meet the palatal shelves in the midline, separating the left and right nasal cavities.

Muscles of the soft palate also evolve from the palatal shelves. The soft palate begins forming during the tenth week of gestation, and fusion of the secondary palate is completed by the end of the twelfth week. Aberrations that prevent fusion of the palatal shelves will result in an isolated cleft of the

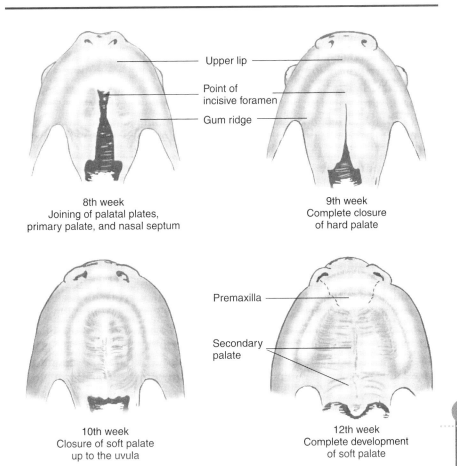

Upper lip

Point of incisive foramen

Gum ridge

8th week
Joining of palatal plates,
primary palate, and nasal septum

9th week
Complete closure
of hard palate

Premaxilla

Secondary
palate

10th week
Closure of soft palate
up to the uvula

12th week
Complete development
of soft palate

FIGURE 11.2
Fusion of the palatal shelves, forming the hard and soft palates.

hard and/or soft palate. As with cleft lip, genetic and nongenetic factors have been identified as causing an isolated cleft of the secondary palate. These factors will be discussed later in this chapter.

CLEFT LIP AND PALATE CLASSIFICATION SYSTEMS

Contemporary cleft palate classification systems are based on the embryological development of the face and palatal structures.

Clefts vary in size and severity, and it is important clinically and for clinical research to accurately classify clefts. At present, there is no universally accepted classification system, but there are some classification systems that are widely used and are useful for clinical reference (Bzoch, 1997).

A cleft lip and palate classification scheme that was developed originally in the 1930s is still in use today. The **Veau system** is useful for a quick general reference regarding the nature and extent of clefts (Bzoch, 1997). Four classes of clefts, identified by Roman numerals, comprise the Veau system and are listed in Table 11.1. More modern clinical classification systems include **Kernahan's Striped Y,** a visual identification system based on location, and one developed by (ACPA), the American Cleft Palate-Craniofacial Association which focuses on the primary and secondary palates.

CLINICAL FEATURES OF CLEFTS

Clefts vary greatly in type and severity, ranging from a small V-shaped notch of the lip to a complete separation of the upper lip, dental arch, and the right and left sides of the hard and soft palate. Clefts are classified commonly as: (1) unilateral or bilateral cleft of the lip, (2) unilateral cleft of the lip and palate, (3) bilateral cleft of the lip and palate, (4) submucous cleft, or (5) bifid uvula. Some of the clinical features of these clefts are discussed below.

TABLE 11.1
The Veau cleft lip and palate classification system

Class	Descriptor
I	Cleft of the soft palate only
II	Cleft of the hard and soft palate to the incisive foramen
III	Complete unilateral cleft of the soft and hard palate and of the lip and alveolar ridge on one side
IV	Complete bilateral cleft of the soft and hard palate and/or the lip and alveolar ridge on both sides

FIGURE 11.3

Unilateral cleft of the lip presurgery (a) and postsurgery (b). Note the "V" shaped notch in the vermilion border of the lip extending toward the left nostril and the flattening of nose and flaring of the nostril on the side of the cleft. (Photographs courtesy of Donald Warren, D.D.S., Ph.D., University of North Carolina, Chapel Hill)

CLEFT OF THE LIP

A cleft of the lip involves the reddish (**vermilion**) portion of the upper lip and may extend through the lip toward the nostril. For example, an **incomplete cleft** of the lip may be a minor V-shaped notch in the vermilion portion of the lip, whereas **complete cleft** of the lip continues through the upper lip into the floor of the nostril. A cleft of the lip has an adverse affect on the shape of the nose characterized by a flattening of the nose and a flaring of the nostril on the side of the cleft. Additionally, the **columella,** the strip of tissue connecting the base and tip of the nose, is short and misaligned. Clefts of the lip may be unilateral or bilateral. When the cleft lip is unilateral (see Figure 11.3), it most commonly occurs on the left side. If the cleft lip is bilateral, it is generally accompanied by a cleft of the palate as well.

An isolated cleft of the lip is rare, accounting for less than 5 percent of all cleft cases (Shprintzen, 1995). Usually, clefts of the lip extend posteriorly through the alveolus. Such clefts may be minor notches in the alveolus, or they may extend completely through the alveolus and involve the premaxilla.

UNILATERAL CLEFT OF THE LIP AND PALATE

A unilateral complete cleft of the lip and palate extends from the external portion of the upper lip, through the alveolus, and through the hard and soft

(a)

(b)

FIGURE 11.4

Unilateral cleft of the lip and palate presurgery (a) and postsurgery (b). Observe that this cleft extends completely through the lip into the left nostril and the alveolus is also cleft. The cleft of the hard and soft palates cannot be seen in this photograph. (Photographs courtesy of Donald Warren, D.D.S., Ph.D., University of North Carolina, Chapel Hill)

palate (see Figure 11.4). The nasal septum attaches to the larger of the two palatal segments.

As was discussed above, a cleft of the secondary palate alone without a cleft lip is sometimes observed. Clefts of the secondary palate alone vary in severity, involving all of the hard and soft palate or only a small portion of the hard or soft palate.

BILATERAL CLEFT OF THE LIP AND PALATE

A bilateral complete cleft of the lip and palate (see Figure 11.5) is the most severe type of cleft due primarily to a severe tissue deficiency. The lip and the alveolus are cleft under both nostrils and the central portion of the lip (**prolabium**), alveolus, and the premaxilla is positioned abnormally at the tip of the nasal septum as a protruding mass of tissue that is sometimes called the free-floating premaxilla (Seagle, 1997; Shprintzen, 1995). In bilateral complete clefts, the columella is usually absent, resulting in the tip of the nose attaching directly to the lip. The nasal septum is not attached to either of the palatal shelves in bilateral clefts.

What are your impressions of the postsurgical results of the clefts you have seen? How do you think these repaired clefts will function during speaking or eating?

THOUGHT QUESTIONS

SUBMUCOUS CLEFT

A submucous cleft is a muscular cleft in the region of the soft palate (see Figure 11.6). The cleft is covered by a thin layer of mucosal tissue that can conceal the underlying lack of muscular fusion. Unlike the clefts discussed above, the submucous cleft may not be discovered until late in childhood. Physical characteristics such as a **bifid uvula** (the uvula appears to be split in half) may indicate the presence of a submucous cleft. However, a bifid uvula may be present in the absence of a submucous cleft. In fact, about one in eighty people has a bifid uvula (Bradley, 1997).

Another symptom of a submucous cleft is a bluish coloration in the middle of the soft palate where the muscles failed to fuse; this may be accompanied by a notch on the posterior border of the hard palate that can be felt. Submucous clefts may lead to velopharyngeal incompetence.

(a)

(b)

FIGURE 11.5

Bilateral cleft of the lip and palate presurgery (a) and postsurgery (b). Note the clefts on both sides of the face and the protruding tissue mass in the central position of the upper lip. (Photographs courtesy of Donald Warren, D.D.S., Ph.D., University of North Carolina, Chapel Hill)

FIGURE 11.6

Submucous cleft. (Photograph courtesy of Donald Warren, D.D.S., Ph.D., University of North Carolina, Chapel Hill)

ETIOLOGIES OF CLEFTS

We have already seen that a cleft of the lip, palate, or both results from a fusion failure among primitive embryonic structures. But what causes such a fusion failure? It is generally accepted that there are four different categories of etiologies that can produce cleft lip, cleft palate, or both cleft lip and cleft palate (Shprintzen & Goldberg, 1995): genetic disorders, chromosomal aberrations, teratogenically induced disorders, and mechanically induced abnormalities.

GENETIC DISORDERS

Genetic disorders account for a substantial percentage of clefting. Clefting is associated with over 400 multiple anomaly **syndromes,** or combinations of symptoms, that occur together in predictable and consistent combinations of traits.[1] Some of the major syndromes that SLPs are likely to encounter include Pierre Robin syndrome (Robin sequence), Treacher Collins syndrome, velocardiofacial syndrome, and Apert syndrome.

The primary symptoms of Pierre Robin syndrome, or, more properly, Robin sequence, include **micrognathia** or an underdeveloped mandible, a retrusion of the tongue into the pharyngeal airway, an isolated cleft of the hard and soft palate, congenital heart problems, digital anomalies, conductive hearing loss, and developmental deficits. Communication deficits are related to cognitive and learning deficits, and severely delayed language de-

---

[1]Another definition for syndromes is "A syndrome may be defined as the presence of multiple anomalies in a single individual with all those anomalies having one primary cause" (Shprintzen, 1995).

velopment is common (McWilliams, Morris, & Shelton, 1990). The small mandible is believed to interfere with the descent of the tongue around the eighth or ninth week of gestation. Position of the tongue between the palatal shelves prevents palatal fusion. The isolated palatal cleft is a result of the tongue's failure to descend.

Treacher Collins syndrome is characterized by **malar hypoplasia,** or an underdevelopment of the cheekbones, underdevelopment of the mandible, malformation of the external ear and the ear canal, conductive hearing loss, cleft palate, and a projection of scalp hair onto the cheek. Brain dysfunction is rare with these individuals, and the major communication problems result from conductive hearing loss and VPI.

Of special interest to the SLP is velocardiofacial syndrome because of the universality of language deficits and learning disabilities in conjunction with a palatal cleft. People with this syndrome are usually of small stature with a broad, flattened nose and have underdeveloped cheekbones and heart problems. A delayed onset of expressive language and persistent language difficulties are primary communication problems among these individuals. The cognitive behavior of individuals with velocardiofacial syndrome is concrete, and they sometimes demonstrate perseverative behaviors (Peterson-Falzone, Hardin-Jones, & Karnell, 2001).

Apert syndrome has an invariable feature called **craniosynostosis** or a premature closing of the sutures of the skull that greatly disfigures the forehead and **syndactyly** or webbing of the fingers and toes with bone fusion. The palate is very high and narrow, giving the appearance of a cleft, but actual clefts occur in only 30 percent of people with Apert syndrome. Conductive hearing loss is frequent, and language development is commensurate with mental ability. Expressive language development is typically delayed.

Before turning our attention to chromosomal aberrations, some mention of general familial inheritance patterns associated with clefting should be made. The risk factors for having a child with a cleft are summarized in Table 11.2.

*P*ut yourself in the position of a parent under each of the conditions listed in Table 11.2. What would you decide about having another child? Would your decision be the same as that of the person sitting next to you in class?

THOUGHT QUESTIONS

CHROMOSOMAL ABERRATIONS

Within the nucleus of human cells are forty-six chromosomes arranged in twenty-three pairs. A chromosomal aberration known as trisomy 13 results in a cleft lip with or without cleft palate in 60 to 70 percent of cases. Trisomy 13 is a rare condition resulting from the appearance of a third #13 chromosome. This condition occurs about once in 6,000 births. Like syndromes, disorders associated with chromosomal aberrations are characterized by multiple congenital abnormalities (Peterson-Falzone et al., 2001).

TABLE 11.2
Risks for cleft lip with or without cleft palate (CL [+/2] CP) and cleft palate (CP)

Situation	(CL [+/−] CP)	(CP)
Frequency of defect in the general population	0.1%	0.04%
My spouse and I are unaffected. We have an affected child. What is the probability that our next baby will have the same condition if:		
We have no affected relatives?	4%	2%
We have an affected relative?	4%	7%
We have two affected children.		
What is the probability that our next child will have the same condition?	9%	1%
I am affected or my spouse is. We have no affected children.		
What is the probability that our next child will be affected?	4%	6%
We have an affected child.		
What is the probability that our next child will be affected?	17%	15%

Source: Adapted from Grabb, Rosenstein, & Bzoch (1971).

TERATOGENICALLY INDUCED DISORDERS

Thalidomide caused thousands of birth defects, including clefting, in the 1960s when the drug was administered to pregnant women. As a result, the drug was outlawed for over thirty years. In 1998, the Food and Drug Administration approved its use for the treatment of certain serious conditions such as leprosy and some cancers associated with AIDS.

Environmental teratogens are agents that interfere with or interrupt normal development of a fetus and create congenital malformations. Recognized teratogens associated with clefting include drugs such as dilantin, an anticonvulsant; thalidomide, a drug that was formerly used as a sedative; excessive use of aspirin, and retinoids, nontopical acne medication. In excessive amounts, ingestion of alcohol, nicotine, and caffeine are also considered to be teratogens responsible for clefting. In addition, X-rays, certain viruses, and some naturally occurring environmental substances have teratogenic properties. The effects of teratogens vary with an individual's unique genetic makeup, the time during pregnancy when the agent was encountered, the amount, and the mother's metabolism (Kummer, 2001; Shprintzen & Goldberg, 1995).

MECHANICALLY INDUCED ABNORMALITIES

Mechanical factors that cause clefts are those that impinge directly on the embryo. With such clefts, the embryo is developing in a normal fashion, and the cleft is induced by something external to the embryo (Shprintzen &

Goldberg, 1995). The most frequent cause of mechanically induced clefts is amniotic rupture (loss of amniotic fluid). Intrauterine crowding as when there is a twin, a uterine tumor, or an irregularly shaped uterus can also result in clefts.

INCIDENCE OF CLEFTS

Clefts occur in approximately one in every 750 live births. Clefts of the lip with or without cleft palate occur more frequently than clefts of the palate alone. Submucous clefts occur in approximately one in every 1,200 births (Peterson-Falzone et al., 2001). There are some indications that the incidence rate for clefts may be increasing because improved prenatal treatment is resulting in the birth of more high-risk fetuses. Additionally, improved postnatal treatment results in adults with clefts who look, speak, and function in a typical manner, making it more likely than it once was that they will have children of their own. Both these factors could serve to increase the size of the genetic pool that carries the cleft trait, resulting in more children being born with clefts (McWilliams et al., 1990; Peterson-Falzone et al., 2001).

GENDER AND RACIAL DIFFERENCES

Clefts of the lip with or without clefts of the palate occur about twice as frequently in males and tend to be more severe. Clefts of the palate alone, however, occur more frequently in females than males. Submucous clefts occur at approximately the same frequency in males and females. In the United States, Native Americans have the highest incidence rates, followed by people of Asian descent, Caucasians, and people of African descent. These incidence differences have been attributed to genetic and environmental factors (McWilliams et al., 1990). Regardless of gender and race, individuals with clefts present many different interrelated problems that require the cooperation of a wide variety of specialists for effective treatment and management (McWilliams et al., 1990; Shprintzen, 1995).

THE CLEFT PALATE TEAM AND GENERAL MANAGEMENT ISSUES THROUGH THE LIFESPAN

The group of specialists working together providing care for persons with cleft palate is referred to as a **cleft palate team.** The concept of a cleft palate team, sometimes called the craniofacial team, was developed originally at the Lancaster Cleft Palate Clinic in Lancaster, Pennsylvania, in the 1930s. Today the Membership-Team Directory of the American Cleft Palate-Craniofacial Association lists 250 cleft palate teams in the United States. Table 11.3 lists the professions that constitute a typical cleft palate team.

TABLE 11.3
Composition of a cleft palate team

Anesthesiologist	Nurse practitioner	Plastic surgeon
Audiologist	Oral surgeon	Prosthodontist
Coordinator	Orthodontist	Psychiatrist
Educator	Otolaryngologist	Psychologist
Endodontist	Parents	Radiologist
Geneticist	Pediatrician	Social worker
Genetic counselor	Periodontist	Speech-language pathologist

Clinical management of people with clefts requires the efficient integration of information among professionals. For example, a surgeon might require information about speech production ability from the SLP when deciding whether to perform a particular operation. Advantages of a team approach include the following:

- The family can see several specialists during one appointment.
- The family associates all aspects of care with one setting.
- Only one contact is required if an emergency arises.
- Follow-up is managed in a controlled manner (McWilliams et al., 1990).

The needs of a person with a cleft and his or her family change during the lifespan, requiring team member compositions and roles to change accordingly.

SLPs, surgeons, dental specialists, and audiologists work closely together on the team. Therefore, the SLP needs to have some familiarity with the specific roles and concerns of the other team members. In the next four sections of this chapter, we will discuss surgical, dental, audiological, and psychosocial concerns regarding clefts. This discussion will be followed by a detailed account of the communicative problems faced by persons with clefts and the SLP's role as a member of a cleft palate team.

SURGICAL MANAGEMENT OF CLEFTS

Although the recorded history of clefts dates back to the Ching dynasty (390 B.C.), surgical repair of clefts did not occur until the nineteenth century. Surgical repair of clefts, or **palatoplasty,** is divided into two stages: primary surgical correction followed by secondary procedures to correct velopharyngeal incompetence.

Primary Surgical Correction

The first stage of primary surgical correction is lip surgery if the child has a cleft of the lip and palate. Lip surgery is performed generally before 3 months of age (Seagle, 1997). Some surgeons prefer to defer surgical correction of the lip until the parents have lived with the baby long enough to understand and accept the cleft. These surgeons hope that during this waiting period, the parents will adjust and develop a realistic attitude about the benefits of surgery and the inevitable scar (Peterson-Falzone et al., 2001).

Surgical correction of a cleft palate is designed to create a velopharyngeal valving mechanism that is capable of separating the oral cavity from the nasal cavity during speech production. Early surgical closure of the palate also improves swallowing function and reduces the number of middle ear and upper respiratory infections. Recent surgical trends advocate closure of the palatal cleft between 6 and 18 months of age. Early closure has a positive influence on velopharyngeal function, midfacial symmetry, and overall appearance (Seagle, 1997).

Secondary Surgical Correction

The efficacy of primary palatal surgery is assessed by the adequacy of the velopharyngeal mechanism for speech production. Approximately one in four individuals who have primary palatal surgery fails to achieve velopharyngeal competence for speech production, requiring additional surgical management to correct the velopharyngeal incompetence (Riski, 1995).

A commonly used secondary surgical procedure designed to correct VPI is called a **pharyngeal flap** operation. A pharyngeal flap is created by cutting a flap of soft tissue from the posterior pharyngeal wall, as shown in Figure 11.7. One end of the flap remains attached to the posterior pharyngeal wall, and the other is sutured to the velum. To permit nasal breathing and the production of nasal speech sounds, small openings are maintained between the flap and the lateral walls of the pharynx. Closure of these openings during swallowing and the production of nonnasal speech sounds is accomplished by active movement of the lateral walls of the pharynx (toward the midline) (Riski, 1995). Pharyngeal flap procedures are performed generally between the ages of 6 and 12, and it has been reported that "normal" speech is realized following the majority of these operations (Peterson-Falzone et al., 2001).

DENTAL MANAGEMENT OF CLEFTS

People with cleft lip and palate have significant dental problems that can interfere with chewing, swallowing, and speech production. During the lifespan, various dental specialists will be involved in care ranging from developing devices to assist the infant's swallowing to treatment focusing on improving the positions of teeth and maxillary bone segments (Peterson-Falzone et al., 2001). **Orthodontists** are crucial members of cleft palate teams who are concerned primarily with the alignment of teeth and dental **malocclusions.** A malocclusion is the improper alignment of the maxillary

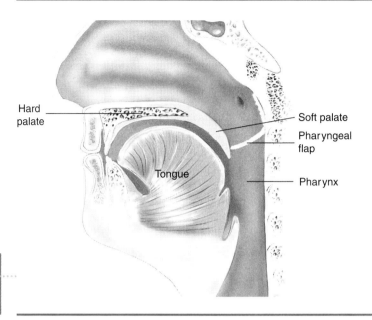

Hard palate

Soft palate

Pharyngeal flap

Tongue

Pharynx

FIGURE 11.7
Stylized drawing of a pharyngeal flap.

and mandibular dental arches. Pressure is applied to the teeth and/or the dental arches with metal bands and various dental appliances.

THOUGHT QUESTIONS

Did you have dental braces as a child? Do you still have braces? Do you remember how your mouth felt after visiting the orthodontist? The discomfort you probably experienced was the pressure being applied to your misaligned teeth.

Abnormal **dentition** based on the kind, number, and arrangement of teeth and malocclusions can have very adverse effects on speech production. Nearly 90 percent of all English consonants are made in the anterior portion of the mouth, the area of the mouth that is most affected by clefts. Missing or misaligned teeth and malocclusions can affect adversely the production of sounds that require accurate tongue placement on the teeth or dental arch, such as /t/, /d/, and /l/. Sounds that require a constriction between the tongue and teeth, such as /s/, /th/, and /sh/, will be adversely affected by the absence or misalignment of teeth (Le Blanc & Cisneros, 1995).

A **prosthodontist,** a dental specialist, is frequently involved in the care of individuals with clefts. Prosthodontics is a dental specialty concerned with the replacement of missing teeth and other oral structures with various appliances. For some individuals with clefts, palatoplasty is not recommended because of other complicating medical conditions, religious beliefs, or simply personal choice. In such circumstances, closure of the cleft can be achieved by a prosthodontic *obturator.* An obturator is a special kind of dental prosthesis designed to occlude or fill the cleft and partition the oral cavity from the nasal cavity. Obturators may be used as primary management of a cleft or as a secondary procedure after unsuccessful palatoplasty (Peterson-Falzone et al., 2001).

Obturators are made of acrylic material and custom built to conform to the general configuration of an individual's oral cavity. The obturator is held in place by clasps that anchor it to the teeth. The palatal portion of the obturator covers the cleft, and the posterior portion extends into the pharynx and terminates in a bulblike structure, called a **speech bulb,** that fills the velopharyngeal space. Velopharyngeal closure is achieved by movement of the lateral pharyngeal walls making contact with the bulb.

AUDIOLOGICAL MANAGEMENT OF CLEFTS

People with clefts exhibit a higher incidence of hearing disorders and middle ear disease than the general population. Middle ear disease is universal during a cleft palate child's infancy, resulting in a conductive hearing loss that may persist into adulthood (Peterson-Falzone et al., 2001). It has been estimated that 58 percent of the cleft palate population has some degree of hearing loss (Kemker, 1995). Later in this section, we will discuss the potential impact of hearing loss on speech and language development, but first we will consider how middle ear disease leads to conductive hearing loss in the cleft palate population.

The middle ear is an air-filled cavity in the temporal bone of the skull bounded on the outside by the tympanic membrane (eardrum) and on the inside by the cochlea, a spiral-shaped structure that contains the nerve endings for hearing. A tube runs from the middle ear down into the nasopharynx (the portion of the pharynx above the velum). This tube, called the **auditory tube,** permits drainage from the middle ear into the pharynx and serves to equalize air pressure in the middle ear with atmospheric pressure.

*Y*ou are a passenger in an aircraft. When the aircraft is taking off or landing, do you feel pressure in your ears? What happens to the sense of pressure when you swallow, yawn, or chew gum vigorously?

THOUGHT QUESTIONS

The auditory tube is normally closed, opening only when one swallows or yawns widely. The tube is opened by contraction of the **tensor veli palatine** muscle of the soft palate. When a cleft of the soft palate occurs, the muscle does not function properly and will not open the tube. Dysfunction of the auditory tube results in poor middle ear ventilation, which, in turn, leads to inflammation and abnormal fluid accumulation. This fluid accumulation is a disease called *otitis media,* which causes mild to moderate conductive hearing loss. Otitis media frequently needs to be treated with a **myringotomy,** which is a surgical puncture of the tympanic membrane and insertion of a ventilating tube for pressure equalization.

TABLE 11.4
Psychosocial concerns during the lifespan of a person with a cleft palate

Developmental Stage	Areas of Concern
Prenatal/Perinatal Period	Parental adjustments to impending birth/birth of a child with cleft palate
Toddler Years	Parental attempts to protect the child from negative reactions of extended family and community members; stress of medical intervention
Preschool Years	Self-concept, peer relationships
Early School and Teen Years	Self-concept, peer relationships, school adjustment, negative judgments by teachers
Adults	Social interactions, life partners, and employment

Source: Adapted from Peterson-Falzone et al. (2001).

You can develop some appreciation of how a mild conductive loss affects your hearing sensitivity by plugging your ears gently with your fingers. Note that you still hear some sounds but not others. In general, loud sounds can be heard, but soft sounds cannot. Try this little experiment with a friend: Have your friend stand behind you and produce a vowel sound such as /a/ for three seconds and then produce /s/ for three seconds. If you have normal hearing, you will hear both these sounds clearly. With your friend still standing behind you, plug your ears gently and have him or her produce those sounds again in the same manner. With your ears plugged, you probably heard the /a/ but not the /s/. If you did hear the /s/, it was very muffled and distorted.

Your little experiment demonstrates that even a mild conductive loss can prevent a listener from hearing many of the sounds of spoken English. Long-standing conductive hearing loss associated with otitis media can have a devastating effect on speech and language development, compounding the already adverse conditions created by the cleft.

The audiologist is a vital member of the cleft palate team who provides critical information to the SLP about an individual's hearing status. For people with clefts, hearing testing should be done routinely every three to six months. During episodes of active otitis media, hearing should be checked more frequently.

PSYCHOSOCIAL MANAGEMENT OF CLEFTS

There is no strong evidence that children with repaired clefts are more mal-adapted psychosocially than their noncleft peers, and they have no documented personality deviations. Frequently, however, these children suffer from social isolation owing to discrimination by peers and teachers who overemphasize the residual evidence of the cleft condition and underestimate the child's real capabilities. Such social isolation may lead to low self-esteem, decreased participation in group activities, inhibited behavior, and lowered expectations on the part of parents, teachers, and peers (McWilliams et al., 1990).

Children with clefts encounter unusual social pressures, and there is a continuing need to ensure their psychological well-being. The SLP needs to be keenly aware of the child's psychological and social needs and "provide treatment or referral as required in individual cases" (McWilliams et al., 1990, p. 144).

Table 11.4 highlights some of the psychosocial concerns as they change during the lifespan of individuals with cleft palate.

COMMUNICATION PROBLEMS ASSOCIATED WITH CLEFTS

Approximately 80 percent of people born with clefts that are not associated with a syndrome and receiving palatal repair by 18 months can be expected to develop reasonably good speech without therapeutic intervention. For the other 20 percent born with clefts and for children with associated syndromes, "the road to normal speech often seems long and arduous" (Golding-Kushner, 1995, p. 327). The child with a cleft palate may have voice disorders, resonance disorders associated with VPI, articulation disorders associated with VPI, dental malocclusions, and possible hearing loss. In addition, children with clefts may exhibit language disorders. In this section, we discuss the presumed causes, assessment, and treatment of these communicative problems.

An SLP who specializes in craniofacial disorders probably has fewer adolescents and adult patients with cleft palate than once was the case. Persons with cleft palate now receive effective treatments earlier in their life and generally speak normally by the time they are adolescents (Peterson-Falzone et al., 2001). Thus, this section of the text will focus on communicative problems that are likely to be diagnosed and treated during childhood.

VOICE DISORDERS

In Chapter 9, we reported that approximately 3 to 6 percent of noncleft children and 3 to 9 percent of noncleft adults exhibit some form of voice disorder. Clinical research indicates that phonatory disorders are much more common in people with clefts, possibly involving over 80 percent of the cleft population. The most common vocal fold pathology is bilateral vocal nodules, which produce a hoarse, breathy vocal quality. The high incidence of individuals with vocal nodules among the cleft palate population is likely related to vocal hyperfunction (Peterson-Falzone, et al., 2001). Vocal hyperfunction is also the presumed cause of vocal nodules in noncleft children, usually associated with excessive yelling and screaming.

Vocal hyperfunction among children with cleft palate appears to be compensatory behavior related to VPI. Children with VPI are unable to increase their vocal intensity in a normal fashion owing to the loss of energy into the nasal cavity. To compensate for this inability, these children position their larynx high in the neck during speaking, and this behavior exerts unusually high tension on the vocal folds, causing the vocal nodules.

Another voice disorder that occurs in children with cleft palates is called **soft-voice syndrome.** Soft-voice syndrome is also a compensatory behavior by which the child purposely reduces vocal intensity to prevent air escape through the nose and reduce hypernasality. Soft-voice syndrome is frequently accompanied by a monotone voice characterized by little variation in pitch.

Assessment of Voice Disorders

Four general steps have been recommended for the assessment of suspected voice disorders associated with clefts (McWilliams et al., 1990). First, a case history should be taken to determine whether the vocal symptoms are of recent origin or longstanding. If the symptoms have been present for a long time, patterns of potential vocal misuse need to be explored in detail.

The second step should explore the individual's personality. Vocal hyperfunction is commonly associated with people who are tense, loud, and/or aggressive. These personality characteristics are not typical of individuals with clefts, but the possibility of such a personality factor contributing to vocal hyperfunction needs to be explored.

A detailed phonation examination to determine the nature of the voice disorder is the third general step. Of interest is the appropriateness of the vocal pitch range, loudness, and vocal quality. Specific techniques and instruments for such assessments have been discussed in numerous texts on voice disorders and in Chapter 9.

The fourth step is to determine whether the person can modify his or her voice. A straightforward procedure to determine an individual's ability to change the voice is to have him or her "sigh" or produce an "um-hum." People who exhibit vocal hyperfunction during connected speech may demonstrate unconsciously the ability to change vocal quality when producing these easy, natural phonations.

As with any suspected disorder of voice, the individual needs to be examined by a physician before commencing therapy. When a hoarse voice quality accompanies a cleft, there is a strong possibility that bilateral vocal nodules exist. Voice therapy is usually the initial treatment of choice with the goal of reducing vocal hyperfunction.

Treatment of Voice Disorders

Therapeutic reduction of vocal hyperfunction is divided generally into three phases: auditory discrimination, establishing a new voice production, and habituating the new voice (Aronson, 1990; McWilliams et al., 1990).

During the auditory discrimination phase, the individual learns to differentiate his or her voice from the voices of people who do not have vocal nodules. A second step in the auditory discrimination phase is to train the individual to recognize differences in quality between their best and poorest vocalizations. This can be accomplished by contrasting connected speech with relaxed production of "um-hum."

A primary goal toward establishing a new voice regards the elimination of **hard glottal attacks.** A hard glottal attack occurs when a client initiates speech using hypertensive vocal fold adduction.

Can you mimic a hard glottal attack? Try this. Inhale deeply and, with your mouth open, trap air in your lungs by approximating your vocal folds. Now say the vowel /a/. What does your voice sound like?

To eliminate hard glottal attacks, the individual is trained to initiate words beginning with vowels using a gentle glottal attack. This strategy is taught by having the individual begin by producing a prolonged /h/ and then gradually moving into the initial vowel in the word. This breathy, relaxed voicing onset can be felt and heard, and the individual is taught to sense the relaxed phonation. Initiating words with the /h/ is gradually phased out, and therapy progresses into two-word combinations, sentences, and finally conversational speech.

Habituating the new voice is divided into two phases: (a) limited habituation; and (b) overall habituation (McWilliams et al., 1990). Limited habituation involves having the individual use his or her new voice only in the presence of the SLP and then in highly controlled situations outside the clinic. Overall habituation involves using the new voice during the entire therapy session, then in specific classes in school, and during certain hours at home. The times and situations are gradually extended. Therapy is terminated when the individual and his or her significant others report a consistent use of the new voice.

RESONANCE DISORDERS

People with VPI are said to have a hypernasal voice quality. Hypernasality is not a problem associated with phonation; rather, it is the result of not partitioning the oral and nasal cavities by actions of the velopharyngeal mechanism. Hypernasality is a resonance problem created by the nasal cavity acting inappropriately as a second "filter" coupled to the oral cavity. Addition of this second filter alters the vocal tract's output in such a way that it sounds as though the individual is talking through his or her nose.

Have you ever used the frequency equalizer on your stereo? Frequency equalizers are filters of a sort. What happens to the sound coming from your speakers when you change the settings on your frequency equalizer?

Several different instruments are commercially available that will obtain nasalance scores. The computation and interpretation of these scores varies according to the instrument.

Some nasal resonance is normal. To illustrate this point, say the sentence "Where were you last year?" aloud. Now pinch your nostrils shut and listen to the difference in your voice quality. Pinching your nostrils shut while speaking reduces normal nasal resonance, and as a result your voice sounds unnatural. This lack of nasal resonance is called **hyponasality.** Your voice may have a hyponasal quality when you experience a bad head cold.

Individuals with VPI exhibit increased nasal resonance and decreased oral resonance, and the voice quality is abnormally nasal sounding, or hypernasal. Hypernasality is associated mainly with vowels. High vowels such as /i/ tend to be perceived as more nasal than low vowels such as /a/, and perceived hypernasality may be greater in connected speech than during the production of isolated words.

Assessment of Resonance Disorders

There are a number of standardized rating scales for assessing vocal resonance. Rating scales permit the assignment of numbers to express increasing severity of the disorder. In general, such rating scales are reliable and valid. Two such rating scales are presented in Table 11.5.

Specially designed instruments are also available to assess resonance disorders. One such instrument, manufactured by Kay Elemetrics, is called a **nasometer.** The nasometer measures simultaneously the relative amplitude of acoustic energy being emitted through the nose and mouth during phonation. A numerical value, the **nasalance score,** is computed that reflects the magnitude of hypernasality. Nasalance scores have been shown to correlate well with rating scales and with the actual degree of velopharyngeal opening (Dalston, 1995; Dalston & Seaver, 1990). Nasometry can also be used as an

---

TABLE 11.5

Two examples of scales used to rate the degree of resonance disorders: (a) a seven-point scale emphasizing hypernasality, and (b) an eight-point scale for rating nasal resonance

(a)

		Hypernasality		
Normal		Mild	Moderate	Severe
1	2	3	4	5	6	7

(b)

		Hypernasality		
Hypo-nasality	Normal	Mild	Moderate	Severe
−1	0	1	2	3	4	5	6

Source: Adapted from McWilliams, Morris, & Shelton (1990).

effective therapeutic feedback technique. Examples of nasometry can be seen on the book's CD-ROM.

The definitive procedure for assessing velopharyngeal function is **multiview videofluoroscopy.** Videofluoroscopy is motion picture X-rays recorded on videotape. Multiview videofluoroscopy permits the imaging of velopharyngeal function from three different perspectives: from the front, from the side, and from beneath. These images provide a complete picture of velopharyngeal closure or the lack thereof.

Treatment of Resonance Disorders

Behavioral treatments designed to improve velopharyngeal functioning and reduce hypernasality have a fifty-year history in the United States. Although for some individuals velopharyngeal closure may be improved without additional surgery (Tomes, Kuehn, & Peterson-Falzone, 1995), those who have anatomical limitations such as a velum that is too short to contact the posterior pharyngeal wall or a velum that is completely immobile will not benefit from behavioral treatments alone. Such individuals will require further surgery or a prosthesis to achieve velopharyngeal competence. The decision to try behavioral treatments to improve velopharyngeal function must be made through careful collaboration of the cleft palate team.

Once the cleft palate team has decided that behavioral management is a viable option for a given individual with VPI, the SLP can choose from several different treatment protocols that are designed to improve velopharyngeal function. Two procedures that show promise for improving velopharyngeal function are the Whistling-Blowing procedure and a relatively new procedure named Continuous Positive Airway Pressure.

The Whistling-Blowing technique (Shprintzen, McCall, & Skolnick, 1975) is a behavioral treatment based on X-ray observations that indicate that velopharyngeal closure patterns during whistling and blowing are similar to closure patterns achieved during normal speech production. This technique can be used with individuals who achieve velopharyngeal closure during whistling and/or blowing, but not during speech production. The general steps of this procedure are outlined in Table 11.6. See Case Study 11.2 on page 337 for an example of the use of whistling-blowing techniques to treat a boy who developed VPI following tonsil and adenoid surgery.

Continuous Positive Airway Pressure (CPAP) therapy is based on the exercise physiology principle of progressive resistance training. Progressive resistance training asserts that when muscles are subjected systematically to weights greater than those to which they are accustomed, they adapt by adding muscle tissue and strength is increased. To continue building muscle tissue, weights are increased systematically until the desired muscle strength is achieved.

Have you tried to increase muscle strength by lifting weights? Did you use progressive resistance training?

<hr>

TABLE 11.6

The general treatment sequence for the Whistling-Blowing therapy designed to improve velopharyngeal functioning

1. Determine whether the individual can achieve closure during whistling or blowing.

2. Teach the individual to blow or whistle and phonate at the same time. Monitor and identify nasal air leakage with a scape-scope.* Reward productions that are free of nasal air emission.

3. Gradually discontinue the use of blowing and whistling during phonation. Reward correct productions and punish nasal air emission during vowel productions.

4. Remove the scape-scope for monitoring and replace with auditory monitoring.

<hr>

*A scape-scope is a simple device that monitors air escaping from the nose. A small hose inserted into the nostrils is connected to a tube. A styrofoam ball inside the tube moves up and down in association with nasal emission.

Source: Adapted from McWilliams, Morris, & Shelton (1990).

The CPAP procedure attempts to strengthen the muscles of the velopharyngeal mechanism by having the velar musculature work against systematic increases of weight. Because it would be quite impractical and probably impossible to use miniature free weights, CPAP uses air pressure in the nasal cavity as a substitute. Heightened air pressure in the nasal cavity is the "weight" that the velopharyngeal mechanism works against (Tomes et al., 1995).

During therapy, the velum works against the increased air pressure in the nasal cavity while producing syllables that contain nasal consonants /n/ or /m/, vowels, and nonnasal consonants. The velum is lowered during production of the nasal consonant and elevated during vowel and nonnasal consonant productions. Nasal air pressure is increased systematically during velar elevation associated with production of the nonnasal consonant.

CPAP is an experimental treatment procedure. The fact that this technique has its roots in physiological principles that are solidly grounded suggests great promise for future development and success.

ARTICULATION DISORDERS

Individuals with clefts are at high risk for disordered articulation. Disordered articulation can be the result of VPI, structural deviations in the oral cavity, misaligned or missing teeth, faulty learning, or combinations of these factors. Sounds that tend to be produced incorrectly more than 60 percent of the time in the cleft population include /s/, /z/, /θ/, /tʃ/, and /ts/ (McWilliams et al., 1990). Vowels and some consonants are produced with a hypernasal quality, as discussed previously.

Case Study 11.2

Personal Story of a Boy with Velopharyngeal Insufficiency

Marty, a 9-year-old boy, was brought to the University Hospital's Communication Disorders Unit by his parents with the concern that after tonsil and adenoid surgery, his speech had deteriorated. At birth, Marty presented with a cleft of the hard and soft palate. The cleft was repaired surgically when he was 11 months old, and the SLP evaluated him regularly for two years after the surgery. On the basis of the SLP's recommendation to the cleft palate team, Marty was enrolled in formal speech training when he was 3½ years old. Speech therapy continued for two years, at which time he was dismissed from the clinic with age-appropriate speech and language skills and normal nasal resonance.

Marty was troubled frequently by throat infections, which caused severe swelling of his tonsils and adenoids that interfered with swallowing. His pediatrician recommended removal of the tonsils and adenoids.

The speech-language evaluation of Marty revealed that his speech was markedly hypernasal with frequent nasal emission. The SLP recommended that

Marty be evaluated by a radiologist with multiview videofluoroscopy to determine the underlying cause of the hypernasal speech and nasal emission.

The videofluoroscopy revealed that Marty's velum was not making adequate contact with the right and left aspects of the pharyngeal walls where the adenoid tissue had been removed. Although adequate velar contact was observed during swallowing, he could not partition the oral and nasal cavities during speech production. A pharyngeal flap operation was the team's recommendation.

After the pharyngeal flap surgery, Marty was evaluated by the SLP and the radiologist. They determined that he was capable of velopharyngeal closure during speech, but he was not achieving closure consistently during speech. The team recommended that Marty receive speech therapy twice weekly for two months. After five weeks of therapy utilizing whistling-blowing techniques, Marty's speech was no longer hypernasal, and there was no evidence of nasal emission.

Production of consonants that require an air pressure buildup in the oral cavity, such as the stop consonants /p/, /t/, and /k/, is frequently accompanied by air escaping inappropriately through the nose. Air escaping through the nose during speech production is called **nasal emission.** Nasal emission is not the same as hypernasal speech quality. Rather, nasal emission is an audible or inaudible leakage of air into the nasal cavity.

People with clefts may also exhibit **compensatory articulation errors** quite apart from the articulation errors discussed here. A compensatory articulation error is a gross sound substitution error that is an attempt to compensate for the physical inability to produce a given sound correctly. A common compensatory articulation error is a **glottal stop** similar to /h/.

Individuals with VPI are unable to build the requisite oral air pressure to produce stops such as /p/, /t/, and /k/ because of air escaping into the nasal cavity, as discussed above. Stop sounds require a brief stoppage of air flow and a buildup of oral air pressure followed by a sudden release of that pressure. The normal production of a /p/ sound, for example, requires a buildup of oral pressure that is accomplished by holding the upper and lower lips together briefly (the stop) followed by a sudden release of that built-up air pressure. The person with VPI is incapable of producing the /p/ in this fashion and compensates by stopping the air at the glottis, approximating the vocal folds. Air is stopped, and pressure is built up beneath the vocal folds instead of behind the lips.

THOUGHT QUESTIONS

Can you produce an acceptable /p/ sound when you purposely open your velopharyngeal portal? What happens when you try?

Ten compensatory articulation substitutions have been identified in the speech of people with clefts and VPI (Witzel, 1995). Some of these compensatory behaviors may become strongly habituated and still be present after the structural deficit that caused them has been corrected. The SLP needs to make a careful inventory of such behaviors during the articulation assessment of people with clefts.

Assessment of Articulation Disorders

A number of widely used articulation tests can be used to assess the sound production skills of people with clefts. Some of these are the *Templin-Darley Test of Articulation,* the *Goldman-Fristoe Test of Articulation,* and the *Fisher-Logemann Test of Articulation Competence.* The *Fisher-Logemann Test* is particularly useful for assessing individuals with clefts because it allows for an analysis of patterns of articulation errors regarding the place, manner, and voicing characteristics of sounds (McWilliams et al., 1990).

Specialized tests of articulation have been developed for use with people who are suspected of having VPI. The *Iowa Pressure Articulation Test* is a subtest embedded in the *Templin-Darley Test of Articulation.* This test is composed of forty-three sounds that have been identified as likely to be misarticulated by people with VPI. The test emphasizes sounds that require the buildup of oral pressure. Individuals who score poorly on this test because of VPI will produce a unique pattern of errors characterized by nasal emission, a lack of oral pressure, and gross compensatory substitutions (McWilliams et al., 1990).

The *Bzoch Error Pattern Diagnostic Articulation Test* is another specialized instrument designed for people with clefts and/or suspected VPI. The test is constructed to facilitate identification of error patterns in speech that are related more to VPI than to functional learning problems.

Phonological process analysis can also be used to assess the sound production skills of people with clefts. Because sound formation difficulties caused by structural anomaly may lead to persistent phonological process simplifications, phonological process analysis should accompany more articulation-based assessment. (Witzel, 1995).

Management of Articulation Disorders

The basic principles that underlie the treatment of deviant articulatory-phonological behaviors in the noncleft population also apply to the treatment of the cleft population. The use of longstanding speech-language pathology techniques for teaching individuals to produce sounds in syllables and words and then to establish the use of those sounds in conversation is recommended (McWilliams et al., 1990). Such techniques include the use of auditory and visual models for imitation, practice, and reinforcement of responses that are appropriate for the individual's capabilities.

Treatment of preschool-age children with repaired clefts should emphasize the development of stop consonant and fricative production. Establishing stopping and frication in a few sounds will contribute to generalization of those features to other sounds. Emphasis is also placed on instructing the child how to direct the air stream in an oral direction rather than a nasal direction.

Articulation-phonology therapy can help many individuals with repaired clefts to achieve normal speech. In some individuals, however, the prognosis for improvement is poor, and therapy must be terminated. The SLP "must have the courage and knowledge to make this decision" (McWilliams et al., 1990, p. 397).

LANGUAGE DISORDERS

In contrast to the communicative problems associated with clefts discussed above, very little attention has been paid to language development and language disorders with this population (Witzel, 1995). Research studies generally have found evidence of mild language delays in children with clefts, particularly children with clefts of the palate only. Unfortunately, these studies are not in agreement regarding the nature and extent of language delays, and the origins of language delays within the cleft population have not been specified (McWilliams et al., 1990).

More research is needed on the relationship among potential contributing factors such as otitis media, learning disabilities, and specific syndromes and language delays in the cleft palate population. Although SLPs need to be aware of the potential for language disabilities among children with clefts, they must also be aware that language disorders are not an invariable consequence of clefting and recognize those children "who are better served if we do not intervene" (McWilliams et al., 1990, p. 244).

Assessment of Language Disorders

Children born with clefts should be routinely examined for potential delays in language development and specific language impairments. Language evaluations should include information about environmental factors, motor and mental development, and hearing acuity. Language assessment of children with clefts is the same as language assessment of other children (McWilliams et al., 1990). Standard tests of receptive and expressive language like those discussed in Chapter 5 can be used effectively with the cleft palate population.

Treatment of Language Disorders

As with language assessment, treating language disorders for children with clefts does not differ substantively from treating language disorders in the noncleft population. In fact, it has been shown that delayed language devel-

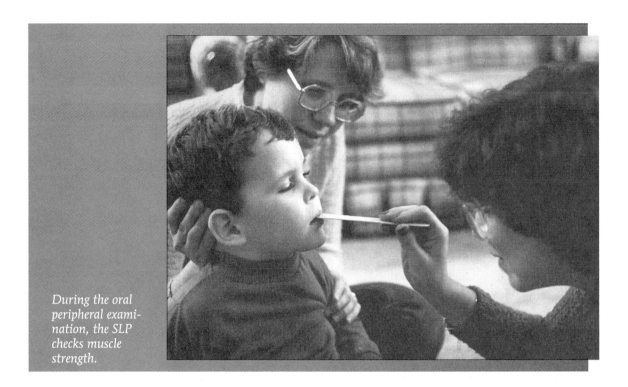

During the oral peripheral examination, the SLP checks muscle strength.

opment can in large part be prevented in this population. Early and repeated family counseling regarding receptive and expressive language development, aggressive treatment of middle ear disease, and language enrichment programs have been shown to prevent language difficulties (Bzoch, 1997).

One last issue regarding language development in children with clefts should be noted. Mothers of cleft children may engage in significantly less verbal play with their child than mothers of noncleft children. The SLP should be mindful of this possibility and counsel new parents about how important early verbal play is to good language development. As the child matures, parents should be encouraged to read to the child and talk about daily events and experiences. Perhaps most important, parents should provide a good language model for their child. The SLP can be invaluable in helping parents to achieve this goal.

Summary

Children with cleft palate face a myriad of problems from early infancy through adulthood. These problems can be treated effectively only when a team of professionals works cooperatively toward their resolution. The speech-language pathologist is an integral member of the cleft palate team who will work in conjunction with surgeons, orthodontists, and other professionals to facilitate the development of normal speech and language for the child with a cleft. Surgical correction of the cleft by reconstruction of the palate and velopharyngeal mechanism must in many cases be followed by long-term therapy to remediate voice, resonance, and articulation disorders.

REFLECTIONS

- Describe the embryological development of the face and palate.
- Describe how clefts of the lip and palate form.
- Describe the clinical features of a cleft of the lip.
- Describe the clinical features of a unilateral cleft of the lip and palate.
- Describe the clinical features of a bilateral cleft of the lip and palate.
- Explain the Veau classification system of cleft types.
- Discuss some of the possible causes of clefts.
- Discuss some of the medical and dental management concerns associated with clefts.
- Explain middle ear disorders associated with clefts.
- Describe some of the communicative problems associated with clefts.

SUGGESTED READINGS

Charkins, H. (1996). *Children with facial differences.* Bethesda, MD: Woodbine House.

Shprintzen, R. J. (1997). *Genetics, syndromes, and communication disorders.* San Diego: Singular.

ONLINE RESOURCES

http://www.cleft.com/   American Cleft Palate-Craniofacial Association.

http://www.widesmiles.org/   Wide Smiles! Cleft Lip and Palate Resource.
   Resources and networking for families of children with clefts.

http://www.cleft.org/   Smiles.
   Stories by families with children born with cleft lip and/or cleft palate, with links to related information.

Neurogenic Speech Disorders

12

12

CHAPTER LEARNING GOALS

When you have finished this chapter, you should be able to:

- Describe the major differences between cerebral palsy, dysarthria, and apraxia of speech

- Explain the causes of neurogenic speech disorders

- Name the types of cerebral palsy and dysarthria

- Explain the general assessment and intervention techniques that are used with neurogenic motor speech disorders

Neurogenic speech disorders are speech difficulties that are related to problems of movement as a result of some neurological disorder or injury. They are sometimes referred to as motor speech disorders. The term "motor" refers to movement.

Neurogenic speech disorders are a heterogeneous group of neurological impairments that affect the planning, coordination, timing, and execution of the movement patterns that are used to produce speech in both children and adults. Any or all of the processes of respiration, phonation, resonation, and articulation, described in previous chapters, may be affected. Although voice and fluency are involved, these are addressed in other chapters. In addition, language disorders often co-occur with neurogenic speech disorders. These are described in Chapter 7, "Adult Language Impairments."

That brief explanation does not begin to hint at the complexity of the disorders that fall within the boundaries of neurogenic speech disorders. So finite and particular are the movements needed for speech that more area in the brain is devoted to control of your vocal folds, tongue, lips, and other articulators than to any other bodily movement, even walking. Given this complexity, it is amazing that the process of producing speech becomes almost automatic and that you give little thought to it when speaking. In fact, we rarely consider the process unless something is wrong.

Case Study 12.1

Case Study of a Teen with a Neurogenic Speech Disorder: Caitlin

Caitlin, a cheerleader and member of the high school theater group, began experiencing slight speech problems in eleventh grade. Her speech became slurred and difficult to understand. Even when she repeated herself to correct her speech, she often made the same errors. Both her parents and teachers noted the difference but assumed that Caitlin was talking too fast. Her parents became worried, however, when their daughter began complaining of severe headaches. After a neurological evaluation including a brain imaging scan, it was determined that she had a tumor that was putting pressure on the left frontal lobe of her brain.

Although surgery was successful, Caitlin still experienced speech difficulties and was referred to a speech-language pathologist who did a complete evaluation of Caitlin's motor speech abilities. The speech-language pathologist coordinated intervention services with a second speech-language pathologist in Caitlin's school district who agreed to provide similar services in the school. Several of Caitlin's friends and teachers were approached by the school SLP and enlisted to talk with Caitlin to ensure that she had to speak in school. Her parents were also part of the intervention team. After eight months, Caitlin's speech has returned to the pretrauma level of performance.

As you read the chapter, think about

- Possible explanations for Caitlin's's difficulties.
- Possible measures of Caitlin's speech that might have been used by her speech-language pathologist.
- Possible reasons for enlisting the help of so many individuals in Caitlins's intervention plan.

THOUGHT QUESTIONS

Do you ever think about producing speech as you're doing it? Have you ever bitten your tongue or choked while talking and eating? Suddenly, you become aware of the movement and the structures. Notice how your mouth moves when you say your name. Production has become automatic. You might never have noticed these movements before.

In this chapter, we limit our discussion to the production of speech. We discuss three types of neurogenic speech impairments: cerebral palsy, dysarthria, and apraxia of speech. In discussing characteristics, such a division is not so simple. Many individuals with cerebral palsy also exhibit dysarthria and apraxia of speech.

It might help you to remember these disorders if we make a somewhat artificial distinction. Because cerebral palsy occurs before, at, or shortly after birth, it is considered a *developmental* neuromotor deficit. In contrast, most but not all cases of dysarthria and apraxia occur after the neuromotor system is fully mature and therefore are considered to be *acquired* disorders.

THOUGHT QUESTION

Suppose a school-aged child had a stroke that resulted in a motor speech problem. Would the disorder be developmental, acquired, or both? Classification is not always clear-cut.

CAUSES OF NEUROGENIC SPEECH DISORDERS

Many conditions can result in disturbances in brain function. Stroke or cerebrovascular accident, discussed in Chapter 7, is the leading cause of neurogenic speech disorders. Certain racial/ethnic and gender differences exist in the incidence of strokes. In the United States, African Americans are more susceptible to strokes and hypertension than are individuals from other ethnic backgrounds (Singh, Cohen, & Krupp, 1996). Although men of all backgrounds have more strokes than women, women seem particularly vulnerable to aneurysms (Leblanc, 1996). Such hemorrhaging is also one of the leading causes of cerebral palsy in infants.

The major causes of neurogenic language and neurogenic speech disorders are similar.

Traumatic brain injury (TBI), also discussed in Chapter 7, is another leading cause of neurogenic speech disorders. Males who experience TBI far outnumber females, and nearly 70 percent of injuries resulting in TBI occur in the under-35 age group.

Brain injury also may result from deprivation of oxygen as in a drowning accident. Greatly reduced oxygen, or **anoxia,** is a more common cause of prenatal, natal, and neonatal brain injury than of adult injury.

*W*hy are fetuses and newborns more susceptible to anoxia than adults?

Brain tumors, or neoplasms, can also lead to neurogenic speech disorders, destroying healthy brain tissue by taking nutrition, impinging on healthy cells, or increasing the pressure within the brain cavity. At any given time, over 60,000 individuals in the United States have tumors of the nervous system. Not all of these affect speech. Some individuals may experience a slow degeneration of their cognitive abilities, while others have a steep decline. Shortly before her death, a friend was reduced to eye blinks and finger squeezes to communicate. Six months earlier, she had little impaired functioning. Some, but not all, tumors are operable or treatable with either chemotherapy or radiation.

Infections and toxins may also cause trauma to the central nervous system (CNS), although the incidence of these causes is changing. Infections such as meningitis and viral and fungal inflammations that once threatened healthy brains are now usually treatable by antibiotics if intervention begins in the early stages. The developing embryo is especially susceptible to infections. Some neural infections, such as those associated with new drug-resistant microbes and the human immunodeficiency virus (HIV), the virus that causes AIDS, offer a challenge to our pharmacological methods of treatment.

The list of brain-injuring toxins is lengthy, and new products are being introduced daily. Obvious neurotoxins are lead, mercury, certain pesticides, and pollution, but the most prevalent culprits are alcohol and drug use by pregnant women. Some toxins can pass the placental barrier between the mother and her infant.

Diseases, either inherited or acquired, can also affect the nervous system. Many are slow, degenerative diseases that gradually rob their victims of muscular control. A "Who's Who" of this rogues' gallery includes, but is not limited to, multiple sclerosis, amyotrophic lateral sclerosis (ALS), Parkinson's disease, Huntington's disease, and myasthenia gravis. Muhammed Ali, former world heavyweight champion boxer; Janet Reno, former Attorney General of the United States in the Clinton administration; and actor Michael J. Fox all have Parkinson's disease. Each of the authors of this text has been touched in some way by a friend or relative with a neurological disease. Maybe you have too.

Whatever the cause, the speech of affected individuals may vary widely. Even individuals with the same etiology may have very different speech problems, depending on the severity of the disorder, the age of the client, the time since the incident, and the extent of the affected area. To the untrained ear, two very different clients may sound the same and both be classified as having speech that is slurred, sloppy, thick, or unclear. Such descriptors do little to differentiate between the various etiologies, and an SLP must describe these behaviors much more thoroughly.

CEREBRAL PALSY

The term *cerebral palsy* describes a heterogeneous group of neurological difficulties resulting from brain injury that occurs very early in fetal or infant development. The disorder is nonprogressive, meaning that the condition does not worsen over time. Affected areas include motor movement, communication, growth and development, locomotion, learning, and sensation. Physical manifestations may range from extreme rigidity and immobility to being ambulatory, or capable of moving about relatively freely. Cerebral palsy may affect one or more limbs and might or might not be accompanied by speech difficulties. The cognitive abilities of people with cerebral palsy range from mental retardation through superior intelligence.

Although the reported incidence is low—1.5 to 3 per thousand births—the data may reflect poor reporting, misdiagnosis, or assignment of other labels, such as mental retardation, because the person has greater disorders in these areas. At present, more than 500,000 individuals in the United States have cerebral palsy; most are under 21 years of age. Anywhere from 30 to 90 percent have some dysarthria (Yorkston, Beukelman, & Bell, 1988).

> Movement patterns are learned from many, many repetitions. Therefore, faulty movement results in faulty patterns being learned. If you have typical motor patterns, you can probably pick up an object without looking at it.

Three characteristics distinguish cerebral palsy from some of the other neurogenic speech disorders that are discussed. First, it is a developmental neurogenic disorder. Most neurogenic speech disorders are considered to be acquired; that is, typical speech patterns were established before the disorder occurred. The insult to the neurological system with cerebral palsy occurs before the neuromotor system has matured. As a result, the child must learn motor movements for which no patterns have been established. Given the neuromotor difficulties of individuals with cerebral palsy, these movements may be learned in an atypical way.

Second, cerebral palsy is not a disease. It is a nonprogressive, noninfectious injury occurring before, at, or shortly after birth. Some children may improve with maturity, especially in the first few years of life as the brain matures rapidly.

Finally, the motor patterns in cerebral palsy are much more predictable than those in acquired neurogenic impairments. Although a person who has suffered a stroke may have severe impairment in an arm and a mild impairment in a leg on the same side, a person with cerebral palsy is more likely to have similar severity in all affected limbs. These may include involvement of the legs (*paraplegia*), all four extremities (*quadriplegia*), one side (*hemiplegia*), or one limb (*monoplegia*).

TYPES OF CEREBRAL PALSY

Not everyone with cerebral palsy is alike. Clients vary in age, culture, education, and type and severity of cerebral palsy. The type of cerebral palsy varies with the areas of the CNS that are affected. Injury may occur in the motor cortex, the pyramidal or extrapyramidal tracts, and the cerebellum.

Most types of cerebral palsy can be classified in one of three ways: spastic, athetoid, or ataxic. Although some infants with cerebral palsy exhibit

Individuals with cerebral palsy are a very heterogeneous group, varying in severity, type, and portion of the body affected. Like all individuals, they also differ in personality, interests, and maturity.

poor muscle tone and weakness, a condition called **hypotonia,** muscle movement and control almost always evolve during infancy into one of the three predominant types discussed here. *Spasticity,* or **hypertonia,** is a condition in which there is too much muscle tone, especially in the muscles that oppose the bending of joints and that help us to stand erect. Tone increases as muscles are stretched. *Athetosis,* or **dyskinesia,** is a slow, involuntary movement of the body. With a change in an individual's emotional state, such as being under stress, excited, angry, or amused, there may be an accompanying increase in muscle tone. **Ataxia** is uncoordinated movement.

Spastic Cerebral Palsy

For approximately 60 percent of individuals with cerebral palsy, the prominent characteristic is spasticity, or increased muscle tone. When a muscle of someone with **spastic cerebral palsy** contracts, the opposing muscle may react abnormally to stretch by increasing muscle tone too much. Rigid opposing muscle groups make movement extremely difficult. Described as "exaggerated stretch reflex," movement is characterized by increased muscle tone in the muscles opposing the movement that is attempted. Because tone increases as these muscles are stretched, muscle movement is described as jerky, labored, and slow. Individuals with spastic cerebral palsy may also exhibit infantile reflex patterns that in nonaffected children typically disappear within a few months of birth.

THOUGHT QUESTION

W*hy would movements in spastic cerebral palsy be jerky? Reach for your pen while trying to pull your arm back. Notice how your arm shakes as it moves.*

Spasticity results from damage to the motor cortex of the brain and/or lower brain areas. Unable to direct and control lower structures, higher centers of functioning cannot block signals to increase muscle tone or rigidity; the result is hypertonicity.

In severe cases, the limbs may be rotated inward with the arms drawn upward and the head drawn to one side. Walking or even standing may be extremely difficult. Figure 12.1a shows the posture of an individual with severe spastic cerebral palsy.

Athetoid Cerebral Palsy

Accounting for approximately 30 percent of individuals with cerebral palsy, athetoid cerebral palsy is characterized by a slow, involuntary writhing, most pronounced when the individual attempts volitional movement. The resultant behavior may be disorganized and uncoordinated. Individuals with athetoid cerebral palsy may also exhibit infantile reflex patterns throughout their lives. In nonaffected children, these typically disappear within a few months of birth.

(a) Spastic cerebral palsy   (b) Athetoid cerebral palsy

FIGURE 12.1

Characteristic posture of severe spastic and athetoid cerebral palsy.

Athetosis is caused by injury to lower brain areas that help to plan motor patterns and modify motor cortex impulses. When damage occurs, cortical impulses cannot be moderated. Inhibitor mechanisms cannot appropriately monitor the excitation mechanisms of the motor cortex. The result is too much muscle activity.

In its most severe form, athetosis causes the individual's feet to turn inward, the back and neck to arch, and the arms and hands to be overextended above the head. The mouth may be open, resulting in drooling. Breathing may also be affected. Figure 12.1b shows the posture of an individual with severe athetoid cerebral palsy.

The severity of athetoid cerebral palsy varies between individuals. In a given person, the moment-to-moment strength of the athetosis varies with the situation. When the individual is quiet or at rest, athetosis might not be evident. Athetoid movements occur or are exaggerated when purposeful movement is attempted and when the individual is excited or emotionally upset.

Ataxic Cerebral Palsy

Ataxic cerebral palsy, accounting for approximately 10 percent of the population with cerebral palsy, is characterized by uncoordinated movement and disturbed balance. The individual with ataxia seems clumsy and awkward. Movements lack direction, and hypotonic muscles lack adequate force and rate and have poor direction control. Walking is particularly difficult for the individual with ataxia and, in the most extreme cases, may be characterized by a wide stance with the head pushed forward and the arms back in an almost birdlike appearance. Even those who are less affected may have a gait resembling that of someone who is intoxicated.

Ataxia results from injury to the cerebellum. Injury to this part of the brain impairs the monitoring of balance information from the inner ears and of proprioceptive information from the muscles regarding the rate, force, and direction of movements. Coordination of muscle movement is difficult without accurate feedback. It is easy to see why walking would be especially problematic.

It may be difficult to keep the types of cerebral palsy clear in your mind. The major features of each are presented on Table 12.1.

TABLE 12.1

Characteristics of cerebral palsy

Type of Cerebral Palsy	Characteristics	Area of Brain Affected
Spastic	Spasticity, increased muscle tone in opposing muscle groups	Motor cortex and/or pyramidal tract
	Rigidity and exaggerated stretch reflex	
	Jerky, labored, and slow movements	
	Infantile reflex patterns	
Athetoid	Slow, involuntary writhing	Extrapyramidal tract, basal ganglia
	Disorganized and uncoordinated volitional movement	
	Movements occur accompanying volitional movement	
Ataxic	Uncoordinated movement	Cerebellum
	Poor balance	
	Movements lack direction, force, and control	

MOTOR SPEECH PROBLEMS ASSOCIATED WITH CEREBRAL PALSY

The different types of cerebral palsy result in differing speech characteristics.

Not everyone with cerebral palsy has motor speech difficulties. For example, individuals might have spastic cerebral palsy that involves primarily their legs (paraplegia). Nearly all people with athetoid cerebral palsy exhibit an accompanying motor speech disorder that affects all aspects of production. Ataxic speech difficulties may be related to cognitive impairment and phonological processing problems (Love, 1992).

Some professionals term the disordered speech of people with cerebral palsy *developmental dysarthria* because it is largely a disorder of motor speech control (Hardy, 1983; Love, 1992). Although adults with acquired motor speech disorders once had typical speech, the developing child did not and consequently may develop atypical motor patterns of production in the process of learning speech using a faulty motor system. In working with individuals with cerebral palsy, the SLP considers both the dysarthric or control dysfunction and the overlaid learning problem.

All aspects of speech production—respiration, phonation, resonation, and articulation, plus prosody—may be affected. Speech may be slow and labored. In severe cases, it may be unintelligible. Swallowing may also be affected, and individuals may exhibit dysphagia (see Chapter 13).

Many individuals with cerebral palsy have breathing difficulties, which, in turn, may affect speech. Breathing may be rapid and shallow. Vital capacity or the total amount of air expelled after a deep inhalation may be decreased, making it difficult for an individual to exhale sufficiently to produce speech. A client's speech may be limited to a word or short phrase.

Inconsistent or inadequate airflow and involvement of the laryngeal muscles will affect phonation. Voice quality may demonstrate hypertonia in several ways, from a breathy voice with puffs of air to a strained voice with hard glottal attack. A breathy voice may indicate a compensatory movement to force air from the lungs.

Resonance difficulties may be characterized by hypernasality resulting from dysfunction of the velopharyngeal mechanism. Inability to seal off the nasal cavity results in loss of air pressure, a critical component for good consonant production.

Why would poor velopharyngeal closure affect consonant production? Is loss of air pressure critical? (See Chapter 10.)

THOUGHT QUESTIONS

Articulation may be extremely difficult if there is involvement of the tongue, lips, and/or jaw. The tongue of an individual with cerebral palsy may move as one unit with limited ability to differentiate its parts. Consequently, consonants, especially those made with the aid of the tip of the tongue—/s/, /z/, /l/, and /r/—will offer a particular challenge. Lip movement may be slow and restricted. Jaw and tongue movements may be unspecified, and they may move together. Articulation problems in athetoid cerebral palsy seem to result from excessive jaw movement, limited tongue mobility, and velopharyngeal insufficency.

The prosodic aspects of speech—pitch, loudness, and duration—may be very monotonous. The client may be unable to perform the subtle oral movements that are necessary to convey shades of meaning or mark grammatical structures or morphological changes. Poor muscle control can make it difficult to initiate phonation and sustain it. The resultant speech may be choppy with short phrases or words and frequent interruptions. Speech may be characterized as nonrhythmic or nonfluent.

In the absence of established motor speech patterns, the child with cerebral palsy may develop abnormal movement patterns, further complicating intervention.

Other factors may also complicate the production of meaningful speech. These include intellectual, auditory, information-processing, and language impairments. Although many individuals with cerebral palsy have average or above-average intelligence, approximately half have some significant cognitive deficits (Bottenberg & Hanks, 1986). Hearing and speech sound discrimination may also be problematic, especially for individuals with athetoid cerebral palsy. Attentional disorders may also be exhibited.

All of these factors plus injury to adjacent areas of the brain account for the language impairment that is found in many individuals with cerebral palsy. This impairment may include delayed language development and immature linguistic structures and use.

ETIOLOGY

It would be impossible to catalogue all the possible prenatal, natal, and neonatal conditions that could result in brain damage for an embryo, fetus, or infant. In general, the younger the developing being, the more rapidly the brain is maturing, and the more susceptible his or her brain is to damage. The incidence of cerebral palsy is higher for extremely high-birthweight and extremely low-birthweight infants, nonwhite babies in the United States, children born to older mothers or in multiple births, and males.

Premature infants account for only 2 percent of all live births but represent a substantially larger percentage of the population of individuals with disability. In some cases, the premature birth is related to prenatal difficulties, including malformation of the CNS. Premature infants are also more susceptible to neonatal complications, including respiratory dysfunction, that can lead to anoxia.

The two most common causes of cerebral palsy are anoxia and hemorrhages in the brain. Anoxia, especially to the neuromotor areas of the brain, which are high oxygen users, can kill neurons in the CNS. Any interruption in the blood supply, as occurs in a hemorrhage in the vascular system, a not uncommon event *in utero,* can cause damage to a developing brain.

Infections and toxins may also disrupt brain development. Bacterial and viral infections, such as HIV, may infiltrate the brain from other bodily organs or be transported within the blood supply. During the first few months of pregnancy, before the development of a placental barrier, the embryo is especially susceptible to infections of the mother, such as influenza, rubella, and mumps, that can damage the developing brain. Toxic agents, such as heavy metals, mercury, and lead, may lodge in the brain and disrupt development. The use of alcohol and illicit drugs by pregnant women can also result in children born with brain dysfunction.

Finally, accidents during pregnancy and in the neonatal period can result in fetal brain injury. The incidence of fetal injury due to automobile accidents has risen in recent years. Sadly, some infants are also physically abused.

LIFESPAN ISSUES

Early symptoms of cerebral palsy may include irritability, weak crying and sucking, excessive sleeping, little interest in surroundings, and persistence of primitive reflexes beyond the newborn stage. Initial parental reactions on learning that their infant has cerebral palsy vary and may include guilt, grief, anger, and denial. One reaction may evolve into another. Typically, parents adjust well to their child but may exhibit *chronic grief,* or the continuing desire for their child to be "normal." The parent-child bonding process may be strained as the child fails to respond in predictable ways. In addition, the care of a child with cerebral palsy may tax the family and introduce stress into the familial relationship.

It may take up to two years to confirm a diagnosis of cerebral palsy among infants with mild involvement. The type of cerebral palsy may change within the first few years, and it is important for the child and family to be in contact with medical and educational professionals. Motor delays associated with cerebral palsy are often the first sign.

Children with cerebral palsy usually begin school or receive intervention services early in life. Training emphasis is on physical movement and communication. Communication training may focus on both speech and language, and augmentative/alternative communication methods, discussed in Chapter 15, may be introduced.

Variables such as severity, associated disorders, parental involvement, and school system flexibility are important in determining the appropriate educational environment. In general, children with average or better intelligence and mild cerebral palsy are more likely to have a more typical educational experience. It is extremely important to assess appropriately the cognitive abilities of people with severe motor disabilities, because a physical handicap may obscure intellectual functioning.

Many individuals, especially those with mild physical and cognitive difficulties, obtain higher education and/or go into competitive employment. Often, physical adaptations are made to improve performance. Other individuals may work and learn in centers run by agencies or the state. Workshops and day treatment programs also provide training in daily living and vocational skills for individuals with severe involvment and/or cognitive impairment. Case Study 12.2 presents the story of a young man with cerebral palsy.

ASSESSMENT

As with many other disorders discussed in this text, assessment and rehabilitation for people with cerebral palsy is a team effort. The team usually includes a pediatrician who often first identifies a disorder; a neurologist who confirms the diagnosis and describes the child's disability; a physical therapist who, along with an orthopedic surgeon, identifies motor patterns and implements muscle training and exercise to increase muscle tone, strength, and timing, and movement accuracy; an otolaryngologist who investigates and makes recommendations about the ear, nose, and throat; and a speech-language pathologist. Over the individual's lifespan, other professionals, including an occupational therapist, special education teacher, clinical psychologist, audiologist, ophthalmologist, rehabilitation engineer, and/or social worker, may also be involved. It is essential that professionals and parents become involved in the intervention process together as soon as possible.

Speech and language problems differ with the type and severity of cerebral palsy and with the age and functioning level of the individual. In addition to the procedures outlined in Chapter 4, the SLP will want to make a more thorough evaluation of the oral mechanism and, in many cases, to assess potential client success with an augmentative/ alternative form of communication. Within the oral peripheral examination, the SLP will note the following with particular interest:

Symmetry, configuration, color, and general appearance of the tongue, palate, lips, teeth, and jaw

Movement of the tongue, soft palate, lips, and jaw

Swallowing (see Chapter 13 for details)

Valving

Lung capacity and control

Phonatory initiation, maintenance, and cessation

Intervention team membership changes in response to the changing life span challenges of the individual with cerebral palsy.

Pitch and volitional pitch variations

Loudness and volitional loudness variations

Volitional pitch-loudness variations

Velophayngeal adequacy

Range, velocity, and direction of tongue, lip, and jaw movement

The specific tasks will be modified for young children, who may be unable to follow directions.

Oral motor abilities will be very important in determining the appropriateness of augmentative/alternative communication (AAC). As the individual matures and develops, the AAC system must be continually reevaluated to determine whether it still maximizes the client's potential for communication (see Chapter 15).

> It is extremely important that the AAC systems evolve with the client's abilities and needs.

Case Study 12.2

Personal Story of a Boy with Cerebral Palsy

Tony was born three months prematurely in a small rural hospital. The delivering obstetrician was concerned about possible oxygen deprivation at the time of birth, although Tony was placed in an incubator shortly after he was born.

Because of their son's prematurity, Tony's parents were counseled to expect developmental delays. They reported that he was irritable and seemed to have difficulty ingesting milk. At 4 months, his pediatrician expressed concern because of the continued presence of some reflexive behaviors, such as the whole-body response to startle, and the lack of motor responding, such as eye-hand coordination. She referred Tony to a developmental team in a large urban hospital.

The interdisciplinary team consisted of a pediatrician, neurologist, physical therapist, occupational therapist, developmental specialist, and speech-language pathologist. They determined that Tony had cognitive and motor delays and moderate dyskinesia or athetoid cerebral palsy.

As a result of the evaluation, it was recommended that Tony participate in a home-based interdisciplinary program with periodic reevaluation at the hospital. During the evaluation and subsequent consultation, Tony's parents heard the term "cerebral palsy" used to describe their child for the first time. The team recommended that the parents receive counseling and participate in a parents' group as a portion of their son's intervention plan.

By age 3, Tony was able to self-feed handheld food with some difficulty. Dressing was limited to completing tasks, such as pulling down a shirt that had been fitted over his arms and head. He could walk with great difficulty and usually needed support to steady himself. His speech consisted of a few words and phrases that were often unintelligible to people other than family. When unsure of his meaning, the family often used the immediate situation for interpretation.

At this time, Tony was enrolled in a special preschool for children with disabilities. On the advice of the school's speech-language pathologist, he began training with AAC. At first, this involved pointing to pictures on a communication board. Although his pointing response was somewhat imprecise, he continued to use the communication board until he entered elementary school. In first grade, Tony began to use a direct selection method of communicating using a computer and a joystick interface. Pictures evolved into words, then to individual letters. Now in third grade, Tony is communicating using a combination of his own speech and selection of pictures, words, and simple spelling on a computer, which he accesses by using the joystick control. He has a computer at home and in school for his use.

The long-term nature of cerebral palsy necessitates the establishment of realistic long-term goals. Limits to motor function improvement exist and must be considered. Once set, goals must be continually reevaluated. Team members can often help each other to set achievable goals.

INTERVENTION

Speech and language training is essential for many individuals with cerebral palsy to correct or compensate for faulty motor speech patterns. Efficient motor patterns are strengthened, and inefficient ones are modified.

Because one motor pattern, such as breathing, may affect another, such as phonation, most SLPs now believe that it is best to use a systems approach, one that targets efficient use of the entire speech production system, rather than one that focuses exclusively on one organ or structure. For example, a systems approach might consider poor lung capacity to be adequate for speech if the client can be taught to use shorter units of production, thus negating the need to strain the breathing system by increasing the demand. In other words, speech production may be possible within the physiological limitations of the individual. In contrast, a focused approach might target lung capacity and efficient breathing alone. In a second example, a clinician using a systems approach might train rate control or the slowing of speech rate to increase overall speech intelligibility. A focused approach might target speech sound production exclusively.

Prosthetic devices and/or intraoral surgery may help to decrease hypernasality. These procedures alone will be insufficient, and the client must be trained with the new or repaired structure (see Chapter 10).

Exercises to improve oral nonspeech movement are usually minimized. Little carryover exists from nonspeech to speech movement patterns (Love, 1992). Likewise, exercising specific muscle groups, such as those for respiration or articulation, does little to improve speech.

Specific sounds will be targeted on the basis of the ease of production. For the child with accompanying language deficits, these sounds and the child's interests will be important in the selection of initial words to be trained. Likewise, the child's interests and the demands of the environment will also be important in content selection with augmentative/alternative communication.

The SLP often works closely with the physical therapist to maximize and facilitate movement patterns. Some employ the *Bobath method,* a procedure using head, body, and limb postures that inhibit reflexive and uncontrolled movements. The child is placed in positions that prohibit certain reflexive movements. For example, the child with athetoid cerebral palsy may be seated with her or his legs bent or flexed and feet firmly supported to inhibit extensor patterns. Once the child can perform desired movements within a reflex-inhibiting posture, the posture is gradually changed to a more functional one while attempting to maintain the desired movement. Even SLPs who do not subscribe to this method of intervention generally accept the notion of using either postural supports or seating systems to improve movement.

Motor performance of individuals with cerebral palsy can often be improved by consideration of positioning and placement of the trunk, neck, and head for maximum facilitation.

Parents must be consulted by the SLP and other professionals regarding their expectations for their child. It is important that parents be realistic about their child's functioning level and the prognosis for change. SLPs must be careful not to mislead parents who have a natural desire for their child to improve. Attempts to reach unattainable goals result in the placing of unrealistic demands on children. Interaction between the family, child, and professionals is essential, and the family should be involved as a fully participating member of the intervention team.

For many individuals with severe cerebral palsy, unaided augmentative and alternative communication (AAC) systems, such as sign, are inappropriate. For these individuals, aided electronic AAC can greatly enhance communication abilities. Recent technological advances have improved intelligible synthetic speech, flexibility of access through increasing variability in devices, and portability. In general, systems with individualized vocabulary and with letter encoding rather than icon or symbol encoding work best and provide optimal flexibility, although individual assessment is needed to determine the optimal system, including the client-device interface or input mode (Angelo, 1992; Light & Lindsay, 1991; Silverman, 1995; Yorkston, Smith, & Beukelman, 1990). See examples on the accompanying CD-ROM.

Much research needs to be done on the effects of AAC on language acquisition in children with cerebral palsy. Research findings suggest that making the process more typical facilitates acquisition (Rhea, 1997). Emphasis on the communication environment of these children is particularly important (Calculator, 1997; Light, 1997). AAC devices may be integrated into a client's technology system. For example, a keyboard that is used for functional communication may also serve as an alternative keyboard for the client's desktop computer.

It is not enough that the client learn symbols—pictures, pictographs, or letters—to be used in communication. Successful use of AAC requires operational, linguistic, social, and strategic competence (Light, 1989). Operational competence enables a client to make maximal use of the device. Linguistic and social competence is needed for the give and take of conversation. Finally, strategic competence includes individual strategies that each client uses to maximize the communication process and make it as typical as possible. These topics are discussed in more detail in Chapter 15.

To be maximally effective, AAC must be integrated into the user's everyday routine, and conversational partners must be trained in its use.

THE DYSARTHRIAS

As was mentioned previously, dysarthria is a group of neuromuscular impairments that may affect the speed, range, direction, strength, and timing of motor movement as the result of paralysis, weakness, or discoordination of the muscles. Motor movements that were previously established may have been lost or modified in some way, though the pattern for that movement still exists. The processes of respiration, phonation, resonation, and articulation all may be affected. Motor function may be excessively slow or rapid, decreased in range or strength, and have poor directionality and coordina-

It might seen strange that movement would be altered but the pattern remain. Have you ever broken a bone? Although movement is altered, you still remember how to make that movement.

tion. It may be more appropriate to speak of *the dysarthrias,* given the wide variety of impairments included under this name.

Speech may be slowed or, in some disorders, be excessively fast or contain involuntary movements. The range of movements may decrease until only tiny, barely discernible ones are possible. Direction may become imprecise and nonrepeatable. Strength may decrease, and timing may become either erratic—fluctuating wildly—or monotonous. Unlike apraxia, a problem of motor planning and coordination, which we discuss later in this chapter, the dysarthrias represent difficulties in motor speech control.

Speech intelligibility is most affected by motoric impairment of the tongue, lips, jaw, and soft palate. A variety of speech features may be affected, and describing them may overwhelm even a seasoned speech-language pathologist. Features that affect articulation, voicing, prosody, and respiration may be intertwined. Accurate description requires the SLP to unweave each speech parameter. The speech pattern presented by a client depends on the location and extent of the neural damage as well as on the etiology. Table 12.2 presents speech dimensions that may be observed in clients with dysarthria. Note that several parameters of voice, mentioned in Chapter 9, are present.

Dysarthria is not a language disorder. The individual with dysarthria but no other complications exhibits good language structure and vocabulary, has good reading comprehension, can participate in the give and take of conversation as well as her or his physical limitations permit, and is able to convey by other means, such as a computer, sentences that she or he seems unable to produce freely through speech. Audio and video speech samples of persons with dysarthia are presented on the accompanying CD-ROM.

TYPES OF DYSARTHRIA AND ASSOCIATED ETIOLOGIES

The muscular disorders that are found in dysarthria represent a variety of neurological diseases. Although individuals with dysarthria share some common symptoms, distinct clusters of neurological and speech characteristics exist that describe particular variations of the disorder.

Different types of dysarthria are the result of lesions to different parts of the CNS and PNS. Certain commonalities exist, as noted in Table 12.3. These include inadequate breath supply; voice deviations, such as pitch variations and breaks and voice quality anomalies; prosodic problems of slow, rapid, or varying speed; nasality; and articulation errors.

Five distinct types of dysarthria can be identified by their speech characteristics and the impaired neuromuscular processes (Bloom & Ferrand, 1997; Darley, Aronson, & Brown, 1975; Rosenbek & LaPointe, 1985). These include **flaccid, spastic, ataxic, hyperkinetic,** and **hypokinetic dysarthria.** Disorders affecting multiple motor systems may yield a mixed dysarthria, as is found in ALS, multiple sclerosis, and Wilson's disease, to name a few. Each type of dysarthria and etiology is discussed briefly below.

> Dysarthria is a group of related motor disorders with a variety of etiologies and sites of lesion.

Flaccid Dysarthria

Flaccid muscles possess a weak, soft, flabby tone, called *hypotonia,* resulting in weakness or paralysis of the affected muscle. Dysarthria of this type usu-

TABLE 12.2
Possible speech dimensions of dysarthria

Respiration

Forced expirations and/or inspirations

Grunt at end of expiration

Audible inspiration

Voice

Pitch

    Inappropriate pitch level

    Monopitch

    Pitch breaks

    Voice tremor

Loudness

    Inappropriate loudness level

    Alternating loudness

    Excess loudness variation

    Monoloudness

    Loudness decay

Quality

    Harsh, strained/strangled, or continuous or transient breathy voice

    Hyponasality or hypernasality

    Nasal emissions

    Voice stoppages

Prosody

Inappropriate rate

    Increased overall or in segments or variable

    Prolonged intervals

    Short rushes of speech

    Short pauses

    Inappropriate silences

    Stress

        Reduced or excess and equal

Articulation

Imprecise consonants

Phonemes repeated or prolonged

Vowels distorted

Source: Adapted from Darley et al. (1975).

ally results from lesions in the cranial and spinal nerves or in the muscle unit itself. Weak muscles tire quickly. Affected muscles may cause reduced vital capacity and shallow breathing, breathy voice and aphonia, reduced pitch and loudness levels, monotone, hypernasality, and imprecise articulation. Bell's palsy, a facial nerve disorder; bulbar palsy; myasthenia gravis; and muscular dystrophy are characterized by flaccid paralysis.

Bulbar Palsy   A flaccid dysarthria, **bulbar palsy** results from involvement at the neuron or nerve cell level or in the synapse or space between neurons. Most likely, the neurons or synapses fail or are slow in chemically resetting after nerve firing. In addition, bulbar palsy is characterized by muscle atrophy and by random and irregular contractions (**vasiculation**) of nerve bundles. These rapid, minute contractions have been described by individuals

TABLE 12.3

Characteristics of the dysarthrias

Type of Dysarthria	Voice Quality	Speech Rate	Articulation
Flaccid dysarthria			
Weak, soft, flabby muscle tone; lesions in the lower motor neurons (cranial and spinal nerves) or in the muscle unit itself	Breathy voice, monopitch/tone, hypernasality, reduced pitch/loudness	Short phrases	Imprecise consonants
Spastic dysarthria			
Stiff and rigid muscles; lesions in the upper motor neurons and the pyramidal tract	Monopitch/loudness, reduced stress, harsh voice, hypernasality, strained/strangled voice	Slow	Imprecise consonants
Ataxic dysarthria			
Damage to the cerebellum; muscle weakness and coordination problems involving accuracy, timing, and direction	Excessive and equal stress, harsh voice	Prolonged pauses and rate	Imprecise consonants, irregular articulatory breakdown
Hyperkinetic dysarthria			
Increased movement from lesions of the extrapyramidal tract and basal nuclei	Monopitch, harsh voice, excess loudness	Variable rate, silences, prolonged intervals	Imprecise consonants, distorted vowels
Hypokinetic dysarthria			
Decrease or lack of appropriate movement from lesions of the extrapyramidal tract and basal nuclei; muscles rigid and stiff	Monopitch/loudness, reduced stress, harsh/breathy voice	Variable rate, silences, prolonged intervals	Imprecise consonants
Mixed dysarthrias			
Severe muscle weakness from diffuse brain damage	Hypernasality, harsh voice, low pitch, monopitch/loudness, excess and equal stress	Slow rate, prolonged intervals	Imprecise consonants, distorted vowels

Source: Adapted from Darley et al. (1975).

with bulbar palsy as feeling like a bubbling under the skin. Tremors may be obvious in the tongue when it is extended. In general, the speech of these individuals is weak, hypernasal, and monopitched with articulation difficulties. A sample of the speech of a person with bulbar palsy is presented on the accompanying CD-ROM.

Myasthenia Gravis   A common disorder, **myasthenia gravis** affects the neuromuscular juncture. The disorder is characterized by a rapid weakening of the muscle due to the inadequate transmission of the nerve impulse. Muscles tire quickly but regain their strength after a short interval of rest. Velar and laryngeal muscles are often affected.

Muscular Dystrophy   In **muscular dystrophy,** the muscles themselves are affected. Muscles may be unable either to contract or to relax. A progressive degenerative disease, muscular dystrophy may eventually affect all aspects of speech.

Spastic Dysarthria

Spastic paralysis—stiff and rigid muscles—is the result of lesions in the lower brain. The most common cause is stroke, and the results may be temporary or permanent. Lesions in the left hemisphere may be accompanied by aphasia and result in mild spasticity (see Chapter 7). More severe spastic dysarthria is bilateral, with the site of lesion in areas such as the brain stem where left and right innervation are in close proximity. Hypertonia makes movement difficult, and speech is characterized as slow with jerky, imprecise articulation and reduction of the rapidly alternating movements of speech.

Pseudobulbar Palsy   *Pseudobulbar palsy* is an example of spastic paralysis. Although individuals with pseudobulbar palsy exhibit the muscle weakness and loss of movement that are found in bulbar palsy, muscle atrophy and vasiculation do not seem to be present. Movement is characterized by hyperflexia, a combination of overreaction and overreach. The voice of individuals with pseudobulbar palsy is strained and strangled-sounding, resulting from intermittent spasticity. The rate is slow, and articulation is imprecise.

Ataxic Dysarthria

Damage to the cerebellum can result in a combination of muscle weakness or reduced tone or hypotonia and problems with muscle coordination, called *ataxia* (Kent, Duffy, Slama, Kent, & Clift, 2001). Ataxic dysarthria is the result of breakdown in motor organization and control (Duffy, 1995). Little or no paralysis exists, and the problem is one involving the accuracy, timing, and direction of movement. Movements overshoot. The signal to start a movement is received, and the accompanying inhibition is impaired. As a result, movements are jerky and imprecise. Congenital ataxia is a form of cerebral palsy that is seen in children.

Speech is characterized by a shift in fundamental frequency and variability in the slow rate of moving between different speech sounds (diadochokinesis) (Kent, Kent, Duffy, Thomas, Weismer, & Stunteberk, 2000).

Energy varies across repeated syllables, respiration is poorly coordinated, and voicing and articulation are inadequate and imprecise.

Hyperkinetic Dysarthria

Hyperkinesia, or increased movement, called tremors and tics, results from lesions of the mid and lower brain. *Tremors* are involuntary, nonpurposeful, rhythmic movements caused by contractions of antagonistic muscles. Several types of tremors exist. **Tics** are involuntary, rapid and repetitive, stereotypic movements. Unlike tremors, tics can be suppressed for short periods of time. One characteristic of hyperkinetic dysarthria is inaccurate articulation. Two disorders, dystonia and chorea, are forms of hyperkinetic dysarthria.

Dystonia   **Dystonia** is characterized by a slow increase and decrease of hyperkinesia involving either the entire body or localized sets of muscles. Excessive movement is slow and sustained, often writhing in nature. Like chorea, dystonia may involve the entire motor system or be localized. As a result, there are excessive pitch and loudness variations, irregular articulation breakdown, and vowel distortions.

Chorea   Unlike dystonia, **chorea** is characterized by rapid or continual hyperkinesia. Chorea movements are characterized as random, irregular, and/or abrupt, usually lasting less than one second (Rosenfield, 1991). Movement may involve the entire body or a particular segment. Hyperkinesia impairs control and reduces coordination, especially in rapid successive movements such as speech. Speech, when affected, may be characterized by inappropriate silences caused by voice stoppage; intermittent breathiness, strained harsh voice, and hypernasality; imprecise articulation with prolonged pauses; and forced inspiration and expiration resulting in excessive loudness variations (Duffy, 1995).

Huntington's Chorea   An inherited progressive disease, also known as Huntington's disease, Huntington's chorea results from a genetic defect on chromosome 4 (American Psychiatric Association, 1994). Initial symptoms include involuntary movements and behavior change. As the disease progresses, movements become rigid with reduced speed and difficulty with coordination. Jerky, irregular movements affect the diaphragm, laryngeal muscles, tongue, and lips. In addition to the speech difficulties, language may be affected as a result of cognitive and memory changes. In general, individuals with Huntington's chorea have the same verbal output as their non-Huntington peers, but they are less informative with their language (Murray, 2000). Their language is characterized by a smaller proportion of grammatical utterances and a larger proportion of simple sentences than both non-Huntington individuals and those with Parkinson's disease. Accompanying personality changes may include depression, paranoia, delusional thoughts, and intellectual decline (Greenamyre & Shoulson, 1994).

Hypokinetic Dysarthria

Like hyperkinetic dysarthria, hypokinetic dysarthria is caused by lesions of the mid and lower brain, though the result is just the opposite: a decrease or lack of appropriate movement. Muscles become rigid and stiff, resulting in restricted motor movement. One form of hypokinetic dysarthria is found in many people with Parkinson's disease.

Parkinson's Disease   In Parkinson's disease, the individual's muscles become rigid as opposing pairs of muscles contract simultaneously. Motor movements become increasingly reduced, a condition called **hypokinesia.** Other characteristics include involuntary shaking or tremors when at rest, slowness of movement, and difficulty initiating voluntary movements. Symptoms reflect the reduced supply of dopamine, a neurotransmitter, a result of loss of dopaminergic neurons. Tremors may be controlled by different neural systems rather than one central tremor generator (Gurd, Bessell, Watson, & Coleman, 1998). Comments by a professional with Parkinson's disease are presented in Case Study 12.3.

The resultant speech is characterized by a rapid rate, a breathy voice, less speech per breath, difficulty initiating motor movement, and reduced loudness, pitch range, and stress. Although speech rate increases, it may be perceived to be even faster that it actually is (Tjaden, 2000). Voice changes may occur early in the course of the disease, although articulation deficits typically do not. Dysarthria is a symptom in the more advanced stages of Parkinson's disease. Speech may become extremely rapid, accompanied by imprecise consonant formation as a result of weak tongue strength and endurance (Solomon, Robin, & Luschei, 2000). Speech deficits may be accompanied by a decrease in nonlinguistic communication, such as gestures and facial expression.

Case Study 12.3

Comments of a Speech-Language Pathologist with Parkinson's Disease

My medication is as helpful as the oil Dorothy used with the Tin Woodsman so that he could move and speak. My oil, pharmacological treatment, temporarily increases the level of dopamine that is reduced by Parkinson's. Unfortunately, the medication does not ensure relief or even last throughout the day. This, coupled with the fact that my schedule as a university professor varies from day to day, makes it challenging to time the medications so that they are at their peak when I need fluid, wide-ranging movement. . . . I live by the clock and I am never without my meds. . . .

One thing that I have learned since I've had Parkinson's is that when we discuss neurological disorders in our class, we so emphasize the effects of these impairments on communication that we underemphasize their broader effects on general health status. As a result, we may inadvertently lead some

students to think that Parkinson's is "just" a movement disorder. There are other aspects of this problem that affect health, nonspeech physiological function, and state of mind. . . .

Interestingly, the reactions of people to my speech and other movements, particularly when I'm having a bad day, have allowed me to relate better to some of my clients who have told me how hard they concentrate on their speech production in an attempt to monitor for maximum intelligibility. Speech has become a more demanding task for me. I am keenly aware of the changes in my speech and work at a high level of consciousness to make online adjustments to preserve normal-sounding articulation.

Source: From Caruso, A. J. (2001, July 24). Parkinson's disease and me. *The ASHA Leader,* 6(13), 7. © American Speech-Language-Hearing Association, reprinted by permission.

Although individuals with Parkinson's have a similar verbal output to their non-Parkinson peers, they are less informative with their language (Murray, 2000). Individuals with Parkinson's disease also have a smaller proportion of grammatical sentences.

The most common form of Parkinson's disease occurs in 1 percent of the population over age 65 (http://www.cdc.gov/nchs/data/factsheets/parkinsons.pdf, 1999). In real numbers, approximately half a million individuals have Parkinson's disease in the United States, and about 50,000 new cases occur annually (http://www.ninds.nih.gov/disorders/parkinsons_disease/parkinsons_disease_backgrounder.htm, 2004). A sample of the speech of a person with Parkinson's disease is presented on the accompanying CD-ROM.

Mixed Dysarthrias

Some dysarthrias are not easily classified within the above system. Called **mixed dysarthrias,** these disorders are characterized by symptoms or areas of brain injury that cross several dysarthrias. Diffuse brain damage may result from degenerative disorders, toxins, metabolic disorders, stroke, trauma, tumors, and infectious diseases. Amyotrophic lateral sclerosis is one example of this category.

Amyotrophic Lateral Sclerosis   Commonly called Lou Gehrig's disease for the baseball player who was afflicted with it in the early twentieth century, **amyotrophic lateral sclerosis (ALS)** is a rapidly progressive degenerative disease that involves both the upper and lower motor neurons and spinal cord.

Mental capacity is not affected, but the individual gradually loses control of her or his musculature. ALS is characterized by fatigue, muscle atrophy (loss of bulk), involuntary contractions, and reduced muscle tone. Speech deficits are common in the later stages of the disorder (Yorkston, Strand, Miller, Hillel, & Smith, 1993). These include a labored, slow rate; short phrasing, long pauses, hypernasality, and severely impaired articulation (Duffy, 1995). The slow rate influences the timing of elements within each sound, distorting its production (Tjaden & Turner, 2000).

ALS combines both flaccid and spastic dysarthria. Dysarthria increases as the disease progresses, and approximately 75 percent of affected people are unable to speak at the time of death. Age of onset is usually in the midfifties. Incidence figures vary but may be as high as 2 per 100,000 individuals. Males are affected more frequently than females. Death usually occurs within five years after the initial diagnosis. A sample of the speech of a person with ALS is presented on the accompanying CD-ROM.

*C*an you imagine the terror of losing motor control while being fully cognizant of the process? Have you ever broken an arm or a leg? If so, you know a little of the frustration faced by those with physical disabilities.

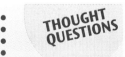

THOUGHT QUESTIONS

LIFESPAN ISSUES

Most acquired dysarthria occurs in adults. Even the individual with mild dysarthria may be reluctant to speak, leading to assumptions by others that the person is frightened, tense, shy, or unfriendly. For some individuals, even a slight speech imperfection can be cause for embarassment or depression. In the more advanced dysarthrias, individuals may be frustrated as loved ones and acquaintances attempt to communicate for them by finishing sentences or ordering for them in restaurants. In turn, the individual may communicate and socialize less. Difficulty communicating may limit the opportunities to participate in social, occupational, and educational activities, leading to feelings of isolation.

Some individuals with dysarthria are unable to live independently and may need daily living assistance or institutional care. The social, physical, psychological, and familial adjustments in this situation can be enormous.

In the later stages of progressive degenerative disorders, the individual may be unable to care for herself or himself. Movement may be very difficult, and the person may be unable to speak. AAC devices may be helpful even for the most severely affected individuals.

> Neuromotor problems are not limited to speech production and may have a profound effect on many aspects of an individual's life.

ASSESSMENT

The SLP is an important member of the diagnostic team. By identifying differing speech patterns characteristic of specific neurological conditions, the SLP provides valuable information on localized neurological conditions to other team members.

The purposes of evaluation for dysarthria are many and include the following:

To determine whether a significant long-term problem exists

To describe the nature of impaired functions, specifically, the types of problems, their extent/severity, and the effect of these impairments on everyday, functional communication

To identify functions that are not impaired

To establish appropriate goals and decide where to begin intervention

To form a well-reasoned prognosis based on the nature of the disorder, the client's age, the age or stage of injury or disease, the presence of other accompanying conditions, client motivation, and family support

As described in Chapter 4, the speech-language pathologist will want to thoroughly evaluate oral peripheral function, conversational speech, and speech in special tasks. The oral-motor mechanism is evaluated as outlined in the section on cerebral palsy. Of particular importance in assessment of dysarthria are the range, speed, and direction of oral movement.

Although very few commercially available test procedures are available, most SLPs working in hospitals or outpatient clinics have a standard assessment protocol that they use for motor speech evaluations. These procedures might or might not rely on the use of instrumental approaches and computerized analysis.

INTERVENTION

Some basic principles underlie intervention for acquired motor speech disorders (Darley et al., 1975):

Compensatory strategies: Maximize individual strengths while working to bypass physical limitations.

Automatic to volitional shift: Foster more purposeful control over automatic and overlearned behaviors.

Behavior change monitoring: Maintain precise records and foster self-monitoring by the client.

An early start: Early intervention forestalls formation of bad habits.

Motivation: Provide information and support.

The SLP begins with this basic foundation.

The type of intervention, its course, and the prognosis will vary with the underlying cause of the dysarthria. Some diseases, such as Parkinson's or Wilson's, are *progressive,* the client's condition degenerating gradually over time. As severity increases or a client becomes less motivated, the prognosis becomes less optimistic. In cases of irreversible disease, therapy goals become holding actions in which the client and the SLP attempt to hold the client's performance at a certain plateau, maintaining the client's speech abilities even as the client's overall function decreases (Yorkston, Miller, & Strand, 1995). Other goals might include teaching compensatory skills, such as the use of an augmentative/alternative form of communication. One young man we know used a keyboard to communicate through his computer. When this became too difficult, he used a joystick to navigate the keyboard. Spelling became too arduous, and electronic picture communication using the joystick was substituted. After several modifications, he now communicates with a combination of eye gazes and hand squeezes.

> Just as the AAC system of the child with cerebral palsy must change as the child matures, so that of the individual with a degenerative disorder must change as the disorder progresses.

Because dysarthria affects all aspects of speech production, intervention must address the client's difficulties in respiration, phonation, resonance, and articulation, as well as prosody. Of concern within each area are muscle timing, strength, and tone. Therapy might focus on sustaining phonation, production of nasal and nonnasal words (*met-pet, neat-beat, king-kid*), and speech-sound production in meaningful words.

Intelligibility of words improves with repeated training, although the mode of presentation of words—audiovisual versus audio only—does not seem to affect production accuracy (Hustad & Cahill, 2003).

Speech supplementation strategies that provide additional information to a listener can also significantly increase speech intelligibility (Hustad & Beukelman, 2001; Yorkston & Beukelman, 2004). The most effective strategies seem to be alphabet cues or combined cues and slower speech (Hustad, Jones, & Dailey, 2003). With alphabet cues, speakers point to the first letter of each word as they say the word. Combined cues include both alphabet cues and topic cues in which the listener is supplied with the topic prior to the speaker's beginning to talk.

Intervention is best when it occurs within a meaningful speech context but may include drill, progressively more complex tasks, and feedback. The SLP works with the physical and occupational therapists to coordinate exercises to increase muscle functioning or to decrease hypertonia through relaxation techniques.

Respiratory exercises emphasize efficient breath control and sustained exhalation. These exercises inevitably lead into sustained phonation. Either vocal fold exercises or relaxation techniques accompanied by easy phonation may also be a part of the intervention regime. Intervention for voice disorders is discussed in Chapter 9. Likewise hypernasality, the primary disorder of resonance, is treated through exercise. In addition, prosthetic devices similar to those discussed with cleft palate (see Chapter 11) may be fitted; the client is then trained to use them properly to achieve either velopharyngeal closure or approximation. Although progress in all these areas will improve articulation, such improvement does not preclude working directly with the client's articulation abilities. Exercises will focus on auditory and proprioceptive feedback and placement of the articulators.

Many individuals with severe dysarthria never regain enough intelligible speech to communicate even simple conversational messages. These clients may benefit from the use of AAC as a substitution for or a complement to oral forms of communication. Even something as seemingly simple as alphabet cues in the form of pointing to the first letter of each word being spoken can greatly increase the intelligibility for severely dysarthric speech (Hustad & Beukelman, 2001). Most of the considerations mentioned in the discussion of cerebral palsy are also applicable.

Unaided AAC systems such as sign may be taught if the client does not have accompanying severe aphasia or severe motor involvement of the hands. Gestures may aid mildly impaired individuals, but involuntary limb movements, such as those found in Parkinson's disease, may interfere with communication (Garcia, Cannito, & Dagenais, 2000). People who have a language disorder in addition to a speech disorder may have some difficulty. Remember that signing is another mode of communication, but language encoding and decoding may still be impaired.

Aided systems, such as communication boards or electronic devices, have been used successfully, although the most common augmentative devices for speakers with dysarthria are speech amplifiers. Communication boards, discussed in detail in Chapter 15, consist of flat, durable surfaces, often attached to a wheelchair. Clients select symbols by touching or looking at them.

As long as there is no accompanying cognitive or language impairment, adults may find spelling of words on an AAC device to be an acceptable substitute for, or accompaniment to, speech.

Mechanical and electronic devices differ widely in their cost, portability, ease of use, symbol systems, and input and output modes. The most common devices are simple, relatively inexpensive handheld printers with keys for each letter. More complex devices may translate pictures or pictographs into simple messages. Only very careful evaluation can help the SLP to determine the appropriate device and symbol system for a client.

Neurosurgical, genetic, and pharmacological interventions hold great promise for individuals with some forms of neurological impairment. For example, surgical placement of an electronic stimulator on the globus pallidus of individuals with Parkinson's disease modifies some abnormal neural activity (Solomon, McKee, et al., 2000). As a result, oral tremors decrease and the amount of voluntary responding increases. Unfortunately, the separately affected centers for speech and nonspeech movement respond differently to intervention (Camicioli, Oken, Sexton, Kaye, & Nutt, 1998).

APRAXIA OF SPEECH

Apraxia is a disorder in volitional or voluntary motor placement and sequencing that is unrelated to muscle weakness, slowness, or paralysis. It is the result of an acquired neurological impairment of the ability to program—organize and plan—and execute movement of the speech muscles for the production of volitional speech. Because apraxia can affect any muscle group, apraxia that affects the initiation and execution of the movement patterns particular to speech is more correctly called *apraxia of speech* or *verbal apraxia*. Apraxia of the mouth area is termed **oral apraxia** and is often, but not always, observed in association with apraxia of speech.

Apraxia of speech is a problem of speech-sound articulation and prosody or rhythm caused by a neurologically based movement disorder (Darley et al., 1975; Haynes, 1985; Kearns & Simmons, 1988; Kent & Rosenbek, 1983; Wertz, 1985; Yorkston et al., 1988). Difficulties are not the result of muscle or linguistic processing deficits, although these disorders may co-occur with apraxia of speech. Individuals with apraxia have difficulty planning and executing the movements to position the articulators for correct sound production.

The speech of individuals with apraxia is characterized by groping attempts to find the correct articulatory position, with great variability on repeated attempts. There are frequent speech-sound substitutions and omissions with sound-sequencing difficulties. Distortions and additions also occur. Unlike the person with dysarthria, who makes predominantly distortions and related substitutions, the person with apraxia makes unrelated substitutions, repetitions, and additions.

Recognizing the errors, the individual with apraxia of speech will make repeated attempts to correct them. As she or he tries to produce the correct sound, there are inordinately frequent pauses and reinitiations of words and sentences (Wertz, LaPointe, & Rosenbek, 1991). Unlike the person with dysarthria, who repeats the same error, the individual with apraxia of speech often produces widely varying productions on repeated attempts. A sample of speech from a person with apraxia follows:

> O-o-on . . . on . . . on our cavation, cavation, cacation . . . oh darn . . . vavation, oh, you know, to Ca-ca-caciporenia . . . no, Lacifacnia, vafacnia to Lacifacnion. . . . On our vacation to Vacafornia, no darn it . . . to Ca-caliborneo . . . not bornia . . . fornia, Bornifornia . . . no, Balliforneo, Ballifornee, Balifornee, Californee, California. Phew, it was hard to say Cacaforneo. Oh darn.

How do you know when you pronounce a word incorrectly? Does it sound wrong? Does it also feel wrong in your mouth?

Consonants and consonant clusters and blends offer a particular challenge, although more frequently used phonemes and words are produced with more accuracy. As you might expect, complex, long, or unfamiliar words are more difficult to produce, although few of the errors that are produced appear to be attempts to simplify the word.

Individuals with apraxia of speech may have no difficulty producing words on one occasion that they struggled to produce on another. In fact, clients may exhibit periods of error-free speech during automatic or emotional utterances. It is not uncommon to have a client struggle with volitional production of a word such as "vacation" only to hear the client easily say later, "Boy, I sure had a lot of trouble with *vacation*!" A sample of the speech of a person with apraxia of speech is presented on the accompanying CD-ROM.

The speaker with apraxia is typically aware of her or his errors and may even anticipate them but is unable to correct them. Monitoring of speech in anticipation of these errors results in a slowed, almost cautious rate with even stress and spacing.

Clients with apraxia of speech frequently report that they know what they want to say but can't initiate the sequence or keep it going. Faced with a naming task, these individuals frequently respond, "I know it, but I can't say it."

Can you imagine how frustrating it would be to be unable to say what you're thinking? Delay even a few seconds when someone speaks to you and note how it disrupts the conversation.

Although apraxia and aphasia often co-occur in an individual, the two are not the same. Aphasia is a language disorder; apraxia is a motor speech problem. The individual with aphasia will have difficulty with word recall in all modalities, while the person with apraxia of speech can recall the word easily when writing but may be unable to say it accurately. In addition, the individual with apraxia of speech has no difficulties with the structure of language. Case Study 12.4 presents the story of a woman with apraxia.

At this point, no doubt, your head is swimming with seemingly overlapping characteristics of the dysarthrias and apraxia of speech. Table 12.4 presents the major differences between the two disorders. As with any attempt to simplify data, individual variations may become lost when presented in a table. The SLP provides the missing data through a thorough diagnostic evaluation adequately describing each person's observable behaviors in detail.

Although we have defined apraxia as a disorder of the mature nervous system, some experts insist that children can also exhibit apraxia of speech, termed *developmental apraxia of speech* (Hall et al., 1993) (see Chapter 10). Data are complicated by causal factors such as TBI and disagreements over the exact characteristics (Thompson, 1988). Most frequently, children who are diagnosed as having developmental apraxia of speech exhibit multiple articulation errors, including addition of speech sounds, sound and syllable repetitions, and sound prolongations.

Case Study 12.4

Personal Story of a Woman with Dysarthria and Apraxia of Speech

Ruth is a 75-year-old female who suffered a stroke in the frontal lobe of the left cerebral hemisphere after surgery. On release from the hospital following her stroke, Ruth began receiving services twice weekly at a rehabilitation center for her speech and for other motor difficulties.

Six months after the incident, her speech is characterized by moderate dysarthria, which is evidenced in poor breath control, decreased loudness, and decreased articulatory precision. In addition, she exhibits apraxia in her ability to initiate and complete functional communication. Her speech is characterized by cluster reduction and inconsistent omission, substitution, and distortion of speech sound and consists primarily of single words. In reading samples, intelligibility decreases with increasingly complex material. Ruth has difficulty begining speech initiation and with sound and syllable sequencing. Her speech seems to improve with preformulation of the message, word-by-word attack, and gesturing.

Auditory comprehension of both conversation and directions and silent reading comprehension of directions are good. Although she reads the newspaper, she seems uninterested in the more substantial pleasure reading that occupied much of her time previously. Ruth's memory and attention seem unaffected.

A retired schoolteacher and widow, Ruth lives alone. She has six children. Her two oldest daughters are attempting to supplement the home health care she receives. Ruth's diet consists primarily of soft foods and semiliquids, which require more time for ingestion than was previously allotted for meals.

ETIOLOGY

In most clients, apraxia of speech is the result of a lesion in the central programming area for speech: Broca's area in the left frontal lobe of the brain (Kent, et al., 2001). Broca's area details and plans the coordination of sequenced motor movements for speech, much as an assembly line computer would organize the various aspects of car production. Breakdown in Broca's area makes speech difficult, just as a glitch in an automobile factory computer might cause a chassis to arrive after the component parts to be installed have already moved on or painting to occur before completion of the body. Without a plan, the person with apraxia of speech has difficulty placing the articulators and sequencing his or her movement. Chewing, sucking, and swallowing may be possible, but speech is inconsistent. The language message is sent from the left temporal lobe, but production through speech is difficult.

In apraxia of speech, it is not the nerves or muscles that are defective but the part of the brain that coordinates and activates them.

TABLE 12.4

Differences between dysarthria and apraxia

Dysarthria	Apraxia of Speech
Speech sound distortions	Speech sound substitutions
Substitution errors related to target phoneme	Substitution errors often not related to target phoneme
Highly consistent speech sound errors	Inconsistent speech sound substitution
Consonant clusters simplified	Schwa (/ə/) often inserted between consonants in a cluster
Little audible or silent groping for a target speech sound	Audible or silent groping for a target speech sound
Rapid or slow rate	Slow rate characterized by repetitions, prolongations, and additions
No periods of unaffected speech	Islands of fluency
Little difference between reactive or automatic speech and volitional speech; both affected	Often very fluent reactive or automatic speech, nonfluent volitional speech

ASSESSMENT

Because of the nature of apraxia of speech, the SLP must pay special attention to additional aspects of assessments. These include the following:

Imitation of single words of varying lengths

Sentence imitation

Reading aloud

Spontaneous speech

Rapid repetition of "puh," "tuh," "kuh," and "puh-tuh-kuh"

Note that a number of the tasks are repetitive or imitative in nature. Recall that in apraxia, performance may vary with repeated performance. Modes of stimulus presentation are also important because the person with apraxia performs better to auditory-visual stimuli than to either auditory or visual stimuli alone.

INTERVENTION

In conjunction with other health professionals, the SLP attempts to increase muscle tone and strength, especially those of the speech mechanism. Increased tone in the body may be accomplished with the use of braces and girdling or by postural adjustments. Prosthetic devices such as slings should be used only with the concurrence of the client's physician. The sequenced production of speech sounds and motor planning that are needed to accomplish this may begin with practice of nonspeech movements

Intervention often begins with sensory bombardment, in which the client hears the correct sound or word repeatedly and sees it in print. Gradually, the client moves to imitation, followed by simultaneous production and finally spontaneous speech. The SLP and the client discuss how the sound or word felt when the articulators were moved. More difficult sounds, consonant clusters, and words are gradually introduced. For clients with severe apraxia of speech, AAC may be introduced (see Chapter 15).

Some individuals will need additional input to be successful. The SLP may provide visual and physical cues and/or aid with physical manipulation. Electromagnetic articulography (EMA), which tracks oral movement, can remediate some articulatory deficits by providing visually guided biofeedback for tongue tip position improvement (Katz, Bharadwaj, & Carstens, 1999).

A decreased rate of production may also improve production. Some clients benefit from the use of carrier phrases that are repeated with each word, such as "I like _____" or "I want _____." Frequently used phrases such as "How are you?" are also practiced and incorporated into the client's verbal repertoire to help the client's speech to sound more normal.

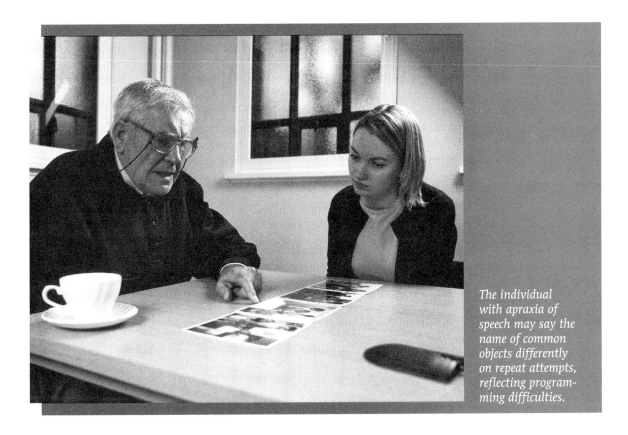

The individual with apraxia of speech may say the name of common objects differently on repeat attempts, reflecting programming difficulties.

SUMMARY

The major types of neurogenic motor speech disorders are cerebral palsy, dysarthria, and apraxia of speech. Cerebral palsy is characterized as a group of developmental, nonprogressive neurological difficulties resulting from brain injury that occurs very early in fetal or infant development and affects motor movement, communication, growth and development, locomotion, learning, and sensation. The three main types of cerebral palsy—spastic, athetoid, and ataxic—result in very different motor patterns and speech difficulties.

Dysarthria is a group of acquired impairments that affect the speed, range, direction, strength, and timing of motor movement as the result of paralysis, weakness, or discoordination of the speech muscles. Unlike apraxia of speech, the dysarthrias represent difficulties in motor speech control. Five distinct types include flaccid, spastic, ataxic, hyperkinetic, and hypokinetic dysarthria. Disorders affecting multiple motor systems may yield a mixed dysarthria.

In contrast, apraxia is an acquired disorder in voluntary motor placement and sequencing that is unrelated to muscle weakness, slowness, or paralysis and results from a lesion in the central programming area for speech in the left frontal lobe. Called Broca's area, it details and plans the coordination of sequenced motor movements for speech.

Neurogenic motor speech disorders, both developmental and acquired, offer a special challenge to the affected individual, family, friends, and the speech-language pathologist. Many clients are in the very frustrating position of being able to formulate the message but unable to produce it intelligibly.

Intervention methods differ greatly. The child with cerebral palsy may be learning to communicate and to acquire language using an augmentative/alternative communication device. Meanwhile, the older adult with a motor speech problem may be relearning or retrieving older speech patterns. Finally, the individual with a progressive degenerative disease, such as Parkinson's disease or ALS, may be attempting to cling to the level of effective communication that was previously possible or exploring additional methods of communication. Changing intervention techniques and promising new surgical procedures and drugs will continue to offer hope to individuals with neurogenic speech disorders.

REFLECTIONS

- What are the major differences between cerebral palsy, dysarthria, and apraxia?
- Name some of the causes of neurogenic speech disorders.
- Describe the main types of cerebral palsy.
- Describe the major types of dysarthria.
- What are the differences between dysarthria and apraxia of speech?

- How do the assessment and intervention techniques used with each neurogenic motor speech disorder differ? How are they similar?

SUGGESTED RESOURCES

Brookshire, R. H. (1997). *Introduction to neurogenic communication disorders* (5th ed.). St. Louis, MO: Mosby.

My Left Foot. (1989). Miramax Pictures.

ONLINE RESOURCES

http://www.alsa.org/　Amyotrophic Lateral Sclerosis Association.
  Official website contains consumer information.

http://www.apple.com/education/k12/disability/
  Apple K–12 resources contains downloadable Mac-compatible files for adapting computers for persons with disabilities.

http://www.asel.udel.edu/at-online/
  Contains links and pointers to a variety of AAC topics including websites.

http://www.asha.org/professionals/multicultural/fact_14.htm
  Neurological/Fluency/Voice Disorders in Multicultural Populations.

http://www.at-center.com/
  Virtual Assistive Technology Center home page provides access to lists of freeware/shareware for AAC use.

http://www.healthtouch.com/level1/leaflets/ASLHA/ASLHA032.htm
  ASHA factsheet on developmental verbal apraxia.

http://www.irsc.org/cerebral.htm
  Links to online information concerning cerebral palsy.

http://www.ninds.nih.gov/healinfo/nindspub.htm
  National Institute of Neurological Disorders and Stroke Web site containing fact sheets and bibliographies on neurological conditions related to speech problems.

http://www.parkinson.org/
  National Parkinson Foundation site contains information and a library with free and online publications.

http://www.ucpa.org/
  United Cerebral Palsy site with search capability and information on advocacy and disability issues.

Disorders of Swallowing   **13**

CHAPTER LEARNING GOALS

When you have finished this chapter, you should be able to:

- Explain why speech-language pathologists are concerned with swallowing

- Describe the basic process of human swallowing

- Identify some causes of swallowing disorders in children and adults

- Describe basic clinical and instrumental assessment techniques

- Explain major concepts in swallowing treatment

You might be puzzled to see a chapter about swallowing in a textbook devoted to communication disorders. In fact, the assessment and management of *dysphagia,* or swallowing disorders, has been of growing interest to speech-language pathologists, and about 50 percent of SLPs who work in hospitals and extended care facilities do some dysphagia assessment or intervention (Clark, 2004, Logemann, 1994). SLPs also often take a leadership position in coordinating services for an individual with swallowing difficulties.

There is also a considerable amount of research regarding normal and abnormal swallowing patterns designed to improve the effectiveness of clinical practice (c.f., Colodny, 2005; Hiss, Strauss, Treole, Stuart, & Boutilier, 2004; Steele & van Lieshout, 2005). In addition, the vast majority of individuals with dysphagia also have communication disabilities (Martin & Corlew, 1990). The SLP is typically responsible for identifying, evaluating, and

Case Study 13.1

Case Study of a Women with Dysphagia: Rhea

Rhea is an 80-year-old woman who lives alone. Her son was concerned about a rapid and noticeable weight loss and approached Rhea's primary care physician with his concerns. A routine physical examination did not reveal anything that could be contributing to the loss of weight. During the doctor-patient interview following the physical examination, Rhea mentioned that she felt a frequent tightness in her throat and that she would sometimes gag when she was eating. Her son also told the physician that Rhea's normally robust appetite has recently become significantly diminished and that she seemed unduly anxious during mealtime. Based on the negative results of the physical examination regarding the cause of Rhea's weight loss and the information presented in the follow-up interview, her physician referred Rhea to the hospital for an evaluation for a potential swallowing disorder.

The staff SLP in charge of swallowing disorders performed the initial portion of Rhea's swallowing examination. Following a review of the case information, the SLP conducted an interview with Rhea and her son. The SLP noted that Rhea was alert during the interview and that she was cognitively intact. During the oral-motor examination, the SLP evaluated head and body posture, the anatomy and general health of Rhea's mouth, and her ability to

produce a strong cough. No problems were found in any of these areas. A modified barium swallow study (videofluoroscopy) showed an efficient swallow. Further testing with variegated textures of liquids and foods revealed that foods that were thick or sticky and hard to chew such as peanut butter or tough cuts of meat increased Rhea's anxiety, often causing her to gag.

Upon reviewing the swallow examination results, the swallowing team agreed that Rhea's difficulty with swallowing was related to life circumstances. The team recommended that Rhea be provided with more opportunities to eat with others rather than alone. Additionally, they recommended modifications to her dietary intake, reducing thick, tough and chewy foods. By following the recommendations of the swallowing team, Rhea has begun to gain weight and her family reports that she experiences less anxiety when eating.

As you read this chapter think about

• How the consistency of a food might affect the person's ability to swallow.
• How a swallowing disorder might affect a person's daily life.
• Conditions other than old age that might adversely affect a person's ability to swallow.

treating people from infancy to old age who are experiencing problems with the ingesting and swallowing of food (ASHA, 1990).

As with much of the work that speech-language pathologists do, they do not function alone. SLPs who treat patients with swallowing problems are generally part of a team consisting of a physician, nurse, nutritionist, radiologist, gastroenterologist, dentist, otolaryngologist, neurologist, occupational therapist, physical therapist, respiratory therapist, and family members. The role of each of these specialists will become clear when we discuss evaluation and treatment later in this chapter.

Swallowing and the efficient intake of food have both medical and psychosocial implications. Eating is essential to physical health. Without proper nourishment, one cannot grow, develop, or survive. Swallowing disorders increase the risk of choking and may lead to *aspiration* of food into the lungs and respiratory illnesses such as pneumonia (Langmore, Terpenning, Schork, et al., 1998). Inadequate swallowing may result in **gastroesophageal reflux (GER),** the movement of food or acid from the stomach back into the esophagus. Eating is also one of our major social activities. Feeding difficulties in children may stress the parent-child relationship. Among older people, dysphagia may lead to isolation, depression, frustration, and diminished quality of life.

The term "dysphagia" comes from the Greek and literally means difficulty with eating. Although it is pronounced both as "dis-FAH-gia" and as "dis-FAY-gia," the former and preferred pronunciation helps to differentiate it from "dysphasia" or "aphasia," which is a language impairment.

What connections can you think of between swallowing, speech, and communication?

THOUGHT QUESTION

In this chapter, we describe the basics of swallowing, characteristics and correlates of disordered swallowing, evaluation, and treatment.

LIFESPAN PERSPECTIVES

Feeding and swallowing problems exist in both children and adults. They may occur at any point in the lifespan. Newborns may be unable to suckle and/or ingest nutriment. As they age, they may refuse food and develop unhealthy food preferences. Neuromotor problems and structural anomalies that are congenital or acquired at any age can interfere with feeding, as can a host of psychosocial factors. Dysphagia may be related to many diverse conditions; therefore, we will describe only some of the more common ones. The correlates of swallowing disorders are not mutually exclusive; for example, an individual may be impaired in swallowing because of mental retardation as well as laryngeal cancer. Whatever the etiology, the outcomes of a swallowing disorder at any age include malnutrition, ill health, weight loss, fatigue, frustration, respiratory infection, aspiration, and even death. Table 13.1 lists common correlates of swallowing disorders in children and adults.

TABLE 13.1
Correlates of swallowing problems in children and adults

Congenital Difficulties	Acquired Conditions
Cerebral palsy	Stroke
Spina bifida	Mouth, throat, laryngeal, or esophageal cancer
Mental retardation/developmental delay	HIV/AIDS
Pervasive developmental disability/autism	Multiple sclerosis
HIV/AIDS	Amyotrophic lateral sclerosis
Cleft lip or palate	Parkinson's disease
Pierre Robin syndrome	Spinal cord injury
Treacher Collins syndrome	Medications and drugs
Pyloric stenosis	Dementia
	Depression and social isolation

THE SWALLOWING PROCESS

Most of us don't typically think about how we swallow food. We know very generally that we put something edible in our mouth, chew for a while, and then swallow. Sometimes, however, we experience difficulty that calls attention to the process. For example, we might eat and cough or feel that the food has "gone down the wrong pipe." Occasionally while drinking, we might laugh and find that fluid comes out of our nose. Once in a while, we feel "all choked up" for an emotional reason and feel unable to eat and swallow. Before we can understand disorders of swallowing, we need to examine the basics of nonproblematic swallowing. Normal swallowing can be described in four phases: anticipatory, oral, pharyngeal, and esophageal. Normal swallowing is presented on the accompanying CD-ROM.

ANTICIPATORY PHASE

Do you occasionally salivate as you pass a candy shop? How about when you're selecting ice cream at your local grocery store? When you do, you are preparing your mouth to take in food. You probably position yourself to eat by sitting down. A pleasant aroma and an attractive presentation stimulate your hunger, and you become physiologically ready to take in food. Many individuals have a ritual that they perform before a meal, such as hand washing, silent or spoken grace, or a sip of water or other beverage that helps to set the stage for eating. Without this premeal interlude, eating might feel rushed and less satisfying.

ORAL PHASE

The oral phase is sometimes considered in two stages: oral preparatory and oral transport.

Oral Preparatory

When you are ready to eat, you put food or beverage into your mouth and close your lips. In the oral preparatory stage of drinking, the tongue forms a cupped position and holds the fluid in a liquid **bolus,** the substance that is to be ingested, against the front portion of the hard palate. In preparation for swallowing solid foods, the tongue and cheeks move the food to the teeth for chewing and mixing with saliva to form a solid bolus. The prepared liquid or solid bolus is held in the mouth by the soft palate, which moves forward and down to touch the back of the tongue and close the passage to the pharynx or throat.

Oral Transport

Once the bolus is formed, oral transport begins. This stage consists of the movement of the bolus from the front to the back of the mouth. When the substance reaches the anterior faucial arch at the rear of the mouth, the pharyngeal swallow reflex is triggered. Oral transport typically takes about 1 second.

PHARYNGEAL PHASE

The soft palate now moves up to meet the rear wall of the pharynx and to prevent the bolus from going into the nasal cavity. The base of the tongue and the pharyngeal wall move toward one another to create the pressure that is needed to project the bolus into the pharynx. While this is occurring, the hyoid bone rises, bringing the larynx up and forward. The larynx prevents the bolus from entering the trachea, or windpipe, by closing the true and false vocal folds and lowering the epiglottis. The pharyngeal phase is complete when the cricopharyngeal sphincter opens and the food or liquid moves into the esophagus. The pharyngeal phase usually lasts about 1 second.

The oral and pharyngeal phases of swallowing involve much of the same anatomy that is used in speaking. There is wisdom to the traditional advice "Don't eat and talk at the same time."

ESOPHAGEAL PHASE

The last stage of the swallowing process occurs when the muscles of the esophagus move the bolus in peristaltic or rhythmic, wavelike contractions from the top of the esophagus into the stomach. This typically takes 8 to 10 seconds in an unimpaired individual.

DISORDERED SWALLOWING

Problems in swallowing can occur in any or all phases of the process. A person may lack appetite or be unable to form a bolus and transport it to the rear of the mouth. In addition, difficulties may arise later if the bolus moves inadequately or is blocked as it passes through the pharynx and esophagus to the stomach.

ANTICIPATORY PHASE

Lack of interest in food may be the result of depression or limited alertness. Sensory impairments involving vision and scent may interfere with a person's readiness to accept food. Some individuals, because of neuromuscular difficulties, cannot position themselves appropriately to take in food or liquid. Infants might not be guided to breastfeed adequately, and their lack of success may lead to a downward spiral culminating in termination of attempts to nurse.

ORAL PHASE

If the lips do not seal properly, drooling can occur. Chewing may be impaired because of poor muscle tone or paralysis involving the mouth or because of missing teeth. Insufficient saliva will impede adequate bolus formation. The muscles of the tongue might not function purposefully or efficiently enough to move the food to the teeth for chewing and to transport the bolus from the front to the rear of the mouth to prepare for the pharyngeal phase.

PHARYNGEAL PHASE

Several serious problems are associated with limitations during the pharyngeal phase. If the swallow is not triggered or is delayed, material may be *aspirated,* or fall into the airway, eventually ending in the lungs. Failure to close the velopharyngeal port, the passageway to the nose, can lead to substances going into and out of the nose. Poor tongue mobility may result in insufficient pressure in the pharynx, which is needed to drive the bolus into the esophagus. Aspiration is presented on the accompanying CD-ROM.

ESOPHAGEAL PHASE

If peristalsis is slow or absent, the complete bolus might not be transported from the pharynx to the stomach. Residue might be left on the esophageal walls, resulting in infection and nutritional problems.

Have you or anyone you know ever experienced a swallowing difficulty? How would you describe it? What was the cause?

PEDIATRIC DYSPHAGIA

Infants and children with swallowing disorders may experience inadequate growth, ill health, fatigue, difficulty learning, and poor parent-child relationships. Their development may be complicated by a broad spectrum of neurodevelopmental impairments (Rogers, 1996). The dysphagia may occur at any phase and may range from mild to severe. Some of the more prevalent correlates of pediatric dysphagia are described below.

Cerebral Palsy

As you'll recall, **cerebral palsy (CP)** is a disorder of motor function that occurring prior to or at birth or soon thereafter. Cerebral palsy is described in greater detail in Chapter 12, "Neurogenic Speech Disorders." A child with spastic cerebral palsy will have excessive muscle tension, exhibit abnormal postures and movements, and might have an exaggerated gag reflex. As an infant, this youngster may not respond well to breastfeeding. The child may be difficult to hold because of increased muscle tone and an arched posture. Once the nipple is in place, the infant may gag and be unable to rhythmically move the tongue to suckle. Gastroesophageal reflux may make ingestion of food painful. The combined unpleasantness of the feeding situation might make the mother not wish to nurse and might result in an infant who refuses to take food (Prontnicki, 1995).

About 25 percent of older children with CP have dysphagia. These youngsters may exhibit infantile bite reflexes, drool, have poor trunk control, be on anticonvulsant medication, and cough or choke during meals. Neither the cause and type of cerebral palsy nor the child's age appears to be related to whether a child with CP has a swallowing disorder order (Waterman, Koltai, Downey, & Cacace, 1992). In addition, difficulty with sucking in infancy does not appear to be a predictor of swallowing problems later in childhood (Selley, Parrott, Lethbridge, et al., 2001).

Spina Bifida

Approximately 1 in 1,000 infants is born with **spina bifida,** a congenital malformation of the spinal column typically involving associated neural damage, resulting in limited sensation and motor control difficulties. A child with spina bifida may experience feeding difficulties in all phases of the process. Sucking and intake of food are often disturbed, owing to sensory impairments and frequently exhibited dyspraxia (difficulty coordinating movement). The pharyngeal and esophageal stages of swallowing may be affected by cranial nerve damage due to the disorder (Prontnicki, 1995).

Mental Retardation and Developmental Delay

About 2 to 3 of every 100 individuals are considered to have intellectual functioning that is enough below average to be labeled as mental retardation. Children with mental retardation are also delayed in mastering motor coordination, and the delay may interfere with self-feeding and the oral phase of swallowing. Communication disorders are common in this population, and children may be limited in their ability to express food desires and preferences, thereby causing disturbances in the anticipatory phase of swallowing. Many people with mental retardation have associated pathologies such as **Down syndrome** or **Prader-Willi syndrome** or a chronic disease such as AIDS that further compounds the dysphagia (Prontnicki, 1995; Rosenfeld-Johnson & Manning, 1997; Sheppard, 1991).

Pervasive Developmental Disorder and Autism

Pervasive developmental disorder (PDD) includes a number of difficulties that impair social interaction in children. You may recall that *autism spectrum disorder (ASD)* is a severe form of PDD that is characterized by social withdrawal, communicative deficits, and repetitive and stereotypic behaviors. Many children with ASD also have disturbances of body posture and muscle tone. They may be hypersensitive to sound, light, pain, smell, and touch. This pattern of symptoms often contributes to eating difficulties. The social withdrawal and communication difficulties may negatively affect the anticipatory phase of swallowing. Infants do not readily snuggle for nursing; older children do not express their food desires. Impaired body posture and tone may interfere with positioning for eating. Hypersensitivity to smell may cause infants to recoil from food. Hypersensitivity to touch and taste may interfere with the oral phase of swallowing. Children with ASD often lick, smell, or attempt to eat nonfood items (Prontnicki, 1995).

HIV/AIDS

HIV (human immunodeficiency virus) causes the illness known as **AIDS (acquired immunodeficiency syndrome).** The white blood cells, the brain, and other parts of the body are affected. In children, HIV/AIDS may have been transmitted while the developing infant was *in utero* and/or through the breast milk of an infected mother. Approximately 14 percent of children with HIV/AIDS have serious feeding problems (Grosz, 1989). These may be largely due to lowered immunity to infections such as oral herpes, which occur with some frequency in this population. These lesions in the mouth may result in pain during eating. Children with AIDS may also exhibit mental retardation, language deficits, and attention deficit disorder resulting in anticipatory swallowing problems (Prontnicki, 1995).

Structural and Physiological Abnormalities

Children born with cleft palate or lip will be impaired in the oral phase of swallowing. Congenital abnormalities of the jaw, as in **Pierre Robin syndrome,** or of the face, as in **Treacher Collins syndrome,** will also negatively affect the ability to use the mouth for intake of food and swallowing. **Esophageal atresia,** which occurs when the esophagus does not have an open connection to the stomach, prevents normal esophageal swallowing and results in choking. This is a life-threatening condition for newborns and must be surgically treated immediately (Prontnicki, 1995).

Similarly life threatening is **pyloric stenosis,** in which the pyloric sphincter at the outlet of the stomach narrows and prevents food from passing to the small intestine. When this is a congenital condition, the infant vomits and cannot ingest milk or water. Prompt surgical intervention usually successfully corrects this difficulty. Pyloric stenosis may also be acquired later in life; it is caused by peptic ulceration or carcinoma.

> Infants who are born today do not spend much time in a hospital. Rapid diagnosis of and attention to congenital defects are essential for the welfare of the child.

DYSPHAGIA IN ADULTS

While most Americans are concerned with excessive weight gain, many aged individuals are at risk for extreme weight loss. Poor nutrition and loss of

weight may result in a failure to thrive, which has been termed "the dwindles" (Egbert, 1996). This situation may be the result of physical ailments,
muscle weakness or incoordination, medications, psychological factors such
as dementia and depression, and/or social isolation. Although most people
as they age experience some reduction in swallowing efficiency and lung
function, severe dysphagic problems are only likely in the presence of some
other disorder such as stroke or the other correlates described in the following paragraphs (Colodny, 2001).

Why do you think some people in their later years experience eating and
swallowing problems? Do you know any older individuals with eating disorders? Have you ever visited a nursing home or adult care facility?

Stroke

In Chapters 7 and 12 we discuss the language and speech implications for
someone who has had a cerebrovascular accident or stroke. Persistent dysphagia is also a serious problem for 5 to 10 percent of these individuals, and
about twice that number may experience swallowing problems during the
first six months after the stroke. Facial paresis (muscle weakness) appears to
be the primary factor associated with dysphagia due to stroke. All phases of
ingestion are likely to be slowed and impaired. Swallowing and breathing are
poorly coordinated, putting the patient at risk for aspiration pneumonia
(Nilsson, Ekberg, Olsson, & Hindfelt, 1998). Pneumonia is the cause for
about one-third of deaths following stroke (Odderson, Keaton, & McKenna,
1995).

Cancer of the Mouth, Throat, or Larynx

Surgery, radiation, and chemotherapy are used to treat tumors of the mouth,
throat, and larynx. Swallowing problems are likely after any type or combination of treatments. Surgery requires removal of the tumor and closing of
the wound. For larger lesions, tissue from another area may be excised and
used to help patch the deficit. The degree of swallowing impairment is
closely related to the size and location of the original tumor and the surgical procedure that is used to close or reconstruct the area. For example, if a
relatively small area of the tongue has been removed, a short-term swallowing problem is likely owing to the swelling following surgery. In more radical surgical procedures in which the tongue is sewn into the mandible to
close the floor of the mouth, oral swallow will be severely affected (Logemann, 1998).

A visit to the dentist
often makes the oral
phase of swallowing
difficult. Imagine
how much more
impaired a person is
after oral surgery or
radiation.

   Radiation therapy may result in diminished salivation, swelling, and
sometimes mouth sores. The swallowing reflex may be reduced. These interferences with normal swallowing may occur during, soon after, or even a
year or two after oral radiation therapy. Chemotherapy may cause nausea,
vomiting, and loss of appetite, which will interfere with the eating process
(Tierney, 1993).

HIV/AIDS

Individuals with AIDS are susceptible to numerous opportunistic infections because of the immune deficiency nature of the disease. A situation was reported in which a 61-year-old man with AIDS complained of swallowing difficulties. The results of the clinical evaluation revealed perforations and growths in the esophagus, which were attributable to Hodgkin's disease, a form of cancer (Gelb, Medeiros, Chen, Weiss, & Weidner, 1997). Esophageal ulcers and esophagitis, or inflammation of the esophagus, were reported in about 16 percent of a group of heterosexual men with AIDS (Yang, Ko, Cheng, et al., 1996).

Multiple Sclerosis

Numbness or a "pins-and-needles" sensation in the extremities or on one side of the face may be an early sign of MS.

Multiple sclerosis (MS), a central nervous system disorder, may affect one or several cranial nerves. Multiple sclerosis is of unknown cause and is typically characterized by periods of both relapse and remission. The major general symptoms are poor coordination, muscle weakness, and often speech and visual disturbances. Delayed swallowing reflex and reduced pharyngeal peristaltic action are the primary forms of dysphagia that are associated with multiple sclerosis (Logemann, 1998).

Amyotrophic Lateral Sclerosis (Lou Gehrig's Disease)

Amyotrophic lateral sclerosis (ALS), discussed in Chapter 12, is a progressive disease that may begin in middle age. It is characterized by muscle atrophy due to degeneration of motor neurons. Poor tongue movement is sometimes an early sign. ALS may interfere with swallowing in several ways. Reduced tongue mobility may result in spillage into the airway before the pharyngeal swallow has been triggered. The larynx might not elevate and close adequately during the pharyngeal phase. Pharyngeal peristalsis is frequently reduced, causing material to remain in the pharynx. Any of these difficulties could result in aspiration of food or liquid (Hardy & Robinson, 1993; Logemann, 1998).

Parkinson's Disease

Tremors and rigidity that are visible in a person's extremities may also occur within the body, resulting in swallowing and other difficulties.

Parkinson's disease (PD), also discussed in Chapter 12, is a progressive disorder, typically of midlife, and is characterized by slowness of movement, muscle rigidity, and tremor. About 30 percent of individuals with PD have been reported to exhibit dysphagia; however, this does not seem to be related to the severity or duration of the disease (Castell, Johnston, Colcher, et al., 2001).

Any or all phases of the swallowing process may be impaired, although in a recent study, only 10 percent of people with PD were found to need dietary aid (Clarke, Gullaksen, Macdonald, et al., 1998). When dysphagia occurs, the bolus is usually formed normally in the oral preparatory stage. However, oral transport may be impaired by a front-to-back rolling pattern until the back of the tongue finally lowers sufficiently to permit the bolus to pass to the pharynx. Pharyngeal swallow may be delayed and laryngeal closure may be impaired in advanced cases of PD. Aspiration sometimes occurs when the patient inhales after a swallow, and material remaining in the pharynx falls into the airway (Logemann, 1998). Esophageal motor abnormalities that impede swallowing may occur in PD even in early stages of the disease (Bassotti, Germani, Pagliaricci, et al., 1998; Johnston, Colcher, Li, et al., 2001).

Spinal Cord Injury

Individuals who have injured their spinal cords because of accidents have a higher incidence of esophageal dysphagia than noninjured people do. Among the problems that they experience are heartburn, chest pain while swallowing, and slow, abnormal peristaltic contractions of the esophagus (Stinneford, Keshavarzian, Nemchausky, Doria, & Durkin, 1993).

Surgery to the front portion of the upper (anterior cervical) spine may result in dysphagia. These swallowing problems may affect any phase of swallowing. Oral preparatory and transport stages are impaired in some postsurgical patients; others experience weakness in the pharyngeal phase or suffer upper esophageal sphincter malfunctioning (Martin, Neary, & Diamant, 1997).

*W*hy might damage to the spinal cord impair swallowing?   :

Medications and Nonfood Substances

While medications are used to cure and manage disease, they may also have negative side effects. Some medications, including decongestants, cough suppressants, and muscle relaxants, might make the patient feel drowsy and/or confused. This condition can interfere with anticipation and the oral phase of swallowing. A dry mouth, or insufficient saliva, has been reported to be a side effect of more than 300 medications (Toner, 1997). High doses of steroids may impede pharyngeal swallowing. Antipsychotic drugs may result in **tardive dyskinesia** (involuntary, repetitive facial, tongue, or limb movements) after a year or more of use. At the extreme, tardive dyskinesia may result in the inability to chew and swallow (Feinberg, 1997).

Behaviors such as smoking and ingesting excessive amounts of caffeine and alcohol may also interfere with normal swallowing. Appetite may be depressed and sensations dulled, resulting in anticipatory phase impairment. Alcohol abuse has been implicated in pharyngeal phase dysphasia (Feinberg, 1997).

*D*id you need another reason to stop or not to start smoking? Have you ever experienced the effects of alcohol, caffeine, or smoking on food intake?

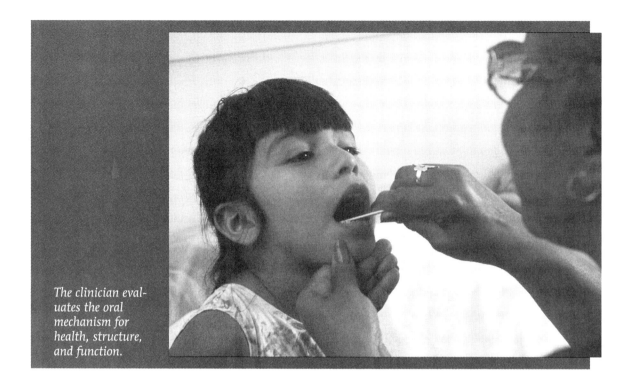

The clinician evaluates the oral mechanism for health, structure, and function.

Dementia

Unlike mental retardation, dementia is an acquired disorder. Although found in some older people, diminution of intellectual function is not an imperative of aging. We all know people in their eighties and nineties whose minds are sharp and capable. As we learned in Chapter 7, dementia is associated with Alzheimer's disease, several small strokes, Parkinson's disease, multiple sclerosis, and other ailments that may occur among older people. The cognitive deficits of dementia may impede attention and orientation to food. Oral preparatory tongue and jaw movements may be lacking in purpose, resulting in poor bolus formation and drooling. Transport of the bolus may be prolonged. Pharyngeal swallow may be delayed and laryngeal elevation reduced, resulting in possible aspiration (Cherney, 1994; Hardy & Robinson, 1993).

Depression and Social Isolation

Life circumstances among the elderly may interfere with several phases of swallowing. Taking a meal is traditionally a social event. We eat with family and friends. As people enter old age, they may find themselves alone and lonely. Spouses and friends have died. Children have moved away. Some may have no experience preparing food and so do not have adequate meals. Others are not motivated to cook just for themselves. Communal meals in retirement homes or long-term care facilities may feature unfamiliar foods and be served in a noisy, hurried environment. For example, mealtime difficulties in one home for the aged were documented in 87 percent of the residents (Steele, Greenwood, Ens, et al., 1997).

Feelings of depression among elderly people are common. Depression is associated with diminished interest in food, restlessness, and fatigue. The throat may feel tight, making swallowing uncomfortable. Some individuals may feel too tired to eat and then are exhausted after they do eat. This may prompt a cycle of inadequate food intake, weight loss, and malnutrition (Toner, 1997).

EVALUATION FOR SWALLOWING

Not everyone with the correlates described in the previous sections will have a swallowing disorder. Furthermore, swallowing problems are not always readily apparent. Patients may not report difficulties, and some may experience **silent aspiration** (lack of cough when food or liquid enters the airway) (Logemann, 1996). Therefore, the first step in evaluation is to identify the individuals who are at risk for dysphagia. Following this screening (refer to Chapter 4, "Assessment and Intervention," for a discussion of screening), the speech-language pathologist will serve on a team to obtain background information and to use clinical and instrumental techniques to assess swallowing. A determination is made about appropriate intervention, and treatment strategies are developed and implemented in coordination with other professionals. Speech-language pathologists are advocates for their clients and help to provide education and counseling to them, their families, and related others (ASHA, 1990).

Some birthing centers have lactation consultants who encourage and assist mothers and infants in the nursing process.

SCREENING FOR DYSPHAGIA IN NEWBORNS AND THE ELDERLY

A primary indication of dysphagia in infants is **failure to thrive.** Infants in a neonatal intensive care unit are carefully monitored for weight gain and development. Full-term infants who are not accepting breast or bottle are signaling feeding problems. The *Non-Instrumental Clinical Evaluation (NICE)* is a systematic way of obtaining clinical and family history and observing the child being fed by a caregiver (Scott, 1998). The child's breathing and physical coordination are evaluated. The child's ability to form a seal and suck are assessed by direct observation and by techniques that enable quantification of nutritive and nonnutritive sucking skill (Lau & Kusnierczyk, 2001). Caregivers can be counseled and instrumental evaluation recommended when warranted.

Checklists to screen for dysphagia in older individuals are also available. The *Burke Dysphagia Screening Test* is a relatively quick way to screen patients who have had a stroke (DePippo, Holas, & Reding, 1992) (see Table 13.2). The 3-ounce water swallow test used in the *Burke* has been found to identify 80 percent of patients who were aspirating as later confirmed by more elaborate tests (DePippo et al., 1992). Table 13.3 outlines this procedure. If oxygen saturation levels in the blood are measured and assessed before and after swallowing water, the accuracy of the water swallow test approaches 100 percent (Lim, Lieu, Phua, et al., 2001).

Additional screening instruments include the *Examine Ability to Swallow (EATS;* Wood & Emick-Herring, 1997) and the *Repetitive Oral Suction*

TABLE 13.2
The Burke Dysphagia Screening Test

Patient Name: _____

ID Number: _____

Date of Evaluation: _____

	Present	Absent
1. Bilateral stroke	____	____
2. Brain stem stroke	____	____
3. History of pneumonia acute stroke phase	____	____
4. Coughing associated with feeding or during a three-ounce water swallow test	____	____
5. Failure to consume one-half of meals	____	____
6. Prolonged time required for feeding	____	____
7. Nonoral feeding program in progress	____	____

Presence of one or more of these features is scored as failing the Burke Dysphagia Screening Test.

Results: Pass   Fail

Source: Used with permission from *Archives of Physical Medicine and Rehabilitation* by W. B. Saunders Co.

TABLE 13.3
Three-ounce water swallow test

Task: Patient drinks three ounces of water from a cup without interruption.

Outcome:

1. No problems.
2. Coughing during swallow.
3. Coughing after swallow.
4. Wet-hoarse voice quality after swallow.

Pass: Outcome 1   *Fail:* Outcome 2, 3, or 4.

Source: Adapted from DePippo, Holas, & Reding (1992).

Swallow (ROSS), which screens swallowing function as individuals sip water through a straw (Nilsson et al., 1998). Stroke patients who, at bedside, exhibit a delay in moving food from the front to the rear of the mouth and incomplete oral clearance signal the likelihood of dysphagic complications (Mann & Hankey, 2001).

For mentally retarded adults and others, inappropriate weight for the person's size may be an indication of nutritional problems that could be due to dysphagia (Sheppard, 1991). All of these measures and indicators have been reported to be useful in identifying serious swallowing difficulties and the need for more complete clinical and instrumental assessment.

CASE HISTORY AND BACKGROUND INFORMATION REGARDING DYSPHAGIA

A parent, caregiver, physician, nurse, or professional from an early intervention program or adult day treatment center may make a referral to a dysphagia team, typically based on three general areas of concern:

- Difficulties have been observed related to feeding and ingestion of food or liquid.
- The client appears to be at risk for aspirating food or liquid into the lungs.
- The client appears not to be receiving adequate nourishment (Rosenthal, Sheppard, & Lotze, 1995).

The swallowing therapist (often an SLP) will then seek answers to questions such as those presented in Table 13.4. The answers to these questions

TABLE 13.4
Important questions pertaining to swallowing

Does the infant accept breast or bottle?	When was the problem first observed?
Does the individual refuse certain foods? Which ones?	Did it worsen slowly or rapidly?
Does the individual appear to chew food?	What exactly happens when the person tries to swallow?
Has drooling been observed?	Does material seem to stop somewhere? Where?
Does the child or adult eat excessively slowly?	What medical diagnoses or conditions may affect the swallow?
Does the child or adult eat excessively rapidly?	Has the person had surgery that may relate to swallowing?
Does coughing or choking occur at mealtimes?	Is the individual using any medications?
Is food or liquid expelled from the nose?	How is the client's respiratory health?
Is food or liquid regurgitated?	How attentive is the client?
Is the child gaining weight?	Is the client able to follow directions?
Is the adult maintaining weight?	

Source: Adapted from Hardy & Robinson (1993).

will give the swallowing therapist preliminary information about the location of the swallowing problem (oral, pharyngeal, or both), the kinds of food substances that are easiest and hardest to swallow, and the nature and severity of the disorder (Logemann, 1998).

CLINICAL ASSESSMENT

Caregiver and Environmental Factors

The swallowing therapist will want to observe feeding as it occurs normally between caregiver and client. The therapist will pay special attention to the following:

- Is the caregiver patient and attentive?
- Does feeding take place in a reasonably quiet environment that is free from distractions?
- What position is the individual in when eating or drinking?
- How does the client express feeding preferences?

The parent or caregiver is an important part of the swallowing team. Careful observation and communication will help the swallowing therapist to assess how best to improve this person's contributions. This is also the opportunity for the SLP to learn about the client's position within the family and cultural and individual factors that may influence therapy. For example, certain foods and spices may be preferred to others. When possible, personal and cultural desires should be respected and accommodated (Logemann, 1998). Case Study 13.2 describes portions of the assessment of a 51-year-old man who was referred for a swallowing evaluation.

Cognitive and Communicative Functioning

Is the client alert and awake during feeding? Can he or she follow directions? What is the client's general level of functioning? Answers to these questions will influence the type of intervention that is most suitable for the client.

Head and Body Posture

The swallowing therapist will observe whether the patient can hold his or her head erect. Does it lean to one side or the other? Does it tend to tilt forward or back? Can the client position the head when asked to do so? The SLP will also note general body posture and tone. Swallowing and ingestion of food and drink involve more than the head, so a complete picture of the individual is important.

Oral-Motor System

The swallowing therapist needs to assess the integrity of the anatomy and health of the mouth. Abnormalities of structure of the lips, teeth, tongue, palate, and velum will be noted. The SLP will look for facial symmetry and will note sagging and imbalances. Motor difficulties such as tremor, flaccidity, excessive muscle tone, and poor coordination will be observed. Oral reflexes will be examined. Certain reflexes such as sucking and rooting

Case Study 13.2

The Personal Story of a Man with Dysphagia

Mr. M. was 51 years of age when he was referred as an outpatient by the Director of Neurology and Rehabilitative Medicine at Municipal Hospital to Ms. R., the staff SLP in charge of swallowing disorders. The referral note read "myotonic dystrophy, dysarthria, dysphagia for solids." Ms. R. recognized her role in ensuring the patient's safety. Difficulty in swallowing foods could result in choking and/or aspiration pneumonia. Ms. R. was also concerned about the dysarthria and wondered to what degree this affected Mr. M.'s communication.

At their first meeting, Ms. R. learned that Mr. M., a recent immigrant from Colombia, had limited English proficiency. Once again, Ms. R. was grateful for her own Spanish language skills; the summer she had spent in Spain after her third year of college had been worthwhile in a multitude of ways. Many of the patients and staff at this inner-city hospital had Spanish as their primary language. Although Mr. M. was mildly dysarthric, his speech was readily intelligible. His responses during the interview were appropriate in form (Spanish) and content. Mr. M. reported that he choked on rice and that this was a staple of his diet. Other foods and liquids did not appear to be a problem. Mr. M. reported that he smoked "a little, just at the Saturday evening dances." A cursory evaluation of the oral mechanism revealed adequate strength and motion of the lips, tongue, velum, and mandible. Although coughing, choking, and gurgling were not observed during trial feeding, an apparent delay in the pharyngeal swallow reflex was noted with both liquids and solids. Ms. R. recommended a modified barium swallow study to confirm and document dysphagia.

Several types of foods were mixed with barium in preparation for the X-ray procedure. Mr. M. ate a spoonful of applesauce and then pudding as the radiologist and Ms. R. watched the X-ray monitor. No difficulties were noted in the oral phase. However, they observed food lingering in the esophagus and building up with each successive swallow. Although the larynx elevated for swallowing, the bolus did not clear, and residue remained on the right **aryepiglottic fold.** Mr. M. was instructed to produce an abdominal cough, but he was unsuccessful, and the food remained on the fold.

Ms. R. made the following recommendations: Mr. M. should not eat alone. He should avoid clear liquids and take only a small amount of food before swallowing. He should try to cough deeply when he feels food stuck in his mouth. At the next appointment, in two weeks, Mr. M. would be instructed in the supraglottic and hard swallow techniques. Because myotonic dystrophy is a progressive disease, Mr. M. requires regular monitoring.

(turning in the direction of a stroke to the cheek) are expected in infants but should disappear as the child matures. The SLP will observe any drooling, which may signal neuromuscular deficits, gum and tooth infections, or upper airway obstruction (Sheppard, 1995). The SLP will also note the client's response to sensation. Does the client accept touch such as face washing? If the client is an older child or adult, is she or he aware of food residue or saliva on the face? (Cherney, 1994).

Laryngeal Function

The SLP cannot directly observe the larynx in the way that he or she can look at the oral mechanism. So the SLP will look for indirect signs of difficulty. In older children and adults, a hoarse, gurgly, or breathy voice quality before, during, or after a swallow may signal laryngeal dysfunction. Other indications of laryngeal problems include the following:

Myotonic dystrophy is a rare, slowly progressive hereditary disease. It is also called Steinert's disease and is characterized initially by poor muscle relaxation following contraction and later by muscle atrophy, especially of the face and neck.

- Inability to rapidly repeat the syllable /ha/ with a clear voiced vowel sound
- Inability to produce vocal tones up and down the musical scale
- An s/z ratio greater than 1.3 (See Chapter 9, "The Voice and Voice Disorders")
- Inability to produce a strong cough (Hardy & Robinson, 1993; Logemann, 1998)

If any difficulties are observed, it is essential that the swallowing therapist refer the client to an otolaryngologist for a thorough laryngeal evaluation.

THOUGHT QUESTION

*W**hy is it important for a medical specialist to evaluate a person who may show signs of laryngeal dysfunction?*

The Swallowing Examination

If the client is alert and does not have a history of aspiration, the swallowing therapist will evaluate the client's ability to swallow. Usually, food or beverage is used, although some SLPs prefer to make the assessment with a piece of gauze that has been soaked in water or juice to prevent aspiration. If real food substances are used, anticipation and the oral phase of swallow can be observed. Pharyngeal phase swallowing efficiency can be judged in part by noting specific behaviors during food or drink intake.

The SLP evaluates the client's reaction to the appearance of food or drink and the associated utensils, observing whether the client's activity level changes and the person appears eager to receive food. A small amount (a quarter of a teaspoon) of thin or thick liquid may be placed in the mouth, and the client is then encouraged to swallow. Oral mechanism function is observed throughout the swallow.

The SLP examines the client's lips to see whether they are together before the taking in of food. The SLP is interested in answering questions such as the following:

> The SLP should observe swallowing on more than one occasion. The nature of the food that is presented and the client's comfort level and hunger will influence the acceptance of foods.

- Do the lips open and then close around the nipple, cup, or spoon?
- Is there sucking activity on the nipple?
- Is food successfully removed from the spoon?
- Is liquid or food dribbled out of the sides of the mouth?

The SLP also observes tongue movement. Again, answers to certain questions are vital:

- When the mouth opens to take in food, does the tongue cup in anticipation?
- Does the client move the tongue to one side of the mouth if food is presented laterally?
- Does the client move the tongue adequately to form a bolus?

- Is the bolus transported efficiently from the front to the back of the mouth?
- Is the tongue used to remove food substances from the lips?

In addition, the SLP notes movements of the jaw and chewing patterns when solid foods are presented:

- Does the client bite food efficiently?
- Does the client isolate tongue and jaw movement?
- Does chewing continue for an adequate period of time?
- Is the jaw clenched?

Several observations pertaining to the adequacy of pharyngeal swallow are performed. If the client is unable to cough, this may suggest difficulty closing the larynx to protect the airway. Nasal regurgitation points to possibly inadequate velopharyngeal closure. The SLP observes the movement of the hyoid bone and thyroid cartilage in the neck by watching and possibly placing a finger gently on this area. These should move up during pharyngeal swallow. The SLP records the number of times the client swallows while ingesting each amount of food or drink. Multiple swallows may suggest inadequate pharyngeal contraction. If vocal quality changes after swallowing this may indicate pooling of liquid (Cherney, 1994).

Of importance to the SLP are which food consistencies appear to cause difficulties and which seem to be swallowed efficiently. Similarly, the SLP notices whether there is a preferential placement in the mouth for food or liquid.

Managing a Tracheostomy Tube

Some clients will have a **tracheostomy tube** in place to facilitate breathing. A swallowing evaluation can still be conducted in most of these cases with the physician's approval. The SLP or nurse deflates the cuff of the tube before assessment and suctions secretions from the mouth and above the cuff. The swallowing evaluation is similar to the one outlined above; however, the patient is instructed to cover the tube with a gauze pad or gloved finger before each swallow to normalize tracheal pressure (Logemann, 1998).

See Online Resource *Aaron's Tracheostomy Page,* referenced at the end of this chapter, for more information.

INSTRUMENTATION

Complete, accurate assessment of the swallowing procedure requires the use of instrumentation. The SLP collaborates with other team members such as the physician, radiologist, and X-ray technologist in the use of diagnostic technology. Some of the more commonly used instrumental procedures are described in the following paragraphs.

Modified Barium Swallow Study

The **modified barium swallow study,** also referred to as **videofluoroscopy,** is an X-ray procedure that has been considered "the gold standard" in dysphagia diagnosis in children or adults (Sonies & Frattalli, 1997).This procedure is used when clinical evaluation or screening suggests

Solid knowledge of anatomy and physiology is essential in order to accurately interpret videofluoroscopic swallowing studies (Wooi, Scott, & Perry, 2001).

dysphagia and/or aspiration. Barium, a substance that can be seen on X-rays, is coated onto or mixed into the food or beverage to be ingested. The SLP typically determines the size, texture, and consistency of the food or beverage to be presented and the head and body position of the patient during the study. A radiologist and an X-ray technologist use fluoroscopic (X-ray) equipment to observe the movement of the barium throughout the swallow. These views are videorecorded for later analysis by the physician and SLP. The study provides real-time visualization of the swallowing process and is highly useful in determining whether the client should be fed orally or nonorally, what food textures are safest, and what types of therapy are appropriate (Hardy & Robinson, 1993; Rogers, Arvedson, Buck, et al., 1994).

Fiber-Optic Endoscopic Evaluation of Swallowing

Fiber-optic endoscopic evaluation of swallowing (FEES) may be used with adult patients who are too ill to be brought to a radiology department for the modified barium swallow study. FEES is not an X-ray procedure. Instead, following topical or localized anesthesia, an otolaryngologist inserts a flexible fiber-optic laryngoscope through the patient's nose and down into the pharynx. A specially trained SLP can also perform this procedure in consultation with a physician. When the scope is in place, the patient may be asked to cough, hold his or her breath, and swallow foods of different textures and thickness that have been dyed for better visualization. The views may be videotaped. FEES may reveal bolus spilling into the pharynx before swallowing and closing of the airway during swallow. Oral and esophageal phases of swallowing are not visible with FEES. Nevertheless, observations with FEES can be performed at the bedside and provide valuable information about desirable body and head posture during feeding, preferred food types, and aspiration. FEES may also be more cost effective than videofluoroscopy, particularly for patients with head and neck cancer (ASHA, 1992; Aviv, Sataloff, Cohen, et al., 2001; Leder, Sasaki, & Burrell, 1998; Sonies, 1997).

> The FEES procedure is increasingly used because of its convenience and portability.

Scintigraphy

Scintigraphy is a computerized technique that is sometimes used with adults for measuring the amount of aspiration during or after a swallow. A specialized physician such as a radiologist, gastroenterologist, or otolaryngologist performs scintigraphy; however, the SLP plays a role in positioning the patient, suggesting swallowing procedures, and interpreting test results. A radioactive tracer is mixed with the food or liquid to be ingested. Radioactive markers may be placed externally on the chin, lip, thyroid notch, and other anatomical landmarks to facilitate measurement. A specialized gamma scintillation camera is used. When scintigraphy is used, it is generally to supplement information obtained from other tests. Scintigraphy provides insight regarding esophageal function and may help in the determination of the safety of oral feedings (ASHA, 1992; Sonies, 1997).

Ultrasound

Ultrasound, or **ultrasonography,** is an imaging technique that uses sound waves at a frequency that is inaudible to human ears, over 20,000 Hz. It is a noninvasive procedure that is safe to use with infants and children as well as adults. A transducer that generates and receives sound waves is placed below the chin for views of the oral cavity and on the thyroid notch for visualizing the laryngeal area. The acoustic images are videotaped. Ultrasonographic real-time measures are particularly helpful in assessing the duration of the oral phases of swallowing as well the structure and movement of the tongue and hyoid bone. One drawback is that ultrasound does not permit visualization of the pharyngeal stage of swallow (ASHA, 1992; Logemann, 1998; Sonies, 1997).

Ultrasound is used in various types of medical assessment. Can you name some? Why is ultrasound used in these situations?

THOUGHT QUESTIONS

YSPHAGIA INTERVENTION AND TREATMENT

Disorders of swallowing present medical, nutritional, psychological, social, and communicative problems, so many individuals are involved in working toward their resolution. As was mentioned earlier, the speech-language pathologist is usually the coordinator of services and the professional who is most likely to implement dysphagia therapy. Nevertheless, input from other team members is essential to a satisfactory outcome.

FEEDING ENVIRONMENT

Whether the patient is an infant, a young child, or an adult, the environment for feeding sets the stage for a satisfactory experience. It is especially important for people with swallowing problems to have their meals in an environment that is conducive to success. Visual and auditory distractions should be minimized. This means that the eating area should not contain nonrelevant objects. Lighting should be comfortable, neither too bright nor too dark. Noise should be reduced and replaced with pleasant familiar music.

The caregiver should have a relaxed, unhurried manner. He or she must be tuned in to the patient's signals regarding feeding speed, food choices, and quantity. When necessary, these communication strategies may be developed and trained. The caregiver should indicate an interest in the person being fed and reinforce his or her healthy, effective eating behaviors. When possible, the goal is the development of self-feeding skills.

Utensils for feeding need to be appropriate to the patient's functioning. For infants, a slow-flow nipple may be helpful in controlling the amount of liquid taken at a time. A Teflon- or latex-covered spoon may be used for children with infantile tonic bite reflex, who will bite hard on any object that is placed on the teeth or gums. Children and adults with motor coordination difficulties may benefit from the use of a shallow-bowled spoon. Special

Whereas children who have excess muscle tone (hypertonia) benefit from low lighting, soft music, and minimal stimulation, children with insufficient muscle tone (hypotonia) often respond better to bright lights, peppy music, and physical stimulation.

cutout cups may help to improve tongue positioning in drinking (Jelm, 1994; Sheppard, 1995).

BODY AND HEAD POSITIONING

Body posture and stability have a strong influence on oral-pharyngeal movements. The basic premise is that controlled mobility stems from a solid base (Woods, 1995). An upright, 90° hip angle, symmetrical position with sufficient postural support to provide stability is generally needed. The individual's head and neck must be positioned and prevented from making extraneous movement.

THOUGHT QUESTIONS

Have you ever observed a parent trying to feed a child who was slumped over in a chair? Why would this interfere with effective feeding?

Occasionally, a child or adult may benefit from a hip angle other than 90°. For example, some infants with severe respiratory and swallowing problems may feed better when placed on their stomach. Some older individuals who have a considerable amount of pharyngeal residue may eat more safely at a bent-over 45° angle to prevent regurgitation of food from the esophagus into the airway (B. J. Martin, 1994; Woods, 1995).

The SLP works closely with the physical therapist and occupational therapist in obtaining optimum positioning for feeding. The **chin tuck** posture is often recommended for patients with delayed pharyngeal swallow. This position will help to prevent food and liquid from entering the airway. The chin tuck posture is presented on the accompanying CD-ROM. The **head-back position** has been found useful for patients with poor tongue mobility if they have excellent airway closure. **Head tilt** and **head rotation** postures are used when an individual has impairment on one side. In these positions, the head may be moved in the direction of (rotation) or away from (tilt) the impairment. Clients who have been found during videofluoroscopy to have residue in the pharynx may be advised to lie on one side while eating (Logemann, 1998; B. J. Martin, 1994).

MODIFICATION OF FOODS AND BEVERAGES

Textures, Quantities, and Temperatures

During the assessment, liquids and foods of varying consistencies, amounts, and possibly temperatures will have been presented to the patient. On the basis of the findings of these tests, appropriate recommendations will be made.

Certain foods that are hard to chew, are small or slick when wet, or are thick and sticky are not recommended for children under age 5 who exhibit neuromotor difficulties. Specific foods for these infants and young children to avoid are listed in Table 13.5.

TABLE 13.5

Specific foods that should be avoided for children under age 5 with neuromotor problems

Frankfurters	Nuts	Chewing gum
Grapes	Seeds	Raw carrots
Popcorn	Hard candy	

Source: Adapted from Lotze (1995).

Clients may exhibit a range of food consistency requirements. They might not tolerate any food by mouth, accept only thin or thick liquids, require a pureed consistency, or be able to ingest the range of normal foods. Table 13.6 lists possible food consistencies.

The amount of food that a client can manage in her or his mouth at a time may be determined by the modified barium swallow study. In general, the goal is to reduce the amount that is presented. Drinking through a straw typically causes too much fluid to enter the mouth, so straws are usually not advised. Spoons with a shallow bowl are helpful in limiting food amounts. Caregivers and patients must avoid placing food in the mouth until the previous bolus has been swallowed. Finally, patients may be encouraged to swallow twice per bite or sip.

Providing foods of varying temperatures may increase the client's sensory awareness of the food and improve swallowing. Cold food or drink sometimes improves tongue movement during the oral transport phase and helps to stimulate pharyngeal swallow, although some patients with respiratory problems prefer all substances to be ingested at room temperature (B. J. Martin, 1994).

Placement

The swallowing therapist places food or drink in the mouth where the patient has intact sensation and adequate muscle strength. For example, an individual who has had oral cancer will have diminished sensation in the region where surgery occurred. Similarly, the ability to feel may be reduced after radiation therapy. Neurological disease and damage may also impair a person's full awareness of foods that are placed in the mouth. Surgery and neurological problems may also compromise muscle tone and make the person less able to move parts of the tongue, lips, or cheeks. Appropriate placement along with the adjustments in texture, quantity, and temperature is critical to successful dysphagia intervention (B. J. Martin, 1994).

ORAL-MOTOR EXERCISES AND SWALLOWING TECHNIQUES

Each of the procedures described below is used only after clinical and instrumental assessment has demonstrated its safety and appropriateness. Clients will also need to be able to follow instructions. All of the techniques

TABLE 13.6
Dietary consistencies

NPO	From the Latin, *non per os,* meaning nothing by mouth. If an individual aspirates more than 10 percent of all foods or is unable to swallow one bolus of food within 10 seconds, alternative means of feeding must be used.
No Liquid by Mouth	Liquids will need to be provided via a nasogastric tube or intravenously for patients who can tolerate pureed or more solid food but are at risk for aspiration of liquids.
Thin Liquid Consistency	This includes foods such as gelatin desserts, which are tolerated by some patients better than thicker consistencies.
Thick Liquid Consistency	Beverages are thickened to the consistency of fruit nectar or tomato juice. A variety of commercial thickeners are available.
Pureed Consistency	Foods are blended to the consistency of mashed potatoes or pudding. This may be recommended for individuals with oral preparatory or oral transport stage difficulties.
Crushed Medication	Pills and capsules are often difficult to swallow, and crushing may facilitate the process. Some medications are time-released, however, and lose effectiveness when crushed. The physician must be consulted before using this approach.
Mechanical Soft Consistency	This consistency is sometimes referred to as *dental soft.* It includes soft foods such as cooked vegetables, fruits, and pasta and may be easier than firmer foods for patients with oral or pharyngeal phase dysphagia to tolerate.
Regular Dietary Consistency	A patient with mild dysphagia may tolerate regular food textures but may need to adjust body or head posture, amount per mouthful, rate of eating, and so on.

Source: Adapted from Hardy, E., & Robinson, N. H. (1993). *Swallowing disorder treatment manual.* Bisbee, AZ: Imaginart. Reprinted by permission.

may be practiced without food. However, the swallowing techniques are specific to improving the actual swallowing process and are described with the use of food or drink.

Muscle Exercises

The motor system that is used in swallowing may be improved through exercise. Clients with impaired swallowing may have restricted mouth opening, tongue or lip movement, and laryngeal elevation. **Range of motion** may be improved by practicing specific exercises. Bite blocks of differing sizes may be used to encourage lowering the mandible. Flavored gauze or a toothette may be placed in various places around the mouth to stimulate tongue and lip movement. A licorice stick or a candy LifeSaver on a string may also be used to improve tongue movement. The client may be instructed in moving her or his lips from pucker to smile and back again. Exercises to facilitate awareness of laryngeal movement may involve placement of the hand on the neck at the level of the hyoid bone. A mirror is often used to provide visual feedback to the patient.

Lip strength and seal may be improved by having the client attempt to hold a tongue depressor with the lips. Pushing the tongue against a tongue depressor is a technique for strengthening that muscle. Improved coordination is taught by asking the client to follow instructions such as moving the tongue to explore the outside, then inside of the upper and lower front teeth. Clark (2004) provides an excellent tutorial regarding neuromuscular treatment of swallowing disorders.

Hard and Double Swallows

A hard or effortful swallow may be helpful for patients whose tongues do not retract enough to trigger pharyngeal swallow. In these cases, the client is instructed to swallow forcefully and try to feel the tongue moving backward. This technique is helpful as swallowing practice with or without food or drink (Logemann, 1997; B. J. Martin, 1994).

Double or multiple **swallows** are advised for individuals who, for whatever reason, retain some food in the oral cavity after a single swallow. Very simply, the client is instructed to swallow two or more times for each bolus (B. J. Martin, 1994).

Supraglottic Swallow

In the normal swallow, the vocal folds are closed to prevent food from entering the airway. The supraglottic swallow may be used for individuals who do not fully close the glottis during swallowing. This technique teaches voluntary closure of the glottal area, and reduces the depth of misdirected swallows (Bulow, Olsen, & Ekberg, 2001). The client is instructed to do the following:

1. Breathe in and hold your breath.
2. Put a small amount of food or liquid in your mouth.
3. Swallow.
4. Cough or clear your throat while exhaling.
5. Swallow again (Hardy & Robinson, 1993; B. J. Martin, 1994).

Mendelsohn Maneuver

The Mendelsohn maneuver is useful for clients who do not have adequate laryngeal elevation during swallowing. The patient is taught to manually hold the larynx at its highest point during the swallow (see Figure 13.1). The instructions are as follows (Hardy & Robinson, 1993; B. J. Martin, 1994):

1. Place a small amount of food or liquid in your mouth.
2. Chew if necessary.

3. Swallow while placing your thumb and forefinger on either side of your larynx.

4. Manually hold the larynx for 3 to 5 seconds during and after swallowing in the highest position it reached during swallowing.

5. Let go of your larynx and let it drop.

During the assessment process, the SLP determines which of the above exercises and techniques are appropriate for a particular client. Evaluation continues, however, and modifications in treatment approaches are often made as therapy proceeds.

MEDICAL AND PHARMACOLOGICAL APPROACHES

Drug Treatments

Neurological patients, such as those with Parkinson's disease and multiple sclerosis who are taking medications to improve their condition, benefit from being medicated with these drugs before eating. In addition, the medication atropine has been reported to control drooling (Logemann, 1998), and nifedipine may be useful in managing dysphagia in individuals who have had a stroke (Perez, Smithard, Davies, & Kaira, 1998). Injections of botulinum toxin have been shown to improve swallowing in individuals with spasticity and hypertonicity of the cricopharyngeal muscle (Shaw & Searl, 2001). As was discussed earlier in this chapter, some medications actually cause or contribute to swallowing disorders. In these cases, the swallowing therapist needs to work with the physician to determine whether alternatives can be used (Feinberg, 1997).

FIGURE 13.1

In the Mendelsohn maneuver, the client manually holds the larynx at its highest position to facilitate swallowing. *Source:* Adapted from Hardy, E., & Robinson, N. M. (1993). *Swallowing disorders treatment manual.* Bisbee, AZ: Imaginart, p. 94. Reprinted by permission.

Prostheses and Surgical Procedures

Patients who lack an intact swallowing mechanism because of malformation, surgery, or another cause may benefit from a prosthetic device. For example, individuals who had oral cancer and have had a significant portion of the soft palate excised may have a **palatal obturator,** a permanent or removable plate, that helps to close this area during speaking or eating (Logemann, 1998). In addition, children with cerebral palsy who exhibit dysphagia have been shown to improve their feeding skills and growth significantly when using an appropriately designed intraoral appliance (Haberfellner, Schwartz, & Gisel, 2001).

If less invasive approaches have been unsuccessful, surgery to improve swallowing and prevent aspiration is sometimes needed. Some techniques attempt to correct organic defects. For example, if the patient has bony growths on the cervical vertebrae that displace the rear pharyngeal wall, these may be reduced surgically. Other surgical procedures are used to increase the dimensions of the vocal folds or elevate the larynx. In severe cases of aspiration, the true or false vocal folds may be sutured closed, and breathing will have to occur through a tracheostomy (Logemann, 1998). For patients with esophageal dysphasia, injection of botulinum toxin is sometimes effective (Sonies, 1997).

Nonoral Feeding

Clients who require more than 10 seconds to swallow a liquid or food bolus or who aspirate more than 10 percent of either will likely require at least some nonoral feeding (Logemann, 1998). Several approaches are used.

Nasogastric tube (NG tube) feeding requires that a tube be placed from the nose to the pharynx, the esophagus, and finally the stomach. Liquefied food and water are inserted through this opening. Unlike the more long-term procedures described below, NG tubes are typically not used for periods of more than five or six months.

In **pharyngostomy,** a feeding tube is inserted into a **stoma,** or hole in the external neck region skin, which extends into the pharynx. **Esophagostomy** is a similar procedure; however, a hole is made into the esophagus from the chest area, and a food tube is inserted through it.

In gastrostomy, a hole is surgically made from the abdomen to the stomach. A soft tube is placed through this, and blended regular food can be inserted into the tube. This procedure is used in cases of severe dysphagia.

A current reference book describing prescription drugs is an essential part of the personal library of the well-informed SLP.

Swallowing disorders may accompany a variety of neuromotor impairments.

PROGNOSES AND OUTCOMES FOR SWALLOWING DISORDERS

The overriding objectives of swallowing therapy are to improve the intake of food and drink and to prevent aspiration of these materials into the lungs. The potential for success of swallowing therapy is determined largely by the cause of the disorder, the severity of aspiration, and the onset of treatment (Denk, Swoboda, Schima, & Eibenberger, 1997). In young children with developmental disabilities, treatment that is based on a careful diagnosis of the feeding disorder results in improved nutrition and generally better health (Schwarz, Corredor, Fisher-Medina, et al., 2001). Early identification and successful intervention for swallowing disorders reduces the risk of aspiration and death following stroke, shortens the length of time patients need to stay in hospital, and improves quality of life (Odderson et al., 1995). While the original causes of swallowing problems may not be remediable, treatment for dysphagia has been reported to be beneficial in at least 80 percent of cases (Johns Hopkins, 2000).

Swallowing specialists have sometimes been successful in preventing dysphagia. Caregivers of youngsters who are at risk are instructed in feeding techniques soon after the child's birth. Well-placed information for the older population is also valuable. Among the elderly, swallowing disorders are sometimes related to poor dentition, which might be corrected by appropriate dental care. Advice to avoid alcohol, caffeine, spicy products, and foods that are extremely hot or cold and may improve swallowing and prevent dysphagia (Toner, 1997).

SUMMARY

Speech-language pathologists who are specially trained often serve as swallowing therapists. They work with infants who are unable to nurse adequately, children with feeding problems, and older people who have dysphagia. The anticipatory, oral, pharyngeal, and/or esophageal phases of swallowing may be impaired. Causes include congenital or acquired neurological problems, stroke, cancer, developmental disability, dementia, and accident. Swallowing affects not only nutrition and health, but also social and personal aspects of life. A team approach is used for both assessment and intervention. Evaluation includes a careful history and direct observation of the client while he or she is feeding. The modified barium swallow study uses videofluoroscopic equipment and is considered the "gold standard" in dysphagia evaluation. Treatment procedures address the feeding environment, the client's body and facial posture, food textures and temperatures, oral-motor mobility, and specific swallowing techniques. Medical, prosthetic, and surgical approaches are used when necessary. Nonoral feeding may be required in severe cases.

REFLECTIONS

- What special skills and knowledge does the speech-language pathologist bring to swallowing therapy?
- Describe the phases of the swallowing process.
- What are some causes of swallowing difficulties in infants and children?
- What are some causes of swallowing problems in older individuals?
- Describe noninstrumental dysphagia assessment.
- Compare the modified barium swallow study and fiber-optic endoscopic evaluation of swallowing.
- What techniques are used to address disorders of swallowing?

SUGGESTED READINGS

Clark, H. M. (2004). Neuromuscular treatment for speech and swallowing: A tutorial. *American Journal of Speech-Language Pathology, 12,* 400–415.

Hall, K. (2000). *Pediatric dysphagia resource guide.* San Diego: Singular.

Logemann, J. A. (1998). *Evaluation and treatment of swallowing disorders* (2nd ed.). Austin, TX: Pro-Ed.

Mills, R. H. (2000) *A clinician's guide to the expanded evaluation of dysphagia in adults.* Austin, TX: Pro-Ed.

ONLINE RESOURCES

http:///www.dysphagia.com Dysphagia Resource Center.
Links to information about swallowing and swallowing disorders; includes anatomy and physiology, tutorials, research references.

http://www.tracheostomy.com Aaron's Tracheostomy Page.
Personal insights from the mother of a child with a tracheostomy tube. Helpful suggestions regarding eating with a tracheostomy and other issues.

Audiology and Hearing Loss

14

Douglas J. MacKenzie, Au.D.

CHAPTER LEARNING GOALS

When you have finished this chapter, you should be able to:

- Describe the psychosocial consequences of hearing loss

- Define audiology and the role of the audiologist in various employment settings

- Describe the mechanics of sound propagation and demonstrate a basic understanding of the anatomy and physiology of the auditory system

- Identify the general types of hearing loss and causes of each

- Name the components of the audiological test battery and explain the general purpose and method used in each test

- Define aural habilitation/rehabilitation and describe the basic techniques that are used to mitigate the effects of hearing loss on communication

For anyone unfamiliar with the topic, there is often the misconception that hearing loss is a condition that afflicts only the elderly as a natural consequence of the aging process. Stereotypical images of elderly individuals having difficulty hearing abound on television and in movies. In reality, hearing loss is prevalent in people of all ages. From newborns to school-aged children, from young adults to seniors, no individual is immune from developing a hearing problem at some point during his or her lifetime. Another common misconception is that hearing loss simply impedes one's ability to hear softer sounds. Although this perception has validity and its consequences should not be downplayed, it is far too simplistic. The impact of a hearing loss can be more far reaching. Hearing loss can have a profound negative impact on speech and language development, educational achievement, vocational performance, social interactions, and psychological well-being. It can also have a

Case Study 14.1

Case Study of an Adult with Sudden Sensorineural Hearing Loss: David

At the age of 22, David was halfway through his senior year at a prominent university, majoring in Political Science/Pre-Law. He had planned to attend law school the following fall with aspirations of becoming a trial attorney. While attending a party one evening, David suffered a skull fracture when the chair he was sitting in gave way as he leaned back. In a matter of hours, David's world was turned upside down as he went from being able to hear normally to being totally deaf in both ears. David's career goals were suddenly in jeopardy, and he began to experience personal isolation due to problems he had communicating with family and friends. "I feel lost," David confided to his audiologist, "because I can't interact with people around me the way I used to."

David's audiologist recommended that he be fitted with hearing aids but they provided minimal benefit. Ten months after his accident, David underwent surgery to obtain a cochlear implant. He worked closely with his audiologist to develop an individualized aural rehabilitation program designed to help him relearn how to make use of sound heard through his cochlear implant. Following intensive auditory training and communication strategy practice, David was now ready to get on with his life and transferred to a college that provided educational support services to deaf and hard-of-hearing students. Unfortunately, David had difficulty developing

new relationships. He no longer felt that he fit into the "hearing world," but at the same time was unable to assimilate into the Deaf Community. He joined a cochlear implant support group and participated in one-on-one auditory therapy with his audiologist to work on specific listening skills. David benefited from these activities and eventually graduated with a degree in Computer Science. Although David's future is once again bright, this case demonstrates the impact a hearing loss can have on all facets of an individual's life. Not only did David have to cope with the emotional consequences of his sudden deafness, he also had to learn how to hear again through his cochlear implant and deal with the various communication, social, academic, and career issues stemming from the hearing loss.

As you read this chapter think about

- Possible explanations for David's communication difficulties.
- The psychological and emotional impact of David's hearing loss.
- Possible evaluation procedures that could be used to measure David's auditory abilities.
- Possible types of intervention that might be considered to help David communicate more effectively.

significant negative impact on family members and close friends. In this chapter, we will take a closer look at how hearing loss occurs, how it impacts people's lives, how it is diagnosed, and how it is treated.

INCIDENCE AND PREVALENCE OF HEARING LOSS

Invariably, one of the first questions asked by those who are unfamiliar with the topic is "How many people are we talking about?" Although this question is difficult to answer precisely, a general estimate is that approximately 28.6 million people in the United States have some degree of hearing loss (Kochkin, 2001). This figure, although significant, may actually be a conservative estimate. Results of a survey conducted by the Educational and Auditory Research Foundation (2004) suggest that nearly half of the U.S. baby boomer generation, a group comprised of adults age 40 to 59, have some degree of hearing loss. When other age groups are factored into the equation, estimates of the number of people suffering from hearing loss are even more staggering.

Relative to children, approximately 1 in every 1,000 births results in a child with a severe or profound degree of hearing loss, or in other words, a child who may be considered "deaf." Approximately 83 in every 1,000 children in the United States exhibit what has been termed an "educationally significant" hearing loss that can have lifelong consequences (National Dissemination Center for Children with Disabilities, 2003).

Over the past decade there has been a concerted effort to mandate universal newborn hearing screening programs in order to identify significant hearing loss in newborn babies. The Joint Committee on Infant Hearing (2000) has recommended that babies who fail a newborn hearing screening and any subsequent rescreening undergo a complete audiological and medical evaluation before the age of 3 months to confirm or rule out the presence of hearing loss. It is equally important that appropriate intervention services be prescribed and treatment promptly initiated once a hearing problem has been identified. Failure to identify hearing loss and provide appropriate intervention can lead to significant difficulties relative to speech-language, social-emotional, and cognitive development, which may ultimately have a negative impact on academic achievement and vocational options (Moeller, 2001; Yoshinaga-Itano, Sedley, Coulter, & Mehl, 1998).

> Although identification of congenital hearing loss is occurring at an earlier age in recent years due to the proliferation of newborn hearing screening programs, it is only the first step, albeit an essential one, in the habilitation process.

HEARING LOSS THROUGH THE LIFESPAN

PSYCHOSOCIAL ASPECTS OF HEARING LOSS

The process of adjusting to and coping with hearing loss can be difficult for those who are afflicted, as well as their families. This period of adjustment can also be frustrating for professionals as clients are often slow to follow through on recommendations for treatment when they have not fully accepted the permanency of their condition. People with hearing impairment

experience a wide range of psychological, social, and emotional consequences (English, 2002). With children who are hearing-impaired, delays in
speech and language may present problems with self-awareness and self-ex-
pression. Ultimately, this may lead to difficulties in the development of social skills. Children with hearing loss, even if only mild in degree, frequently
exhibit lower self-esteem and reduced self-worth that may ultimately impact
interpersonal relationships with peers and family members (Bess, Dodd-
Murphy, & Parker, 1998).

The psychosocial consequences of hearing loss may not only manifest in
children who are afflicted, but also in their parents. A somewhat staggering
statistic is that greater than 90 percent of hearing-impaired children have
parents with normal hearing. Most parents have little knowledge, let alone
experience, pertaining to hearing loss and the challenges it presents. The
birth of a child is one of the most joyous times in the lives of parents. Feelings of euphoria, however, can quickly turn to feelings of despair and helplessness upon receiving word that their newborn baby is hearing-impaired.
Parents may feel as if their lives are spiraling out of control as they face the
reality of raising a child who has a disorder that they are unprepared to handle. Parents often go through various stages of grief, experiencing shock, denial, anger, and depression before they are finally able to accept the reality
of the situation (Tanner, 1980).

Adults who have acquired hearing loss over the course of their lifetime,
whether gradually or suddenly, are equally susceptible to psychosocial problems. Many go through the same stages of grief as parents of hearing-impaired children. The reality of no longer being able to enjoy social activities
to the same degree as in the past, or not being able to understand conversations on the phone, at meetings, or during family gatherings, may cause an
adult with hearing loss to experience a variety of emotions including anger
and frustration, which may ultimately lead to depression (Mullins, 2004).
Having to rely on others to answer the phone or clarify messages that were
misunderstood can lead to feelings of inadequacy, guilt, reduced self-suffi-
ciency, and reduced self-worth. Family relationships may become strained as
a hearing-impaired member is increasingly excluded from conversations due
to frequent requests for repetition. The spouse of a hearing-impaired person
may become particularly vulnerable to stress imposed by having to assume a
greater responsibility for assisting with the partner's daily communication
requirements. Spouses may also face the likelihood of reduced social interactions with friends and acquaintances as their hearing-impaired partners
withdraw from activities that were once routinely engaged in as a couple. It
is imperative that professionals identify and explore these psychosocial issues
in order to determine the full impact of the hearing loss on a client and his
or her significant other.

THOUGHT QUESTIONS

*Does someone in your family have a hearing loss? What impact has the
hearing loss had on his or her psychosocial well-being? What impact has it
had on other members of the family?*

CLASSIFICATION OF IMPAIRMENT, DISABILITY, AND HANDICAP

When it comes to describing the affects of hearing loss, terminology can be confusing. The terms "impaired," "disabled," and "handicapped" are tossed about freely. The World Health Organization (WHO) classification system is used extensively in the disciplines of education, sociology, anthropology, speech-language pathology, and audiology. The WHO defines **impairment** as a loss of structure or function. Relative to the auditory system, impairment can occur due to trauma to the eardrum or the tiny bones of the middle ear, a loss of sensory cells in the inner ear, or compression of the auditory nerve due to a tumor. Simply because an impairment exists, however, does not necessarily mean it will have a significant impact on a person's ability to communicate. The functional consequences associated with a particular impairment are referred to as activity limitation or **disability.** For those with hearing loss, the resulting disability may be an inability to understand speech in the presence of background noise, difficulty understanding conversations on the phone, or difficulty hearing low-intensity speech sounds. It is important to determine one's degree of disability in order to determine an appropriate course of treatment.

Impairment and disability may lead to participation restriction or **handicap,** which is defined as the psychosocial consequence of the hearing loss. As we have already seen, hearing loss can have a profound negative affect on one's ability to cope. It may lead to reduced self-concept and self-worth, social isolation, and strained family relationships. Simply put, all people with hearing loss experience impairment. Many of these individuals will experience disability. Not all who experience disability, however, will necessarily experience handicap. Despite problems hearing on the phone or understanding conversations in noisy settings, many hearing-impaired people are well-adjusted, independent, fully participating members of society. In contrast, others are completely debilitated by the same degree, or in some cases, a lesser degree of hearing loss. Professionals need to be cognizant of the full spectrum of psychosocial consequences that often result, while at the same time never losing sight of the fact that not all people with hearing loss are impacted to the same degree in terms of communication handicap. As we will see later, counseling is a critical process in helping clients realize and understand the psychosocial implications of their hearing problem.

DEAFNESS, THE DEAF COMMUNITY, AND DEAF CULTURE

Many severely to profoundly hearing-impaired individuals view deafness not as a disability or handicap, but as a cultural trait. These individuals make up what is referred to as the **Deaf Community,** a group who views deafness with a sense of pride that serves to unite its members and positively shapes their sense of self-identity and self-concept.

An important distinction needs to be made between the labels "deaf" with a lowercase "d" and "Deaf" with an uppercase "D." Individuals who are "deaf" share a common physiological condition of severe-to-profound hearing loss. In contrast, "Deaf" refers to individuals who are members of the

Deaf Community. Simply having a hearing loss, however, does not automatically indoctrinate one into the Deaf Community. There must be a concomitant identification with what is known as **Deaf Culture.**

A culture is created when a group of people share in a common background of language, traditions, mores, and values. Those in the United States who identify with Deaf Culture share a common language, **American Sign Language (ASL),** which is considered the natural language of the Deaf and serves to foster group cohesion and identify. Deaf Culture is further characterized by its rich history, traditions, folklore, and various contributions to the arts including poetry, dance, and theater.

The continued existence of any culture is dependent on the perpetuation of its native language and traditions. Within the Deaf Community, this is usually accomplished through education and marriage. Residential schools for the deaf provide a means for deaf children to freely interact using ASL. Through the socialization process, pride in their identity as a Deaf person is fostered. Upon reaching adulthood, members of the Deaf Community often marry others who share the same cultural ideals. The desire to have children who are deaf to whom they can pass on their traditions and values is very strong.

Needless to say, growing up within the Deaf Community is not without its struggles. A deaf person faces many challenges in trying to compete or simply coexist with members of the "hearing world." Because ASL is the primary language of the Deaf, they are faced with the prospects of learning English as a second language and thus encounter many of the same challenges as other non-native speakers. Since most hearing people have no knowledge of sign language, the limited English skills of those who are deaf inhibit their ability to effectively communicate with the vast majority of non-signing people with whom they come into contact. Certainly, for a young person, this can lead to isolation and loneliness. For an adult, poor written and spoken English skills may significantly limit employment opportunities. Many settle for lower paying jobs with little or no opportunity for advancement.

In an effort to improve the quality of life for Deaf individuals, the town of Laurent, South Dakota, was recently established as an exclusive "signing community." Frustrated by municipalities designed by and for hearing people, developers of the Laurent township have designated sign language as the primary mode of communication among residents and businesses including schools, restaurants, government offices, and public safety agencies. While some believe that a community of this type will be a haven, others view it as simply an attempt by the Deaf Community to insulate themselves from the reality of living in the hearing world.

Those who are considering a career in speech-language pathology or audiology should be aware that some members of the Deaf Community view professionals in these disciplines in a negative light. Speech-language pathologists and audiologists may be viewed as being paternalistic or oppressive by emphasizing the need to develop spoken language skills or promoting the use of amplification. Professionals have been accused of profiting from deafness and focusing on how people who are deaf are different from

> Those who embrace Deaf Culture share common beliefs and customs that have been passed on from one generation to the next.

the norm and thus require treatment to overcome what they perceive to be a disabling or handicapping condition.

Two issues that are particularly volatile within the Deaf Community are those surrounding cochlear implants (to be discussed later in this chapter) and gene therapy. Many within the Deaf Community believe that the cochlear implant and efforts to regenerate damaged hair cells in the human cochlea pose a serious threat to the future of their culture and their language. These scientific advancements lead them to wonder whether their culture can survive if the incidence of deafness is significantly reduced. Some have even gone so far as to label these efforts as "cultural genocide." Cochlear implant programs in particular have been criticized by the Deaf Community for their efforts to discourage the use of American Sign Language by children who have been implanted in order to provide greater opportunities for auditory stimulation and the development of spoken language skills.

Although it would be unfair to suggest that all individuals who are deaf identify with the Deaf Community and its strong cultural values, speech-language pathologists and audiologists must be cognizant of these issues. Having a firm understanding of Deaf Culture and the unique perspective of the Deaf Community can serve to positively shape the direction and success of services provided to those who are severely and profoundly hearing impaired.

*G*o *to your local library and see if you can check out the documentary* Sound & Fury. *Why are so many members of the Deaf Community opposed to cochlear implants, particularly for children? Do you think this technology poses a threat to Deaf Culture?*

THOUGHT QUESTIONS

WHAT IS AUDIOLOGY?

We have already alluded to the fact that some speech and language disorders are the direct result of significant hearing loss. While SLPs are able, under their scope of practice, to conduct basic hearing screenings, the detailed information provided by a comprehensive audiological evaluation is critical to the development and implementation of an appropriate intervention plan. Additionally, the complementary nature of habilitative/rehabilitative services provided by each of these disciplines requires speech-language pathologists and audiologists to closely work together. It is appropriate, therefore, that we consider the discipline of audiology in the overall scope of communicative disorders.

The American Speech-Language-Hearing Association (ASHA) defines audiology as the discipline involved in "the prevention of and assessment of auditory, vestibular, and related impairments as well as the habilitation/rehabilitation and maintenance of persons with these impairments" (ASHA,

A key point contained within this definition is that audiology consists of professional efforts related to assessment *and* habilitation/rehabilitation.

2004, p. 2). All too often, students new to the area of communication disorders perceive audiology as a discipline that deals strictly with the diagnosis of hearing loss. While assessment is a critical component, what is subsequently done in terms of treatment and management of a client diagnosed with a hearing problem is equally important. Audiologists are not simply technicians. They must be adept in providing habilitative/rehabilitative services including counseling, the fitting of **amplification,** and various therapeutic services designed to facilitate communication and improve one's overall quality of life.

Audiology is a relatively new field of study, with its roots dating back only to the mid 1940s. It is the product of two disciplines; speech pathology, which by now you are quite familiar with, and otology, a medically based discipline concerned with the diagnosis and treatment of disorders of the auditory system. At the end of World War II, service personnel returning home were in need of rehabilitative services to overcome communication difficulties associated with battle-related hearing loss. Rehabilitation centers were established by medical departments within the military to provide medical and aural rehabilitation services. Eventually, these services were extended to the general civilian population through community-based clinics, and audiology began to distinguish itself from speech pathology and otology as a unique and separate discipline.

Today, audiology continues to be an exciting, ever-changing profession with employment opportunities in a wide range of settings. A recent survey of ASHA-certified audiologists revealed that more than half work in nonresidential health care settings (e.g. private practices, community speech and hearing centers, physician's offices), with 26 percent employed in hospital settings, 11 percent in schools, and a small percentage in colleges and universities and residential health care facilities (ASHA, 2003). There is a tendency for audiologists to specialize depending on where they work and the population(s) they serve. For example, audiologists in private practice typically specialize in the fitting and dispensing of hearing aids, while educational audiologists specialize in the fitting of personal and classroom amplification systems and the diagnosis, treatment, and management of auditory processing disorders. Some audiologists in medical settings even participate as members of surgical teams by conducting interoperative monitoring of auditory nerve function during surgery.

FUNDAMENTALS OF SOUND

It is unlikely that you have spent much time pondering the question "What is sound?" However, in order to fully appreciate the process of hearing, a brief overview of the fundamentals of sound may be helpful.

Several conditions must exist in order for sound to occur and be perceived. For the purpose of this discussion, let's focus specifically on the speech signal. As described in Chapter 3, there must be an available energy source, such as exhalation of air from the lungs; an object for the energy source to act upon that is capable of vibrating, such as the vocal folds of the larynx; and a medium available that is capable of conducting the resulting vibrations, such as air. Finally, there needs to be a receptor in place to receive, decode, and interpret the sound. The remainder of this chapter will focus exclusively on the human auditory system as the receptor.

How is it that sound is able to travel great distances through the air to reach our ears? Let's first consider how an object, such as a simple guitar string, vibrates. Vibration can be thought of as a series of rhythmic back-and-forth movements. As the guitar string is plucked, it vibrates to and fro. As it moves in one direction, an increase in pressure occurs as air molecules lying in close proximity are compressed or packed tightly in relation to one another. As the guitar string moves in the opposite direction, the air molecules that were initially compressed begin to rebound or spread apart, creating a subsequent decrease in pressure referred to as a rarefaction. Sound is a series of compressions and rarefactions that move outward from a vibrating source. It is important to note that the individual air molecules themselves do not travel to the ear from their original position near the sound source. Rather, it is the sound wave resulting from changes in pressure that propagates to the ear.

Because a vibrating object moves back and forth relative to its normal resting position, it takes on some special qualities. First, the vibrator travels a measurable distance in either direction. This is referred to as the amplitude or **intensity** of the vibration and is measured in *decibels (dB)*. Second, this back-and-forth movement regularly repeats itself, resulting in a certain number of cycles during a specified period of time. This is referred to as the **frequency** of the vibration and is expressed in *Hertz (Hz)*. The amplitude of a sound is generally associated with the perception of loudness while the frequency is associated with the perception of pitch. This information is decoded by your auditory system, enabling you to differentiate the infinitesimal number of sounds that occur throughout the course of the day.

> Every sound can be described in terms of its characteristic intensity and frequency.

AUDIBILITY VERSUS INTELLIGIBILITY

When discussing hearing and hearing loss, it is important to differentiate the concepts of **audibility** and *intelligibility*. Audibility is the ability to detect the presence of a given sound through your sense of hearing. In contrast, intelligibility refers to your ability to understand what you hear. Not only can you detect a stimulus such as speech, you also are able to identify the individual phonemes that are critical for understanding words and sentences.

As we shall see, hearing loss affects intelligibility as well as audibility. Sounds are softer than usual or may be inaudible altogether. Obviously, this will impede one's ability to understand speech unless audibility can be improved through the use of amplification. One complaint, however, that is common among many hearing-impaired persons is that they are able to hear people talking (i.e., speech is audible), but they can't figure out what the person is saying. In other words, speech is unintelligible. You may have found yourself in a situation where you were able to hear a TV or radio playing in a neighboring room. The sound was audible but too muffled to make out what was being said. This is similar to what is experienced by many hearing-impaired individuals during everyday conversations. Unfortunately, for some individuals, even if we are able to make speech audible though amplification, intelligibility may not improve significantly due to distortion imposed by damage to the auditory system.

ANATOMY AND PHYSIOLOGY OF THE AUDITORY SYSTEM

Before we can delve into a discussion of the various types and causes of hearing loss, a general understanding of the anatomy and physiology of the auditory system is essential. Anatomically, the auditory system can be divided into several general areas. They include the outer ear, the middle ear, the inner ear, the vesibulocochlear nerve, the auditory brainstem, and the auditory cortex of the brain. The first four areas (Figure 14.1) are commonly referred to as the peripheral auditory system, while the remaining two comprise the central auditory system. In general, damage to structures within the peripheral system results in a loss of sensitivity while damage to the central auditory system results in deficits related to the processing of sound. We will begin our discussion at the point where sound enters your auditory system—the area referred to as the outer ear.

THE OUTER EAR

The **outer ear** is comprised of the **pinna** or auricle, and the **external auditory meatus** or external auditory canal. The pinna is composed of flexible cartilage covered with skin. Although somewhat simple in appearance, the various ridges and depressions associated with the pinna serve to enhance and funnel sound into the ear canal while also serving as a natural res-

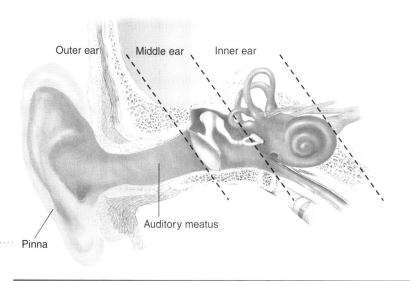

FIGURE 14.1
The peripheral auditory system.

onator. In addition, they facilitate determining where sound originates in space, a process called **localization.**

The external auditory meatus is an elliptical tube lined with skin that extends from the bowl-like depression of the pinna to the **tympanic membrane** or **eardrum.** Approximately one inch in length in adults, the canal has a slight S-shaped contour and narrows slightly as it progresses toward the eardrum. The outer region is marked by a proliferation of hair follicles and glands that produce a substance called **cerumen** or ear wax. Since the external auditory meatus is essentially a tube, it functions as a resonator, much like a musical instrument, naturally amplifying high frequency (2700 Hz to 3400 Hz) sounds.

THE MIDDLE EAR

The external auditory canal leads to the tympanic membrane, which marks the boundary between the outer ear and the **middle ear.** The tympanic membrane is a thin, concave-shaped structure that is highly elastic and responds much like a stereo speaker, vibrating in response to sound waves that travel down the canal. Most of the surface area of the tympanic membrane is composed of three distinct layers of tissue. A healthy eardrum is often described as appearing pearl gray in color. It is highly vascular, and, due to its semitransparent nature, it is often possible to observe some of the structures of the middle ear when conducting a visual examination.

Located behind the tympanic membrane is the **middle ear space,** or **tympanic cavity.** This air-filled cavity, housed within the temporal bone of the skull, is roughly cube-shaped and lined with mucous membrane. Located near the bottom of the anterior wall is the opening to a structure called the **Eustachian tube,** which connects the middle ear with the **nasopharynx.** Usually closed, the Eustachian tube opens periodically, providing a passageway for air to ventilate the middle ear space and equalize air pressure on each side of the eardrum.

Spanning the length of the middle ear cavity, much like a suspension bridge, is a chain formed by three small bones, called the **malleus, incus,** and **stapes** and collectively referred to as the **ossicles** or **ossicular chain** (see Figure 14.2). The first and largest bone in the chain, the malleus, is embedded in the fibrous layer of the eardrum. The upper portion articulates with the incus, which in turn, articulates with the stapes, the smallest bone in your body. Resembling a stirrup, the stapes contains two curved arms that terminate in a flat, bony disc called the footplate. The footplate rests against the **oval window,** a thin membrane that marks the entrance to the inner ear. Attached to the neck of the stapes is the tendon of the **stapedius muscle,** which when contracted, dampens the transmission of energy through the middle ear.

THE INNER EAR

The **inner ear** is a complex structure that serves two important roles. One major component, the **cochlea,** is responsible for providing auditory input

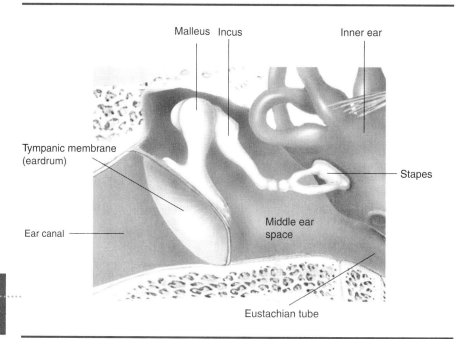

Malleus Incus   Inner ear

Tympanic membrane
(eardrum)

Stapes

Ear canal

Middle ear
space

Eustachian tube

to the central auditory nervous system. The other major component, the **vestibular system,** is responsible for supplying information regarding balance and spatial orientation. Deficits in the vestibular system often result in problems related to dizziness, imbalance, and **vertigo** or the sensation of spinning.

The cochlea, a coiled structure that resembles a snail's shell, spirals two and one-half times around a central core of bone and is the portion of the inner ear that contains the auditory sensory receptor cells. The cochlea is comprised of two concentric labyrinths. The outer labyrinth is composed of bone and filled with a fluid called **perilymph,** while the inner labyrinth is composed of membrane and contains a fluid called **endolymph.**

Running along the center of the membranous labyrinth is an intricate structure called the **organ of Corti** (see Figure 14.3). The base of the organ of Corti is formed by the **basilar membrane.** The portion of the basilar membrane closest to the stapes responds best to high-frequency sounds while the portion nearest the apex of the cochlea responds best to low-frequency sounds. Forming the roof of the organ of Corti is a gelatinous, tongue-shaped structure called the **tectorial membrane.** The tectorial membrane is fixed at one end, while the opposite end is free to move up and down in response to displacement of the surrounding fluid.

Situated on the basilar membrane are thousands of tiny **hair cells,** which are the sensory receptor cells for the auditory system. Located on the top of each cell are small hairlike projections called **stereocilia.** As the hair cells are bent and sheared through the movement of the tectorial and basi-

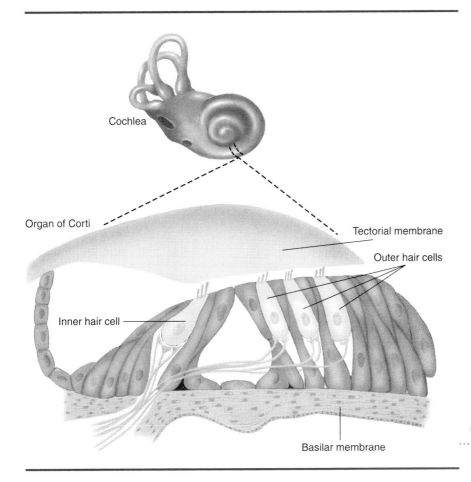

Cochlea

Organ of Corti

Tectorial membrane

Outer hair cells

Inner hair cell

Basilar membrane

lar membranes, neuroelectrical energy is generated. Innervating the base of the hair cells are auditory nerve fibers that collectively form the acoustic branch of the **vestibulocochlear** or **VIIIth nerve.**

Before we end our discussion of the inner ear, a brief mention of the vestibular system is in order. The vestibular system is also comprised of bony and membranous sections and contains two important features: the **semicircular canals** and the **otolith system.** There are a total of three semicircular canals positioned at right angles to one another. Sensory receptor cells located within each canal sense angular acceleration such as up-and-down head movement. The otolith system senses linear acceleration, such as that occurring when riding in a car or an elevator. Nerve fibers innervating the sensory cells of the vestibular system collectively form the vestibular branch of the VIIIth nerve. Given the interrelationship between the auditory and vestibular systems, it is considered within the audiologist's scope of practice to conduct vestibular testing and provide nonmedical intervention of balance disorders (ASHA, 2004).

THE VESTIBULOCOCHLEAR NERVE

Fibers that originate in the vestibular and cochlear portions of the inner ear traverse through a bony canal called the **internal auditory meatus.** Upon exiting the canal, they join the brainstem at a region referred to as the **cerebellopontine angle,** which marks the juncture of the peripheral and central auditory systems.

THE CENTRAL AUDITORY NERVOUS SYSTEM

The central auditory nervous system is highly complex. It consists of ascending and descending pathways comprised of nuclei, nerve fibers, nerve tracts, and their associated connections. Only a grossly simplified overview of the ascending auditory pathways will be presented in this section. Although it may appear that the anatomical structures leading to the brain serve merely as relay centers for the transmission of neural impulses, they actually play a key role in the extraction, enhancement, and processing of auditory signals (Bellis, 2003a).

Nerve fibers from the cochlear branch of the VIIIth nerve enter the brainstem and synapse at the cochlear nucleus. Beyond this point, nerve fibers from each ear divide into two distinct branches. Some nerve fibers ascend to the brain on the same side of the brainstem, while the majority cross over and ascend on the opposite side. From the cochlear nucleus, the majority of fibers ascend to the superior olivary complex located in the pons. The superior olivary complex plays a significant role in localization and activation of the stapedius muscle reflex. From there, nerve fibers generally progress subcortically to the pons, the midbrain, and the thalamus. Beyond this level, the auditory nerve fibers fan out and proceed to the primary auditory cortex in the temporal lobe. In most individuals, the left hemisphere is the primary area where linguistic information is processed, while the right hemisphere is responsible for processing nonlinguistic auditory cues such as rhythm and stress.

Now that we have a general understanding of the anatomical structures of the auditory system, let's briefly review the process of how sound is transmitted to the brain. Sound waves generated by a vibrating object go through a series of energy transformations as they pass through the auditory system. As acoustic energy travels down the external auditory meatus, it is transformed into mechanical energy by the movement of the tympanic membrane and ossicular chain. The resulting mechanical energy, in turn, is converted to hydraulic energy through the motion of the stapes footplate in and out of the oval window. Displacement of the cochlear fluids results in movement of the tectorial and basilar membranes, which, in turn, leads to the bending and shearing action of the stereocilia located on the tips of the hair cells in the organ of Corti. This process converts the hydraulic energy into neuroelectrical impulses that are transmitted to the auditory cortex of the brain via the auditory branch of the vestibulocochlear nerve and ascending auditory pathways. Amazingly, this complex process takes place within matter of milliseconds, making it a truly remarkable system.

TYPES OF HEARING LOSS

The previous section described the ear from an anatomical and physiological standpoint. Functionally, the outer and the middle ear serve to collect, amplify, and conduct sound to the cochlea. The outer and middle ear, therefore, are referred to as the conductive system. The cochlea is the actual sensory organ of hearing and the auditory branch of the VIIIth nerve is responsible for transmitting the resulting neural signal to the brainstem and ultimately to the auditory cortex for processing. The cochlea and auditory nerve, therefore, make up the sensorineural system. In describing peripheral hearing loss, it is most common to describe the loss from a functional perspective. That is, conductive versus sensorineural. Deficits relative to the central auditory nervous system can be functionally described, as well, in terms of their impact on auditory processing abilities. As we shall see in the next section, each of these general types of hearing loss can present unique challenges for people of all ages.

CONDUCTIVE HEARING LOSS

A *conductive hearing loss* occurs as a result of a deformation, malfunction, or obstruction of the outer or middle ear. It is important to note that not all disorders of the outer and middle ear will necessarily result in a loss of hearing. In many cases, however, problems in these areas reduce or eliminate the ear's natural conduction and amplification function, impeding sound reaching the cochlea. The result is that the intensity of sound arriving at the inner ear is reduced, thus the primary consequence of conductive hearing loss is a loss of loudness or audibility. If sound can somehow be made loud enough for the individual, it will be heard without difficulty as long as the sensorineural system remains intact.

While conductive hearing loss can have a significant impact on audibility, it does not result in a total loss of hearing. In other words, a person who is considered to be "deaf" would not have lost his or her hearing solely as a result of a conductive deficit. Fortunately, most conductive losses are not permanent. Some resolve spontaneously while most others are medically treatable. In those instances, however, where treatment of the underlying disease does not completely resolve the hearing loss, use of amplification may be warranted.

THOUGHT QUESTIONS

Curious as to what it is like to have a mild conductive hearing loss? Purchase a set of inexpensive foam earplugs from your local department or drug store and insert them in your ears. Leave them in for a few hours and go about your daily routine (within reason — don't wear the earplugs where it is unsafe to do so, such as while driving). What effect do they have on audibility and intelligibility? What effect do they have on your ability to communicate? How do others react to you? How does it impact your ability to go about your daily activities?

Disorders of the Outer Ear

Starting with the outer ear, several conditions can occur owing to the malformation of structures during embryonic development. The first, **microtia,** refers to a small, malformed pinna. By itself, microtia does not result in a loss of hearing sensitivity. When observed, however, the audiologist is alerted to the possibility of other congenital conditions, such as **atresia.** Atresia is a disorder in which there is complete closure of the external auditory meatus. Since sound cannot travel through the ear canal in the usual manner, significant hearing loss is likely. **Stenosis,** a severe narrowing of the external canal, may occur in some individuals. Unlike atresia, however, stenois does not result in hearing loss unless debris or earwax becomes trapped in the narrow opening.

A much more common cause of conductive hearing loss in the outer ear is due to either impacted cerumen or foreign object. It may be hard to believe but cerumen or ear wax actually serves several useful purposes. Cerumen naturally cleanses the external canal as it migrates outwards and provides lubrication to prevent the skin that lines the canal from drying out. It also provides a chemical barrier to bacterial and fungal infection and protects the ear from invasion of insects and other foreign bodies.

Some populations, such as young children and the elderly, are more prone to problems resulting from excessive cerumen production or entrapment in the canal. This can create a mild to moderate degree of hearing loss, necessitating medical intervention to remove the cerumen plug. In some states cerumen management (removal) is considered within the audiologist's scope of practice, although it should be conducted with extreme caution and only after extensive training.

> These conditions most frequently occur in conjunction with other craniofacial disorders (see Chapter 11) as in the case of Down syndrome or Treacher Collins syndrome.

Disorders of the Middle Ear

Several causes of conductive hearing loss can be traced to the middle ear. For example, the tympanic membrane may be perforated as a result of disease, trauma, or sudden change in pressure or become thickened as a result of calcium plaque formation. Likewise, the bones of the ossicular chain may become disarticulated due to a blow to the head, or their movement may be impeded by a tumor in the middle ear.

Cholesteatoma is a tumor-like mass composed of epithelial (skin) cells, keratin, and fat that migrates into the middle ear cavity, usually through a perforated eardrum. The resulting mass can grow in size and has a propensity to erode bone, including the ossicles and bony walls of the middle ear space. Left untreated, this can lead to irreversible damage to the inner ear, facial nerve, and structures of the cranial cavity. Due to its destructive nature and the potential for serious complications, prompt surgical removal is required.

Otosclerosis is a disorder that afflicts primarily young adults, particularly females, and in the majority of cases is linked to genetic factors. It is characterized by the formation of spongy bone in the vicinity of the stapes footplate, resulting in partial or complete fixation. Since normal movement of the stapes in and out of the oval window is impeded, hearing loss is a likely consequence. Treatment of otosclerosis usually consists of surgical removal of part or all of the fixated footplate and insertion of a prosthetic device that acts as an artificial stapes.

One of the most common causes of conductive hearing loss, particularly in children, is otitis media, an inflammation of the mucous membrane lining the middle ear cavity. In fact, otitis media is the most frequently diagnosed disorder in the United States in children under 15 years of age. Almost 95 percent of children experience at least one episode by the age of 6 years, with peak incidence generally occurring during the period from birth to 2 years of age. Children who experience longstanding or frequently reoccurring episodes are of particular concern since their timing tends to coincide with the period that is most crucial for speech, language, and cognitive development (Gravel & Wallace, 1999).

A number of factors place certain children at risk for otitis media. They include the presence of craniofacial anomalies such as cleft palate and those associated with Down syndrome, daycare placement, and exposure to second-hand smoke. Heredity, race, and gender are also contributing factors. Although it is significantly more prevalent in children, adults are not immune to otitis media. Despite its prevalence, there is a great deal of confusion and controversy surrounding the disorder, particularly when it comes to terminology and treatment.

Otitis media generally results from Eustachian dysfunction, which prevents proper ventilation of the middle ear cavity. A normal functioning Eustachian tube opens periodically as one chews, yawns, or swallows, allowing for the equalization of air pressure between the middle ear and the external environment. In children, the Eustachian tube is shorter, oriented more in the horizontal plane, and more pliable than in adults, making it less efficient in ventilating the middle ear. If adequate ventilation cannot be provided by the Eustachian tube due to enlarged adenoids or swelling of the tissue lining the nasopharynx, oxygen is absorbed into the mucous membrane lining the middle ear cavity, forming a vacuum. This, in turn, results in a reduction in air pressure within the middle ear compared to the pressure in the ear canal. This pressure imbalance causes the eardrum to retract into the middle ear cavity, diminishing its ability to freely vibrate. If normal ventilation of the middle ear is not restored, further retraction of the eardrum into the middle ear cavity will continue. At this point, the person may experience a sensation of his or her ear(s) feeling plugged or even slightly uncomfortable.

THOUGHT QUESTIONS

Have you ever had difficulty hearing on an airplane flight or felt your ears "pop" when in an elevator or driving in a mountainous region? What do you think causes these temporary problems?

The resulting vacuum within the middle ear can lead to the secretion of fluid, a condition referred to as **otitis media with effusion (OME).** As fluid fills the cavity, further stiffening the eardrum and the ossicular chain, sound must be conducted through a less efficient fluid-filled medium instead of the usual air-filled environment. If the fluid is sterile, the condition is classified as **serous otitis media.** However, when pathogens are present and make their way from the nasopharynx through the Eustachian tube, infection of the middle ear cavity is likely. Pus forms within the middle ear cavity as a direct result of the infection of the mucous membrane. This condition is referred to as **purulent** or **suppurative otitis media.** Symptoms associated with an active infection include restlessness, irritability, ear pain, fever, and vomiting. During this process the tympanic membrane may appear reddish in color or bulging. Spontaneous rupturing of the tympanic membrane may occur along with concomitant fluid discharge.

Otitis media can be further classified based on the general time course of the disease process. **Acute otitis media** is characterized by rapid onset, with resolution within approximately three weeks. When the condition persists for longer than eight weeks, it is referred to as **chronic otitis media.** Episodes lasting between three weeks and eight weeks are referred to as **subacute otitis media.**

Treatment of otitis media is a complex process, since an active infection may or may not be involved. In some cases the recommended course of treatment is to simply monitor the situation to see whether it will resolve spontaneously. Decongestants and antihistamines may be prescribed to resolve the underlying problem of inadequate Eustachian tube function. Antibiotics are frequently used in cases of acute otitis media to prevent the development of chronic disease and reduce the risk of complications such as damage to the structures of the middle and inner ear and meningitis. There is strong concern expressed regarding the increased resistance of certain pathogens to antibiotics that in the past have been successful in treating acute otitis media (Smith, Pearson, Wilcox, et al., 1998).

Surgical treatment is sometimes warranted and involves a relatively simple procedure called a *myringotomy,* whereby an incision is made in the tympanic membrane and fluid within the middle ear cavity is drained. Another type of surgical treatment is the insertion of a **pressure equalization (PE)** or **tympanostomy tube** into the tympanic membrane. The tube or grommet is very small in diameter and serves the same purpose as the Eustachian tube, allowing air to pass into the middle ear space. However, instead of passing from the nasopharynx, air enters the middle ear from the external auditory.

SENSORINEURAL HEARING LOSS

A second general type of hearing loss, sensorineural hearing loss, results from the absence or malformation of, or damage to the structures of the inner ear, most notably the hair cells within the cochlea. Sensorineural hearing loss may be present at birth or develop over the course of one's life. It may be sudden in onset, occurring over a matter of hours, or gradual, manifesting over a period of years. Some forms of sensorineural hearing loss have a genetic basis while other forms are acquired, resulting from factors external to the individual. Hearing may remain stable, become worse, or fluctuate. It is in many ways the direct opposite of conductive hearing loss since sensorineural losses are usually permanent. Recent breakthroughs, however, in auditory hair cell regeneration in animals through gene therapy hold promise as they may one day become a viable means of restoring hearing in humans who have experienced hair cell damage (Izumikawa, Minoda, Kawamoto, et al., 2005).

While sensorineural hearing loss may affect any range of frequencies, most cases are characterized by hearing loss predominantly in the higher frequency range, while sensitivity in the lower frequencies often remains unaffected. Unlike conductive hearing loss where the problem stems from sound not being loud enough, sensorineural hearing loss presents an additional problem, that being the lack of clarity. Not only are certain sounds inaudible or softer than normal; but sounds that are audible are often perceived as being distorted. To illustrate this point, let's consider a conventional AM/FM radio. When a radio is tuned to a particular station but is set at a very low volume level, it simulates a conductive hearing loss. That is, sound is softer than normal, making it difficult to perceive the signal being broadcast. If, however, the volume is increased (i.e., the conductive disorder is overcome), the radio signal not only becomes easier to hear, its clarity remains true and easy to understand. If we now take the same radio, but this time adjust the tuner slightly so that it is no longer centered directly on the desired station, the signal remains audible but is distorted and harder to understand. Increasing the volume does little to improve the signal's clarity. This simple demonstration reveals how sensorineural hearing loss is not simply a problem of reduced audibility, but reduced clarity as well, which may negatively impact intelligibility.

Because of its permanency and corrupting effect on the quality of the auditory signal, sensorineural hearing loss can be expected to have a negative impact on speech, language, and cognitive development. To what degree depends on several factors including the cause of the hearing loss, the person's age when the hearing loss occurred (age of onset), when it was discovered, and the type and quality of intervention provided.

Age of onset is usually described in terms of being either congenital, present at birth, or **adventitious,** occurring sometime after birth. Another way of looking at this is to consider whether the hearing loss occurred **prelingually,** that is, before speech and language skills have developed, or **postlingually,** after the person has acquired spoken language skills. There is no precise age that delineates the two, although generally, hearing loss that occurs prior to the age of 2 years is considered to be prelingual in onset while hearing loss that occurs after the age of 5 years is considered to be postlingual. If a congenital hearing loss goes undetected until a child is 4 or 5 years of age, it will have a far more adverse effect on speech and language development than if it is discovered as a newborn and appropriate early intervention services are provided. In the latter case, the prognosis for development of age-appropriate speech and language skills is much more encouraging.

Disorders of the Inner Ear.

Now that we have a general understanding of sensorineural hearing loss, let's take a look at some of the causes starting with those that are congenital and hereditary. When a hearing loss is due to the absence or malformation of inner ear structures during embryonic development, it is referred to as **aplasia.** There are several types of aplasia, depending on which part of the inner ear is affected. Very often, congenital hereditary sensorineural hearing loss is a component of a group of disorders associated with a syndrome. For example, **Usher syndrome** is a genetic disorder characterized by sensorineural hearing loss ranging from severe to profound in degree, and retinitis pigmentosa, a degenerative visual impairment that results in night blindness and reduced peripheral vision (see Case Study 14.2 on page 426). **Waardenburg syndrome** is another genetic disorder characterized by mild to severe sensorineural hearing loss, pigmentary discoloration of the irises and hair, and craniofacial malformation of the nasal area. **Alport syndrome** is marked by sensorineural hearing loss and kidney disease.

Although sensorineural hearing loss may be present at birth, it is not always the result of genetic factors. Instead, an illness or toxic agent experienced by the mother during pregnancy may be the cause. The most notorious example is hearing loss resulting from **maternal rubella** or German measles. During the early to mid 1960s, an outbreak of rubella resulted in an estimated 10,000 to 20,000 children being born with handicapping conditions. Over 50 percent of these children had severe to profound hearing losses. Fortunately, development of a vaccine has significantly reduced the incidence of rubella. Other viruses, however, such as the Human Immunodeficiency Virus (HIV) and cytomegalovirus (CMV), continue to be a major cause of congenital sensorineural hearing loss when contracted by the mother during pregnancy. Sexually transmitted bacterial diseases such as syphilis can cause various degrees of central nervous system disorders, mental retardation, and hearing loss in the developing fetus. Aside from infections, complications during pregnancy, such as Rh incompatibility and anoxia (oxygen deprivation), can also result in sensorineural hearing loss.

Sensorineural hearing loss can occur as a result of circumstances encountered at any point during one's lifetime. Acquired hearing loss may be due to viral infections such as mumps, rubeola, and herpes zoster oticus, or due to a bacterial infection such as meningitis. **Meningitis** is an inflammation of layers of tissue covering the brain and frequently leads to a severe or profound hearing loss in young children and adults. The structures of the inner ear are susceptible to damage either from the bacteria that cause the disease or from the high fever that often accompanies the illness. Moreover, because bacterial meningitis is potentially life-threatening, it requires treatment with high doses of potent antibiotics that can be toxic **(ototoxic)** to the structures of the inner ear. In this case, it may be the cure rather than the disease that causes the hearing loss.

Specific drugs that are known to be ototoxic include aminoglycocides, particularly those belonging to the -mycin family, cisplatin and carboplatin used to treat cancer, loop diuretics, aspirin taken in large doses, and drugs used to treat HIV and AIDS. Hearing loss resulting from ototoxicity may be permanent or reversible. Frequent monitoring of hearing is often recommended for individuals being treated with these medications so that drug type and dosage can be adjusted as needed.

Although the majority of sensorineural hearing losses are gradual in terms of their onset and progression, sudden hearing loss is possible, occurring in approximately 10 to 20 per 100,000 individuals (Wilson, 1994). This can be a particularly tenuous situation for those afflicted, most of whom are adults between the ages of 30 and 60 years, as they go from being able to hear normally to having a significant hearing loss in a matter of hours or days. In the vast majority of cases only one ear is affected. Although some can be traced to a specific incident involving trauma to the head, many cases of sudden hearing loss occur seemingly without cause or advanced warning. It is thought that the majority of these cases are due to either viral infection or vascular insult. Individuals who experience sudden hearing loss frequently complain of vertigo, **tinnitus** (ringing), or fullness in the ear. It is critical that these individuals be referred for prompt treatment as this condition constitutes a medical emergency. Surprisingly, hearing recovers spontaneously in the majority of cases (Byl, 1984). When it fails to do so, however, various treatments are employed including the administration of steroids, vasodilators, anticoagulants, and histamines. Inhalation of carbogen, a combination of carbon dioxide and oxygen, is also recommended in some cases. Case Study 14.1 (on page 406) presents the story of one young man who experienced sudden hearing loss.

Ménière's disease is another disorder that can produce hearing loss that is rather sudden in onset. First described by Prosper Ménière in 1861, Ménière's disease is caused by pressure resulting from the buildup of endolymph within the membranous labyrinth of the inner ear. The classic symptoms associated with Ménière's disease are fluctuating and progressive sensorineural hearing loss, roaring or ringing tinnitus, vertigo, and a feeling of fullness in the ear. It should be noted, however, that not all of these symptoms will be experienced by all who are afflicted. In addition, the disorder is episodic in nature whereby symptoms intensify and abate over a matter of hours of days. This can be particularly disconcerting to those afflicted since they may have little or no warning of an impending attack of vertigo that may leave them incapacitated. Treatment may include drug therapy, surgical intervention, or regulation of one's diet to alleviate symptoms.

Although quite rare, an **acoustic neuroma** or auditory nerve tumor may develop in some individuals. These tumors, found mostly in adults, are typically benign and slow growing and tend to form on only one side. Most tumors originate from cells that form the outer covering of the vestibular branch of the VIIIth nerve. Pressure exerted by the tumor can disrupt blood flow, which may ultimately affect the function of the vestibulocochlear and facial nerves. Symptoms of an acoustic neuroma include dizziness, tinnitus, and hearing loss marked by significant difficulty understanding speech. Treatment involves surgical removal of the tumor, since it can compromise other structures and possibly result in death. Unfortunately, surgical removal often necessitates severing part of or all of the auditory nerve, resulting in permanent hearing loss.

Case Study 14.2

A Person with Usher's Syndrome

Although Marie was born with a hearing loss in both ears, it was not identified until the age of 6 years. At that time she was fitted with hearing aids. At the age of 15, Marie began to experience periodic episodes of dizziness and feelings of being "off balance." She also noticed a steady decline in her ability to hear. While attending college, Marie began to experience problems with her vision. Initially, she noticed difficulty only at night and simply attributed this to being "clumsy." Over time, however, Marie began to experience difficulty with greater frequency. A follow-up medical evaluation revealed that Marie was suffering from Usher's syndrome, a progressive genetic disorder of the auditory and visual systems.

From the time Marie graduated from college until she reached her early 30s, she continued to experience a steady decline in her ability to hear and understand speech. In addition to her night blindness, she began to experience "tunnel vision." Although her primary mode of communication up to this point had been spoken language, a continued decline in hearing prompted her to learn sign language in order to supplement auditory and visual speech cues.

Marie currently works as a guidance counselor at a residential school for the deaf. She continues to use hearing aids to help her hear important environmental sounds, identify talkers, and facilitate lipreading, but finds them to be bothersome in noisy environments. At age 50, Marie has begun mobility training to learn how to use a cane to help her navigate her home and work environments in preparation for the day when she will lose her vision completely. For assistance in identifying important sounds around the home, she recently acquired a trained "hearing dog." As her ability to hear continues to decline, Marie's next step in the rehabilitative process is to investigate getting a cochlear implant to facilitate listening.

Even children are not immune to the potential negative effects of noise exposure—many of today's toys, electronic games, and personal stereos produce sounds at levels that are potentially hazardous.

Let's now turn our attention to a cause of sensorineural hearing loss that in most cases is avoidable—that is, hearing loss resulting from excessive exposure to high levels of sound (noise). We live in an age where we are inundated with ever-increasing amounts of noise. From machines at factories and construction sites to common everyday items such as power tools, motorcycles, and musical instruments, it is almost impossible to escape the constant bombardment of noise associated with occupational and recreational activities. And what about loudly playing that MP3 player of yours? It should come as no surprise, then, that **noise-induced hearing loss** is one of the leading causes of acquired sensorineural hearing loss in young and middle-aged adults. Exposure to high levels of noise subjects the delicate structures housed within the cochlea to considerable stress that may inevitably lead to irreversible damage.

Hearing loss that occurs from exposure to high levels of noise can be temporary or permanent. **Temporary threshold shift (TTS)** is a term used to describe hearing loss that results from short-term exposure but recovers spontaneously. Most people are familiar with this effect. After attending a loud party or rock concert, it is not uncommon to experience a reduction in hearing accompanied by tinnitus. After several hours of rest, the ringing ceases and hearing returns to normal. Of course, if short-term exposure involves sound that is sufficiently intense, such as that resulting from an explosion, immediate and irreversible hearing loss can result.

Frequent exposure to high levels of noise for extended periods of time may eventually lead to **permanent threshold shift (PTS).** A PTS is typically characterized by a loss of sensitivity in the high-frequency range (between 3000 and 6000 Hz), with better hearing for frequencies on either side. As damage resulting from long-term exposure increases, the range of frequencies affected widens. Increased difficulty understanding speech, particularly in the presence of background noise, is often associated with noise induced sensorineural hearing loss.

What is particularly disconcerting about PTS is that in most cases it is preventable. The risk of experiencing PTS is a function of how long a person is exposed relative to the intensity of the sound. The Occupational Safety and Health Administration (OSHA) has established regulations for employment settings that limits daily exposure by workers (OSHA, 1983). Not all persons are equally susceptible to the potential risks of noise exposure. Factors such as age, genetics, medication use, and exposure to certain chemicals can all influence one's susceptibility.

Finally, the reality is that most of us will eventually experience some degree of sensorineural hearing loss in our lifetime, and sadly we have little control over it. Hearing loss that occurs through the aging process is referred to as **presbycusis** (Willot, 1996). Although included in our discussion of sensorineural hearing loss, it is important to note that the aging process may not only result in dysfunction of the structures of the inner ear, such as hair cells and acoustic nerve fibers, but other structures of the peripheral auditory system such as the tympanic membrane and ossicular chain. The aging process can also affect the central auditory nervous system. As a result, the consequences of presbycusis may involve not only reduced hearing sensitivity, particularly for high-frequency sounds, but deficits in auditory perception as well. Some individuals with presbycusis experience difficulty understanding speech that is far greater than one would expect based on their degree of hearing loss. This condition is referred to as **phonemic regression** and may be attributed to deficits beyond the inner ear (Gaeth, 1948). What makes these cases particularly challenging is that the use of amplification, while helpful in improving the audibility of speech, may not significantly improve intelligibility. Approximately 45 percent of adults between the ages of 48 and 92 years have some degree of hearing loss, with males demonstrating a higher prevalence than females (Cruickshanks, Wiley, Tweed, et al., 1998). Given that the elderly population is one of the fastest growing segments within the United States, it is imperative that speech-language pathologists and audiologists have a good understanding of presbycusis and its associated consequences, including those related to psychosocial adjustment.

MIXED HEARING LOSS

The third general type of hearing loss, mixed hearing loss, is the simultaneous presence of conductive and sensorineural hearing loss. For example, a person with a sensorineural hearing loss resulting from noise exposure might also develop otitis media or impacted cerumen, which further depresses his or her hearing sensitivity. In most cases the conductive component can be medically treated, leading to some improvement in overall hearing sensitivity. However, since the sensorineural component remains, the person's hearing cannot be fully restored to normal levels.

AUDITORY PROCESSING DISORDERS

The three types of hearing loss described in the preceding sections refer to damage sustained to the peripheral auditory system or the structures of the ear spanning from the pinna to the auditory nerve. The function of the peripheral auditory system is what is routinely assessed during the course of a comprehensive audiological evaluation. Audiologists, however, must consider the entire auditory system, including problems that affect the central auditory nervous system. This can generally be thought of as the auditory structures, pathways, and neural synapses that span from the level of the brainstem to the cortex of the brain (see Figure 14.4). Problems associated

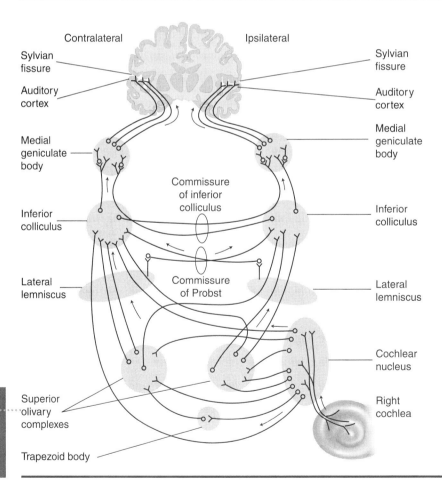

FIGURE 14.4
Schematic representation of the central auditory nervous system.

with the central auditory nervous system do not typically result in a loss of hearing sensitivity. Instead, they are characterized by an inability to efficiently and effectively use and interpret auditory information. This is often reflected in problems associated with sound localization and lateralization, auditory discrimination and temporal (timing and order) processing of speech, and understanding speech in background noise or other acoustic conditions that significantly degrade the quality of the speech signal. Such deficiencies are collectively referred to as **auditory processing disorders (APD)** or central auditory processing disorders (CAPD).

Despite a significant rise in awareness among professionals over the last decade, establishing a consensus in terms of how to define APD has been difficult and at times controversial. Deficits associated with the central auditory nervous system manifest in a variety of ways, with the associated signs and symptoms often similar to those exhibited by individuals with higher order language impairments, learning disabilities, attention-deficit hyperactivity disorder (ADHD), and autism, to name a few. Although APD can coexist with these other disorders, it is not an outcome. The ASHA Working Group on Auditory Processing Disorders has defined APD as "difficulties in the perceptual processing of auditory information by the central nervous system" (ASHA, 2005, p. 2).

Auditory processing disorders are prevalent in children and adults and may be the result of delayed neuromaturation of the central auditory nervous system, neurologic disorders, diseases, or insults such as a stroke, tumor, head trauma, complications resulting from surgery, or neurologic changes associated with the aging process (Chermak & Musiek, 1997). Some forms of APD may have a genetic link (Bellis, 2003b) or develop as a result of auditory deprivation suffered as a consequence of chronic otitis media (Hall & Grose, 1993). It has been estimated that APD occurs in 2 to 3 percent of children, with males outnumbering females by a ratio of 2 to 1. In older adults, prevalence estimates range anywhere from 10 to 20 percent, up to as high as 70 percent (Chermak & Musiek, 1997; Stach, Spretnjak, & Jerger, 1990). With children, we are usually concerned with how APD impacts language development and learning, which naturally has significant implications for academic achievement. With adults, APD may have greater implications for communication in social situations or in the workplace.

A variety of behavioral characteristics have been identified that raise suspicion concerning the possible presence of an auditory processing disorder. For example, individuals with an APD may be easily distracted and demonstrate difficulty comprehending rapid speech or understanding speech in poor acoustic environments such as settings with competing noise or **reverberation** (echo) caused by reflected sound. Difficulty localizing sounds in space, following complex auditory directions, or differentiating speech sounds that are acoustically similar are also common characteristics. Individuals with APD may demonstrate difficulty paying attention or frequently request repetition when they misunderstand spoken information. Other characteristics include responding slowly or inconsistently to verbal messages, increased dependency on visual cues, or a tendency to intently watch the speaker's face when engaged in spoken communication. It is im-

> Differentiating APD from problems related to other higher order processes poses a significant challenge.

portant to note that individuals with APD do not necessarily demonstrate all of these characteristics. It is also important to remember that these characteristics are often associated with other disorders. It is critical, therefore, that one does not automatically jump to the conclusion that a person has an auditory processing disorder if he or she exhibits one or more of these tendencies. Only by administering a comprehensive battery of appropriate tests can an audiologist diagnose the presence of an auditory processing disorder, not through the use of checklists or observation of an individual's behavior.

DEGREES OF HEARING LOSS

When describing a person's hearing loss, audiologists use terminology such as conductive, sensorineural, mixed, and so forth to specify the "site of lesion" or region of the auditory system that is affected. Although this is a critical part of the diagnostic process, it is equally important to quantify the degree of hearing loss. Quantitatively, the degree of hearing loss is expressed in units called decibels (dB). A decibel is a mathematically derived unit based on the pressure exerted by a particular sound. The lowest decibel level at which a given sound is barely audible represents a person's auditory threshold. The greater the decibel value required to reach a person's threshold, the greater the degree of hearing loss. As we will later see, this type of measurement can be conducted using tones that vary as a function of frequency. It is important to remember that an individual's degree of hearing loss may not be the same at all frequencies. In other words, there may be a greater degree of hearing loss for high-frequency sounds, for example, compared to sounds in the low-or mid-frequency range. This can have significance in terms of which speech sounds are audible and which need to be amplified.

Audiologists have adopted the terms presented in Table 14.1 to apply descriptive labels corresponding to the degree of hearing loss. In very general terms, individuals whose degree of hearing loss falls within the mild to moderately severe range are classified as **hard of hearing.** These individuals depend extensively on their **residual hearing** for receptive communication and the learning of new concepts. For people whose auditory thresholds fall in the severe to profound range, however, the auditory system provides limited or no access to speech without the use of amplification. As was previously mentioned, these individuals are usually referred to as deaf, which presents challenges that are radically different from people who are born with normal hearing or even those who are hard of hearing.

AUDIOLOGICAL ASSESSMENT PROCEDURES

Having described the basic principles of sound, the anatomy and physiology of the auditory system, and the various types and causes of hearing loss, we are now ready to take a look at how this information is used clinically in the

TABLE 14.1
Degrees of hearing loss

Decibel Range	Degree of Loss	Description
0 dB–20 dB	Normal hearing	
21 dB–40 dB	Mild	Difficulty with distant or faint speech.
41 dB–55 dB	Moderate	Difficulty following conversational level speech.
56 dB–70 dB	Moderately severe	Can hear only loud speech.
71 dB–90 dB	Severe	Difficulty understanding even loud speech; may require alternative communication system.
91 dB +	Profound	Usually considered "deaf"; cannot depend on auditory system alone to obtain information.

assessment of hearing. It is important to stress that no single test can accurately represent the full extent of a person's hearing loss or the effect it has in terms of overall communication function or psychosocial well-being. Instead, the audiologist must rely on a battery of tests to obtain an accurate picture of an individual's hearing problem. A battery approach also enables the audiologist to cross-check the results of each test to determine if there are any trends or inconsistencies.

Before continuing, now is a good time to differentiate "assessment," as we will discuss in this section, from "screening," which was referred to earlier in this chapter. Screening is the process that is used to determine which individuals, whether children or adults, are *likely* to have a hearing loss. If you ever had your hearing tested as part of a schoolwide program, it is likely that you participated in a screening. As previously mentioned, newborn hearing screening programs are increasing in order to identify those infants who are likely to have a congenital hearing impairment. Those who pass the screening in all likelihood have normal hearing, although periodic monitoring should continue, since hearing loss can occur at any point afterwards. However, it cannot be definitively concluded that those who fail the screening are indeed hearing-impaired. Failure of a hearing screening simply indicates that additional in-depth assessment is warranted to determine if a hearing loss is present, and if so, to quantify the type and degree. The remainder of this section will focus on the types of tests available for inclusion in a comprehensive audiological assessment battery.

ASSESSING INFANTS AND CHILDREN VERSUS ADULTS

The special skills of the pediatric audiologist are called into play when assessing infants and young children since obtaining reliable information

As with speech and language, auditory behavior is developmental and, as long as the audiologist is familiar with the different stages of auditory development, in most cases age-appropriate response can be elicited.

from this population can be challenging, to say the least. In addition to information gained from behavioral, electroacoustic, and electrophysiological tests, there are a number of commercially available instruments that can be used with younger children to assess progress relative to functional auditory development (Anderson, 2002; Stredler-Brown & Johnson, 2003).

Assessing adult clients can also present challenges to the audiologist. Adults with developmental, neurogenic, language, or cognitive disorders frequently require modifications to the test battery, test materials, and administration procedures. Cases of **nonorganic hearing loss** are particularly challenging and at times frustrating. Nonorganic hearing loss is a term used to describe the condition where an individual portrays having a hearing loss when one does not exist or exaggerates the degree of a true organic impairment (Martin & Clark, 2003). The audiologist must be skilled in identifying these individuals and obtaining an accurate measure of their true auditory function. Finally, geriatric clients often present challenges during testing due to fatigue and slower reaction time. Fortunately, modifications to test procedures can be made to address these issues.

COUNSELING

Although not a test per se, counseling is an essential component of any audiological service. Counseling is usually thought of as the process of imparting information. In this somewhat narrow view, the audiologist provides information while the client listens, perhaps interjecting a pertinent question from time to time. For example, the audiologist might explain the results of individual tests, provide technical information on the anatomy of the ear, or explain how hearing loss occurs so the client can better understand the nature of his or her problem. The audiologist might also present possible courses of treatment, including amplification and rehabilitation options designed to facilitate spoken communication. This type of counseling, referred to as **informational counseling,** is critical and requires great skill on the part of the clinician so that information is communicated in a manner that is understood and remembered. It has been reported that only 50 percent of the information conveyed by healthcare providers is actually retained by clients, and that approximately half of this information is remembered inaccurately (Kessels, 2003; Margolis, 2004). Although important, informational counseling is only one facet of the counseling process.

As discussed earlier in this chapter, hearing loss can have a significant impact on a person's psychological, social, and emotional well-being. Clients may struggle as they try to come to terms with feelings of anger, anxiety, fear, frustration, and despair that are a direct result of their hearing loss. It is important to remember that these feelings are not limited to the hearing-impaired client. They often transcend to others who are in close contact with the individual such as parents or a spouse. Unless these individuals receive support from an empathetic clinician, they cannot proceed with efforts to remediate the problem. The process of assisting the client and the family in dealing with the emotional consequences of hearing loss is referred to as **personal adjustment counseling.** As part of this process, the audiologist must pay close attention to a client's affective statements and questions in order to uncover any personal adjustment issues. This involves listening intently and encouraging clients to "tell their story" of what it's like to live with a hearing loss. Clients need to accept and assume ownership of their hearing loss before any efforts to remediate the condition can proceed. Simply telling clients what they should do will not lead to compliance if they do not first acknowledge and accept the fact that a problem exists. The audiologists needs to be adept at determining when a client is asking for "information" as opposed to seeking acknowledgment of an affective or emotional concern that conveys personal feelings about their hearing problem (English, 2002).

Several key points regarding the counseling process must be stressed. First, clinicians must be cognizant of the client's and the family's cultural background and linguistic needs to ensure appropriate communication (Scott, 2000). Second, audiologists should seize the moment by providing counseling whenever the opportunity presents itself, not only at the conclusion of the session. Additionally, clinicians need to remember that clients and family members process information at different rates. Some want as much information as possible at the time of the diagnosis, while others need time to deal with the initial shock before they can move on and consider various treatment options. Finally, clinicians should always be aware of their professional boundaries relative to counseling. When potential psychological or mental health issues arise, clinicians should not hesitate to refer clients to a qualified professional counselor.

REFERRAL AND CASE HISTORY

Referral for audiological testing may originate from a variety of sources including physicians, school nurses, speech-language pathologists, psychologists, teachers, and family members, to name a few. Self-referral may also occur. The referring source may be able to provide important background information, such as the results of previous tests, that is helpful in gaining a better understanding of the client's problem.

Before conducting any testing, the audiologist will spend time interviewing the client and collecting case history information. This process provides an opportunity to obtain background information from the client's perspective and helps the audiologist map out an appropriate assessment plan. It is important to know why the client has come in for the evaluation, whether there is a family history of hearing loss, if the client has sustained a recent head injury or is taking medication, whether he or she has been exposed to noise, and so on. The audiologist will ask the client to describe the situations in which he or she is having difficulty or any symptoms that may be present such as tinnitus, ear pain, or dizziness. A complete case history can often provide the audiologist with a strong indication of what the problem is even before any tests are administered. An audiological interview can be seen on the book's CD-ROM.

Formal self-assessment questionnaires are available that can assist the audiologist in obtaining the client's perspective on the types of communication problems he or she is experiencing, including measures of hearing disability or activity limitation, and handicap or participation restriction. For example, a particular item might ask the client to rate the degree of difficulty experienced when listening in a noisy restaurant. Several of these questionnaires contain a companion version that can be completed by the client's significant other. Obtaining input from someone close to the client can shed additional light on the particular problems encountered as a result of the hearing loss. As an added benefit, these self-assessment instruments facilitate the counseling process by providing a vehicle for promoting self-reflection, self-disclosure, and discussion of one's attitudes and feelings about their hearing problem.

OTOSCOPIC EXAMINATION

One of the first procedures performed during an evaluation is a visual or otoscopic examination. The examination is conducted using a small, handheld device called an **otoscope** that illuminates the external auditory meatus and allows the audiologist to visually inspect the canal and tympanic membrane. The audiologist will also visually inspect the external surface of the pinna for any signs of abnormality. This is a critical first step in the assessment process because it promptly calls attention to any conditions that may impede sound during testing, such as excessive cerumen, or warrant immediate medical referral, such as drainage from the ear. A newer version of this device, called a video-otoscope, projects the image of the ear onto a television or computer monitor, allowing the client and family members to simultaneously observe. In addition to enhancing the counseling process, this technology enables the audiologist to print images to facilitate communication with medical personnel.

ELECTROACOUSTIC AND ELECTROPHYSIOLOGICAL TESTING

Over the past thirty years, advances in technology and in our understanding of the hearing process have led to the development of specialized electroacoustic and electrophysiological tests of the auditory system. These tests evaluate the integrity of the peripheral and central auditory systems without the need for an overt behavioral response on the part of the client. While they are not true "hearing" tests since hearing requires the person to be able to recognize and use sound, they represent a major step forward in the early diagnosis and comprehensive evaluation of the auditory system.

Electroacoustic measures record acoustic signals from within the client's external auditory canal using specialized equipment. Two types of electroacoustic measures commonly performed on children and adults are tests of acoustic immittance and otoacoustic emissions.

Acoustic immittance measures are useful in the diagnosis of conductive pathology and can be completed in a relatively short period of time. No behavioral response is required, making it an excellent tool for children, including infants, as well as adults. All that is necessary is for the client to remain relatively still and refrain from vocalizing.

Acoustic immittance testing is performed using an electronic device that consists of a small probe containing a microphone, air-pressure pump, and sound generator connected to a recording instrument. The probe is inserted in the external auditory meatus, creating an airtight seal. During testing, a continuous tone is emitted into the canal as the air pressure is automatically increased and decreased. This change in pressure sets the eardrum into motion. The microphone measures any changes in the intensity of the tone as it flows through the canal and is reflected by the tympanic membrane. The result is a graph called a **tympanogram** that plots the compliance of the middle ear as a function of changes in ear canal pressure (see Figure 14.5). Quantitative data obtained as part of this process, as well as the overall shape of the resulting tympanogram, can assist in identifying the presence of conductive pathology and determining whether it is due to otosclerosis, a break in the ossicular chain, otitis media with effusion, or a perforation of the eardrum.

Frequently included as a part of the acoustic immittance battery is a test involving the acoustic reflex. As previously discussed, the stapedius muscle contracts in response to high-intensity sounds, causing the ossicular chain and tympanic membrane to stiffen. The same device used to generate a tympanogram is capable of measuring the contraction of the stapedius muscle in response to different stimuli. By analyzing whether the reflex is present, and if so, at what intensity level, the audiologist is able to make important inferences as to the possible site of the disorder. A demonstration of acoustic immittance testing can be seen on the book's CD-ROM.

Otoacoustic emissions (OAEs) are a second type of elecroacoustic measure that has received considerable attention during the past decade. Discovered by David Kemp (1978), otoacoustic emissions are low-intensity

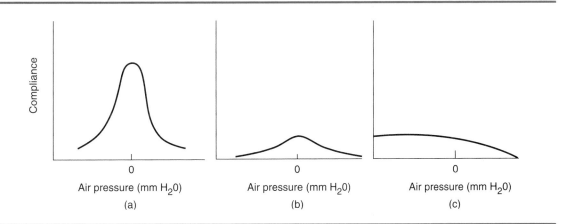

FIGURE 14.5
Schematic of three common tympanogram patterns: (a) normal middle ear function, (b) somewhat reduced compliance due to otosclerosis, (c) minimal compliance due to otitis media with effusion.

sounds, commonly referred to as "echoes," that are generated within the cochlea as a result of movement of the outer hair cells. These echoes propagate outward from the cochlea, through the middle ear, to the external auditory canal. They occur spontaneously in some individuals, but for clinical purposes they are evoked by presenting a moderate-intensity acoustic stimulus by way of a small probe placed in the ear canal. The stimulus used to generate these emissions consists of a series of clicks or pairs of tones that are closely spaced in terms of their frequency. The same probe is capable of recording the low-level emissions. Results are interpreted by analyzing the absolute amplitude of the resultant waveform relative to the frequency of the stimulus as in Figure 14.6, by analyzing the amplitude relative to the noise level measured in the ear canal, and by analyzing how reproducible the responses are over repeated trials.

Generally, when OAEs are present, hearing sensitivity is normal or no worse than a mild loss (Prieve & Fitzgerald, 2002). In contrast, reduced or absent OAEs are indicative of outer hair cell dysfunction. Caution must be exercised, however, when interpreting "absent" results since conductive pathology can impede the return path of the emission in the same manner that it attenuates sound that naturally enters the auditory system.

OAE testing has several important clinical applications. Since OAEs measure the integrity of the outer hair cells, they are a powerful tool in dif-

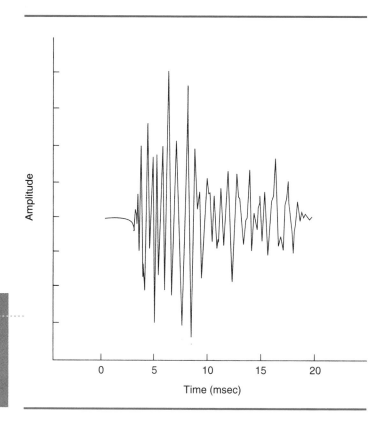

FIGURE 14.6

Example of a transient-evoked otoacoustic emission generated by a click stimulus to a normal ear.

ferentiating disorders that are cochlear in origin from those that occur beyond the cochlea, as well as differentiating disorders of the outer hair cells from those of the inner hair cells. OAEs are also useful in monitoring outer hair cell function for clients being treated with potentially ototoxic drugs such as those used in chemotherapy. Frequently, early signs of cochlear damage are revealed during OAE testing before they show up on more traditional behavioral hearing tests. This may also be the case for those who demonstrate early signs of outer hair cell damage due to excessive noise exposure (Lonsbury-Martin, 2005). Finally, since the measurement of OAEs is noninvasive and can be accomplished while a child sleeps, this powerful tool is used extensively in newborn hearing screening programs.

In addition to electroacoustic tests, several electrophysiological tests are available to the audiologist. Electrophysiological tests record neuroelectric responses (nerve impulses) generated by the auditory system in response to acoustic stimulation. These responses are collectively referred to as **auditory evoked potentials,** or **AEPs,** and can be further classified based on the anatomical site(s) where they are generated, and when they occur (measured in milliseconds) following presentation of a stimulus. Neuroelectric responses are recorded by electrodes placed at strategic points on the surface of the head while a stimulus is delivered to the ear. These tiny responses are extracted from the greater ongoing electrical brain activity using specialized computer equipment. Once the resulting waveform is recorded and displayed, analysis can occur by measuring the amplitude or height of specific peaks associated with the response, and the latency or number of milliseconds it takes to generate the various peaks following presentation of a stimulus.

Several unique types of AEPs can be recorded and evaluated by the audiologist. Through a process called **electrocochleography (ECoG),** the audiologist is able to measure auditory potentials from the cochlea and the VIIIth nerve. Recordings are made using an electrode that is either surgically placed on or near the cochlea, or positioned in the external auditory meatus. Electrocochleography has many useful applications including the monitoring of cochlear and VIIIth nerve function during surgery, and the evaluation of those suspected of having Ménière's disease.

A second type of auditory evoked potential, the **auditory brainstem response (ABR),** measures the neuroelectric activity of the auditory nerve and the brainstem. In normal ears this response is characterized by 5 to 7 distinct peaks in the waveform that occur within the first 10 milliseconds after stimulation. Although varying somewhat from person to person, these waves have a typical form with regard to their amplitude and latency that allows them to be used for diagnostic purposes (see Figure 14.7). It is thought that the first two waves reflect neuroelectric activity generated by the cochlea and VIIIth nerve, whereas the remaining waves are generated by sites within the brainstem (Jewett, Romano, & Williston, 1970). ABR testing is most useful in the estimation of auditory threshold in those who are unable or unwilling to be evaluated using conventional behavioral techniques, such as infants and young children. Testing can be conducted while the child sleeps, or in some cases under mild sedation, making this an ideal tool for early identification of hearing loss. Other applications of the ABR include neurological assessment of the central auditory nervous system including suspected cases of acoustic neuroma and multiple sclerosis.

Other types of auditory evoked potentials include the middle latency (MLR) and late responses. The middle latency responses occur approximately 10 to 80 milliseconds after stimulation while the late responses occur anywhere from 80 to 500 milliseconds after stimulation (Hood, 1998). The MLR evaluates anatomical sites spanning from the brainstem to the cortex and is more effective than the ABR in estimating auditory sensitivity for low- and mid-frequency signals. Unlike the ABR, however, the MLR is more affected by the individual's sleep state, particularly in children. Measurement of the late responses can be performed using a variety of signals including tones and speech. Responses are highly affected by the client's attention and are more effective in evaluating higher level auditory processing functions than other types of AEPs.

BEHAVIORAL TESTING

An audiometer contains numerous controls that allow for the selection, manipulation, and presentation of various stimuli used to assess hearing.

A fundamental limitation of electroacoustic and electrophysiological measures is that while they yield information about the integrity of the auditory system, they do not provide information about how the individual responds to sound. Therefore, behavioral data are necessary to fully define a hearing loss.

Most behavioral tests are administered using a specialized piece of electronic equipment called an **audiometer.** Testing is usually carried out in a specially treated sound booth that limits the penetration of extraneous noise that can interfere with hearing and thus confound the results.

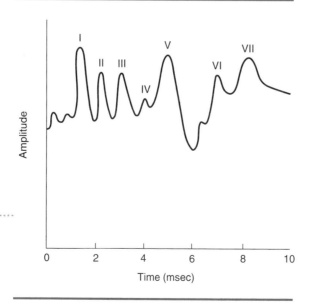

FIGURE 14.7

Schematic drawing of a typical auditory brainstem response (ABR) waveform for a normal ear.

The most basic form of behavioral assessment used with infants is a process referred to as **behavioral observation audiometry (BOA).** As the term implies, the audiologist presents a stimulus such as speech or tones through a loudspeaker and observes the child's reaction. Basic responses the audiologist looks for in response to sound are gross body movements such as startling, widening of the eyes, and facial grimacing. Cessation of movement may also indicate a response to loud sounds. Although fairly simple to administer, BOA is wrought with problems that call into question its reliability and validity (Hicks, Tharpe, & Ashmead, 2000). Making judgments as to whether a child's bodily movement was a direct response to the stimulus or haphazard in nature can be a difficult task, and the child may quickly habituate to the task, ceasing to respond after only a few presentations. Given these limitations, electroacoustic and electrophysiological tests are a better choice when assessing children younger than 5 months of age.

As a child reaches the age of 5 to 6 months, the natural ability to localize, or turn toward a sound, emerges, and the audiologist can begin to employ a technique called **visual reinforcement audiometry (VRA)** to assess behavioral responses to speech and frequency-specific tones. With VRA, the child is rewarded for a head-turn response toward the stimulus by way of an appealing visual display such as an animated or lighted toy. VRA is more reliable and less prone to problems related to habituation than BOA and has been shown to be an effective tool for accurately assessing hearing sensitivity in young children (Diefendorf, 1988).

By 2½ years of age, a child should be able to engage in testing procedures that approximate those used with an adult. The child should be able to wear earphones and can be taught to respond to pure tones using various techniques. A popular technique, referred to as **conditioned play audiometry (CPA),** involves the use of toys such as blocks, puzzle pieces, or stacking rings to engage the child in a listening game. The child is conditioned to put a block in the bucket, a ring on the post, or the like each time the test signal is heard. After a few demonstrations, most children are able to comply with the task, allowing the audiologist to obtain frequency-specific results for each ear. Conditioned play audiometry can be used until a child is able to be tested via conventional pure tone audiometry, which usually occurs somewhere around the age of 5 to 8 years.

Pure Tone Audiometry

A great deal of information can be obtained about a person's hearing through **pure tone audiometry.** In fact, the pure tone test is considered to be one of the, if not the most, fundamental behavioral tests in the standard audiometric assessment battery. **Pure tones** are sounds that contain energy only at a single frequency. Those that are routinely used in evaluating hearing sensitivity are octave frequencies ranging from 250 Hz to 8000 Hz. By following this progression from low frequency to high frequency, the integrity the cochlea spanning a broad range from apex to base is evaluated.

The purpose of pure tone testing is to determine a person's threshold at each test frequency for the right and left ears. **Threshold** is defined as the lowest (quietest) intensity level, measured in decibels, at which a person can

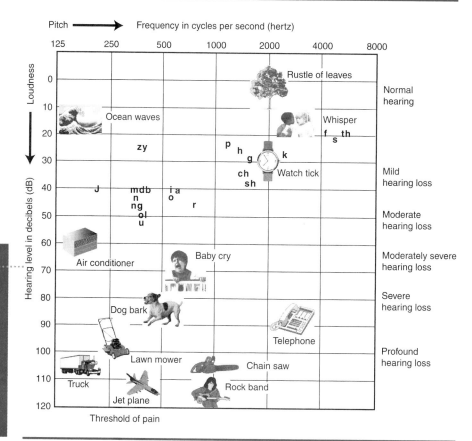

just barely detect a stimulus approximately 50 percent of the time. The audiologist measures a client's threshold by presenting a single pure tone (e.g., 1000 Hz) for approximately one second and looking for a response from the client indicating whether it was heard. Adult clients are typically instructed to raise their hand or finger or press a button to signal when they have heard the tone. Each time the tone is detected, the intensity level is reduced by 10 decibels and presented again. This process continues until the tone becomes inaudible as it reaches a level below the client's auditory threshold. Once the tone can no longer be heard, the audiologist reverses the process by increasing the intensity in 5 decibel increments until once again it becomes audible. This process of raising and lowering the intensity continues until the audiologist finds the lowest presentation level at which the person is just barely able to detect the tone approximately 50 percent of the time for a specific number of trials. Once the threshold is established for a 1000 Hz tone, the audiologist repeats the procedure at 2000 Hz, then 4000 Hz, and so forth until all of the octave frequencies ranging from 250 Hz to 8000 Hz have been tested. Under some circumstances, additional frequencies such as 125 Hz, 750 Hz, 1500, 3000 Hz, and 6000 Hz may be evaluated. Pure tone

FIGURE 14.8

Audiogram showing typical frequency range and intensity of common environmental and speech sounds. *Source:* Adapted from: J. Northern & M. Downs, 1976. *Hearing in children* (2nd ed.). Baltimore, MD: Williams and Wilkins.

threshold results are recorded by placing symbols on a graph, called an **aud-iogram.** An example of an audiogram is shown in Figure 14.8. The presence or absence of hearing loss is determined by comparing the client's thresholds to normative values for each frequency.

Auditory thresholds are established by delivering pure tones in two different ways: through **air conduction** and **bone conduction.** Air conduction testing is administered while the client wears either insert phones or earphones. Presentation by air conduction results in transmission of sound to the cochlea via the outer and middle ear. Hence, hearing loss resulting from disorders occurring within the outer, middle, or inner ear are identified in this manner. Once air conduction testing is completed, the process is repeated using a **bone oscillator;** a small vibrating device that is positioned against the skull, either on the forehead or the mastoid located directly behind the pinna. When a stimulus is presented through the oscillator, the bones of the skull are set into vibration at the same frequency. This vibration directly stimulates the cochlea by displacing the fluids encased within its two concentric labyrinths. Consequently, the person is able to hear the stimulus even though it has not directly passed through the outer or middle ear.

THOUGHT QUESTIONS

Have you ever listened to your voice on an audiotape or CD? Does it sound different to you in comparison to way you normally perceive your own speaking voice? What might explain this difference?

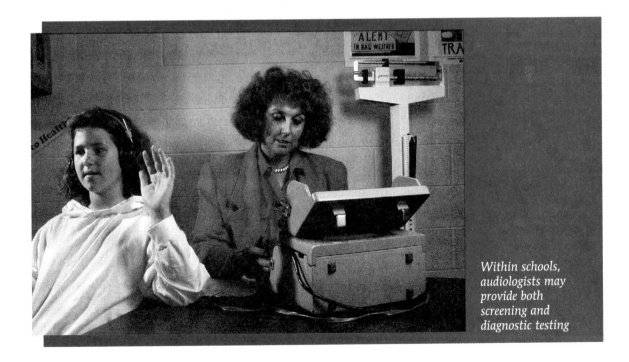

Within schools, audiologists may provide both screening and diagnostic testing

By comparing the results of air conduction testing to those obtained from bone conduction testing, it is possible to identify the type of hearing loss. Consider the audiograms in Figures 14.9 and 14.10. In Figure 14.9, the right ear air conduction thresholds (represented by the circles) fall within the moderate hearing loss range. However, the bone conduction thresholds (represented by the brackets) fall within the normal range of hearing. From this, the audiologist can infer that the client has difficulty hearing sound when it is introduced in the conventional manner through the external auditory meatus. Notice, however, that the client has no difficulty hearing sound if the outer and middle ear are bypassed and the cochlea is stimulated directly. Therefore, the conclusion can be drawn that the client is suffering from a conductive hearing loss occurring in the outer or middle ear. In Figure 14.10, both the air and bone conduction thresholds fall outside the normal limits to within the severe range. Since the results are unchanged when the inner ear is stimulated directly via bone conduction, the audiologist can conclude that the inner ear itself must be damaged. Therefore, this client is suffering from a sensorineural hearing loss.

In Figure 14.11, again both the air and bone conduction thresholds fall outside the normal range. However, the degree of hearing loss represented by

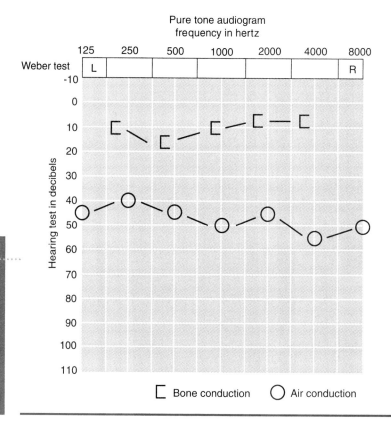

FIGURE 14.9

Audiogram representing a moderate conductive hearing loss in the right ear. (Note: The symbol used to denote bone conduction thresholds is dependent on the method used to assess it.)

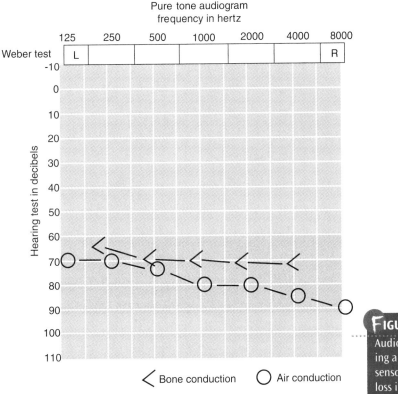

Pure tone audiogram
frequency in hertz

Weber test	125	250	500	1000	2000	4000	8000
	L						R

Hearing test in decibels

< Bone conduction   ○ Air conduction

FIGURE 14.10
Audiogram representing a severe sensorineural hearing loss in the right ear.

the air conduction thresholds is greater than the degree of hearing loss represented by the bone conduction thresholds. In this case, the audiologist concludes that while there is obvious damage to the inner ear as evidenced by the bone conduction results, the person has the potential to hear better if the outer and middle ear are bypassed. Consequently, there is evidence that both a sensorineural and a conductive hearing loss exist simultaneously. In other words, the client has a mixed hearing loss.

Speech Audiometry

Although pure tone audiometry is often considered to be the most fundamental component of an audiological evaluation, we must keep in mind that clients typically seek the services of an audiologist because they are having difficulty understanding speech, not pure tones. There are numerous tests available to assess a client's auditory skills for speech. Most are commercially available on tape or compact disc and can easily be routed through the audiometer. Use of recorded materials ensures consistency of the signal from one administration to the next, which is essential when making comparisons of an individual's performance over time or from one clinical facility to another. In some cases, such as when testing young children, the audiol-

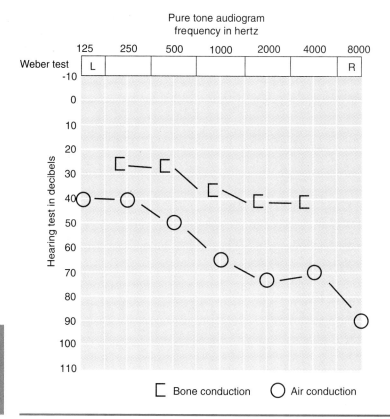

Pure tone audiogram
frequency in hertz

FIGURE 14.11

Audiogram representing a moderate to severe mixed hearing loss in the right ear.

ogist may opt to use his or her own voice to administer a test. This process is referred to as monitored live voice testing and requires the audiologist to speak into a microphone connected to the audiometer. As with any type of assessment, it is critical to select tests and materials that are age-appropriate, have normative data, and tap the specific auditory skills necessary to diagnose the problem and make appropriate recommendations for treatment and management.

It is only natural that we evaluate a client's ability both to hear and to understand speech as part of the assessment battery.

Two measures that are typically included in the speech audiometry battery are the speech recognition threshold and the word recognition test. The **speech recognition threshold (SRT)** is a measure of the lowest intensity where a person can recognize approximately 50 percent of the words presented. The speech stimuli that are used for this test are a special group of words called **spondees.** Spondees are two-syllable compound words, such as "hotdog," "birthday," or "cowboy," that are spoken with equal stress on both syllables. As the words are presented, the intensity level is systematically adjusted until the audiologist finds the lowest level where the client is able to correctly repeat approximately half of the words for a specified number of trials. The intensity level where this occurs is recorded as the SRT for a given ear. The decibel value of the SRT should closely agree with the average of the pure tone threshold values for 500 Hz, 1000 Hz, and 2000 Hz. When there is poor agreement between the pure tone data and the SRT, the audiologist may begin to question the accuracy of the results. The SRT may also be used as an estimate of overall hearing sensitivity when pure tone results cannot be obtained or are incomplete, such as with younger children and adults who are unable to comply with the pure tone test protocol. A demonstration of SRT testing can be viewed on the book's CD-ROM.

A second measure routinely conducted as part of the speech audiometry battery is the **word recognition test (WRT).** The WRT is different from the other procedures discussed so far in that it is not a measure of sensitivity, per se. Instead, the WRT assesses how well the client is able to identify words presented at some level above threshold. The speech stimuli that are used in the WRT are also different from those used to assess a client's SRT in that they are taken from lists of one-syllable, **phonetically balanced (PB)** words. Each speech sound is incorporated into the word list in the same proportion in which it appears in everyday language.

The intensity level at which the WRT is administered will vary depending on the type of information that is of interest. It is often desirable to determine maximal word recognition performance because this may be helpful in determining the potential for improvement if the client is ultimately fitted with hearing aids that amplify the speech signal.

Obviously, most conversational exchanges consist of connected discourse rather than single-syllable words that are unrelated to one another. To address these limitations, a variety of speech tests have been developed that incorporate sentence-length stimuli. Several have been recorded with competing background noise to evaluate those who complain of difficulty hearing in noisy places, or they contain sentence lists recorded with and without visual cues to determine how much a client benefits when listening and speechreading are combined compared to listening alone. These types of tests hold considerable promise in presenting an overall picture of how an individual functions under conditions that are more representative of real-world settings.

Auditory Processing Assessment.

Although the audiologist is the professional responsible for the diagnosis of auditory processing disorders, assessing an individual for a possible auditory processing disorder requires a multidisciplinary approach. Typically, personnel involved in the assessment process include the audiologist, who administers specific auditory tests of the peripheral and central auditory pathways; the speech-language pathologist, who assesses the individual's expressive and receptive oral language skills; the psychologist, who assesses cognitive function; and when dealing with children, various school personnel, who provide input on academic performance and the functional impact of the problem.

Numerous auditory tests are available, both behavioral and electrophysiological, to evaluate a variety of auditory processes. The overall goal is not just simply to determine whether an auditory processing disorder exists, but to analyze the nature of the disorder in order to recommend appropriate strategies for treatment and management. In each case, therefore, it is critical to design an individualized assessment plan that taps the specific characteristics or deficits demonstrated by the individual. No single test can adequately assess all levels of the central auditory system or all aspects of auditory processing. Instead, a battery approach is necessary. Unfortunately, because of the high degree of variability associated with the maturation of the auditory system in younger children, most behavioral tests for APD are generally not appropriate for those under the age of 7 years. In addition, impairment of the peripheral auditory system may affect the results obtained on some auditory processing tests; therefore, assessment of the peripheral system is a prerequisite.

While it is beyond the scope of this chapter to present all of the tests available for inclusion in an individualized assessment battery, it is helpful to discuss some of the general types of measures frequently administered in the evaluation of the central auditory nervous system. One general type consists of what are called **dichotic** measures. Dichotic tests involve the simultaneous presentation of different stimuli to each ear. Depending on the specific test, stimuli may consist of digits (numbers), consonant-vowel pairs, words, or sentences. The individual may be asked to direct his or her attention to only one ear and identify what is heard, or attend to and identify what is heard in both ears. These types of tasks assess the person's ability to separate or integrate the competing signals.

A second general type of measure includes tests of temporal processing. These tests are used to evaluate a client's ability to process timing cues associated with speech, such as ordering and sequencing. Specific tests may require the individual to identify differences in the duration pattern (e.g., long-long-short, or long-short-long) for a series of three tones or clicks, differences in the frequency pattern (e.g., high-high-low, or high-low-high) for a series of three tones, or the presence of short gaps separating pairs of tones or clicks.

A third general type of auditory processing measure involves what is referred to as monaural low-redundancy speech. These tests are termed "monaural" because the stimulus is directed to only one ear. Low-redundancy means that the stimulus has been altered to reduce the speech signal's inherent redundancy and to tax the auditory system of clients with auditory processing deficits who often demonstrate increased difficulty in the ability to fill in the missing information when the signal is compromised. For example, acoustic energy above a specific frequency is filtered out, rate of speech is altered, or speech is presented in various levels of background noise or reverberation.

The final general type of measure are those that assess **binaural integration,** which is the process of assimilating different information presented to each ear into a single unit. For example, a portion of a one- or two-syllable word may be presented to the left ear while another portion is presented to the right ear. The individual must combine the two components in order to identify the target word.

While behavioral tests such as those mentioned above are the most popular means of assessing auditory processing function, the incorporation of electrophysiological measures such as the auditory brainstem response and the middle and late responses into the assessment battery can be extremely useful. Due to neuromaturation of the central auditory nervous system and the contributions of learning, it is critical that any test administered be scored according to age-appropriate normative data. Also, it is critical that all data collected be interpreted in conjunction with the test results obtained by the other specialists within the multidisciplinary team.

AURAL HABILITATION/REHABILITATION

Once the audiological assessment has been completed and the test results analyzed, it is time to recommend and implement an appropriate course of treatment. This may entail referral to a physician for a medical evaluation. It may also entail various therapeutic services referred to as **aural habilitation/rehabilitation,** which can be defined as "intervention aimed at minimizing and alleviating the communication difficulties associated with hearing loss" (Tye-Murray, 2004, p. 2).

Before discussing the specific intervention options available, it is important to differentiate the terms *aural habilitation* and *aural rehabilitation*. The term *aural habilitation* refers to intervention that is conducted with individuals whose hearing loss occurred at an early age and therefore prevented the normal development of auditory and spoken language skills. In general, this refers to services and therapies used primarily with children who are prelingually hearing-impaired. The focus of aural habilitation is to teach those skills that are missing. In contrast, *aural rehabilitation* refers to services and therapies provided to individuals who have lost their hearing later in life, after spoken language skills have fully developed. In this case, the focus is on preservation and restoration of communication skills that have been negatively impacted by a loss of hearing. Despite these differences, the term *aural rehabilitation* is frequently used by professionals to refer to both habilitative and rehabilitative aspects of intervention and for the sake of convenience, will be used during the remainder of this section.

No discussion of aural rehabilitation should begin without also mentioning an important concept that has received considerable attention in recent years. That is the concept of **evidence-based practice.** Evidence-based practice is the process whereby a clinician makes important decisions regarding individual client care and specific courses of treatment based on current, well-designed research pertaining to the therapeutic options under consideration. Failure to adhere to the principles of evidenced-based practice may lead to inappropriate recommendations regarding treatment, which in turn may limit the individual's progress, waste time and money, and ultimately cause him or her to question the competency of the professional.

An important first step in the aural rehabilitation process is to identify, describe, and clarify the individual's communication problems resulting from his or her hearing loss. This can usually be accomplished by synthesizing information obtained from the case history interview, self-assessment questionnaires, and results of the audiometric test battery. By identifying the

Before recommending any form of intervention, clinicians must be confident that current research supports the efficacy of such measures in the treatment of hearing loss.

specific needs of the individual and selecting treatment methods using principles of evidence-based practice, both the client and the clinician can feel confident that the rehabilitation process will proceed based on the best available information.

Audiologists may find themselves working closely with professionals from other areas in the development of a comprehensive aural rehabilitation program. Depending on the specific needs of the individual, this may include medical personnel, speech-language pathologists, special education teachers, teachers of the deaf and hard of hearing, psychologists, and vocational rehabilitation counselors.

The overall goal of most aural rehabilitation programs is to improve functional communication. Typically, key areas considered when designing an individualized program include amplification, assistive listening devices, auditory training, communication strategy training, and communication methodology, to name a few. Depending on the degree to which the hearing loss affects communication, goals will be developed relative to one or more of these areas. We will address each of these separately, but it should be emphasized that many of these areas are routinely attended to at the same time since work in one area may have implications for performance in others.

AMPLIFICATION

Amplification is often considered to be the heart of most aural rehabilitation plans. The success of other treatment strategies incorporated into the plan is often predicated on the use of appropriate amplification. Therefore, one of the first steps in the aural rehabilitation process is the selection, fitting, and evaluation of amplification. In most cases amplification consists of personal **hearing aids,** although as we will later see, other amplification options are available.

Hearing Aids

Hearing aids come in a variety of styles and sizes ranging from tiny custom models that fit entirely within the external auditory canal to larger instruments that are worn behind the ear (see Figure 14.12). Regardless of the style, every hearing aid contains three basic components: a microphone, an amplifier, and a receiver. The microphone picks up acoustic energy from the environment, converts it to an electrical signal, and sends it to the amplifier. The amplifier increases the voltage of the electrical signal and sends it to the receiver, which, in turn, converts it back into acoustic energy and routes it to the user's ear canal.

The majority of hearing aids dispensed today incorporate sophisticated digital signal processing. Sound entering the hearing aid is converted into a digital code that can be uniquely processed by applying a series of mathematical formulas. These formulas allow the signal to be manipulated in various ways to improve audibility while maintaining comfort, reduce background noise, and eliminate acoustic feedback.

Most modern hearing aids are adjusted, or programmed, using a computer and special software. Many new hearing aids contain directional mi-

FIGURE 14.12
Styles of hearing aids.
(Photos courtesy of
Siemens Hearing
Instruments.)

crophone technology consisting of two or more microphones that automatically suppresses background noise originating from in back of, or to the side of, the user. Some hearing aids even incorporate a handheld remote control that allows the user to adjust the volume or turn the hearing aid on and off.

The primary goal in most hearing aid fittings is to make speech audible to the user in order to improve intelligibility. This is not a simple task since people often have greater hearing loss at some frequencies compared to others. In addition, some frequencies, such as those in the higher range, are more critical in making speech intelligible and may require more amplification. These factors must be taken into account when determining how much amplification to provide. Additionally, while the overall goal is to make speech audible, it is essential that the amplified signal never becomes uncomfortably loud for the user or cause additional trauma to the auditory system.

Unlike eyeglasses, which can restore a person's sight to 20/20, a hearing aid will not return hearing to normal. Although audibility for speech should improve, the amplified signal may not necessarily restore its clarity. When a person is considering amplification, it is critical that he or she be counseled on this point so as not to develop unrealistic expectations. It usually takes time, training, and practice before a person can become a successful, full-time hearing aid user. As part of the counseling process, the audiologist will also instruct the client on hearing aid care and maintenance and how to properly adjust the controls for different listening situations. Specific strategies designed to facilitate listening are also reviewed. If the audiologist does not take the time to cover this information, more than likely the hearing aids will end up in the dresser drawer. A demonstration of hearing aid counseling can be seen on the book's CD-ROM.

It has been estimated that only 20 percent of those who may possibly benefit from hearing aids actually use them. Why do you think this is the case? Why are people more willing to wear eyeglasses than hearing aids?

THOUGHT QUESTIONS

One alternative to traditional hearing aids is a device called a **middle ear implant.** Components of this device are implanted into the middle ear cavity and attached to the ossicular chain. The implant amplifies sound by mechanically "driving" the ossicular chain. The amplified signal is transmitted to the inner ear and processed in the usual manner. Compared to traditional hearing aids, middle ear implants may provide users with improved sound quality, reduced acoustic feedback, greater comfort, and greater cosmetic appeal.

Those with conductive hearing losses that are not medically treatable, such as atresia, may benefit from a bone conduction hearing aid. This device consists of a headband and bone vibrator coupled to a conventional hearing aid. With the bone vibrator placed firmly against the skull, sound is converted to mechanical vibration that stimulates the inner ear, bypassing the impaired outer or middle ear. A newer version of this device, called a **bone anchored hearing aid (BAHA),** functions in the same manner but consists of a small titanium screw that is surgically implanted into the skull behind the pinna. A small, external device containing the microphone and other electronic components attaches to the screw and converts sound to mechanical vibration that stimulates the cochlea via bone conduction.

Cochlear Implants.

Some people with severe-to-profound hearing losses receive little or no benefit from traditional hearing aids. For this select group, a cochlear implant (Figure 14.13) may be an option. A cochlear implant is a neural prosthesis designed to bypass the damaged hair cells of the cochlea and directly stimulate the surviving auditory nerve fibers with electrical energy.

A cochlear implant consists of externally worn and internally implanted components. The external components consist of the microphone, speech processor, and external transmitter. The internal components include the receiver-stimulator that is surgically coupled to the skull and the electrode array that is inserted approximately 22 to 30 mm into the cochlea. In the past, only one ear was implanted. Today, many individuals are being considered for bilateral implantation.

Let's take a closer look at how a cochlear implant works. The microphone is typically positioned on the head, at or near the pinna. It picks up sound, converts it to electrical energy, and transmits it to the speech processor. The speech processor is a sophisticated microcomputer that is custom programmed for each user to maximize reception of the speech signal. Only certain aspects of the input signal are sent to the cochlea. These are defined by the processing scheme, or coding strategy, incorporated into the device. The intent is to send the impaired ear those features of the speech signal that are critical to intelligibility. Most of the newer speech processors are worn behind the ear. The coded signal is sent through a cable to the external transmitting coil that is magnetically secured to the head. Using FM radio waves, the signal is transmitted across the skin to the internal receiver-stimulator and finally to the individual electrodes implanted in the cochlea. Modern cochlear implants contain multiple electrodes that provide electrical stimulation to many sites along the basilar membrane, taking advantage

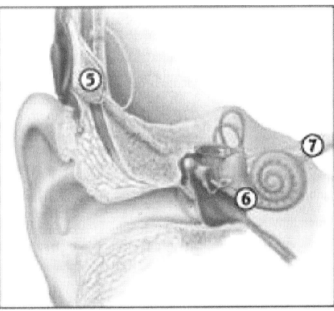

FIGURE 14.13

Schematic depicting the components of an ear-level cochlear implant (1) microphone, (2) speech processor, (3) transmitting cable, (4) transmitting coil, (5) receiver-stimulator, (6) electrode array, (7) VIIIth nerve. (Courtesy of Cochlear Corporation, Inc.)

of the way the cochlea naturally codes frequency information. The resulting neural impulses are transmitted to the brain in the usual manner via the ascending auditory pathways.

Originally, only adults who were postlingually deafened were candidates. Today, however, cochlear implant surgery is routinely conducted on severely to profoundly hearing impaired children as young as 12 months and adults of all ages, including those with prelingual as well as postlingual hearing losses. Postlingually deafened adults tend to benefit extensively because they can more readily make use of the auditory cues provided by the device. Children who are implanted at an early age and receive intensive auditory therapy also demonstrate significant gains relative to speech perception (Waltzman & Cohen, 1998).

It is important to understand that a cochlear implant will not restore a person's hearing to normal and that the degree of benefit will vary significantly from one recipient to another. Some rely on the device strictly to provide greater awareness of environmental sounds. Others find that the device provides sufficient auditory cues to enhance their ability to speechread. Some individuals are able to understand connected speech without visual cues including over the phone. The degree of benefit obtained from a cochlear implant depends on many factors, including when the person became deaf (prelingually or postlingually), the amount of time between when they became deaf and received an implant, the number of surviving auditory nerve fibers available for stimulation, and the scope and quality of aural rehabilitation services administered following implantation, to name just a few. Given the impressive results demonstrated by many recipients—young children in particular—it is clear that the number of individuals receiving cochlear implants will continue to grow significantly over the next decade. Speech-language pathologists and audiologists must be prepared to provide aural rehabilitation services to these individuals in order to maximize their spoken language skills.

THOUGHT QUESTIONS

Are you curious what it sounds like to hear through a cochlear implant? Go to www.ucihs.uci.edu/hesp/simulations/simulationsmain.htm to listen to some simulations. What does it sound like? Are you able to understand what is being said? What factors might influence someone's performance with this device?

ASSISTIVE LISTENING DEVICES

Assistive listening devices (ALDs) are another category of amplification that is routinely incorporated into the aural rehabilitation plan. While hearing aids and cochlear implants provide benefit in many situations, it is not uncommon for users to experience difficulty in certain environments. Use of an assistive listening device can be helpful in overcoming these problems in settings such as classrooms, restaurants, meeting rooms, and auditoriums.

The principle behind most ALDs is to position the microphone of the device in close proximity to the desired sound source. For example, the microphone can be clipped to the talker's lapel or placed in the center of a conference table, increasing the intensity of the desired signal compared to unwanted noise in the background. Using various types of wired or wireless technology, the signal is delivered directly to the listener via headphones or to their hearing aid or cochlear implant. In many cases, use of an ALD allows the listener to be seated at a significant distance, yet be able to hear as if positioned right next to the talker.

One type of ALD that is very popular, particularly in educational settings, is the personal **FM system.** The talker speaks into a small lapel or headset microphone that is attached to a body-worn transmitter and "broadcasts" on a designated frequency or channel. The hearing-impaired listener wears a receiver tuned to the same FM frequency as the transmitter. In cases where the person uses a hearing aid or cochlear implant, the FM receiver can be coupled to the instrument using a special audio cable or through an electromagnetic induction device called a **telecoil** that is located inside the hearing aid or speech processor. A few manufacturers have introduced hearing aids that contain a built-in FM receiver or accept a small FM "boot" receiver that plugs into the hearing aid, eliminating the need for cumbersome cords and conspicuous body-worn devices.

Another type of ALD that is also widely used in schools is **sound field amplification.** Similar to personal FM, sound field amplification consists of a lapel or boom microphone that is worn by the talker (often a teacher) and a wireless transmitter. The main difference, however, is that instead of broadcasting the signal to individual receivers, the signal is sent to loudspeakers that are strategically placed around the room. Small, portable desktop speakers are also available. The primary advantage of sound field amplification over other types of systems is that all students in the room can benefit.

A variety of ALDs are available for specialized applications such as TV and telephone listening. For those who have losses so severe that they do not benefit from amplification, specialized devices are available that alert the user, usually by way of a flashing light, of important sounds in the environment. For example, devices are available that visually alert the person of a ringing phone, alarm clock, smoke detector, or baby cry. For phone communication, deaf callers often rely on a portable keyboard called a **teletypewriter (TTY)** that allows text conversations to be conducted over regular phone lines. In recent years the Internet has played a significant role in expanding communication options for those who are deaf by allowing them to converse through email, instant messaging, synchronous chat, and videoconferencing. Last but not least, many deaf people look to the assistance and companionship of a "hearing dog" to facilitate receptive communication. Similar to guide dogs for the visually impaired, a hearing dog is trained to alert its master to important sounds in the environment such as the doorbell, microwave, or smoke alarm.

> The FM system operates on the same principle as traditional FM radio.

AUDITORY TRAINING

Once a client has been fitted with an appropriate amplification device, he or she may need to be taught or retaught how to use his or her remaining hearing through some type of structured listening practice. This process is referred to as auditory training. The goal of auditory training is to maximize a person's use of their residual hearing to enhance the perception of speech and nonspeech cues (Schow & Nerbonne, 2002). Improvements in auditory perceptual skills should lead to progress in other areas, including speech and language development and academic achievement.

When developing an individualized auditory training plan, it is important to consider the individual's degree of hearing loss and whether he or she is prelingually or postlingually hearing impaired. In most cases, intensive auditory training activities are conducted with children, particularly those who have recently received hearing aids or cochlear implants. Prelingually hearing-impaired adults, particularly those with severe to profound losses who have begun using amplification for the first time or are resuming amplification after many years of nonuse, may also benefit from structured listening practice.

Development of an individualized training program usually begins with a thorough assessment of the person's auditory perceptual skills. This type of assessment goes beyond what is routinely conducted as part of the basic audiological evaluation previously described. Several commercially available tools are available that assess a wide variety of perceptual skills, ranging from simple phoneme awareness to comprehension of connected discourse. In some cases it is helpful to administer speech perception tests that evaluate how well a person makes use of visual as well as auditory cues to determine how well he or she is able integrate the two modalities to facilitate receptive communication.

Many of the instruments that assess auditory perceptual skills are components of larger, comprehensive auditory training curricula. Some of these programs have been designed specifically for hearing-impaired children, including infants with severe to profound losses. These curricula are developmentally based and are designed to be integrated into the child's overall speech and language treatment plan. Many of these programs are designed specifically for the home, with the child's family assuming an active role in the training process.

Although there is no universally recommended approach to auditory training, one of the most widely used models is appropriate for children and adults and can be used for visual as well as auditory perceptual training (Erber, 1982). The general framework of this model is a matrix comprised of two distinct variables: the complexity of the training stimulus and the complexity of the perceptual task. Stimulus complexity is arranged in hierarchical order from environmental sounds and suprasegmental aspects of speech to consonants and vowels, syllables, words, phrases, sentences, and ultimately more complex forms of connected discourse. The most basic perceptual task is detection or awareness—that is, being able to determine the presence or absence of a stimulus. The basic premise is that a stimulus cannot be processed unless it can be detected. Therefore, at this level the task is to determine which environmental (e.g., telephone ring, smoke alarm) or speech sounds are audible to the individual. Auditory awareness is followed by the next level, auditory discrimination, whereby a person makes judgments as to whether pairs of stimuli are the same or different. For example, when presented with the syllable pair /pa/ - /sa/, the client must determine whether they sound the same. This can be done for environmental sounds, words, phrases, and sentences as well. At the next level, training focuses on identification, whereby the client must label what he or she hears, such as by repeating or pointing to a picture representing the target. The final level, comprehension, focuses on the person's ability to understand the meaning of the spoken message.

This model is highly flexible in that it can be adapted for use in a variety of settings, and training activities can be infused into many facets of an individual's daily routine such as listening in the classroom or on the phone. In addition, it can accommodate a variety of materials that are geared specifically to the individual, making the process both interesting and relevant. Although some levels of this model are characterized by significant drill and practice, it is flexible enough to allow clinicians to incorporate listening activities that are less formal.

COMMUNICATION STRATEGY TRAINING

Most adults with hearing loss can improve their conversational interactions through the use of specific strategies designed to facilitate communication or repair breakdowns that occur during the course of a conversation (Tye-Murray, 2004). Demonstrating and practicing how to implement these strategies is a major component of most adult aural rehabilitation programs. The ultimate goal is for clients to efficiently and effectively manage communication problems that arise during their daily activities.

As part of the training process, clients must first increase their awareness of the various environmental barriers that may preclude successful communication, including background noise, poor lighting, and distance. Clients are taught to recognize these obstacles and assertively, yet tactfully, request appropriate modifications such as turning off a radio in the background, adjusting the lighting, or moving to another location. In addition, the hearing-impaired listener may need to ask the talker to modify his or her speaking behavior by slowing down, speaking louder, or facing them in order to facilitate speechreading. Simply revealing one's hearing loss to the talker can facilitate communication since it raises awareness that accommodations may be necessary.

Another critical component of communication strategy training is to teach clients to anticipate or predict what is likely to be said during a conversation. Walking into your favorite fast food restaurant, you can probably guess the types of questions, statements, and vocabulary the person behind the counter will use. By anticipating what is likely to be said based on the context of the conversation and the environment, clients can eliminate vocabulary that is unlikely to be spoken, allowing them to better predict the message and fill in any missing pieces. Having a good handle on the English language is extremely helpful as it allows the hearing-impaired person to predict a missed word by analyzing the grammatical structure of the utterance. For example, if the talker says "Let's go to the movies" but the hearing-impaired person misses the final word, knowing the grammatical rules of English enables the listener to realize that the missed word must be a noun, limiting the number of possible choices to some degree. Having a good understanding of semantics limits the number of choices even further.

For most of us, when we miss what someone has said, we usually respond with "what?" or "pardon?" to indicate that we would like the talker to repeat the message. Although not very instructive, this type of response is quick to implement and fairly effective for those with normal hearing. Asking for repetition, however, is usually not as effective for a hearing-impaired person, since it tends to elicit a rote response that provides no additional information. A more effective strategy is for the hearing-impaired individual to ask for the message to be rephrased, which may provide enough additional information to facilitate comprehension. Other effective repair strategies include asking the talker to provide a key word, identify the topic of the conversation, provide additional information, or restate the message using less complex syntax and terminology. Gestures and writing may also be helpful in repairing a breakdown. The end result is likely to be a more fluent conversational exchange between the hearing-impaired person and those with whom he or she interacts with on a regular basis.

TREATMENT AND MANAGEMENT OF AUDITORY PROCESSING DISORDERS

> The treatment and management of APD must be based on the findings obtained as part of a comprehensive evaluation.

As you recall from our earlier discussion, auditory processing disorders refer to deficits of the central auditory nervous system that affect one's ability to efficiently and effectively use and interpret auditory information. No single form of treatment is appropriate for all cases. It is therefore necessary to develop an individualized intervention plan. Treatment generally encompasses three general areas: environmental accommodations, compensatory strategies, and direct skills remediation.

Environmental accommodations provide the individual with greater access to auditory information. This may be accomplished by acoustically treating a room to reduce noise and reverberation, seating the individual closer to the sound source, fitting the individual with a personal FM or sound field system, or providing written notes to supplement verbal information. Accommodations may also include a variety of instructional techniques such as speaking clearly at a moderate rate, providing clear and concise directions, using familiar vocabulary and simple sentence structure, breaking utterances into smaller segments, and having the individual repeat critical information to ensure comprehension.

Compensatory strategies are introduced to strengthen higher order resources including attention, language, and cognition. This may include the use of memory and organizational techniques such as chunking, reauditorization, mnemonics, visualization, and written reminders. It may also focus on making use of linguistic and contextual cues to predict what is likely to be said in order to facilitate auditory closure.

Finally, direct skills remediation involves intensive auditory training designed to eliminate or reduce auditory deficits. Activities are selected that address the specific auditory deficits identified and may include formal exercises involving auditory discrimination, localization, temporal sequencing, sound blending, and understanding speech in noise, to name a few. Direct skills remediation may take place during individual sessions with the audiologist or speech-language pathologist. Various curricula and computer-based programs are also available for individualized training outside the clinic environment, including the home.

COMMUNICATION MODALITY

Communication options for people with hearing loss can be generally divided into two major categories: those that utilize spoken communication or speaking and listening and those that utilize manual communication or sign language. A third category, referred to as total communication, combines features common to both. Proponents of spoken communication advocate for the use of speech and audition to facilitate adjustment to the hearing world. It is their feeling that learning to communicate orally provides hearing-impaired children with a greater number of social, educational, and vocational options during the course of their lifetime. In contrast, proponents of manual communication argue that children who learn to sign are able to communicate more quickly without frustration and therefore are able to learn at a faster pace. Advocates of manual communication also believe that signing serves to facilitate socialization with, and acceptance by, a child's hearing-impaired peers, which ultimately has a positive impact on self-concept and self-esteem.

The decision regarding which method of communication to embrace is one of the most difficult involved in the treatment and management process, especially for those with losses in the severe-to-profound range. Many factors need to be considered, such as the amount of residual hearing, the individual's language and cognitive abilities, manual dexterity, and personal preference. The preference of the family is especially important when working with hearing-impaired children because there are numerous complex personal and philosophical issues that must be considered. As previously discussed, for a deaf child of Deaf parents, language is not just a means of communication; it is also a cultural trait. Some Deaf families actively oppose the use of speech or total communication, firmly believing that ASL is the best option for their deaf children. On the other hand, many parents aspire for their children to communicate using speech and don't want to pursue a method of communication that will cause them to appear different from their normal-hearing peers. Since family support is critical to the success of either method, speech-language pathologists and audiologists may need to counsel the family as to the various options available. Consequently, professionals must be sensitive to all aspects surrounding the communication issue and be prepared, if necessary, to advocate in the best interests of the child. It is beyond the scope of this chapter to discuss these issues with the depth required to do them justice. Rather, a brief overview of the nature of spoken and manual communication will be provided.

Spoken Communication Options

The vast majority of people with hearing loss communicate through spoken language. This is not so much an indication that spoken communication is superior to manual forms of communication as it is a recognition that the majority of hearing losses are no worse than moderately severe in degree and most of these individuals have sufficient residual hearing to be able to use this modality both receptively and expressively.

The best candidates for this option are those who are consistent users of amplification. Speechreading skills are also taken into consideration. There are differing opinions on this issue, however. Some professionals believe that speechreading ability is an inherent skill and therefore should not be a determining factor in choosing a communication mode. Others believe that speechreading can be taught through formal instruction, and therefore speechreading training is incorporated into the overall goals of the aural rehabilitation plan.

In terms of communication methods designed to promote the development of spoken language skills, there are currently two approaches that have received considerable attention. The primary goal of each is to develop speech and communication skills necessary for successful integration into the hearing world.

The overall goal of the **auditory/verbal** approach is the development of spoken language through audition by focusing on the use of residual hearing with amplification. Since this approach strives to maximize an individual's listening skills, no forms of manual communication are used and the individual is discouraged from relying on speechreading. During training activities this is accomplished by having parents and therapists eliminate the use of visual cues in order to promote reliance on listening alone. This approach has been used extensively with children by way of one-on-one therapy and family-centered teaching activities designed to facilitate the early, consistent, and successful use of amplification.

Similar to the auditory/verbal approach, the **auditory/oral** approach teaches the individual to make maximum use of his of her residual hearing through amplification. Where it differs, however, is that it also emphasizes the use of visual cues such as speechreading to facilitate receptive communication. The use of any forms of manual communication, other than natural gestures, is strongly discouraged.

Both approaches require extensive training and practice. The individual must be immersed in a speech-intensive environment both at home and at school, with the consistent use of appropriate amplification strictly enforced. Therefore, a strong commitment on behalf of the family is essential.

Manual Communication Options

For those whose residual hearing is insufficient to make use of the acoustic speech signal, even through amplification, some form of manual communication is usually necessary. Manual communication or sign language allows information to be conveyed visually by way of the hands and has long been used by large numbers of deaf individuals to communicate with each other.

Manual communication can occur in isolation or in combination with speech, a process referred to as **simultaneous communication.** Individual signs are formed through the combination of four distinct parameters: hand shape, location of the hands relative to the body and to each other, palm orientation, and movement. Simply by altering any one of these parameters can significantly change the meaning of a sign. In addition, the meaning can be changed by varying the size, intensity, speed, and duration of the sign. Also of importance in conveying meaning are nonmanual cues such as facial expression, body position, head tilt, and eye gaze. These cues are particularly important for expressing feelings and emotions, for conveying spatial relationships between people and objects, and for differentiating statements, questions, and commands.

ASL is a language unto itself rather than a visual representation of an existing language such as English.

When attempting to distinguish the array of manual communication systems available, it is helpful to view them along a continuum bounded by forms of manually coded English (e.g., Signing Exact English) at one end and American Sign Language (ASL) at the opposite end (see Table 14.2). The origin of ASL can be traced to France, and it was subsequently introduced to the United States in 1815 by Thomas Gallaudet. It is very much a conceptual

TABLE 14.2
Sign-language continuum

Manually Coded English Signing Systems ⟶		American Sign Language (ASL)
Signed Exact English (SEE)	Pidgin Signed English (PSE)	
Word meaning is NOT considered (e.g., the word "right" will have the same sign regardless of context).	Signs used are more conceptual. One word may have many signs depending upon meaning.	Has its own vocabulary, grammar, and sentence structure. One sign may represent an entire thought.
All grammatical markers (articles, auxiliary verbs, plurals, etc.) are signed.	Grammatical markers may or may not be signed.	Does not have specific signs for grammatical markers.
	Facial expression and gestures are incorporated.	Facial expression, body position, space, and repetition are used extensively.

language with a single sign having the capability of conveying an entire thought, and since ASL and English are distinct languages with different grammatical structures, one cannot simultaneously speak syntactically correct English sentences while using ASL. An interesting aspect of ASL is that unlike most primary languages, it is usually learned from deaf peers since only 10 percent of children who are born deaf have deaf parents.

Pidgin Signed English (PSE) is an intermediate variety of the languages of ASL and English. In general, PSE is characterized by the use of ASL signs with English word order, thus preserving the conceptual integrity of ASL while integrating English syntax. PSE is usually the type of manual communication taught in basic sign curricula for hearing people interested in learning to sign.

Other forms of manual communication, referred to as **manually coded English,** have been developed for use with deaf children in educational settings to more accurately replicate spoken English. Unlike natural languages, these sign systems are contrived and operate under the premise that competency in spoken and written English is critical for academic achievement. Manually coded English uses two types of gestures: sign vocabulary, most of which comes from ASL, to visually represent English words and sign markers that visually represent English grammatical principles including common affixes (e.g., -ly and -ing). Signs are produced in the exact order in which they are spoken, which allows English to be modeled using visual and auditory modalities. Several systems have been developed, and although there are subtle differences among each, their main purpose is to accurately represent spoken English in a manual form.

Two additional forms of manual communication are **fingerspelling** and **Cued Speech.** Fingerspelling consists of distinct handshapes used to vi-

Preschool children may pose a special challenge for the audiologist.

sually represent each of the twenty-six letters of the English alphabet. Although not very efficient, since each letter of a word must be manually produced, fingerspelling is routinely incorporated into ASL, PSE, and Signed English systems to make reference to proper names, technical vocabulary, English words that have no corresponding sign, and words and concepts where the signer does not know the formal sign.

Cued Speech is a manual communication system designed to overcome the ambiguity associated with speechreading. One's dependence on visual cues provided through speechreading tends to increase as the degree of hearing loss becomes more severe. Unfortunately, by itself, speechreading is not an efficient means of receptive communication because approximately 50 percent of speech sounds are visually indistinguishable. For example, consider the sounds /p/, /b/, and /m/. If you look in the mirror and produce all three, you will notice that visually there are no differences. These sounds are referred to as **homophenous** because they look alike on the lips. Likewise, the words "palm," "bomb," and "mom" are visually indistinguishable and would be difficult to differentiate without the use of audition. This is the type of problem people encounter when their hearing loss prevents them from making fine distinctions between sounds that look alike.

Cued Speech was developed by Dr. Richard Orin Cornett in 1966 as a means of helping hearing-impaired persons identify speech sounds that are visually similar, as well as those that are not readily visible such as /g/ and /k/. Cued Speech combines the natural movements of the mouth produced while speaking with "cues" formed using eight unique hand shapes and four hand positions relative to the face. This system is designed to facilitate speechreading and the development of language and literacy skills. Users must have a good grasp of phonetics in order to effectively use Cued Speech, which may be why it is not as popular as other forms of manual communication.

*W*hy is knowledge of ASL useful for both audiologists and speech-language pathologists? Does your college offer courses in ASL? Do you think they should fulfill foreign language requirements? Why or why not?

SUMMARY

The profession of audiology is a richly diverse field that offers the opportunity to work with many populations in a wide variety of settings. The audiologist has the responsibility for assessing auditory and vestibular function and for providing aural habilitation/rehabilitation services. A hearing loss is caused by an interruption at one or more points along the auditory pathway. The three types of hearing loss that affect the peripheral auditory system are conductive, sensorineural, and mixed. Audiologists are also concerned with problems affecting the central auditory nervous system, including the brainstem, the subcortical auditory pathways, and the auditory cortex of the brain. Problems along these pathways generally result in an inability to efficiently and effectively use and interpret auditory information, referred to as an auditory processing disorder.

When describing a hearing loss, audiologists use terminology such as conductive, sensorineural, mixed, and central to identify the portion of the auditory system that has been affected. Another important set of terms describe the degree of hearing loss measured in decibels. Each degree of hearing loss refers to a specific decibel range. Individuals with hearing loss in the mild to moderately severe range are often referred to as hard of hearing and depend as much as possible upon the use of residual hearing for communication. For people with a severe to profound hearing loss, often referred to as "deaf," the auditory system provides little or no access to sound without proper amplification.

When evaluating the auditory system, audiologists rely on electroacoustic, electrophysiological, and behavioral measures. A battery of tests is administered to identify the presence of a hearing loss, determine its type, quantify its degree, and determine its impact on communication. Informational and personal adjustment counseling are critical to the entire process.

Aural habilitation/rehabilitation refers to the services and procedures that are designed to minimize and alleviate communication difficulties presented by a hearing loss. Aural habilitation alludes to therapies that are used primarily with children to teach missing communication skills, while aural rehabilitation refers to services provided to those who have lost their hearing later in life, after spoken communication skills have been established. The focus of aural rehabilitation is to help the person recover lost skills and to effectively use compensatory strategies. Areas typically considered in creating an individual aural rehabilitation program are the evaluation and fitting of amplification and assistive listening devices, auditory training, communication strategy training, and determination of an appropriate mode of communication.

REFLECTIONS

- In what settings are audiologists employed?
- What are the main functions of the outer, middle, and inner ear?
- Explain the differences between conductive, sensorineural, and mixed hearing loss.
- Explain how disorders of the peripheral auditory system differ from those of the central auditory system.
- What are some causes of different types of hearing loss?
- What affects can hearing loss have on communication and psychosocial well-being?
- Identify the methods used in evaluating hearing in children. How do these compare with methods used with adults?
- What are the goals of aural habilitation and rehabilitation?
- Explain the types of intervention considered when developing an individualized aural habilitation/rehabilitation plan.

SUGGESTED READINGS

Bellis, T. J. (2003). *Assessment and management of central auditory processing disorders in the educational setting: From science to practice.* San Diego: Singular Publishing Group.

Clark, J. G., & English, K. (2004). *Audiologic counseling in clinical practice: Helping clients and families adjust to hearing loss.* Boston: Allyn and Bacon.

Martin, F. N., & Clark, J. G. (2003). *Introduction to audiology* (8th ed.). Boston: Allyn and Bacon.

Tye-Murray, N. (2004). *Foundations of aural rehabilitation: Children, adults, and their family members* (2nd ed.). Clifton Park, NY: Delmar Learning.

ONLINE RESOURCES

http://www.asha.org/ American Speech-Language-Hearing Association. General information about audiology.

http://www.audiology.org American Academy of Audiology. General information about audiology.

http://www.audiologyonline.com
General information about audiology.

http://ctl.augie.edu/perry/perry.htm
Perry C. Hanavan of Augustana College has created a virtual tour of the ear.

http://www.nidcd.nih.gov National Institute on Deafness and Other Communication Disorders.
General information about hearing loss.

http://www.betterhearing.org Better Hearing Institute.
General information about hearing loss.

http://www.hearnet.coml Hearing Education and Awareness for Rockers.
Information about noise/music-induced hearing loss for musicians and music lovers.

http://www.ncapd.org National Coalition on Auditory Processing Disorders, Inc.
Information about auditory processing disorders.

http://www.acoustics.org/press/133rd/2paaa2.html Acoustical Society of America.
Simulated hearing loss recordings.

http://www.colorado.edu/slhs/mdnc Marion Downs National Center Website.
Information about infant hearing.

http://www.healthyhearing.com
Information about hearing aids.

http://www.cochlear.com Cochlear Corporation.
Information about cochlear implants.

http://www.signingonline.com
Interactive web-based instruction in American Sign Language.

http://www.cuedspeech.org National Cued Speech Association.

http://www.dogsforthedeaf.org Dogs for the Deaf.
Information about hearing dogs.

http://tap.gallaudet.edu Technology Access Program, Gallaudet University.
Information about assistive technologies for the deaf.

http://www.rcsullivan.com/www/ears.htm
Roy Sullivan developed this website, which provides video-otoscopic images of various outer and middle ear disorders.

Augmentative and Alternative Communication

15

Laura Piché, MA, SLP

Case Study 15.1

Case Study of a Child Requiring an Augmentative and Alternative Communication (AAC) System: Nicky

Nicky is an 8-year-old girl who is nonverbal, is diagnosed as having a developmental disability, and has difficulty with fine motor skills. She attends second grade in a blended classroom. When Nicky was a preschooler, she received early intervention services in her home where she was seen by a speech-language pathologist and an occupational therapist. Nicky is able to make some sounds, she approximates the words *mom* and *dog;* in addition, she nods her head for yes and no. Although the speech-language pathologist working with Nicky has not ruled out the possibility that she could someday talk, at this stage, Nicky needs an alternative method of communication to supplement her few words, sounds, and gestures.

Last year, Nicky's speech-language pathologist tried teaching her sign language; however, given Nicky's fine motor issues, signing was difficult for her. In addition, none of the students in Nicky's class knew sign. Given the motor requirements of signing, Nicky's team elected to begin using a symbol-based system. Nicky learned to use several symbols to communicate a variety of messages including such things as "Hi," "My name is Nicky," "My favorite color is purple," "I love to swim," "Let's play a game," "I want a cookie," and "That's yucky!"

The speech-language pathologist worked with Nicky's classroom teacher, other school personnel, and Nicky's parents to ensure that new symbols added to Nicky's repertoire reflected priority needs across her environments. In addition, her team is now exploring the use of a voice output communication aid (VOCA) so that when Nicky touches a symbol, a girl's voice would speak the messages out loud—giving Nicky a voice.

As you read the chapter, think about:

- Why sign language was not the best choice for a communication system for Nicky.
- How you would begin to decide which symbols/messages should be added to Nicky's device.
- What type of VOCA would be most appropriate for Nicky at this point in time.

Throughout this text, individuals have been mentioned who have severe speech and language impairments and might need either some additional support or an alternative method of communication. These forms of communication, referred to as **augmentative and alternative communication (AAC),** include everything: gestures, signing, pictures, photographs, print, computerized communication, and voice production (Glennen & De-Coste, 1997). The American Speech-Language-Hearing Association (ASHA) defined AAC by saying,

> AAC is, foremost, a set of procedures and processes by which an individual's communication skills (i.e., production as well as comprehension) can be maximized for functional and effective communication. It involves supplementing or replacing natural speech and/or writing with aided (e.g., picture communication symbols, line drawings, Blissymbols, and tangible objects) and/or unaided symbols (e.g., manual signs, gestures, and finger spelling). (ASHA, 2002b, p. 98)

Use of the term AAC can be further clarified by understanding the difference in meaning and clinical approach between the words augmentative and alternative. *Augmentative* communication can be thought of as the process of augmenting, or supplementing, existing speech abilities, whereas *alternative* refers to some method that becomes a substitute, or replacement, for speech (Glennen, 1997; Lloyd, 1985).

The importance of AAC as an intervention in the field of speech-language pathology can easily be seen when one considers that "approximately 12 of every 1000 people are unable to meet their daily communication needs through speech. . . . Unless these individuals receive effective AAC interventions and supports they will not have a 'voice' and will remain silenced" (Light, Beukelman, & Reichle, 2003, p. ix).

Individuals who might benefit from AAC include, but are not limited to, those with deafness, mental retardation (MR), autism spectrum disorder (ASD), aphasia, traumatic brain injury (TBI), motor speech problems, cerebral palsy (CP), glossectomy, laryngectomy, dysarthria, and apraxia of speech, to name a few. More than at any time in human history, people with disabilities are meeting new challenges, participating in life to the fullest, and demanding that their voices be heard. As mentioned in Chapter 2, legislation, adaptations, and technology are helping to ensure this participation. Individuals are overcoming what were considered only a few years ago to be insurmountable barriers to independence.

In this chapter, we will explore AAC, describing what it is and how it works, and then focusing on assessment and intervention considerations. Most chapters in this book discuss specific types of communication disorders, whereas this chapter discusses an intervention approach—AAC—that benefits people with many different types of communication disorders.

The goals for AAC intervention vary with each individual user; however, general treatment aims typically include one, or more, of the following:

1. Assist individuals with their daily communication needs.
2. Help facilitate the development of speech and language.
3. Help facilitate the return of speech and language. (Blackstone, 1989)

Only careful and ongoing evaluation of a client's abilities, his or her needs, and the environment can ensure that these goals will be met effectively and efficiently.

> All typical communicators augment speech with other means of communication, such as gestures and facial expression.

TYPES OF AAC

AAC systems can be separated into two primary categories: aided and unaided. Aided systems involve the use of some type of equipment or device and range from very simple to extremely sophisticated options. Unaided systems do not involve any external equipment and rely only on the individual's body (Lloyd, Fuller, & Arvidson, 1997).

UNAIDED AAC

All of us use gestures to communicate. We shake our head, shrug our shoulders, point, and reach. Gesturing is a form of unaided AAC, as are signing, fingerspelling, Cued Speech, and writing.

Signing is a highly developed form of communication, as is speech. Because signing is other than speech, it is considered to be a form of AAC. The sign system is the code or the language. As noted in Chapter 14, "Audiology and Hearing Loss," American Sign Language or ASL, the language of the Deaf Culture in the United States, is a language with its own vocabulary and syntax. Other sign systems in use in the United States are translations of English into sign and include Signed English, Signing Essential English (SEE-I), and Signing Exact English (SEE-II). Signed English is the most frequently taught sign system in the United States.

American Indian gestural or hand communication, called AmerInd, is a gestural system used with some nonspeaking individuals. It is a relatively grammar-free, nonsign system of 250 concept signals. Almost all gestures in AmerInd can be made with one hand, making it easier for those with hemiplegia, paralysis on one side of the body, or hemiparesis, weakness on one side.

Individual signs can be classified based on their ease of production or comprehension. In general, it is easier to produce signs that touch the body and that use both hands, and, when both hands are used, it is easier to produce signs that are symmetrical (both hands produce the same movement).

Some signs are easy to comprehend because they look like what they represent. These signs are called *iconic*. For example, the sign for "drink" in most systems is made by miming drinking. Unfortunately, few signs are of this type. Signs that are easily guessable, explainable, and memorable are called *transparent*. In most sign systems "America" is made by interlocking the fingers, palms in, and moving them in a circle. Definitely not iconic, but consider the explanation. When the early Europeans came to the Western Hemisphere they were impressed by the abundance of timber; so much that it could be stacked to make fences that resemble the hand shape for "America." Whether this is the derivation of the sign or not, it makes sense, thus the sign is easy to remember. Many signs are transparent. AmerInd has a high proportion of transparent signs. Signs, such as "apple," which are difficult to interpret, are called *opaque*. Examples of iconic, transparent, and opaque signs are presented in Figure 15.1.

THOUGHT QUESTIONS

Might the degree of sign transparency differ across individuals, cultures, and ability levels? "Milk" is signed by miming milking a cow. Does every child know where milk comes from?

Gestural communication systems can be differentiated based on their grammatical structure. As we have discussed, sign languages, like ASL, have their own syntax or grammar, while sign systems like Signed English, SEE-I, and SEE-II are based on, and follow, the rules of American English grammar; thus, they are not separate languages.

For most Deaf signers, fingerspelling is mixed with signs and used for new words or names. Fingerspelling, or the manual alphabet, may be a good alternative for older clients with both good cognitive and fine motor abili-

ICONIC

coat

Make an "A" shape with both hands. With thumbs, trace shape of jacket lapels.

cold *(adj.)*

Make an "S" shape with both hands. Draw hands close to body and shiver.

TRANSPARENT

boy

With hand by forehead, snap a flat "O" shape twice, indicating the brim of a baseball cap.

girl

Make an "A" shape with right hand. Place thumb by right earlobe and move down jaw line.

OPAQUE

gray

Make a "5" shape with both hands, thumbs up, palms facing body. Move hands back and forth with Ⓡ fingers passing between Ⓛ ones.

more

Make a flat "O" shape with both hands, fingertips facing each other. Tap fingertips together twice.

FIGURE 15.1

Examples of Iconic, transparent, and opaque signed English signs.

ties. The client has ultimate flexibility because any word in the language can be spelled for transmission.

AIDED AAC

Unaided systems are not appropriate for every individual who needs either to enhance or replace his or her current method of communicating. For example, an individual with severe motor involvement in the limbs as in some forms of CP may be unable to make the fine motor adjustments necessary for many signs. Another problem with gestural communication systems has to do with the number of possible communication partners available. Unfortunately, many individuals in the community (e.g., outside of a signer's home or school environments) are not familiar with sign and may not be able to understand what the signer is trying to communicate. For these individuals, a communication board or an electronic mode of communication may be more appropriate. These devices are collectively called **assistive technologies,** a broad term that includes aids for daily living, communication aids, environmental controls, prosthetic and orthotic devices, sensory aids, seating and positioning systems, and mobility/transportation aids.

Aided systems differ in the type of system, the graphic means of representation, and the input and output modes. Selection of each is determined by ongoing careful assessment.

Aided AAC Systems

Aided AAC systems vary from "no-tech" to "low-tech" to "high-tech" and can be represented by a continuum of technology (see Figure 15.2). No-tech systems are those that do not involve the use of any technology and use readily available materials (e.g., paper and pencil, writing the letters of the alphabet on a piece of paper so the user can spell out a message). Low-tech systems are those that are fairly simple and contain few moving parts (Mann & Lane, 1991). Examples of low-tech AAC systems include such devices as BIGmack™, Step-by-Step™, and VoicePal Max™ to name a few. High-tech AAC systems are those electronic devices that are considerably more sophisticated, many of which are based on computer technology. Examples would include such devices as a DynaVox™, a Lightwriter™, or a Pathfinder™. See Figure 15.3 for examples of some of these AAC systems.

FIGURE 15.2
Continuum of aided AAC technology with examples of each.

No-Tech	Low-Tech	High-Tech
Alphabet board	Communication board	DynaVox™
Word board	BIGmack™ communication device	Lightwriter™
Paper and pencil	VoicePal Max™	Pathfinder™

No-Tech

Alphabet board

Client points to letters to communicate message.

Eye gaze systems

Client communicaties by looking at the desired symbol.

Low-Tech

BIGmack™, manufactured by AbleNet, Inc.

Client touches plate switch to transmit prerecorded message.

Voice Pal Max™, manufactured by Adaptivation

Client selects picture to transmit a prerecorded message.

High-Tech

DynaVox and DynaMyte Series 4, manufactured by DynaVox Systems, inc.

Client selects picture/letter to generate a message for transmission.

FIGURE 15.3
Examples of aided AAC systems.

Graphic Means of Representation

Whether on a communication board or an electronic device, graphic symbols are just as important to aided AAC as words are to speech or signs to signing. Symbols may include pictures, various representational systems, and/or printed words, grouped together to form symbol systems. Some symbol systems have been specifically designed for AAC use.

Graphic symbol systems include iconic representations, such as Picture Communication Symbols (PCS) and some Rebus Symbols, less iconic representations, such as Picsyms and Pictogram Ideogram Communication (PIC), and opaque symbol systems, such as Blissymbolics. Symbolic systems are more rule-governed and generative, allowing for symbol combination and the creation of new symbols.

Graphic symbol systems may use a variety of means to express different referents. Rebus symbols are line drawings of both concrete and abstract concepts and of sound sequences, originally developed as an aid for teaching reading. Picsyms and PIC contain ideograms used to represent an idea rather than the way a referent, or the concept it refers to, appears in the real world. Ideograms and symbols, such as those used in Blissymbolics, can be used for abstract concepts just as words can. Blissymbols consist of 100 pictographic representations and arbitrary symbols that can be combined to create words.

With very young children or more severely cognitively impaired individuals, SLPs may choose to use actual objects, product packaging, photographs, or drawings. These are very concrete and may not represent anything beyond the immediate referent. A system called Tangible Symbols (Rowland & Schweigert, 1989) attempts to bridge the gap between actual objects and graphic representations by using objects or pictures with a clear relationship to the referent. For example, a key or a shoelace might represent *car* or *shoe* respectively.

> Graphic symbols may be selected directly by the AAC user or scanned, when each symbol is highlighted in turn until the desired one is reached.

Aided System Input

Input, or access method, is especially important, and great care must be exercised in choosing the appropriate interface between the client and the device. The two primary means of symbol selection are direct selection and scanning. The client may select the symbol directly by pointing with a finger, hand, head pointer, optical head pointer, or by operating a joystick. The client might point directly at the symbol or touch the keys on a keyboard. In cases of severe neuromuscular involvement, eye gaze, sometimes referred to as eye pointing, may be used to select symbols. Most users of communication boards indicate their message by pointing.

Pointing may be aided by the use of either hand splints or pointing sticks that strengthen, or enable, the client's response. Optical head pointers may be used with both electronic and nonelectronic systems. For example, something as simple as a small flashlight or penlight attached by a headband to an individual's head communicates when the individual shines the light onto the desired symbol or message. Some electronic communication devices have sensors built into the device itself. The optical head pointers used with these devices typically utilize infrared (IR) technology. As the optical head pointer moves across the symbol display, the device's sensors light up, indicating to the user what symbol it is on. When the individual gets to the desired symbol, he or she stops there for a predetermined period of time (called dwell time). Once the user has rested on that location for that period of time, the device knows that the user is "selecting" that symbol. The dwell time on most devices can be set depending on the needs of each individual. Some individuals can use a short dwell time, others, as a result of significant motor issues, may require a longer dwell time.

Individuals using eye gaze look at symbols on a clear acrylic board located between the user and the communication partner. The user gazes at desired symbols, which appear on both sides of the board.

Another access method for individuals with limited motor abilities is scanning. In scanning, the choices are presented to the user, and the user signals when the desired symbol has been presented (Piché & Reichle, 1991; Quist & Lloyd, 1997). This can be done by another person's pointing to symbols on a communication board and the user's vocalizing when the symbol/message he or she wants to communicate has been presented. While this form of manual scanning can be and is used, a more common form of scanning is electronic scanning, or scanning that occurs on a communication device. In this case, the device presents (or menus) the choices to the user, and the user responds or signals by using some type of switch when the desired symbol has been menued.

People with motor limitations can use many different types of switches—everything from simple pressure switches to pneumatic "sip and puff" switches to switches that can be activated with the blink of an eye. The type of switch an individual uses depends upon his or her particular needs and abilities. Often, an SLP, along with an occupational therapist (OT), will be involved in selecting the most appropriate type of switch for an individual to use to access his or her AAC system. When scanning, an individual activates a switch to start the scanning process. The device then presents the choices. When the symbols are presented visually, either by a LED in a corner of the symbol lighting up or by the appearance of an illuminated frame around the symbol, it is referred to as visual scanning. Auditory scanning works in a similar way, but in addition to the symbols being presented visually, there is also an auditory cue present. For example, imagine a lunch page on which the device has the symbols hamburger, hotdog, and pizza present. For visual scanning, when those symbols were presented, an illuminated frame would appear first around the hamburger. If no selection was made, the frame would move to the hotdog, and then if this selection was not made, it would move to pizza. To select pizza, when the pizza symbol was highlighted, the individual would activate his or her switch, and a message that said "I'd like pizza for lunch today" would be spoken by the device. If the individual was an auditory scanner, the device would work as described above, but with the addition of an auditory cue. So when the hamburger symbol was highlighted, the device would say "hamburger." If no selection was made, the illuminated frame would move to hotdog, and the device would say "hotdog." If no selection was made again, the illuminated frame would move to pizza and the device would say "pizza." If the individual activated his or her switch to select pizza, the device would speak the message that had been programmed into that location: "I'd like pizza for lunch today."

Scanning is a very effective option for individuals with significant motor limitations. However, it is an extremely slow and laborious process. The majority of an individual's time is spent waiting while extraneous things are presented (Vanderheiden, 1984). Scanning requires extended concentration and has the potential to be very frustrating, especially when symbols are missed and the process must be repeated.

Efficiency can be enhanced by placing symbols so that the most frequently used symbols are scanned most frequently. For example, if the cursor begins at the top of the display and returns there after each symbol selection, then the most frequently used symbols would be placed at the top. Obviously, such an arrangement requires constant monitoring by those in the user's environment to ensure peak efficiency.

Various scanning methods can also increase efficiency (Venkatagiri, 2000). For example, in linear scanning each possible selection is presented in sequence. In contrast, both row-column and block scanning enable the user to scan larger areas, then refine the scan once the desired area has been highlighted. As an example, the user might press the switch to begin the scan. Rows are lighted in sequence until the desired one is found. The user presses the switch again and individual symbols within that row are highlighted one at a time.

Obviously, the type of access method is as important as the symbol system used. In general, the SLP and client will determine the most efficient and accurate access method given the client's cognitive and physical abilities and the environmental demands. Several individuals are presented using AAC deviced on the accompaying CD-ROM.

Aided System Output

As in unaided AAC, with communication boards the partner interprets the message directly. With electronic AAC devices, a wide range of outputs are possible. Electronic output or transmission may be as simple as a light over or behind a symbol or as elaborate as a voice and printed message. SLPs help the client to find the most appropriate output for his or her needs. Several types of output options exist. In some situations, an individual may need written or printed output. For example, at school a device user may need to submit a hard copy of a speech he or she delivered in class, necessitating written output. In many other situations, spoken output (often referred to as voice output) would be the most natural and appropriate.

Voice output can be either recorded (also called digitized), synthesized, or a combination of both. Because digitized output is actually recorded by a person, it is much more natural sounding, and it is relatively easy to age and gender match the voice on the device for the individual using it. However, a disadvantage to digitized speech is that the only output an individual can produce on his or her device is messages that have already been anticipated and programmed, or stored, in the system's memory. Synthesized speech has more flexibility but often sounds mechanical or robotic. Instead of recording actual words or phrases, the speech synthesizer contains sounds and rules for combining them. Generally, messages are programmed into a device with synthesized speech by simply typing in the words and phrases/messages. The speech synthesizer then converts that text string into spoken output using the sounds and rules for combining them contained in its program. Many times, people and place names are problematic for synthesized speech devices. However, virtually every device that uses synthesized speech contains a pronunciation dictionary, which is a place where you can correct the pronunciation of words and/or names that the device mispronounces.

Computers sometimes use synthetic speech. When you have heard synthetic speech, did it seem artifical to you? Would you want this voice to be yours in communication?

THOUGHT QUESTIONS

Compared to natural speech, comprehension of synthesized speech requires increased focused attention by the partner. When attention is divided, partners comprehend significantly less synthesized speech (Drager & Reichle, 2001). Partners tend to respond more slowly to synthesized speech (Reynolds & Jefferson, 2000).

Decisions on the appropriate type of AAC are made only after careful evaluation. As the user's abilities or needs change, that decision may need to be revisited. Users may also employ multiple types of AAC communication. Training of both the user and others in the user's environment is essential for maximum efficacy.

SPEECH AND AAC

Obviously, AAC is not the same as speech. There are some important distinctions that may not be readily apparent. First, with the exception of expert signers, the typical AAC user is much slower than the typical speaker. This has implications for users as well as their communication partners. Communication partners may feel compelled to complete the message for the users or take more responsibility for the communication than during speech. The untrained communication partner may take control away from the AAC speaker unintentionally.

AAC use can change the communication process in ways that are not always predictable.

Second, some AAC communication will be less face to face. Both participants may be attending to the device in aided systems. In unaided systems, such as signing, it is easier to glance from hands to face and back but eye contact will still be less than in speaking situations. With less face-to-face communication, shades of meaning may be missed.

Caregivers sometimes worry that learning a different means of communication will adversely affect an individual's natural speech. People often mistakenly believe that ". . . if a person produces manual signs, points to graphic symbols, and/or uses a speech-generating device (SGD) (also known as voice output communication aid or VOCA), his or her natural speech will diminish or fail to develop" (Blischak, Lombardino, & Dyson, 2003, p. 29). In reality, the opposite is true. As you will see in the following section, learning to use an AAC system often enhances other aspects of communication, and many times it actually facilitates production of natural speech.

*T*HEORY AND REALITY

Use of AAC has been documented to increase conversational participation, speech intelligibility, and conversational initiations (Dattilo & Camarata, 1991; Glennen & Calculator, 1985; Hunter, Pring, & Martin, 1991; Spiegel, Benjamin, & Spiegel,1993). Training conversational partners as well as the client results in increased reciprocity in turn taking and initiations (Light, Dattilo, English, Gutierrez, & Hartz, 1992).

THOUGHT QUESTIONS

*W*hy is it important to train conversational partners to use AAC systems? How might your conversational behaviors be affected if your partner used an AAC device that was considerably slower than speech?

In short, AAC facilitates the development of both communication and language. None of these positive statements about AAC suggests that it is the great panacea for "curing" all communication ills, but, as with any good intervention method, AAC works very well with certain clients.

Several factors can explain the effects of AAC. These are presented in Table 15.1. When others in the user's environment also use AAC, they increase the user's comprehension by producing the symbols at a slower rate than speech, by reducing the number of symbols and grammatical structures used, and by eliminating many irrelevant or wordy comments that often accompany speech. For the user, production may be easier than speech because of reduced physical demands, removal of the pressure to speak, hand-over-hand shaping and modeling, and increased involvement of the right hemisphere.

The use of AAC does not relieve the SLP of his or her responsibilities to follow good clinical practice. Even the best of methods must be monitored

TABLE 15.1
Why AAC facilitates communication as compared to speech

Simplification of input

    Irrelevant and parenthetical comments eliminated.

    Slower rate permits more processing time.

Response production advantages

    Pressure to speak removed.

    Physical demands decreased compared to speech.

    Physical manipulation of client's hands or other parts of body by trainer is possible.

    Client observation of physical manipulation facilitated.

Advantages for individuals with severe cognitive impairment

    Limited and functional vocabulary.

    Individual's attention easier to maintain.

Receptive language/auditory processing advantages

    Structure of language is simplified.

    Auditory short-term memory and/or auditory processing problems minimized.

Simultaneous processing/stimulus association advantages

    Visual nature of the symbol makes it more obvious.

    Visual symbols have more consistency.

    Duration of symbol is greater than spoken word.

    Visual symbols more easily associated with visual referents.

Symbolic representation advantages

    Supplement speech symbols.

    Symbols visually represent referents.

Source: Adapted from Lloyd, L. L., & Kangas, K. A. (1994). Augmentative and alternative communication. In G. H Shames, E. H. Wiig, & W. A. Secord (Eds.), *Human communication disorders* (4th ed.). Boston: Allyn and Bacon.

for progress and use within the everyday environment of the client. Sometimes AAC methods fail, especially when they are not a good match for the client's abilities and needs and the needs of the environment. For example, if no one in the client's home or school is willing to learn sign, sign usage will not generalize to these situations. Several other factors may account for lack of progress or failure to generalize. These include the lack of functional client-centered content, the precedence of training over communication, nonuse in the environment, and inflexibility in the use of the means of communication. Inflexibility is an insistence by either the SLP or the client on the exclusive use of only one means of communication.

Why might a client decide to use one AAC method exclusively? Can you imagine a situation in which this might occur?

Generally, communication is best when multiple means can be used. For example, the client may have some usable speech, a few easily recognizable signs, and a communication board with symbols in various stages of maturity from photos through black and white drawings to Blissymbolics. Most SLPs would not recommend training with such a variety of AAC systems, but clients with a history of AAC use may have acquired some symbols in a few different systems. Generally, the user has some vocalizations, some speech, nonlinguistic behaviors such as gestures and body language, and AAC. If the client can easily produce a verbal "no," it seems inflexible to ignore that word and insist on the sign or symbol equivalent.

LIFESPAN ISSUES

AAC users may have other needs that call for the use of additional assistive technologies.

Severe communication impairments, whether developmental or acquired, often affect many aspects of an individual's life. In addition, those with severe communication deficits also may have a wide array of other disabling conditions.

Children with evident syndromes or impairments, those at risk, or those failing infant measures, such as hearing screenings, will be candidates for early intervention (EI). For some of these children, especially those with CP or deafness, exposure to augmentative communication may begin within the first few months. Caregivers will talk to the infant, but supplement this input with sign or other visual input. AAC may or may not become the primary means of communication and the SLP will continue to work on oral motor skills and sound production. Case Study 15.2 presents the story of one young woman whose life was changed by AAC.

Just as a developmental continuum exists for speech, so it does for AAC (Cress, 2001). Communication begins with an infant prior to development of speech, language, and AAC use. Experiencing AAC signs and symbols prior to using them directly facilitates a child's understanding of their nature and function (Romski & Sevcik, 1996; Rowland & Schweigert, 2000).

Later, the child may begin to use AAC to produce language. If exposed to signs, children with deafness will begin to sign their first words at about 8 months. Unfortunately, some infants and toddlers with deafness live in nonsign environments and do not begin to learn sign until they attend a special preschool.

Some children may not be identified as having a communication impairment until later. As you will recall, children with autism spectrum disorder (ASD) are often identified as toddlers. AAC can provide initial communication and a motivation for learning language. For example, using behavior chain interruption, a technique in which the SLP stops a pleasurable activity and prompts the child to signal beginning again, the SLP can establish initial meaningful communication with the child. Communication can then be expanded as new desires by the child are identified.

Case Study 15.2

Jean's Story

Her parents eagerly anticipated Jean's birth. She was their first child. Although her motor behavior seemed rigid at birth, the pediatrician assured them that her behavior was typical reflexive behavior for an infant. They were saddened and confused when Jean was later diagnosed with spastic cerebral palsy.

Although her parents tried to give Jean a typical childhood, their task was complicated by her motor impairment. Jean was enrolled in a preschool, but her lack of speech and language inhibited her interactions with other children. She was later enrolled in a special preschool where she received speech and language services, daily living skills training, and academic preparation.

Unfortunately, Jean's SLP chose to emphasize speech intervention and AAC was not attempted. When she began first grade, Jean had only a few words that were understood by her immediate family, teacher, and the SLP. Her new SLP decided to use AAC with Jean but opted for signing primarily because other children in the school signed. Signing was not a good match for Jean because of the motor involvement of her hands.

Finally, after several frustrating years of less than adequate communication, Jean's new SLP suggested combined use of an electronic communication board, plus some of Jean's easily recognizable signs and words. Using creative funding and a state grant, the SLP was able to purchase an electronic device. The manual board was used when Jean was between these two sites or when she traveled in the car with her family. Although she used direct selection on her manual board, it was a slow, frustrating process. Her elctronic board was accessed through the use of a joystick that enabled Jean to go to the desired symbol.

Now a young adult, Jean lives at home with her parents and attends vocational training at the local United Cerebral Palsy Association workshop. She continues to receive speech-language pathology services and has a large repertoire of graphic symbols at her disposal. She is able to request, to ask and answer questions, and to make conversational comments. Her life has become more fulfilling thanks to the many means she can use to communicate. It is hoped that soon she will be able to attempt an assisted living arrangement.

Inevitably, some children and adolescents will experience acquired communication impairments because of accidents or illness. Many children and adolescents with TBI benefit from short-term or long-term use of AAC. In one case, a young man who had lost speech and language as the result of a gun-related suicide attempt was able to retrieve language and some speech by learning signs. His new communication system consists of vocalizations, verbalizations, gestures, and signs.

As AAC users mature, communication needs change. Approximately 20 percent enjoy full- or part-time employment (Balandin & Morgan, 2001). Adults with CP are less likely to marry and own a home, two factors that are important for continued independent living in old age. Nursing home staffs rarely are knowledgeable in AAC use. Changes in hearing and vision with age may also affect AAC use. Good communication skills can positively affect health, well-being, and safety (Straus, Cable, & Shavelle, 1999).

How might the potential changes in your life affect your communication needs? Suppose that you are an AAC user and think about this question again.

THOUGHT QUESTION

For both children and adults with degenerative disorders, aided AAC may provide continued communication when speech is no longer possible. For one young man, it was extremely important to his family that he be able to express his needs and thoughts for as long as possible. Although he became less able to control his body's movements, he continued to communicate. His computer was modified and modified again as his ability to interface changed. Typing letters gave way to touching pictures, which in turn changed to scanning the same pictures. When he could no longer use his computer, a yes/no signal system and eye gaze were used. Throughout this process, the SLP worked closely with the family and the visiting caretakers.

In the early stages of intervention with individuals with degenerative neuromuscular conditions, intervention focuses on maintaining natural communication (Doyle & Phillips, 2001). During the middle stages, as motor function deteriorates, the individual may begin to use AAC in specific situations. As motor control and speech become severely impaired, the individual may rely on AAC. The SLP continually monitors the progress of the disease and modifies the AAC system and/or the interface between the client and the AAC device. As devices have become more sophisticated, many now affer the option of utilizing both digitized (recorded) and synthesized speech, and a process known as "voice banking" has begun to emerge. Before an individual loses his or her ability to speak (and before speech is too compromised), he or she records and stores voice samples in an AAC system that uses both digitized and synthesized speech. This person may not need the AAC system yet, but has preserved his or her own voice for the day when it will no longer be usable. There are many benefits of voice banking, not the least of which is that ". . . it enables communication in his or her own voice, tone, and intonation pattern, which helps to preserve a part of his or her personality . . ."(Costello, 2000, p. 141).

Adults may also experience accidents and illness. As with children, they may benefit from AAC use. Those with apraxia of speech may have very good hand coordination and may be primary candidates for augmentative use. Individuals with aphasia may benefit from the use of graphic symbols or signs. Much visual information is interpreted in the right hemisphere. By tapping into this area of the brain, it is possible with some clients to build a "bridge" to the damaged areas of the left hemisphere and to improve access to language. It may be more difficult for an adult who once spoke typically to accept AAC. Embarrassment and shame may accompany the loss of speech or language. The SLP must stress the positive benefits of AAC use.

As noted in other assessments of communication impairment, assessment for AAC use is a team effort.

ASSESSMENT CONSIDERATIONS

As in other areas of speech-language pathology, careful thorough assessment of a client's abilities and needs is essential for determining the appropriate AAC system and the course of intervention services. Assessment should include not only the client's speech, language, and communication abilities and needs but also motor and perceptual skills, preferences, and the willingness of the environment to support AAC use. This data will be collected through the help of a team of professionals who will be identified as we discuss each element of the evaluation.

Speech considerations include the types of sounds and sound combinations produced, intelligibility, and connected speech. Spontaneous speech and imitative speech samples should be collected and analyzed. In addition, an oral peripheral examination with attention to different motor behaviors, swallowing, and oral movement imitation is essential.

Hearing is extremely important for speech production and feedback and should be assessed thoroughly by an audiologist. Seniors may have hearing loss that is unrelated or related to the acquired speech and/or language impairment. Individuals with developmental speech and/or language impairments may have hearing, perceptual, or central auditory processing impairments related to various syndromes or disorders.

Language and prelanguage skills, both receptive and expressive, will be important for programming content and selection of symbol systems, especially graphic. Although certain cognitive abilities seem to be needed for some types of symbol use, clients should not be excluded from AAC consideration because these abilities are still developing. Prelinguistic skills can be taught at the same time the client is learning to communicate with the AAC system.

Communication skills are very important. The desire to communicate or to communicate better forms the basis for AAC intervention and the motivation for learning. Although individuals with severe disabilities have great difficulty making clear and intentional signals, they often create their own individualistic gestures (Iacono, Carter, & Hook, 1998; Yoder & Munson, 1995). The multimodal nature of AAC necessitates a systematic exploration of the role these gestures play in communication (Hunt-Berg, 2001; Reichle, Halle, & Drasgow, 1998).

It is very difficult not to communicate. Consequently, one of the SLP's roles is to determine the communication method, or methods, currently used by the client. This is often more difficult than it sounds because sometimes the manner in which an individual is communicating is not always recognized as communication. For example, a young girl with severe disabilities was frequently observed to tap her cheek after coming in from the playground. It was not until the SLP began to look at that behavior more closely that people realized she was using that cheek tapping to indicate that she wanted a drink. Communication is often demonstrated when an individual engages in a consistent behavior (e.g., cheek tapping) in the same situations over time (e.g., after coming in from the playground). The SLP should also attempt to determine the current and future communication needs of the client.

Can you not communicate? Do some behaviors communicate information even when we do not intend them to do so?

An occupational (OT) and/or physical therapist (PT) can aid in motor assessment. Of interest is ambulation or the ability to move about, fine motor dexterity for signing or pointing, range of movement especially of the upper limbs, motor imitation skills, and the consistency and accuracy of motor responses. This data will be extremely important in deciding the appropriate aided or unaided system and the placement and size of graphic symbols.

Visual and auditory acuity and perception will be important for system selection and intervention. Vision, along with motor skills, will be used to decide the size of graphic symbols. A vision specialist will be an invaluable member of the team in assessing these abilities.

Occasionally, the environment will not support the use of AAC. Caregivers may be uncomfortable, feel inadequate, or just not want to be involved. The SLP may need to educate caregivers about the benefits of AAC to the client and to the home or school. Explaining the likely course of intervention may increase caregiver comfort levels.

Intervention will be maximally effective if caregivers also use AAC along with speech. Caregivers can be taught a few simple signs, or they can learn to use an individual's communication board and point to a symbol while speaking their message. For individuals using an electronic device, caregivers can and should learn to use the device, and again, pair what they are saying with using the voice output of the device. This is referred to as augmented input, and it serves as a model for use of the communication device (Romski & Sevcik, 1996).

Caregivers are sometimes fearful that they will be expected to sign as if interpreting for a deaf audience. Nothing could be further from reality with most clients. Signs or graphic symbols can be used as gestures for important words in an utterance as the caregiver continues to speak.

Last, the SLP is interested in collecting a list of client preferences and of possible symbols to train. Likes and desires of the client will be important for intervention. This information can be gathered from client responses or choices, from caregiver suggestions, or through observation of the client. This portion of the assessment can be very positive with the focus on communication potential rather than on impairment. It is especially important for those with acquired communication disabilities (Klasner & Yorkston, 2001). With these disabilities, such as dysarthria, the focus tends to be on loss rather than potential, so a positive shift is welcome.

It is not always clear whether a client will benefit from AAC use. If the SLP believes that AAC support may be beneficial in the future, the topic should be introduced early in the assessment and intervention process. Need becomes apparent if the client's communication abilities are being constrained by slowly recovering or developing speech. The following recommendations can help families accept AAC use (Zangari, 2001):

- Provide honest information
- Honor their concerns and provide information that addresses those concerns
- Recognize the emotional impact in realizing that a loved one may use AAC and try to address concerns that are stated and those that are not

> Caregivers are part of the AAC intervention team.

- Address the client's strengths and the way in which AAC enhances them
- Provide specific rationales for your recommendations

The actual assessment is only a first step. The SLP, in coordination with the family and other professionals, such as the OT, PT, audiologist, vision specialist, psychologist, rehabilitation engineer, and/or classroom teacher, uses the data from the assessment to make decisions on the appropriate AAC method, AAC symbol system, and potential vocabulary. These decisions will be adjusted and modified as the client progresses.

AAC SYSTEM SELECTION

In deciding on the appropriate AAC system or method, the SLP will consider the client's motor and cognitive abilities, the potential size of the client's lexicon, the ease in learning and using the system, the acceptability of the system to the user and potential communication partners, and the flexibility and intelligibility of the system. For example, unaided systems are very portable and can be expanded easily without concern for limited storage or display space but allow for no permanent record, thus necessitating use of some graphic system for purposes such as homework. Many graphic symbols appear with the printed word, making them easy for communication partners to use, but these same symbols require the partner to concentrate on the graphic message to the exclusion of the user's face.

The potential user's motor abilities are very important in determining the best system to use. Individuals with severe motor impairments in their upper extremities may be poor candidates for unaided systems. However, poor pointing skills need not deter the individual from using a communication board or a device and accessing it via head pointing, eye gaze, or with an assistive device like a T-stick (a "T"-shaped stick that allows the individual to hold the stick; the bottom leg of the "T" serves to point to the desired symbol or location). In addition, poor motor abilities may dictate the use of certain selection methods (e.g., scanning) to access an electronic communication device.

Those in the potential user's communication environment must find the AAC system acceptable. Lack of portability or embarrassment concerning use may lead to nonuse in certain situations or by some potential partners.

The selection of the AAC system can lead to further questions. For example, if the SLP decides to use a communication board, several considerations influence its final design. These include, but are not limited to, the construction material, overall size, arrangement and size of the symbols, placement and organization of the symbols, and the mounting of the board if necessary.

AAC SYMBOL SELECTION

Decisions on the appropriate symbol system will flow naturally from the method of communication chosen. If signing is deemed to be the appropriate method, the SLP must make decisions on the best gestural or sign system

AAC system selection is much more than merely matching the client and the system.

to use. In addition to the cognitive and motor abilities of the potential user, the SLP might consider the gestural or signing system used most frequently in the client's school or workplace and in the local community, the availability of teaching materials, and the ease in using these materials.

Selection of aided symbol systems may be guided by the potential user's cognitive abilities, the ease of learning different graphic AAC systems, and the willingness of potential communication partners. Aided symbols form a continuum from actual objects, which may represent only themselves, to letters that can be used to spell words. As we move from concrete objects to abstract symbols and letters, the client gains increased communication flexibility. Although not all clients can spell or use an encryption code, potential partners may be uneasy with interpretation of pictures, photographs, or other symbols. If we expect the client to use the system at home or in school, then partner concerns are important.

THOUGHT QUESTIONS

Is it important to include home, school, leisure, and work environments in AAC intervention? Why? Why not?

Vocabulary should reflect the client's current needs and communication potential.

AAC VOCABULARY SELECTION

The vocabulary chosen will have a great impact on future communication. Decisions about potential vocabulary will continue to be made as long as the client uses AAC. The best guideline is to select vocabulary that reflects the user's needs, desires, likes, and preferences and is functional or useful based on observation of the client and the communication environment. The resultant vocabulary should be highly individualized.

Several lists of potential vocabulary are available and may serve as a guide when matched with the client's communication needs. These lists may also suggest various communication intentions and semantic categories of language that are important for early language development with presymbolic clients. Individuals with acquired speech and language impairments may have very different needs and rarely must relearn language.

The order of teaching signs or symbols must also be guided by the client's immediate needs. In addition, the iconicity and transparency of different signs/symbols must be considered. Selecting appropriate and useful vocabulary can make or break how successful an AAC system will be for an individual. "Poorly selected or inappropriate vocabulary may be one of the primary deterrents to successful communication" (Yorkston, Honsinger, Dowden, & Marriner, 1989, p. 101). The impact of vocabulary selection on AAC use cannot be underestimated.

INTERVENTION CONSIDERATIONS

Although intervention will be a team effort, it is important for services not to become fragmented (Beukelman & Mirenda, 1992). Rather, a coherent, holistic approach is needed—one that includes the user's natural environment and communication partners. Family members, whether parents of a child with a developmental communication impairment or spouses and children of an adult with an acquired communication impairment, must be integral members of the intervention team.

The SLP must be concerned with linguistic and communicative competence as well as operational competence for the AAC system being trained. Intervention must include both the short-range and long-range needs of the client (Beukelman & Mirenda, 1997). The good intervention practices described in Chapter 4 will be just as important when working with individuals using AAC (Zangari & Kangas, 1997).

Some intervention considerations apply more specifically to AAC. These include but are not limited to the following:

- Establish an environment of AAC
- Use everyday experiences as the training context
- Individualize the content as discussed earlier
- Train others to modify their interactional style
- Consider positioning for those with severe motor impairments
- Make communication real

Each of these will be discussed in some detail.

An environment of augmentative communication is very important and highlights the need to have others, such as caregivers and teachers, involved. The AAC system should be used by others and aided systems should always be available for the user. We are reminded of one teacher who constructed a huge communication board on one wall of her classroom so that she could use it when addressing the entire class. Naturally, integration into the classroom requires a collaborative strategy involving both the classroom teacher and the SLP. AAC training for the entire educational team—teachers, instructional aides, SLPs, and parents—is a key element in success with children (Soto, Muller, Hunt, & Goetz, 2001).

As much as possible we want to program so that the client has multiple partners in multiple situations to increase social integration, especially among peers. In one classroom, we trained partners to interact with AAC users and reinforced them when they did. Educators can also organize clubs and experiences, such as an integrated dramatic arts program, to promote AAC use (McCarthy & Light, 2001).

In short, the SLP must identify opportunities for communication, create a need for communication, and maximize the instructional benefit of these opportunities (Sigafoos, 2000). Partners will need instructional support if they are to function as effective communication partners for AAC users.

Clients with acquired communication impairments may elect, if possible, to continue to work. Self-reports indicate that access to appropriate AAC

Simple props are often used to elicit language in a nonthreatening way.

All members of the intervention team should use the AAC system to provide multiple partners and multiple situations.

systems is an important factor in facilitating continued employment (McNaughton, Light, & Groszyk, 2001).

Everyday events and routines provide *scripts* or personalized event sequences that enable each of us to participate. When circumstances are modified as in the use of AAC, we rely heavily on the script to help us. Use of the script frees "cognitive energy" to be applied to other aspects of the situation. In addition, the use of everyday events teaches the client to use AAC as the need arises. The SLP must use instructional strategies that integrate AAC into the different communication environments of the user (Ball, Marvin, Beukelman, Lasker, & Rupp, 2000; Rainforth, York, & MacDonald, 1992). Even children using low-tech communication boards can have ample opportunities to use their AAC systems to communicate during the school day in greetings, academics, snack, sharing, and recess (Downey, Daugherty, Helt, & Daugherty, 2004).

THOUGHT QUESTIONS

*A*re some communication situations easier than others for you? Are more familiar situations easier? Can you think of the script that helps you in these situations?

Acceptance of AAC is the degree to which the system is integrated into the life of the user (Lasker & Bedrosian, 2000). Optimal use occurs when AAC is used willingly and at every opportunity. Community-based training approaches in which the client becomes more comfortable and efficient using AAC in public may lead to optimal use (Lasker & Bedrosian, 2001). In these approaches, venues, such as the post office, grocery store, and fast food outlets, are identified. Training begins with scripted interactions that are modified gradually to more spontaneous communication.

Unless trained, well-meaning communication partners may assume too active a role in their interaction with the AAC user. Partners need to offer real choices, to acknowledge the user's communication attempts, and to allow time for the user to express the message. Because communication partners may be unfamiliar with AAC, it is important that systems and their purpose be explained carefully (Cress, 2001). Partners should also be trained to use AAC expressively, not because they need AAC to be understood, but because they can help the user acclimate to this new method of communication. Finally, partners should be consulted for their observations, suggestions, and ideas for intervention. As members of the intervention team, they become invested in the outcomes for the client.

For clients with severe motor impairments, such as CP, positioning is very important and can often be the determining factor in successful motor movement. Control of the head, shoulders, spine, and hips and alignment along the midline is essential.

Finally, the user of AAC must be involved in real communication with meaningful outcomes. It is all too easy for intervention to evolve into touching objects or pictures with no real outcome except a reinforcing word by the

SLP or other partner. Training must include real communication choices, not just performance of a sign or locating a symbol. With meaningful communication, the grief and sense of loss that accompanies acquired communication impairments and laryngectomy and glossectomy can be replaced by a sense of empowerment (Fox & Rau, 2001).

Issues of efficacy or the effective use of AAC intervention methods must still be explored (Calculator, 2000). AAC is a relatively new area—only since the late 1970s for most methods—and much clinical research remains to be accomplished.

SUMMARY

Augmentative and alternative communication (AAC) includes many forms and the strategies and methods to assist individuals in using them to meet their communication needs. AAC may enhance or augment an individual's speech or may become the primary means of communication. Individuals who might benefit from AAC include those with deafness, MR, ASD, aphasia, TBI, motor speech problems, CP, glossectomy, laryngectomy, dysarthia, and apraxia of speech.

Although the specific goals of AAC intervention vary with each individual user, treatment aims include the following:

1. Assist individuals with their daily communication needs.
2. Help facilitate the development of speech and language.
3. Help facilitate the return of speech and language.

Caregivers sometimes worry that learning a different means of communication will adversely affect speech. In reality, learning to use AAC enhances all other aspects of communication.

AAC systems can be roughly divided into unaided, those requiring no external devices, and aided, those that do. Unaided AAC includes includes signing, gesturing, fingerspelling, Cued Speech, and writing. These systems are not appropriate for every individual, and an aided system, such as a communication board or an electronic communication device, may be more appropriate. Aided systems differ in the type of system, the graphic means of representation, and the input and output modes. Selection of each is determined by ongoing careful assessment.

Decisions on the appropriate type of AAC may need to be revised as the user's abilities or needs change. Users may also employ multiple types of AAC communication. Training of both the user and others in the user's environment is essential for maximum efficacy.

A careful, thorough assessment of a client's abilities and needs is essential for determining the appropriate AAC system and the course of intervention services. Assessment should include not only the client's speech, language, and communication abilities and needs but also motor and perceptual skills, preferences, and the willingness of the environment to support AAC use. The SLP, in coordination with the family and other professionals, uses the data from the assessment to make decisions on the appropriate AAC method, AAC symbol system, and potential vocabulary.

The SLP must be concerned with linguistic and communicative competence as well as operational competence for the AAC system being trained. Intervention must include both the short-range and long-range needs of the client. Intervention considerations include but are not limited to the following:

- Establish an environment of AAC.
- Use everyday experiences as the training context.
- Individualize the content as discussed earlier.
- Train others to modify their interactional style.
- Consider positioning for those with severe motor impairments.
- Make communication real.

REFLECTIONS

- What are the major types of unaided and aided AAC systems?
- How do AAC needs change throughout the lifespan?
- What are the major concerns in client assessment for AAC?
- What are the major elements of intervention with AAC?

SUGGESTED READINGS

Lloyd, L. L., Fuller, D. R., & Arvidson, H. H. (1997). *Augmentative and alternative communication: A handbook of principles and practices.* Boston: Allyn and Bacon.

Reichle, J., Halle, J. W., & Drasgow, E. (1998). Implementing augmentative communication systems. In A. Wetherby, S. Warren, & J. Reichle (Eds.), *Transitions in prelinguistic communication* (pp. 417–436). Baltimore: Paul H. Brookes.

ONLINE RESOURCES

http://www.aacintervention.com/
Julie Maro and Caroline Musselwhite of AAC Intervention offer ideas and products for teaching AAC.

http://apple.com/disability/language/ Apple Computer site.
Contains downloadable files (Mac compatible) for adapting computers for use with persons with disabilities.

http://www.at-training.com/ University of Buffalo.
Assistive technology training online.

http://www.augcominc.com Augmentative Communication Inc.
Newsletter site with on-line tutorials and article synopses.

http://www.closingthegap.com/
Delores and Budd Hagan founded this internationally recognized source of information on innovative applications of computer technology in special education.

http://www.creative-comm.com Creative Communicating, Inc.
Teaching ideas and materials.

http://www.mrtc.org/~duffy/yaack/ AAC Connecting Young Kids site.
Useful information on how to get started, to assess, and to teach for AAC with references to professional articles.

http://www.trace.wisc.edu/ Trace Center, University of Wisconsin.
AAC research site offering materials on research and products at the center.

http://www.unl.edu/ University of Nebraska-Lincoln.
Device tutorials and resources.

http://www.aacprodeucts.org
Communication Aid Manufacturers Association (CAMA). Provides information about AAC devices and other assistive technology equipment.

Glossary

Acoustic immittance   The term used to refer to either the flow or opposition to the flow of energy through the middle.

Acoustic neuroma   A tumor of the vestibulo-cochlear (VIIIth) nerve.

Acquired   Occurring after birth.

Acquired immunodeficiency syndrome (AIDS)   A viral disease in which a person becomes susceptible to an assortment of other illnesses.

Acute laryngitis   Temporary swelling of the vocal folds, resulting in a hoarse voice quality.

Acute otitis media   Inflammation of the middle ear characterized by rapid onset, with resolution within approximately three weeks.

Addition   In articulation, the insertion of a phoneme that is not part of the word.

Adventitious   Occurring sometime after birth.

Affricate   A combination of a stop and fricative phoneme.

Agnosia   Sensory deficit accompanying some aphasias that make it difficult to understand incoming sensory information.

Agrammatism   Omission of spoken and written grammatical elements found in some aphasias in which individuals omit short unstressed words and morphological endings.

Agraphia   Writing difficulty accompanying some aphasias and characterized by mistakes and poorly formed letters.

AIDS   See *Acquired immunodeficiency syndrome.*

Air conduction   A method of evaluating hearing by transmitting sound to the inner ear via the outer and middle ear.

Alexia   Reading difficulties found in some aphasias in which the client may be unable to recognize even common words that he or she says.

Allophone   A phonemic variation.

Alport syndrome   A hereditary disorder characterized by kidney disease and bilateral progressive sensorineural hearing loss.

ALS   See *Amyotrophic lateral sclerosis.*

Alveolar   Refers to the alveolar or gum ridge of the mouth. In speech, alveolar consonants are those that are produced with the tongue on the alveolar ridge.

Alveolus   Area of the mandible and maxilla that houses the teeth.

Alzheimer's disease   A cortical pathology that affects primarily memory, language, or visuospatial skills as a result of diffuse brain atrophy; presenile dementia.

American Sign Language (ASL)   A complex non-vocal language containing elaborate syntax and semantics. Proficiency in its use is one of the primary methods by which a deaf individual becomes part of the Deaf Community.

Amplification   Technology such as hearing aids, cochlear implants, and assistive listening devices that improve access to sounds by electronically increasing their intensity.

Amyotrophic lateral sclerosis (ALS)   Commonly called Lou Gehrig's disease, ALS is a rapidly progressive degenerative disease in which the individual gradually loses control of her or his musculature. It is characterized by fatigue, muscle atrophy or loss of bulk, involuntary contractions, and reduced muscle tone. Speech in the later stages is labored and slow with short phrasing, long pauses, hypernasality, and severely impaired articulation.

Anatomy   The study of the structures of the body and the relationship of these structures to one another.

Aneurysm   A type of hemorrhagic stroke resulting from the rupture of a sac-like bulging in a weakened artery wall.

Ankyloglossia   Tongue-tie; a relatively short lingual frenum.

Anomia   Difficulty naming entities.

Anomic aphasia   A fluent aphasia characterized by naming difficulties and mild to moderate auditory comprehension problems.

Anoxia   Deprivation of oxygen.

Aphasia   An impairment due to localized brain injury and affecting understanding, retrieving, and formulating meaningful and sequential elements of language.

Aplasia   Hearing loss due to the absence or malformation of the inner ear structures during embryonic development.

Approximant   Sometimes called a semivowel; an oral consonant that is produced with less constriction than the obstruents, includes glides and liquids.

Apraxia or **verbal apraxia**   A neurological impairment of the ability to program—organize and plan—and execute movement of the speech muscles, unrelated to muscle weakness, slowness, or paralysis.

Arteriovenous malformation   A poorly formed tangle of arteries and veins that may result in a rare type of stroke in which arterial walls are weak and give way under pressure.

Articulation   Rapid and coordinated movement of the tongue, teeth, lips, and palate to produce speech sounds.

Articulatory/resonating system   Structures used during sound production including the oral cavity, nasal cavity, tongue, and soft palate.

Aryepiglottic folds   The membrane and muscle that connect the sides of the epiglottis to the arytenoid cartilages in the larynx.

Asperger's syndrome   Mild form of pervasive developmental disorder (PDD) characterized by normal intelligence and typical language development with deficits in social and communication skills.

Aspiration   Inhaling; used to mean the inhalation of fluid or food into the lungs; in phonology, a puff of air that is released in the production of various allophones.

Assessment of communication disorders   The systematic process of obtaining information from many sources, through various means, and in different settings to verify and specify communication strengths and weaknesses, identify possible causes, and make plans to address them.

Assistive Listening Devices (ALD)   The general term applied to electronic devices designed to enhance the reception of sound by those who are hearing-impaired.

Assistive technologies   Aids for daily living, communication, environmental controls; prosthetic or orthotic devices; sensory aids; seating and positioning systems; and mobility/transportation aids.

Ataxia   Disorder of muscle coordination.

Ataxic cerebral palsy   A congenital disorder characterized by uncoordinated movement and disturbed balance. Movements lack direction, and hypotonic muscles lack adequate force and rate and have poor directional control.

Ataxic dysarthria   A motor speech disorder involving a combination of muscle weakness or reduced tone or hypotonia and problems with muscle coordination. Little or no paralysis exists, and the problem is one involving the accuracy, timing, and direction of movement. Speech is characterized by excessive and equal stress and imprecise articulation, especially in repetitive movements.

Atresia   Congenital disorder resulting in complete closure of the external auditory meatus.

Attention deficit hyperactivity disorder (ADHD)   Hyperactivity and attentional difficulties in children who do not manifest other characteristics of learning disabilities.

Audibility   The ability to detect the presence of sound.

Audiogram   A graph on which results of pure tone audiometry are recorded.

Audiologist   A professional whose distinguishing role is to identify, assess, manage, and prevent disorders of hearing and balance.

Audiometer   A device used to regulate and deliver pure tone and speech stimuli during audiometric testing.

Auditory bombardment   In phonological therapy, the repeated presentation of target phonemes at a slightly amplified level.

Auditory brainstem   Nuclei and colliculi located in the brain stem that are related to audition.

Auditory brainstem response (ABR)   A type of electrophysiological testing that records neural responses along the ascending auditory pathways occurring within the first 10 milliseconds following stimulus presentation.

Auditory cortex   Heschel's gyri, located in the temporal lobe, that is concerned with the analysis and elaboration of speech.

Auditory evoked potentials (AEPs):   Small neuroelectic responses to auditory stimulation by the ascending auditory pathways leading from the cochlea to the cortex of the brain.

Auditory oral approach   A training method for hearing-impaired persons that emphasizes the use of residual hearing and speechreading (lipreading).

Auditory processing disorder (APD)   Deficits of the auditory structures, pathways, and neural synapses spanning from the brainstem to the cortex of the brain that inhibit one's ability to efficiently and effectively use and interpret auditory information. Also referred to as central auditory processing disorder (CAPD).

Auditory tube A tube connecting the middle ear cavity with the nasopharynx with the principal function of equalizing atmospheric and middle ear cavity air pressures.

Auditory training Listening activities designed to maximize a hearing-impaired person's ability to detect, discriminate, identify, and comprehend auditory information.

Auditory verbal approach A training method for hearing-impaired persons that emphasizes the use of residual hearing rather than vision.

Augmentative and alternative communication (AAC) Gestures, signing, picture systems, print, computerized communication, and voice production used to complement or supplement speech for persons with severe communication impairments.

Aural habilitation/rehabilitation: Services and procedures designed to improve communication deficits that result from hearing loss.

Authentic data Information about an individual that is based on real life.

Autism spectrum disorder (ASD) Term used to characterize individuals at the severe end of the pervasive developmental disorder (PDD) continuum. ASD is an impairment in reciprocal social interaction with a severely limited behavior, interest, and activity repertoire that has its onset before 30 months of age.

Automaticity The ease with which a person uses a particular skill without apparent thought.

Babbling Single-syllable nonpurposeful consonant-vowel (CV) or vowel-consonant (VC) vocalizations that begin at about 4 months of age.

Baseline data Information about client performance before intervention begins.

Basilar membrane The membrane that forms the floor of the organ of Corti. It is nonuniform in width and thickness, allowing it to respond differently to different frequencies of sound (tonotopically). The basilar membrane contains thousands of hair cells, the receptor cells for the auditory system.

Behavior modification A systematic method of changing behavior through careful target selection, stimulation, client response, and reinforcement.

Behavioral observation audiometry (BOA) A method of assessing infant hearing by presentation of different stimuli and watching for any changes in activity that signals a response.

Bifid uvula A uvula that is split in half.

Bilabial Pertaining to two lips, as phonemes produced with both lips.

Bilateral Both sides.

Binaural integration The process of assimilating different information presented to each ear into a single unit.

Blending Creating a word from individual sounds and syllables.

Bolus A chewed lump of food ready for swallowing.

Bone anchored hearing aid (BAHA) A type of amplification in which some of the components are surgically implanted into the temporal bone of the skull, stimulating the cochlea via bone conduction.

Bone conduction A method of evaluating hearing by transmitting sound to the inner ear by mechanically vibrating the bones of the skull.

Bone oscillator A small, vibrating device that is positioned against the skull behind the pinna in bone conduction testing.

Bony hard palate Anterior two-thirds of the roof of the mouth.

Booster treatment Additional therapy, based on retesting, offered after treatment has been terminated.

Bound morpheme A morpheme that must be attached to a free morpheme to communicate meaning; grammatical morpheme.

Breathiness Perception of audible air escaping through the glottis during phonation.

Broca's aphasia A nonfluent aphasia that is characterized by short sentences with agrammatism; anomia; problems with imitation of speech because of overall speech problems; slow, labored speech and writing; and articulation and phonological errors.

Bulbar palsy A progressive neurological condition resulting in flaccid dysarthria characterized by muscle atrophy and by rapid, random, irregular, and minute contractions (vasiculation) of nerve bundles.

Carryover Transference or generalization; the use of the corrected form outside of the clinical setting.

Case history Background information on a client.

Central auditory processing disorder (CAPD) Problems along the brainstem pathways and the auditory cortex of the brain resulting in an inability to efficiently utilize and interpret auditory information, although hearing is within the normal range.

Cerebellopontine angle: The area of the brainstem formed by the junction of the cerebellum, medulla, and pons.

Cerebral arteriosclerosis   A type of ischemic stroke resulting from a thickening of the walls of cerebral arteries in which elasticity is lost or reduced, the walls become weakened, and blood flow is restricted.

Cerebral palsy (CP)   A heterogeneous group of neurogenic disorders that result in difficulty with motor movement; were acquired before, during, or shortly after birth; and affect one or more limbs.

Cerebrovascular accident (CVA)   Stroke, the most common cause of aphasia, results when the blood supply to the brain is blocked or when the brain is flooded with blood.

Cerumen (earwax)   A substance produced by glands in the ear canal that provides lubrication and protects the ear from the invasion of insects and other foreign objects.

Chin tuck   A posture with the chin down that is helpful with some patients who have a swallowing disability.

Cholesteatoma   A tumor-like mass of epithelial (skin) cells, keratin, and fats such as cholesterol that migrate into the middle ear cavity.

Chorea   A form of hyperkinetic dysarthria characterized by rapid or continual, random, irregular, and/or abrupt hyperkinesia. Speech, when affected, may be characterized by inappropriate silences caused by voice stoppage; intermittent breathiness, strained harsh voice, and hypernasality; imprecise articulation with prolonged pauses; and forced inspiration and expiration resulting in excessive loudness variations.

Chronemics   The study of the effect of time on communication.

Chronic laryngitis   Vocal abuse during acute laryngitis that leads to vocal fold tissue damage.

Chronic otitis media   Inflammation of the middle ear lasting longer than eight weeks.

Cleft   An abnormal opening in an anatomical structure.

Cleft palate team   A team of professionals including a surgeon, orthodontist, a speech-language pathologist, and one additional specialist according to the requirements of the American Cleft Palate-Craniofacial Association.

Closed syllable   A syllable, or basic acoustic unit of speech, that ends in one or more consonants.

Cluttering   Disfluent speech that is characterized by overuse of fillers and circumlocutions associated with word-finding difficulties, rapid speech, and word and phrase repetitions. Cluttering does not seem to contain the fear of words or situations found in stuttering.

Cochlea   The portion of the inner ear that contains the sensory cells for the auditory system. It is composed of two concentric labyrinths; the outer one is made of bone, the inner one of membrane.

Cochlear implant   An electronic amplification device that is surgically placed in the cochlea and provides electrical stimulation to the surviving auditory nerve fibers.

Code switching   Process in which bilingual speakers transfer between two languages based on the listener, context, or topic.

Cognitive rehabilitation   A treatment regimen for individuals with TBI that is designed to increase functional abilities for everyday life by improving the capacity to process incoming information.

Columella   A strip of tissue connecting the tip of the nose to the base.

Communication   An exchange of ideas between sender(s) and receivers(s).

Communication disorder   An impairment in the ability to receive, send, process, or comprehend concepts of verbal, nonverbal, or graphic symbol systems.

Compensatory articulation error   Gross sound substitution errors that are an attempt to make up for the physical inability to produce a given sound correctly.

Complete cleft   A total separation of a normally fused structure.

Conditioned play audiometry (CPA)   A method of assessing the hearing of children ages $2\frac{1}{2}$ to 3 years and older by instructing them to put a block in a bucket, a ring on a peg, or other action whenever they hear the test signal.

Conduction aphasia   A fluent aphasia in which the individual's conversation is abundant and quick. Characterized by anomia, mildly impaired auditory comprehension if at all, extremely poor repetitive or imitative speech, and paraphasia.

Conductive hearing loss   A loss of auditory sensitivity due to malformation or obstruction of the outer and/or middle ear.

Congenital   Present at birth.

Congenital laryngeal webbing   Extraneous tissue on the anterior aspects of the vocal folds that can interfere with breathing; present at birth.

Consistent aphonia   Persistent absence of voice.

Consonant   A phoneme that is produced with some vocal tract constriction or occlusion.

Contact ulcer   A benign lesion that may develop on the posterior surface of the vocal folds.

Conversion aphonia   Psychologically based loss of voice.

Conversion disorder   Condition in which emotion is suppressed and transformed into a sensory or motor diability.

Correlate   Something that tends to exist in the presence of something else or be associated with it, but without a demonstrated causal relationship.

Craniofacial anomalies   Congenital malformations involving the head (*cranio:* above the upper eyelid) and face (*facial:* below the upper eyelid).

Craniosynostosis   Premature closing of the sutures of the skull, which greatly disfigures the forehead.

Critical literacy   Reader's ability to actively interpret between the lines, to analyze, and synthesize information and to be able to explain content.

Criterion referenced   An evaluation of an individual's strengths and weaknesses with regard to specific skills.

Cued Speech   A visual communication system that combines the mouth movements of speech with manual cues designed to facilitate the identification of speech sounds that are visually similar, as well as those that not readily visible.

Cycles approach   A method of phonological therapy in which the same target processes are addressed in several training periods, or cycles.

Deaf Community   A group of persons who share a common means of communication (American Sign Language) that facilitates group cohesion and identity.

Deaf Culture   A view of life manifested by the mores, beliefs, artistic expression, understandings, and language (ASL) that are specific to Deaf people.

Decibel (dB)   A mathematically derived unit based upon the pressure exerted by a particular sound vibration.

Decoding   Breaking or segmenting a written word into its component sounds and then blending them together to form a recognizable word.

Decontextualized   Outside of a conversational context. When we write, we construct the context with our writing rather than having it constructed by our conversational partner(s).

Dementia   An acquired pathological condition or syndrome that is characterized by intellectual decline, especially memory, due to neurogenic causes. Additional deficits include poor reasoning or judgment, impaired abstract thinking, inability to attend to relevant information, impaired communication, and personality changes.

Dentition   The number, type, and arrangement of teeth.

Developmental apraxia of speech (DAS)   An impairment in programming the musculature for speech without apparent muscle weakness or paralysis. Apraxia of speech in children is characterized by multiple articulation errors including addition of speech sounds, sound and syllable repetitions, and sound prolongations.

Developmental disfluency or developmental stuttering   Whole-word repetitions and other self-conscious nonfluency that is apparent in many young children.

Developmental verbal dyspraxia (DVD)   See *Developmental apraxia of speech.*

Diagnosis   A statement distinguishing an individual's difficulties from the broad range of possibilities.

Diagnostic therapy   Ongoing assessment and evaluation as intervention takes place.

Dialect   A linguistic variation that is attributable primarily to geographical region or foreign language background. It includes features of form, content, and use.

Dichotic   The simultaneous presentation of different stimuli to each ear.

Diphthong   Two vowels that are said in such close proximity that they are treated as a single phoneme.

Diplophonia   The perception of two vocal frequencies.

Disability   The functional consequence of an impairment.

Distinctive features   The attributes of phonemes that differentiate one from another on the basis of a binary principle.

Distortion   In articulation, a deviant production of a phoneme.

Double swallow   A technique in which the patient swallows more than once per bolus.

Down syndrome   A congenital condition that is characterized by multiple defects and varying degrees of intellectual deficit.

Dynamic   Characterized by energy or effective energy, changing over time.

Dynamic literacy   Reader's ability to interrelate content to other knowledge through both deductive and inductive reasoning.

Dysarthria   One of several motor speech disorders that involve impaired articulation, respiration, phonation, or prosody as a result of paralysis, muscle weakness, or poor coordination. Motor function may be excessively slow or rapid, decreased in range or strength, and have poor directionality and timing.

Dysgraphia   A disability that is characterized by difficulty producing written symbols.

Dyskinesia   Impairment in the ability to control voluntary movement; sometimes due to prolonged use of certain medications.

Dyslexia   A disability that is characterized by difficulty comprehending printed symbols and recognizing words. Children with dyslexia often exhibit delayed language development, listening comprehension problems, and poor phonological awareness.

Dysphagia   A disorder of swallowing.

Dystonia   A form of hyperkinetic dysarthria that is characterized by a slow, sustained increase and decrease of hyperkinesia involving either the entire body or localized sets of muscles. As a result, there are excessive pitch and loudness variations, irregular articulation breakdown, and vowel distortions.

Eardrum   See *Tympanic membrane.*

Ear training   The first stage in the Van Riper approach to articulation therapy. It involves identification, localization, stimulation, and discrimination of the target phoneme.

Echolalia   An immediate imitation of another speaker. Among children with ASD, it may represent the storage and production of unanalyzed whole units of language.

Edema   Swelling due to an accumulation of fluid.

Electrocochleography (ECoG)   A type of electrophysiological testing that records neural responses occurring within 2 milliseconds following stimulus presentation.

Electrolarynx   Battery-powered device that sets air in the vocal tract into vibration.

Embolism   A blood clot, fatty materials, or an air bubble that may travel through the circulatory system until it blocks the flow of blood in a small artery. If it travels to the brain, it may cause a stroke.

Endolymph   The fluid that fills the membranous labyrinth of the cochlea and vestibular system.

Endoscope   A lens coupled with a light source used for viewing internal bodily structures, including the vocal folds.

Episodic aphonia   Uncontrolled and unpredictable occasional loss of voice.

Esophageal atresia   The absence of a normal open passageway from the esophagus to the stomach.

Esophageal speech   Speech that is produced by using burping as a substitute for the laryngeal voice.

Esophagostomy   A surgical hole in the esophagus through which a feeding tube may be inserted.

Etiology   Cause or origin of a problem; also the study of cause.

Eustachian tube or **auditory tube**   The tube that connects the middle ear space with the upper portion of the pharynx and provides a passageway for air to move in and out, maintaining equality of air pressure on either side of the eardrum and ensuring its maximum mobility.

Evidence-based practice   The process of making decisions regarding individual client care and specific courses of treatment based on current, well-designed research.

Examination of the peripheral speech mechanism   Sometimes called *oral peripheral exam;* assessment of the structure and function of the visible speech system.

Executive function   An aspect of metacognition used in self-regulation and including the ability to attend; to set reasonable goals; to plan and organize to achieve each goal; to initiate, monitor, and evaluate your performance in relation to that goal; and to revise plans and strategies based on feedback.

Explicit   Clearly defined.

External auditory meatus or canal   The tubular structure that extends from the concha of the pinna to the tympanic membrane.

External error sound discrimination   Perceiving differences in the production of the target phoneme in another person's speech.

Failure to thrive   The absence of healthy growth and development.

Fast mapping   Process in which a child infers the meaning of a word from context and uses it in a similar context at a later time. A fuller definition evolves over time. Fast mapping enables preschool children to expand their vocabularies quickly by being able to use a word without fully understanding the meaning.

FEES   See *Fiberoptic endoscopic evaluation of swallowing.*

Fetal alcohol syndrome (FAS)   Overuse of alcohol during pregnancy, which severely impairs the neurological and physical development of the fetus, resulting in growth deficiencies, craniofacial disorders, central nervous system dysfunction, limited cognitive development, and, in some cases, sensorineural hearing loss.

Fiberoptic endoscopic evaluation of swallowing (FEES)   A laryngoscopic technique for viewing swallowing.

Figurative language   Nonliteral phrases consisting of idioms, metaphors, similes, and proverbs.

Filler   Utterances such as "er," "um," and "you know" that are used within productions. Sometimes characteristic of dysfluent speech and/or stuttering.

Fingerspelling   A form of manual communication system consisting of 26 distinct handshapes that visually represent each letter of the English alphabet.

Flaccid dysarthria   Speech disorder caused by weak, soft, flabby muscle tone, called hypotonia. May result in hypernasality, breathiness, and imprecise articulation.

Fluency   Smoothness of rhythm and rate.

Fluent   Speech that is relatively smooth and free of disruptions.

Fluent aphasia   Speech characterized by word substitutions, neologisms, and often verbose verbal output. Also called Wernicke's aphasia.

FM system   A type of assistive listening device that transmits sound to a hearing-impaired person via FM radio waves. The system consists of a microphone, transmitter, and a wireless receiver.

Follow-up testing   Assessment after dismissal from therapy to ensure that skills have been maintained.

Free morpheme   The portion of a word that can stand alone and designate meaning; root morpheme.

Frequency   An acoustical term that refers to the number of sound wave cycles that are completed within a specific time period. Subjectively, it is perceived as the pitch of the sound.

Fricative   A consonant phoneme that is produced by exhaling air through a narrow passageway.

Frontonasal process   Embryonic structure that develops into the nasomedial processes and the lateral nasal processes during the fifth week of gestation.

Functional   Having no known organic cause; perhaps psychogenic or learned.

Fundamental frequency   The lowest frequency component of a complex vibration.

Gastroesophageal reflux (GER)   Movement of food or acid from the stomach back into the esophagus.

Genderlect   Variations in language associated with males or females; gender-based dialect.

Generalization   The extending of a skill learned in a clinical setting to other "natural" environments or skills; carryover or transference.

Generative   Capable of being freshly created; refers to the infinite number of sentences that can be created through the application of grammatical rules.

Glide   Phoneme in which the articulatory posture changes from consonant to vowel.

Global or mixed aphasia   A profound language impairment in all modalities as a result of brain damage.

Glossectomy   The surgical removal of the tongue.

Glottal   Relating to, or produced in or by the glottis, the space between the vocal cords.

Glottal stop   A compensatory behavior where a stoppage of air occurs at the level of the glottis rather than in the oral cavity.

Grammar   The rules of a language.

Granuloma   A nodular lesion due to injury or infection. May occur on the vocal folds and be caused by a breathing tube placed through the glottis.

Habitual pitch   The basic frequency level that an individual uses most of the time.

Hair cells   Auditory receptor cells located in the organ of Corti that are responsible for encoding auditory information.

Handicap   The psychosocial consequence of a disability.

Hard glottal attacks   Abrupt initiation of voicing using hypertensive vocal fold adduction.

Hard of hearing   Mild to moderately severe hearing loss. Hard-of-hearing individuals usually depend as much as possible on their hearing for communication and learning of new concepts.

Harmonics   Frequencies in a complex sound that are integer multiples of the fundamental frequency.

Head-back position   A posture with the head held back that is useful for some clients with a swallowing disability.

Head rotation   A posture with the head toward the impairment, used for some clients with a swallowing disability.

Head tilt position   A posture with the head away from the impairment, used for some individuals with a swallowing disability.

Hearing aid   Personal amplification device ranging from tiny, completely-in-the-canal models to those worn behind the ear.

Hematoma   Blood trapped in an organ or skin tissue owing to injury or surgery.

Hemianopsia   Blindness in the left or right visual field of both eyes caused by lesions on the temporal or lower parietal lobe.

Hemiparesis   Muscle weakness on one side of the body, resulting in reduced strength and control.

Hemiplegia   Paralysis on one side of the body.

Hemisensory impairment   Loss of the ability to perceive sensory information on one side of the body.

Hemorrhagic stroke   A type of stroke resulting from the weakening of arterial walls that burst under pressure.

Hertz (Hz)   Number of complete vibrations per second.

Hesitation   A pause before or between parts of utterances. If used excessively, it may be considered a sign of dysfluency or stuttering.

HIV/AIDS   See *Human immunodeficiency virus* and *Acquired immunodeficiency syndrome*.

Hoarseness   A voice quality that is characterized by a rough, usually low-pitched quality.

Holistic   Pertaining to the whole; multidimensional.

Homophenous   Refers to phonemes that are visually indistinguishable when spoken, such as /p/ and /b/.

Human immunodeficiency virus (HIV)   The organism responsible for AIDS.

Huntington's chorea   An inherited progressive disease also known as Huntington's disease, resulting from a genetic defect on chromosome 4.

Hyperadduction   Excessive movement toward the midline, often resulting in a tense voice quality.

Hyperfluent speech   Very rapid speech found in people with fluent aphasia and characterized by few pauses, incoherence, inefficiency, and pragmatic inappropriateness.

Hyperkinetic dysarthria   A speech disorder characterized by increased movement, such as tremors and tics, and by inaccurate articulation.

Hyperlexia   A mild form of pervasive developmental disorder (PDD) characterized by an inordinate interest in letters and words and by early ability to read but with little comprehension.

Hypertonia   A condition in which there is too much muscle tone, especially in those muscles that oppose the bending of joints and that help us to stand erect. Also called spasticity.

Hypoadduction   Reduced movement toward the midline of the vocal folds, often resulting in a breathy voice quality.

Hypokinesia   Abnormally decreased motor function or activity.

Hypokinetic dysarthria   A speech disorder that is characterized by a decrease or lack of appropriate movement as muscles become rigid and stiff, resulting in monopitch and monoloudness and imprecise articulation.

Hyponasality   A lack of nasal resonance.

Hypotonia   Poor muscle tone and weakness.

Idiolect   An individual's unique way of speaking, a personal dialect.

Impairment   A loss of structure or function.

Implicit   Assumed but not directly expressed.

Inappropriate pitch   Pitch judged to be outside the normal range for age and/or sex.

Incidental teaching   Using a natural activity to train targets.

Incomplete cleft   A separation of a normally fused structure that involves only a portion of the structure.

Incus   The middle bone of the ossicular chain in the middle ear. It articulates with the malleus at the top and has a projection that is joined to the stapes at the bottom.

Infarction   Death of bodily tissue due to deprivation of the blood supply.

Inferior longitudinal muscle (tongue)   Intrinsic muscle of the tongue that shortens the tongue.

Informational counseling   The process of imparting information to patients and their families.

Inner ear   The interior section of the ear containing the cochlea and vestibular system. It supplies information to the brain regarding balance, spatial orientation, and hearing.

Intelligibility   The ability to understand what has been detected auditorily.

Intensity   A measure of loudness generally expressed in decibels.

Intentionality   Goal directedness in interactions. It is first demonstrated at about 8 months of age primarily through gestures.

Interdental   Between the teeth; see *Linguadental.*

Internal auditory meatus   The bony canal housing the vestibulocochlear (VIIIth) nerve that runs from the cochlea to the brainstem.

Internal error sound discrimination   Judging the accuracy of one's own phoneme production; intrapersonal error sound discrimination.

Interpersonal error sound discrimination   See *External error sound discrimination.*

Intonation   Pitch movement within an utterance.

Intrapersonal error sound discrimination   See *Internal error sound discrimination.*

Ischemic stroke   A cerebrovascular accident resulting from a complete or partial blockage or occlusion of the arteries transporting blood to the brain.

Jargon   In infancy, long strings of unintelligible sounds with adultlike intonation that develop at about 8 months of age and exhibit the pitch and intonational pattern of the language to which the child is exposed. Jargon may sound like questions, commands, and statements. In some aphasias, jargon refers to meaningless or irrelevant speech, characterized by typical intonational patterns and frequently correct syntax.

Kernahan's Striped Y   A visual classification system for cleft lip and palate.

Kinesics   The study of bodily movement and gesture. Also known as body language.

Labiodental   Pertaining to lips and teeth; phonemes produced with lip and tooth contact.

Language   A socially shared code for representing concepts through the use of arbitrary symbols and rule-governed combinations of those symbols.

Language impairment   A heterogeneous group of deficits and/or immaturities in the comprehension and/or production of spoken or written language.

Language-learning disability   Term used to describe the approximately 75 percent of children with learning disability (LD) who have difficulty primarily with learning and using symbols.

Language sample   A systematic collection and analysis of a person's speech or writing. Sometimes called a corpus; used as a part of language assessment.

Laryngeal cancer   Carcinoma of supraglottal, glottal, or subglottal structures.

Laryngeal papilloma   Wartlike growth on the vocal folds.

Laryngeal system   Structures of the larynx used for sound production.

Larynx   The superior termination of the trachea that protects the lower airways and is the primary sound source for speech production.

Lateral nasal processes   Primitive embryological tissue that gives rise to the nasal alae.

Lexicon   An individual's personal dictionary of words and meanings.

Limited English proficiency (LEP)   Language differences that are found in some individuals learning English as a second language. Differences do not in themselves constitute language impairments.

Linguadental   Pertaining to tongue and teeth; phonemes produced with tongue and tooth contact.

Linguist   A scientist who studies the nature and structure of language(s) and often child language acquisition.

Linguistic intuition   A language user's underlying knowledge about the system of rules pertaining to his or her native language; linguistic competence.

Liquid   Refers to the oral resonant consonants /r/ and /l/.

Literacy   Use of visual modes of communication, specifically reading and writing.

Localization   The process of determining where sound originates in space.

Loudness variation   Speaking too loudly or too softly for a particular vocal situation.

Maintaining cause   The perpetuating cause that keeps a problem from self-correcting; for example, parents of an 8-year-old considering a lisp "cute."

Malar hypoplasia   Underdevelopment of the cheek bones.

Malleus   The largest of the ossicles. It is fastened to the eardrum and articulates with the incus, the next bone in the chain.

Malocclusion   Improper alignment of the maxillary (upper) and mandibular (lower) dental arches.

Mandibular processes   Primitive embryological tissue that gives rise to the mandible.

Manually coded English   Sign communication systems designed to manually duplicate spoken English for teaching children who are deaf.

Maternal rubella   German measles contracted during pregnancy, which may result in various disorders in the developing fetus.

Maxillary processes   Primitive embryological tissue that gives rise to the lateral aspects of the maxilla and palatal shelves.

Maximal contrast   A minimal pair in which the differing phonemes differ in more than one distinctive feature; for example, "say" (/se/) and "bay" (/be/).

Maximal opposition   See *Maximal contrast*.

Mean length of utterance (MLU)   The average length of utterances measured in morphemes. In English, this is an important measure of preschool development, because language becomes more complex as it becomes longer.

Ménière's disease   A condition resulting from excessive endolymph in the inner ear, resulting in vertigo, tinnitus, aural fullness, and sensorineural hearing loss.

Meningitis   An inflammation of the meninges, or layers of tissue covering the brain and spinal cord.

Mental retardation/developmental disabilities   A disorder characterized by substantial limitations in intellectual functioning, concurrent related limitations in adaptive skill areas, and manifestation before age 18.

Metacognition   Knowledge about knowledge and cognitive processes, including self-appraisal.

Metalinguistic skills   Abilities that enable a child to consider language in the abstract, to make judgments about its correctness, and to create verbal contexts, such as in writing.

Metaphon   An approach to phonological therapy that is based on the premise that phonological disorders in children are developmental language learning disorders.

Micrognathia   Underdeveloped mandible.

Microtia   Congenital disorder resulting in a small, malformed pinna or ear canal.

Middle ear   The section of the ear containing the ossicles. It is bounded laterally by the tympanic membrane and medially by the cochlea.

Middle ear implant   A type of amplification device that is partially or fully implanted into the middle ear cavity to assist those with sensorineural hearing loss.

Middle ear space or tympanic cavity   The cube-shaped area between the outer and middle ear containing the ossicles.

Minimal contrast   A minimal pair in which the differing phonemes differ in a single distinctive feature; for example, "lope" (/lop/) and "lobe" (/lob/).

Minimal pair   Two words that differ in a single phoneme; for example, "say" (/se/) and "bay" (/be/).

Mixed dysarthrias   Symptoms or areas of brain injury that cross several dysarthrias as a result of degenerative disorders, toxins, metabolic disorders, stroke, trauma, tumors, or infectious diseases.

Mixed hearing loss   Combination of a sensorineural hearing loss with a conductive component.

Modified barium swallow study   An X-ray procedure that is used to visualize the swallowing process. Also known as *videofluoroscopy*.

Monoloudness   Voice lacking normal variations of intensity that occur during speech.

Monopitch   Voice that lacks normal inflection in tone.

Monotone   Voice that is produced without varying the fundamental frequency.

Morpheme   The smallest meaningful unit of language.

Morphophonemic contrast   Change in pronunciation as a result of morphological changes.

MS   See *Multiple sclerosis*.

Mucosal tissue   Pinkish tissue lining the inside of the mouth.

Multiple sclerosis (MS)   A progressive disease characterized by demyelinization of nerve fibers of the brain and spinal cord.

Multiview videofluoroscopy   Motion picture X-rays recorded from various angles.

Muscular dystrophy   A group of genetic diseases characterized by progressive weakness and degeneration of the muscles that control movement. Forms differ in the pattern of inheritance, age of onset, rate of progression, and distribution of muscle weakness.

Myasthenia gravis   A disorder characterized by fatigability and rapid weakening of muscles, a cause of flaccid dysarthria.

Myelination   Development of a protective myelin sheath or sleeve around the cranial nerves.

Myofunctional disorder   See *Tongue thrust*.

Myringotomy   A small surgical incision made in the surface of the tympanic membrane.

Nasal   Phoneme that is produced with nasal resonance.

Nasal alae   Lateral flaring of the nostrils.

Nasalance score   A numerical score that reflects the magnitude of hypernasality when measured by a nasometer.

Nasal cavity   Cavity above the oral cavity related to the nose.

Nasal emission   Air escaping through the nose during speech production.

Nasogastric tube (NG tube) A tube placed into the nose then through the pharynx and esophagus by which liquefied food may be fed.

Nasomedian processes Primitive embryological tissue that gives rise to the anterior portion of the upper lip and premaxilla.

Nasometer A commercially available device that is used to measure nasality.

Nasopharynx The space within the skull that is behind the nose and above the roof of the mouth.

Neologism A novel word that does not exist in the language. Neologisms are created and used quite confidently by some individuals with aphasia.

Neonate Newborn.

Neurogenic stuttering Disorder of fluency associated with some form of brain damage.

Noise-induced hearing loss Hearing impairment resulting from exposure to high levels of occupation or recreational noise.

Nonfluent aphasia A language disorder that is characterized by slow, labored speech and struggle to retrieve words and form sentences.

Nonorganic hearing loss A condition where a patient portrays having a hearing loss when one does not truly exist or exaggerates the degree of a true auditory deficit.

Nonverbal Without words.

Nonvocal Without voice.

Norm referenced A comparison that is usually based on others of the same gender and similar age.

Obstruent In articulation refers to speech sounds that are produced with a significant amount of constriction in the vocal tract (stops, fricatives, affricates); also called nonresonant phonemes.

Obturator A prosthetic device that forms an artificial palate. It is used to cover a cleft palate.

Olfactory pits Depressions between the nasomedian and lateral nasal processes that will ultimately become the right and left nasal cavities.

Omission In articulation, the absence of a phoneme that has not been produced or replaced.

Open syllable A syllable, or basic acoustic unit of speech, that ends in a vowel.

Optimal pitch level A particularly suitable pitch level for an individual largely determined by vocal fold structure.

Oral apraxia A neurological impairment in programming and executing speech and nonspeech movements of the mouth.

Oral cavity The mouth, housing the teeth and tongue.

Oral-motor training Exercises and activities that train volitional control over movements needed for speech. Also known as motor programming.

Organ of Corti The intricate structure that runs along the center of the membranous labyrinth of the cochlea and contains the auditory sensory receptor cells.

Organic Physiological.

Orthodontist A dental specialist who is concerned primarily with alignment of the teeth.

Ossicles or Ossicular chain Small bones within the middle ear, including the malleus, the incus, and the stapes.

Otitis media Inflammation of the middle ear.

Otitis media with effusion (OME) Inflammation of the middle ear with fluid.

Otoacoustic emissions (OAEs) Measurable low-level sounds or echoes, occurring either spontaneously or in response to acoustic stimulation, due to outer hair cell motility within the cochlea.

Otolith system The portion of the vestibular system responsible for sensing linear acceleration.

Otosclerosis A disorder characterized by the formation of spongy bone in the region of the stapes footplate, resulting in a progressive conductive hearing loss.

Otoscope A small, handheld device used to visually inspect the external auditory canal and tympanic membrane.

Ototoxic Refers to drugs and chemical agents that may damage the inner ear.

Outer ear The section of the ear comprised of the pinna and the external auditory meatus or ear canal.

Oval window A small, oval membrane located on the lateral wall of the cochlea, behind the stapes footplate.

Palatal Refers to the front area of the roof of the mouth. In speech, palatal consonants are produced with the tongue touching or approximating the hard palate.

Palatal obturator A plate that covers a portion of the soft palate. It is useful for individuals who have had palatal surgery.

Palatal shelves Wedge-shaped tissue masses that will become the bony hard palate.

Palatoplasty Surgical correction of a cleft palate.

Paraphasia Word substitutions that are found in some individuals with aphasia who may talk fluently and grammatically.

Paresis Muscle weakness, partial paralysis.

Parkinson's disease   A progressive neurogenic disorder that is characterized by resting tremors, slowness of movement, and difficulty initiating voluntary movements. Speech may be rapid, breathy, and reduced in loudness, pitch range, and stress.

Pedunculated polyp   Polyp that appears to be attached to the vocal fold by a stalk.

Perceptual training   See *Ear training.*

Perilymph   The fluid that fills the bony labyrinth of the cochlea and vestibular system.

Perpetuating cause   See *Maintaining cause.*

Permanent threshold shift (PTS)   a permanent change in hearing acuity associated with exposure to high-intensity noise.

Personal adjustment counseling: The process of assisting patients and their families in dealing with the emotional consequences of hearing loss.

Pervasive developmental disability (PDD)   Any of several disorders of childhood that are characterized by markedly atypical behaviors and severe impairment in the ability to relate to others, including infantile autism and childhood schizophrenia.

Pharyngeal cavity   The throat.

Pharyngeal flap   A secondary surgical procedure to correct velopharyngeal incompetence.

Pharyngostomy   A surgical hole in the pharynx through which a feeding tube may be placed.

Pharynx   The anatomical passageway connecting the nasal and oral cavities.

Phonation   Production of sound by vocal fold vibration.

Phonemic awareness   Ability to manipulate sounds, such as blending sounds to create new words or segmenting words into sounds.

Phonemic regression   Difficulty understanding speech that is far greater than expected based on the degree of hearing loss.

Phonetically balanced (PB)   Refers to words used in auditory word recognition testing where each phoneme is represented in the same proportion in which it occurs in everyday English.

Phonetically consistent forms (PCFs)   Consistent vocal patterns that function as meaningful "words" for the infant. These are a transition to words.

Phonics   Sound-letter or phoneme-grapheme correspondence.

Phonological awareness   Knowledge of sounds and syllables and of the sound structure of words.

Phonological process   A simplification of adult phonology; a system of describing children's articulatory patterns.

Phonology   The study of the sound systems of language.

Phonotactic   The study of the way in which phonemes are combined and arranged in syllables and words of a particular language or dialect.

Physiology   The branch of biology that is concerned with the process and function of parts of the body.

Pidgin Signed English (PSE)   A sign system that incorporates ASL signs while maintaining English word order.

Pierre Robin syndrome   A congenital condition resulting in a small mandible, cleft lip, cleft palate, and other facial abnormalities.

Pinna   The funnel-shape outermost part of the ear, which serves to collect the sound waves and channel them into the ear.

Pitch   The perceptual counterpart to fundamental frequency associated with the speed of vocal fold vibration.

Pitch breaks   Sudden uncontrolled upward or downward changes in pitch.

Postlingually   After the development of speech and language.

Posttherapy testing   Assessment following intervention.

Prader-Willi syndrome   A congenital condition characterized by obesity and intellectual deficit.

Pragmatics   The use, function, or purpose of communication; the study of communicative acts and contexts.

Precipitating cause   Factors that trigger a disorder; for example, a stroke.

Predisposing cause   Underlying factors that contribute to a problem; for example, a genetic basis.

Prelingually   Prior to the development of speech and language.

Premaxilla   The anterior portion of the hard palate to the incisive foramen.

Presbycusis   Hearing loss incurred as a result of the aging process.

Pressure equalization (PE) tube   A small-diameter tube that is surgically placed in the eardrum and provides ventilation of the middle ear space via the external auditory meatus.

Prevalence   The total number of cases of a disorder at a particular point in time in a designated population.

Print awareness   Knowledge of the meaning and function of print, including recognition of words and letters and terminology, such as letter, word, or sentence.

Production training   In the Van Riper approach to articulation, therapy that involves teaching the client to say the target phoneme in isolation, then syllables, words, phrases, and sentences.

Prognosis   An informed prediction of the outcome of a disorder.

Prolabium   Central prominence of the lip; also isolated soft tissue mass in unrepaired bilateral clefts.

Prolongation   In fluency analysis, the process of holding a phoneme longer than is typical; for example, "sssssso."

Prosody   The rate and rhythm of language; the melodic pattern of speech.

Prosthodontist   A dental specialist who is concerned with the replacement of missing teeth and other oral structures with various appliances.

Proxemics   The study of physical distance between people.

Pseudobulbar palsy   A condition that resembles progressive bulbar palsy, characterized by spastic dysarthria and dysphagia.

Psychogenic   Caused by psychological factors.

Pure tone audiometry   A procedure that is used to assess hearing sensitivity at discrete frequencies.

Pure tones   Sounds that contain energy at only a single frequency, usually 250 Hz, 500 Hz, 1000 Hz, 2000 Hz, 4000 Hz and 8000 Hz, and are used in pure tone audiometry.

Purulent otitis media   Pus formation and discharge by the tissue of the middle ear cavity.

Pyloric stenosis   A narrowing of the sphincter connecting the stomach to the small intestine, resulting in a blockage to the intestines.

Range of motion   The extent of movement of a joint from maximum extension to maximum flexion.

Rate   The speed at which something occurs. In speech this may be the number of words or syllables in a given period of time.

Recurrent branch   Branch of the tenth cranial nerve that innervates muscles of the larynx.

Reduplicated babbling   Long strings of consonant-vowel syllable repetitions, such as "ma-ma-ma-ma-ma."

Reinforcement   A procedure that follows a response with the intent of perpetuating or extinguishing it; used in conditioning.

Repetition   In fluency analysis, the process of repeating a word or a part of a word, as in "the-the-the" or "b-b-ball."

Representation   Process of having one thing stand for another, such as a piece of paper used as a blanket for a doll.

Residual hearing   Any hearing that remains following the onset of hearing loss.

Resonant   A consonant phoneme that is produced with resonance occurring throughout the vocal tract; refers to nasals, liquids, and glides.

Respiratory system   Stuctures, including the lungs, bronchi, trachea, larynx, mouth, and nose, that are used in breathing for life and speech.

Reverberation   The short, echo effect caused by the reflection of sound waves off of solid surfaces within a confined space.

Reverse swallow   See *Tongue thrust.*

Right hemisphere injury or syndrome (RHI)   A group of neuromuscular, perceptual, and/or linguistic deficits that result from damage to the right hemisphere of the brain and may include epilepsy, hemisensory impairment, and hemiparesis or hemiplegia.

Scintigraphy   A computerized technique for measuring aspiration during or after a swallow.

Segmentation   Creating a word when a phoneme or syllable is deleted.

Self-monitoring   The ability to recognize one's own errors and correct them.

Sensorimotor training   Articulatory training that emphasizes tactile and proprioceptive sensations and sound, syllable, and word production.

Semantic features   The pieces of meaning that come together to define a particular word.

Semantic-pragmatic disorder   A mild form of pervasive developmental disorder characterized by limited vocabulary, concrete definitions, and poor conversational skills.

Semantics   The study of word and language meaning.

Semicircular canals   Series of three canals located in the inner ear that senses angular acceleration.

Sensorineural hearing loss   Permanent hearing loss as the result of the absence, malformation, or damage to the structures of the inner ear.

Serous otitis media   Inflammation of the middle ear with sterile fluid.

Sessile polyp   Polyp with a broad-based attachment to the vocal fold.

Silent aspiration   Lack of coughing when food or liquid enters the airway.

Simultaneous communication   The use of sign language in combination with speech.

SLP   See *Speech language pathologist.*

Sociolinguistics   The study of influences such as cultural identity, setting, and participants on communicative variables.

Soft-voice syndrome   Compensatory behavior in which a child with velopharyngeal incompetence purposely reduces vocal intensity to prevent air escape through the nose and reduce hypernasality.

Somatogenic   Coming from the body; organic or physiological.

Sound field amplification   A type of assistive listening whereby sound is transmitted via a microphone to loudspeakers that are strategically placed within a room.

Spastic cerebral palsy   A congenital disorder that is characterized by increased muscle tone, such that when a muscle contracts, the opposing muscle may react abnormally to stretch by increasing muscle tone too much. Muscle movements are described as jerky, labored, and slow.

Spastic dysarthria   Speech that is characterized as slow with jerky, imprecise articulation and reduction of the rapidly alternating movements of speech because of stiff and rigid muscles.

Spastic dysphonia   A voice disorder that is characterized by hyperadduction of the vocal folds resulting in a strained/strangled voice production with intermittent stoppages.

Speech bulb   An obturator that fills the velopharyngeal space, closing the velopharyngeal portal.

Speech community   A group of people who share a common understanding of the rules and restrictions that govern communicative situations.

Speech-language pathologist (SLP)   A professional whose distinguishing role is to identify, assess, treat, and prevent speech, language, communication, and swallowing disorders.

Speech recognition threshold (SRT) test   A test procedure used in speech audiometry that measures the lowest (quietest) level at which a person can recognize approximately 50 percent of the spondee words presented for a given number of trials.

Speech sample   A systematic collection and analysis of a person's speech, a corpus; used in language assessment.

Spina bifida   A congenital malformation of the spinal column.

Spondees   Two-syllable compound words that are spoken with equal emphasis on both syllables and used in speech recognition threshold testing.

Spontaneous recovery   A natural recovery process that proceeds without professional intervention.

Stabilization   In the Van Riper approach to articulation therapy, reinforcement and maintenance of the corrected phoneme.

Stapes   The third and smallest of the ossicles in the middle ear.

Stapedius muscle   The small muscle that attaches to the neck of the stapes and contracts in response to high-intensity sound.

Stenosis   Narrowing of the external auditory meatus.

Stereocilia   Small, hair-like projections situated on the top of the hair cells in the organ of Corti.

Stimulability   The ability to imitate a target phoneme when given focused auditory and visual cues.

Stimulus   Anything that is capable of eliciting a response.

Stoma   A small opening; for example, a surgical hole in the external neck region extending into the pharynx to permit breathing following laryngectomy.

Stop   Consonant phoneme produced by building air pressure behind the point of constriction.

Story grammar   Common elements and event sequences in narratives.

Strain and struggle   Difficulty initiating and maintaining voice.

Stridor   Noisy breathing or involuntary sound that accompanies inspiration and expiration.

Stroke   Cerebrovascular accident (CVA), the most common cause of aphasia, resulting when the blood supply to the brain is blocked or when the brain is flooded with blood.

Stuttering   A disorder of speech fluency characterized by hesitations, repetitions, prolongations, tension, and avoidance behaviors.

Subacute otitis media   Inflammation of the middle ear lasting between three and eight weeks.

Subcortical aphasia   Fluent aphasia as the result of lesions in the thalamus and basal ganglia below the level of the cortex.

Subglottal pressure   Pressure beneath the vocal folds that sets them into vibration.

Substitution   In articulation, the production of one phoneme in place of another.

Support group   Individuals with similar problems who meet together to share feelings, information, and ideas.

Suppurative otitis media: Pus formation and discharge by the tissue of the middle ear cavity.

Suprasegmental   Features such as loudness, rate, and intonation that affect more than a single phoneme and add meaning to an utterance.

Syndactyly   Webbing of the fingers and toes.

Syndrome   A combination of symptoms that occur together in predictable and consistent combinations of traits.

Syntax   How words are arranged in sentences.

Symbolization   Using an arbitrary symbol, such as a word or sign, to stand for something.

Tactiles   Touching behaviors.

Tardive dyskinesia   Involuntary, repetitive facial, tongue, or limb movements that sometimes occur as a side effect of certain medications.

TBI   See *Traumatic brain injury.*

Tectorial membrane   The gelatinous, tongue-shaped structure that forms the roof of the organ of Corti.

Telecoil   A device located inside a hearing aid or speech processor of a cochlear implant that picks up sound via electromagnetic induction.

Teletypewriter (TTY)   A portable keyboard used for remote text conversations over regular phone lines by those who are deaf.

Temporary threshold shift (TTS)   A temporary change in hearing acuity followed by spontaneous recovery that is associated with short-term exposure to high-intensity noise.

Tensor veli palatini   Muscle of the soft palate that opens the auditory tube.

Teratogens   Chemical or environmental agents that produce congenital abnormalities.

Threshold   The lowest (quietest) presentation level (measured in decibels) at which a person can barely detect a stimulus 50 percent of the time it is presented.

Thrombosis   A blood clot within a blood vessel of the body. It may result in an ischemic stroke.

Tics   Involuntary, rapid and repetitive, stereotypic movements.

Tidal breathing   Breathing to sustain life.

Tinnitus   The perception of sound (ringing, buzzing) in the ears or head where there is no external source present.

Tongue thrust   Swallowing with a forward movement of the tongue, resulting in misarticulation of various phonemes. Also known as *myofunctional disorder.*

Tracheo-esophageal shunt (TEP)   A device that directs air from the trachea to the esophagus for esophageal speech.

Tracheostomy tube   A tube that is inserted into the trachea to relieve a breathing obstruction.

Transcortical motor aphasia   A nonfluent aphasia that is characterized by impaired conversational speech, good verbal imitative abilities, and mildly impaired auditory comprehension.

Transcortical sensory aphasia   A rare fluent aphasia that is characterized by word substitutions, lack of nouns and severe anomia, and poor auditory comprehension, but the ability to repeat or imitate words, phrases, and sentences.

Traumatic brain injury (TBI)   Damage to the brain resulting from bruising and laceration caused by forceful contact with the relatively rough inner surfaces of the skull or from secondary edema or swelling, infarction or death of tissue, and hematoma or focal bleeding.

Treacher Collins syndrome   An inherited disorder that is characterized by excessive muscle tone in the face and jaw.

Tympanic cavity   See *Middle ear space*

Tympanic membrane or eardrum   The thin, cone-shaped structure composed of three layers of tissue located at the end of the external auditory meatus. It is set into vibration as acoustic energy strikes its surface.

Tympanogram   The graph generated during acoustic immittance testing that depicts compliance of the eardrum relative to changes in air pressure.

Tympanostomy tubes   See *Pressure equalization (PE) tubes*

Ultrasonography   Ultrasound.

Ultrasound   A technique that uses high frequency sound waves to visualize internal bodily organs.

Unilateral hearing loss   Loss of hearing on one side.

Usher syndrome   A hereditary disorder characterized by sensorineural hearing impairment and progressive blindness.

Uvula   Fleshy mass termination of the soft palate.

Variegated babbling   Long strings of consonant-vowel syllables, in which adjacent and successive syllables in the string are not identical.

Vasiculation   Rapid, random, irregular, and minute contractions of nerve bundles.

Veau system Roman numeral classification system for describing clefts of the lip and/or palate.

Velar Refers to the posterior area of the roof of the mouth. In speech, velar consonants are produced with the tongue touching or approximating the velum or soft palate.

Velopharyngeal incompetence (VPI) Inability of the velopharyngeal mechanism to separate the oral and nasal cavities during swallowing and speech.

Velopharyngeal mechanism Velum (soft palate) and walls of pharynx (back of throat), used to close the velopharyngeal portal.

Velopharyngeal portal Opening or the conduit connecting the oral and nasal cavities.

Verbal stereotype An expression that is repeated over and over; characteristic of some individuals with aphasia.

Vermilion Pinkish to brown coloration of the lips.

Vertigo The sensation of spinning relative to one's surroundings.

Vestibular system Structures of the inner ear responsible for supplying information to the brain regarding balance and spatial orientation.

Vestibulocochlear nerve or VIIIth nerve The cranial nerve that runs from the base of the cochlea to the cochlear nucleus of the brainstem. It is comprised of the vestibular and the cochlear branches.

Videofluoroscopy See *Modified barium swallow study.*

Visual reinforcement audiometry (VRA) A method of hearing assessment in which a child is rewarded for localizing to a test signal through the use of moving toys and/or flashing lights.

Vocal abuse Any of several behaviors, including smoking and yelling, that can result in damage to the laryngeal mechanism.

Vocal fold paralysis Immobilized vocal fold usually due to nerve damage.

Vocal hygiene Proper care of the voice.

Vocal nodules Localized growths on the vocal folds that are associated with vocal abuse.

Vocal polyp A fluid-filled lesion of the vocal fold that results from mechanical stress.

Vocal tremor Variations in the pitch and loudness of the voice that are involuntary.

Voice Vocal tone and resonance.

Vowel Any of several voiced phonemes that are produced with a relatively open vocal tract.

Waardenburg syndrome A hereditary disorder characterized by pigmentary discoloration, particularly in the irises and hair; craniofacial malformation of the nasal area; and severe to profound hearing impairment.

Wernicke's aphasia A fluent aphasia that is characterized by rapid-fire strings of sentences with little pause for acknowledgment or turn taking. Content may seem to be a jumble and may be incoherent or incomprehensible, though fluent and well articulated.

Word recognition test (WRT) A test procedure used in speech audiometry to measure an individual's ability to recognize single-syllable words presented at a predetermined level above their auditory threshold.

References

Air, D. H., Wood, A. S., & Neils, J. R. (1989). Considerations for organic disorders. In N. A. Creaghead, P. W. Newman, & W. A. Secord (Eds.), *Assessment and remediation of articulatory and phonological disorders* (2nd ed.). Columbus, OH: Merrill.

Ambrose, N., Yairi, E., & Cox, N. (1993). Genetic aspects of early childhood stuttering. *Journal of Speech and Hearing Research, 36,* 701–706.

American Association on Mental Retardation. (1992). *Mental retardation: Definition, classification, and systems of support* (9th ed.). Washington, DC: Author.

American Psychiatric Association. (1987). *Diagnostic and statistical manual of mental disorders* (3rd ed. rev.) Washington, DC: Author.

American Psychiatric Association. (1994). *Diagnostic and statistical manual of mental disorders* (4th ed.). Washington, DC: Author.

American Speech-Language-Hearing Association (ASHA). (1990). Skills needed by speech-language pathologists providing services to dysphagic patients/clients. *Asha, 32* (Suppl. 2) 7–12.

American Speech-Language-Hearing Association (ASHA). (1992, March). Instrumental diagnostic procedures for swallowing. *Asha, 34* (Suppl. 7), 25–33.

American Speech-Language-Hearing Association (ASHA). (1993). Definitions of communication disorders and variations. *Asha, 35* (Suppl. 10), pp. 40–41.

American Speech-Language-Hearing Association (ASHA). (1995a). Characteristics of state licensure laws. *Asha, 37*(3), 84–94.

American Speech-Language-Hearing Association (ASHA). (1995). *Guidelines for the training, credentialing, use, and supervision of speech-language pathology assistants.* Rockville, MD: Author.

American Speech-Language-Hearing Association (ASHA). (1997). *Preferred practice patterns for the profession of speech-language pathology.* Rockville, MD: Author.

American Speech-Language-Hearing Association (ASHA). (2000a). Council on Professional Standards. Background information for the standards and implementation for the certificate of clinical competence in speech-language pathology. (Effective date: January 1, 2005) [Online] http://professional.asha. org/library/slp_standards.htm

American Speech-Language-Hearing Association (ASHA). (2000b). Council on Professional Standards. Background information for the standards and implementation for the certificate of clinical competence in audiology. (Effective date: January 1, 2007) [Online] http://professional. asha.org/library/audiology_standards htm

American Speech-Language-Hearing Association (ASHA). (2000c). Fact Sheet: Speech-Language Pathology. Online at http://professional. asha.org/students/careers/slp.htm

American Speech-Language-Hearing Association (ASHA). (2000d). Speech-Language Disorders and the Speech-Language Pathologist. Online at http:// professional.asha.org/ students/careers/sld.htm

American Speech-Language-Hearing Association (ASHA). (2001a, December 26). Code of ethics (revised). *ASHA Leader, 6*(23), 2.

American Speech-Language-Hearing Association (ASHA). (2001b). Council on Academic Accreditation. Standards for accreditation of graduate education programs in audiology and speech-language pathology. [Online] http://professional.asha.org/students/ caa_programs/standards.htm

American Speech-Language-Hearing Association (ASHA). (2001c). Fact Sheet: Audiology. [Online] http://professional.asha.org/students/ careers/audiology.htm

American Speech-Language-Hearing Association (ASHA). (2001d). *Roles and responsibilities of speech-language pathologists with respect to reading and writing in children and adolescents* (position paper, technical report, and guidelines). Rockville, MD: Author.

American Speech-Language-Hearing Association (ASHA). (2002a). About ASHA: mission statement. [Online] http://professional.asha.org/ services/ about_asha.cfm

American Speech-Language-Hearing Association (ASHA). (2002b). Augmentative and alternative communication: Knowledge and skills for service delivery. *ASHA Supplement 22*, 97–106.

American Speech-Language-Hearing Association (ASHA). (2003). *2003 Omnibus survey: Practice trends in audiology.* Rockville, MD: Author.

American Speech-Language-Hearing Association (ASHA). (2004). Scope of practice in audiology. *ASHA Supplement, 24.*

American Speech-Language-Hearing Association (ASHA). (2005). *(Central) auditory processing disorders.* [Online] http://www.asha.org/members/ deskref-journals/deskref/default

Anderson, K. L. (2002). Early Listening Function: Discovery tool for parents and caregivers of infants and toddlers. [Online] http://www.phonak.com

Anderson, R. C., Hiebert, E., Scott, J. A., & Wilkenson, J. A. (1985). *Becoming a nation of readers.* Washington, DC: National Institute of Education.

Andrews, G., Craig, A., Feyer, A. M., Hoddinott, S., Howie, P., & Neilson, M. (1983). Stuttering: A review of research findings and theories circa 1982. *Journal of Speech and Hearing Disorders, 48,* 226–246.

Andrews, G., Guitar, B., & Howie, P. (1980). Meta-analysis of the effects of stuttering treatment. *Journal of Speech and Hearing Disorders, 45,* 287–307.

Angelo, J. (1992). Comparison of three computer scanning modes as an interface method for persons with cerebral palsy. *American Journal of Occupational Therapy, 46,* 217–222.

Apel, K., & Masterson, J. (2001). Theory-guided spelling assessment and intervention: A case study. *Language, Speech, and Hearing Services in Schools, 32,* 182–194.

Apel, K., & Self, T. (2003). Evidence-based practice: The marriage of research and clinical practice. *The ASHA Leader, 8*(16), 6–7.

Aram, D. M. (1997). Hyperlexia: Reading without meaning in young children. *Topics in Language Disorders, 17*(3), 1–13.

Aram, D. M., & Eisele, J. A. (1994). Limits to a left hemisphere explanation of specific language impairment. *Journal of Speech and Learning Research, 37,* 824–830.

Aronson, A. E. (1990). *Clinical voice disorders.* New York: Thieme.

Aviv, J. E., Sataloff, R. T., Cohen, M., et al. (2001). Cost effectiveness of two types of dysphagia care in head and neck cancer: A preliminary report. *Ear, Nose, and Throat Journal, 80,* 553–558.

Azuma, T., & Bayles, L. A. (1997). Memory impairments underlying language difficulties in dementia. *Topics in Language Disorders, 18*(1), 58–71.

Baken, R. J., & Orlikoff, R. F. (2000). *Clinical measurement of speech and voice* (2nd ed.). San Diego, CA: Singular Thompson Learning.

Baker, L., & Brown, A. I. (1984). Metacognition and reading. In P. D. Pearson, M. Kamil, R. Barr, & P. Moesenthal (Eds.), *Handbook of reading research* (pp. 353–394). New York: Longman.

Balandin, S., & Morgan, J. (2001). Preparing for the future: Aging and alternative and augmentative communication. *Augmentative and Alternative Communication, 17,* 99–108.

Ball, L. J., Marvin, C. A., Beukelman, D. R., Lasker, J., & Rupp, D. (2000). Generic talk use by preschool children. *Augmentative and Alternative Communication, 16,* 145–155.

Bankson, N. W., & Bernthal, J. E. (1990). *Bankson-Bernthal Test of Phonology.* Austin, TX: Pro-Ed.

Bankson, N. W., & Bernthal, J. E. (1998a). Factors related to phonologic disorders. In J. E. Bernthal & N. W. Bankson (Eds.), *Articulation and phonological disorders* (4th ed.). Boston: Allyn and Bacon.

Bankson, N. W., & Bernthal, J. E. (1998b). Phonological assessment procedures. In J. E. Bernthal & N. W. Bankson (Eds.), *Articulation and phonological disorders* (4th ed.). Boston: Allyn and Bacon.

Barron, S. (2001, September 25). A personal story. *The ASHA Leader, 6*(17), 5, 7, 17.

Bass, P. M. (1988, November). *Attention deficit disorder: Management in preschool, adolescent, and adult populations.* Paper presented at the Annual Convention of the American Speech-Language-Hearing Association, Boston.

Bassotti, G., Germani, U., Pagliaricci, S., Plesa, A., Giulietti, O., Mannarino, E., & Morelli, A. (1998). Esophageal manometric abnormalities in Parkinson's disease. *Dysphagia, 13*(1), 28–31.

Baumann-Waengler, J. (2000). *Articulatory and phonological impairments: A clinical focus.* Boston: Allyn and Bacon.

Bayles, K. A., & Kazniak, A. W. (1987). *Communication and cognition in normal aging and dementia.* Boston: Little, Brown.

Bayles, K., & Tomoeda, C. K. (1994). *Functional Lin-*

guistic Communication Inventory. East Aurora, NY: Slosson.

Bear, D. R. Invernizzi, M., Templeton, S., & Johnston, F. (2000) Words their way: Word study for phonics, vocabulary, and spelling instruction (2nd ed.). Upper Saddle River, NJ: Prentice Hall.

Bear, D. R., Invernizzi, M., Templeton, S., & Johnston, F. (2004). Words their way: Word study with phonics, vocabulary, and spelling instruction (3rd ed.) Upper Saddle River, NJ: Merrill/Prentice-Hall.

Bedore, L. M., & Leonard, L. B. (2001). Grammatical morphological deficits in Spanish-speaking children with specific language impairment. Journal of Speech, Language, and Hearing Research, 44, 905–924.

Beebe, S. A., Beebe, S. J., & Redmond, M. V. (1996). Interpersonal communication: Relating to others. Boston: Allyn and Bacon.

Behrman, A., & Orlikoff, R. F. (1997). Instrumentation in voice assessment and treatment: What's the use? American Journal of Speech-Language Pathology, 6, 9–16.

Bellis, T. J. (2003a). Assessment and management of central auditory processing disorders in the educational setting: From science to practice. San Diego, CA: Singular Publishing Group.

Bellis, T. J. (2003b). Auditory processing disorders: It's not just kids who have them. The Hearing Journal, 56, 10–19.

Bello, J. (1994). Prevalence of speech, voice, and language disorders in the United States. Communication facts, 1994 ed. Rockville, MD: American Speech-Language-Hearing Association.

Ben-Yishay, Y., & Diller, L. (1993). Cognitive remediation in traumatic brain injury: Update and issues. Archives of Physical Medicine and Rehabilitation, 74, 204–213.

Bernhardt, B. H., & Holdgrafer, G. (2001). Beyond the basics I: The need for strategic sampling from in-depth phonological analysis. Language, Speech, and Hearing Services in Schools, 32, 18–27.

Berninger, V. W. (2000). Development of language by hand and its connections with language by ear, mouth, and eye. Topics in Language Disorders, 20(4), 65–84.

Berninger, V. W., Abbott, R. D., Billingsley, F., & Nagy, W. (2001). Processes underlying timing and fluency of reading: Efficiency, automaticity, coordination, and morphological awareness. In M. Worf (Ed.), Dyslexia, fluency, and the brain (pp. 383–413). Timonium, MD: York.

Berninger, V. W., Cartwright, A., Yates, C., Swanson, H. L., & Abbott, R. (1994). Developmental skills re-

lated to writing and reading acquisition in the intermediate grades: Shared and unique variance. Reading and Writing: An Interdisciplinary Journal, 6, 161–196.

Berninger, V. W. Vaughan, K., Abbott, R., Brooks, A., Abbott, S., Reed, E., Rogan, L., & Graham, S. (1998). Early intervention for spelling problems: Teaching spelling units of varying size within a multiple connections framework. Journal of Educational Psychology, 90, 587–605.

Bess, F. H., Dodd-Murphy, J., & Parker, R. A. (1998). Children with minimal sensorineural hearing loss: Prevalence, educational performance, and functional status. Ear and Hearing, 19, 339–354.

Beukelman, D. R., & Mirenda, P. (1992). Augmentative and alternative communication: Management of severe communication disorders in children and adults. Baltimore: Paul H. Brookes.

Beukelman, D., & Mirenda, P. (1997). Augmentative and alternative communication: Management of severe communication disorders in children and adults (2nd ed.). Baltimore, MD: Paul H. Brookes.

Bienemann, L. L. (1989). Psychological implications of right hemisphere injury. In P. A. Pimental & N. A. Kingsbury (Eds.), Neuropsychological aspects of right brain injury (pp. 65–72). Austin, TX: Pro-Ed.

Bird, J., Bishop, D. V., & Freeman, N. H. (1995). Phonological awareness and literacy development in children with expressive phonological impairments. Journal of Speech and Hearing Research, 38, 446–462.

Blackstone, S. (1989). Augmentative communication services in the schools. Asha, 31(1), 61–64.

Blalock, J., & Johnson, D. (1987). Adults with learning disabilities: Clinical studies. New York: Grune & Stratton.

Blischak, D., Lombardino, L., & Dyson, A. (2003). Use of speech-generating devices: In support of natural speech. Augmentative and Alternative Communication, 19(1), 29–35.

Blood, G. W., & Blood, I. M. (2004). Bullying in adolescents who stutter: Communicative competence and self-esteem. Contemporary Issues in Communication Science and Disorders, 31, 69–79.

Bloodstein, O. (1995). A handbook on stuttering. San Diego, CA: Singular Publishing Group.

Bloom, L. (1970). Language development: Form and function of emerging grammars. Cambridge, MA: MIT Press.

Bloom, R. L., & Ferrand, C. T. (1997). Neuromotor speech disorders. In C. T. Ferrand & R. L. Bloom (Eds.), Introduction to organic and neurogenic disorders of communication: Current scope of practice. Boston: Allyn and Bacon.

Boburg, E., & Kully, D. (1995). The comprehensive stuttering program. In C. W. Starkweather & H. F. M. Peters (Eds.), *Stuttering: Proceedings of the First World Congress on Fluency Disorders* (pp. 305–308). Munich: International Fluency Association.

Bonita, R. (1992). Epidemiology of stroke. *Lancet, 339*–320.

Boone, D. R., & McFarlane, S. C. (2000). *The voice and voice therapy* (4th ed.). Boston: Allyn and Bacon.

Boshart, C. A. (1998, April). *Oral-motor techniques.* Short course presented at the New York State Speech-Language-Hearing Association Annual Convention, New York.

Bosman, A., & van Orden, G. (1997). Why spelling is more difficult than reading. In C. Perfetti, L. Riebert, & M. Fayol (Eds.), *Learning to spell: Research, theory, and practice across languages* (pp. 173–194). Mahwah, NJ: Lawrence Erlbaum Associates.

Boswell, S. (2004). International agreement brings mutual recognition of certification. *The ASHA Leader, 9*(19), 1, 22.

Bottenberg, D. E., & Hanks, J. M. (1986). Language and speech of physically handicapped children. In V. A. Reed (Ed.), *An introduction to children with language disorders* (pp. 201–219). New York: Macmillan.

Boudreau, D. M., & Chapman, R. (2000). The relationship between event representation and linguistic skills in narratives of children and adolescents with Down syndrome. *Journal of Speech, Language, and Hearing Research, 43*, 1146–1159.

Boudreau, D. M., & Hedberg, N. L. (1999). A comparison of early literacy skills in children with specific language impairment and their typically developing peers. *American Journal of Speech-Language Pathology, 8*, 249–260.

Boudreau, D. M., & Larson, J. (2004). *Strategies for teaching narrative abilities to school-aged children.* Paper presented at the Annual Convention of the American Speech-Language-Hearing Association, Philadelphia.

Brackenbury, T., & Pye, C. (2005). Semantic deficits in children with language impairments: Issues for clinical assessment. *Language, Speech, and Hearing Services in Schools, 36*, 5–16.

Bradley, D. P. (1997). Congenital and acquired velopharyngeal inadequacy. In K. R. Bzoch (Ed.), *Communicative disorders related to cleft lip and palate* (4th ed., pp. 223–243). Austin, TX: Pro-Ed.

Bradshaw, M. L., Hoffman, P. R., & Norris, J. A.

(1998). Efficacy of expansions and cloze procedures in the development of interpretations by preschool children exhibiting delayed language development. *Language, Speech, and Hearing Services in Schools, 29*, 85–95.

Brand Robertson, S., & Ellis Weismer, S. (1999). Effects of treatment on linguistic and social skills in toddlers with delayed language development. *Journal of Speech, Language, and Hearing Research, 42*, 1234–1248.

Brinton, B., & Fujiki, M. (2004). Social and affective factors in children with language impairment: Implications for literacy learning. In C. A. Stone, E. R. Silliman, B. J. Ehren, & K. Apel (Eds.), *Handbook of language and literacy: Development and disorders* (pp. 130–153). New York: Guilford.

Brinton, B., Fujiki, M., & Powell, J. M. (1997). The ability of children with language impairment to manipulate topic in a structured task. *Language, Speech, and Hearing Services in Schools, 28*, 3–11.

Bryan, K. L. (1989). *The right hemisphere language battery.* Leicester, UK: Far Communications.

Bulow, M., Olsson, R., & Ekberg, O. (2001). Videomanometric analysis of supraglottic swallow, effortful swallow, and chin tuck in patients with pharyngeal dysfunction. *Dysphagia, 16*, 190–195.

Burns, M. M., Halper, A. S., & Mogil, S. I. (1985). *Clinical management of right hemisphere dysfunction.* Rockville, MD: Aspen.

Butkowsky, I. S., & Willows, D. M. (1980). Cognitive-motivational characteristics of children varying in reading ability: Evidence of learned helplessness in poor readers. *Journal of Educational Psychology, 72*, 408–422.

Byl, F. M. J. (1984). Sudden hearing loss: Eight years experience and suggested prognostic table. *Laryngoscope, 94*, 647–651

Bzoch, K. R. (1997). Introduction to the study of communicative disorders in cleft palate and related craniofacial anomalies. In K. R. Bzoch (Ed.), *Communicative disorders related to cleft lip and palate* (4th ed., pp. 3–44). Austin, TX: Pro-Ed.

Caccamise, D., & Snyder, L. (2005). Theory and pedagogical practices of text comprehension. *Topics in Language Disorders, 25*(1), 1–20.

Calculator, S. (1997). Fostering early language acquisition and AAC use: Exploring reciprocal influences between children and their environments. *Augmentative and Alternative Communication, 13*, 149–157.

Calculator, S. N. (2000). AAC outcomes for children and youths with severe disabilities: When seeing is believing. *Augmentative and Alternative Communication, 16,* 4–12.

Calvert, D. (1982) Articulation and hearing impairments. In Lass, L., Northern, J., Yoder, D., & McReynolds, L. (Eds.), *Speech, language, and hearing* (Vol. 2). Philadelphia: Saunders.

Calvin, W. H., & Ojemann, G. A. (1980). *Inside the brain.* New York: New American Library.

Camicioli, R., Oken, B. S., Sexton, G., Kaye, J. A., & Nutt, J. G. (1998). Verbal fluency task affects gait in Parkinson's disease with motor freezing. *Journal of Geriatric Psychiatry and Neurology, 11,* 181–185.

Carlson, V., Cicchetti, D., Barnett, D., & Braunwald, K. B. (1989). The development of disorganized/disoriented attachment in maltreated infants. *Developmental Psychology, 25,* 525–531.

Carlsson, G. S., Svardsudd, K., & Welin, L. (1987). Long-term effects of head injuries sustained during life in three male populations. *Journal of Neuropsychology, 67,* 197–205.

Caruso, A. J. (2001, July 24). Parkinson's disease and me. *The ASHA Leader, 6*(13), 7.

Casby, M. W. (1997). Symbolic play of children with language impairment: A critical review. *Journal of Speech, Language, and Hearing Research, 40,* 468–479.

Castell, J. A., Johnston, B. T., Colcher, A., et al. (2001). Manometric abnormalities of the oesophagus in patients with Parkinson's disease. *Neurogastroenterology and Motility: The Official Journal of the European Gastrointestinal Motility Society, 13,* 361–364.

Castrogiovanni, A. (1999a). Incidence and prevalence of hearing impairment in the United States. *Communication facts, 1999 ed.* Rockville, MD: American Speech-Language-Hearing Association.

Castrogiovanni, A. (1999b). Incidence and prevalence of speech, voice, and language disorders in the United States. *Communication facts, 1999 ed.* Rockville, MD: American Speech-Language-Hearing Association.

Castrogiovanni, A. (1999c). Special populations: Dysphagia. *Communication facts, 1999 ed.* Rockville, MD: American Speech-Language-Hearing Association.

Catts, H. W. (1996). Defining dyslexia as a developmental language disorder: An expanded view. *Topics in Language Disorders, 16*(2), 14–29.

Catts, H. W. (1997). The early identification of language-based reading disabilities. *Language, Speech, and Hearing Services in Schools, 28,* 86–89.

Catts, H. W., Fey, M. E., Zhang, X., & Tomblin, J. B. (1999). Language basis of reading and reading dis-

abilities: Evidence from a longitudinal investigation. *Scientific Studies in Reading, 3,* 331–361.

Catts, H. W., Fey, M. E., Zhang, X., & Tomblin, J. B. (2001). Estimating the risk of future reading difficulties in kindergarten children: A research-based model and its clinical implementation. *Language, Speech, and Hearing Services in Schools, 32,* 38–50.

Catts, H. W., & Kamhi, A. (2005a). Causes of reading disabilities. In H. W. Catts & A. G. Kamhi (Eds.), *Language and reading disabilities* (2nd ed.; pp. 94–126). Boston: Allyn and Bacon.

Catts, H. W., & Kamhi, A. (2005b). Classification of reading disabilities. In H. W. Catts & A. G. Kamhi (Eds.), *Language and reading disabilities* (2nd ed.; pp. 72–93). Boston: Allyn and Bacon.

Causino Lamar, M. A., Obler, L. K., Knoeful, J. E., & Albert, M. L. (1994). Communication patterns in end-stage Alzheimer's disease: Pragmatic analysis. In R. L. Bloom, L. K. Obler, S. DeSanti, & J. L. Ehrlich (Eds.), *Discourse analysis and application: Studies in adult clinical populations* (pp. 217–235). Hillsdale, NJ: Lawrence Erlbaum Associates.

Chapman, S. B. (1997). Cognitive-communication abilities in children with closed head injury. *American Journal of Speech-Language Pathology, 6*(2), 50–58.

Chapman, S. B., Watkins, R., Gustafson, C., Moore, S., Levin, H., & Kufera, J. A. (1997). Narrative discourse in children with closed head injury, children with language impairment, and typically developing children. *American Journal of Speech-Language Pathology, 6*(2), 66–76.

Chermak, G. D., & Musiek, F. E. (1997). *Central auditory processing disorders: New perspectives.* San Diego: Singular Publishing Group.

Cherney, L. R. (1994). Dysphagia in adults with neurologic disorders: An overview. In L. R. Cherney (Ed.), *Clinical management of dysphagia in adults and children.* Gaithersburg, MD: Aspen.

Chomsky, N. (1965). *Aspects of the theory of syntax.* Cambridge, MA: MIT Press.

Chomsky, N., & Halle, M. (1968). *The sound patterns of English.* New York: Harper & Row.

Choudhury, N., & Benasich, A. A. (2003). A family aggregation study: The influence of family history and other risk factors on language development. *Journal of Speech, Language, and Hearing Research, 46,* 261–272.

Clark, H. M. (2004). Neuromuscular treatment for speech and swallowing: A tutorial. *American Journal of Speech-Language Pathology, 12,* 400–415.

Clarke, C. E., Gullaksen, E., Macdonald, S., et al. (1998). Referral criteria for speech and language therapy assessment of dysphagia caused by idiopathic Parkinson's disease. *Acta Neurologica Scandinavica, 97*(1), 27–35.

Clarke, L., & Witte, K. (1991). Nature and efficacy of communication management in Alzheimer's disease. In R. Lubinski (Ed.), *Dementia and communication* (pp. 238–256). Philadelphia: B. C. Decker.

Cleave, P. L., & Fey, M. E. (1997). Two approaches to the facilitation of grammar in children with language impairments: Rationale and description. *American Journal of Speech-Language Pathology, 6*(1), 22–32.

Coelho, C. A. (1997). Cognitive-communicative disorders following traumatic brain injury. In C. T. Ferrand & R. L. Bloom (Eds.), *Introduction to organic and neurogenic disorders of communication: Current scope of practice* (pp. 110–137). Boston: Allyn and Bacon.

Coelho, C. A., Liles, B. Z., & Duffy, R. J. (1995). Impairments of discourse abilities and executive functions in traumatically brain injured adults. *Brain Injury, 9,* 471–477.

Coffin, J. M., Baroody, S., Schneider, K., & O'Neill, J. (2005). Impaired cerebellar learning in children with prenatal alcohol exposure: A comparative study of eyeblink conditioning in children with ADHD and dyslexia. *Cortex, 41,* 389–398.

Colodny, N. (2001). Effects of gender, age, disease, and multisystem involvement on oxygen saturation levels in dysphagic persons. *Dysphagia, 16,* 48–57.

Colodny, N. (2005). Dysphagic independent feeders' justifications for noncompliance with recommendations by a speech-language pathologist. *American Journal of Speech-Language Pathology, 14,* 61–70.

Colton, R. H., & Casper, J. K. (1990). *Understanding voice problems: A physiological perspective for diagnosis and treatment.* Baltimore, MD: Williams & Wilkins.

Colton, R. H., & Casper, J. K. (1996). *Understanding voice problems: A physiological perspective for diagnosis and treatment* (2nd ed.). Baltimore, MD: Williams & Wilkins.

Connell, P. J., & Stone, C. (1992). Morpheme learning of children with specific language impairments under controlled conditions. *Journal of Speech and Hearing Research, 35,* 844–852.

Conti-Ramsden, G., & Botting, N. (2004). Social difficulties and victimization in children with SLI at 11 years of age. *Journal of Speech, Language, and Hearing Research, 47,* 145–161.

Conture, E. G. (1990a). Childhood stuttering: What is it and who does it? In J. Cooper (Ed.), *Research needs in stuttering: Roadblocks and future directions* (ASHA Reports 18, pp. 2–14). Rockville, MD: American Speech-Language-Hearing Association.

Conture, E. G. (1990b). *Stuttering* (2nd ed.). Englewood Cliffs, NJ: Prentice-Hall.

Conture, E. G. (1996). Treatment efficacy: Stuttering. *Journal of Speech and Hearing Research, 39,* S18–S26.

Conture, E. G., & Guitar, B. (1993). Evaluating efficacy of treatment of stuttering: School-age children. *Journal of Fluency Disorders, 18,* 253–287.

Convit, A., deLeon, J. J., Tarshish, C., DeSanti, S., Tsui, W., Rusinek, H., & George, A. (1995). *Hippocampal volume in pre-clinical and early Alzheimer's dementia: Relationship to cognitive function.* Austin, TX: Pro-Ed.

Cooper, E. B. (1984). Personalized fluency control therapy: A status report. In M. Peins (Ed.), *Contemporary approaches to stuttering therapy* (pp. 1–38). Boston: Little, Brown.

Costello, J. (2000). AAC intervention in the intensive care unit: The Children's Hospital Boston model. *Augmentative and Alternative Communication, 16,* 137–153.

Crago, M. B., Eriks-Brophy, A., Pesco, D., & McAlpine, L. (1997). Culturally based miscommunication in classroom interaction. *Language, Speech, and Hearing Services in Schools, 28,* 245–254.

Craig, A., & Calvert, P. (1991). Following up on treated stutterers: Studies of perception of fluency and job status. *Journal of Speech and Hearing Research, 34,* 279–284.

Crary, M. A. (1993). *Developmental motor speech disorders.* San Diego, CA: Singular.

Cress, C. J. (2001). Language and AAC intervention in young children: Never too early or too late to start. *American Speech-Language Hearing Association Special Interest Division 1, Language Learning and Education Newsletter, 8*(1), 3–4.

Crites, L. S., Fischer, K. L., McNeish-Stengel, M., & Siegel, C. J. (1992). Working with families of drug-exposed children: Three model programs. *Infant-Toddler Intervention: The Transdisciplinary Journal, 2*(1), 13–23.

Cruickshanks, K. J., Wiley, T. L., Tweed, T. S., Klein, B. E. K., Klein, R., Mares-Perlman, J. A., et al. (1998). Prevalence of hearing loss in older adults in Beaver Dam, Wisconsin: The epidemiology of hearing loss study. *American Journal of Epidemiology, 148*(9), 879–885.

Culatta, R., & Goldberg, S. A. (1995). *Stuttering therapy: An integrated approach to theory and practice.* Boston: Allyn and Bacon.

Cummings, J. L., & Benson, D. F. (1992). *Dementia:*

A clinical approach (2nd ed.). Boston: Butterworth-Heinemann.

Cupples, L., & Iacono, T. (2000). Phonological awareness and oral reading skill in children with Down syndrome. *Journal of Speech, Language, and Hearing Research, 43,* 595–608.

Dale, P. S., Price, T. S., Bishop, D. V. M., & Plomin, R. (2003). Outcomes of early language delay: I. Predicting persistent and transient language difficulties at 3 and 4 years. *Journal of Speech, Language, and Hearing Research, 46,* 544–560.

Dalston, R. M. (1995). The use of nasometry in the assessment and remediation of velopharyngeal inadequacy. In K. R. Bzoch (Ed.), *Communicative disorders related to cleft lip and palate* (4th ed., pp. 331–346). Austin, TX: Pro-Ed.

Dalston, R. M., & Seaver, E. J. (1990). Nasometric and phototransductive measurements of reaction times in normal adult speakers. *Cleft Palate Journal, 27,* 61–67.

Daly, D., Simon, C., & Burnett-Stolnack, M. (1995). Helping adolescents who stutter focus on fluency. *Language, Speech, and Hearing Services in Schools, 26,* 162–168.

Damico, J. S. (1997, April). *Authentic classroom assessment for the speech-language pathologist.* Workshop presented at annual convention of the New York State Speech-Language-Hearing Association, Buffalo.

Darley, F., Aronson, A., & Brown, J. (1975). *Motor speech disorders.* Philadelphia: W. B. Saunders.

Dattilo, J., & Camarata, S. (1991). Facilitating conversation through self-initiated augmentative communication treatment. *Journal of Applied Behavior Analysis, 24,* 369–378.

Davis, A. (1993). *A survey of adult aphasia and related language disorders.* Englewood Cliffs, NJ: Prentice-Hall.

Dawson, G., Carver, L., Meltzoff, A. N., Panagiotides, H., McPartland, J., & Webb, S. J. (2002). Neural correlates of face and object recognition in young children with autism spectrum disorder, developmental delay, and typical development. *Child Development, 73,* 700–712.

Deevy, P., & Leonard, L. B. (2004). The comprehension of wh- questions in children with specific language impairment. *Journal of Speech, Language, and Hearing Research, 47,* 802–815.

Denk, D. M., Swoboda, H., Schima, W., & Eibenberger, K. (1997). Prognostic factors for swallowing rehabilitation following head and neck cancer surgery. *Acta Otolaryngolica, 117*(5), 769–774.

Dennis, M. (1992). Word finding in children and adolescents with a history of brain injury. *Topics in Language Disorders, 13*(1), 66–82.

DePippo, K. L., Holas, M. A., & Reding, M. J. (1992). Validation of the 3-oz water swallow test for aspiration following stroke. *Archives of Neurology, 49*(12), 1259–1261.

DeSanti, S. (1997). Differentiating the dementias. In C. T. Ferrand & R. L. Bloom (Eds.), *Introduction to organic and neurogenic disorders of communication: Current scope of practice* (pp. 84–109). Boston: Allyn and Bacon.

Deutsch, G. K., Dougherty, R. F., Bammer, R., Siok, W. T., Gabrieli, J. D., & Wandell, B. (2005). Children's reading performance is correlated with white matter structure measured by diffusion tensor imaging. *Cortex, 41,* 354-363.

Diefendorf, A. (1988). Pediatric audiology. In J. Lass, L. McReynolds, J. Northern, & D. Yoder (Eds.), *Handbook of speech language pathology and audiology* (pp. 1315-1338). Toronto, Ontario, Canada: B. C. Decker.

Dollaghan, C. (2004). Evidence-based practice: Myths and realities. *The ASHA Leader, 9*(7), 4-5, 12.

Donahue, M. L., & Foster, S. K. (2004). Social cognition, conversation, and reading comprehension: How to read a comedy of manners. In C. A. Stone, E. R. Silliman, B. J. Ehren, & K. Apel (Eds.), *Handbook of language and literacy: Development and disorders* (pp. 363-379). New York: Guilford.

Dore, J., Franklin, M., Miller, R., & Ramer, A. (1976). Transitional phenomena in early language acquisition. *Journal of Child Language, 3,* 13–28.

Downey, D., Daugherty, P., Helt, S., & Daugherty, D. (2004). Integrating AAC into the classroom. *The ASHA Leader, 9*(17), 6-7, 36.

Downey, D. M., & Snyder, L. E. (2000). College students with LLD: The phonological core as risk for failure in foreign language classes. *Topics in Language Disorder, 21*(1), 82–92.

Doyle, M., & Phillips, B. (2001). Trends in augmentative and alternative communication use by individuals with amyotrophic lateral sclerosis. *Augmentative and Alternative Communication, 17,* 167–178.

Drager, K. D. R., & Reichle, J. E. (2001). Effects of age and divided attention on listeners' comprehension of synthesized speech. *Augmentative and Alternative Communication, 17,* 109–119.

Dromi, E., Leonard., L. B., Adam, G., & Zadunaisky-Ehrlich, S. (1999). Verb agreement morphology in Hebrew-speaking children with specific language impairment. *Journal of Speech, Language, and Hearing Research, 42,* 1414–1431.

Duchan, J. F. (2002). What do you know about the history of speech-language pathology? And why is it important? *The ASHA Leader, 7*(23), 4–5, 29.

Duffy, J. R. (1995). *Motor speech disorders; Substrates, differential diagnosis, and management.* St. Louis: Mosby Year Book.

Duvoisin, R. C. (1991). *Parkinson's disease: A guide for patient and family* (3rd ed.). New York: Raven Press.

Eckert, M. A., Leonard, C. M., Wilke, M., Eckert, M., Richards, T., Richards, A., & Berninger, V. (2004). Anatomical signatures of dyslexia in children: Unique information from manual and voxel based morphometry brain measures. *Cortex, 41,* 304–315.

Educational and Auditory Research Foundation (2004, October 14). *New study indicates half of baby boomers experiencing hearing loss.* Retrieved April 29, 2005, from http://www.earfoundation.org

Edwards, H. T. (1997). *Applied phonetics: The sounds of American English* (2nd ed.). San Diego, CA: Singular.

Edwards, M. L. (1983). Selection criteria for developing therapy goals. *Journal of Childhood Communication Disorders, 7,* 36–45.

Egbert, A. M. (1996). The dwindles: Failure to thrive in older patients. *Nutrition Review, 54* (1, Pt. 2), pp. S25–S30.

Ehri, L. C. (2000). Learning to read and learning to spell: Two sides of a coin. *TLD, Topics in Language Disorders.* 20(3), 19–36.

Ehri, L. C., & McCormick, S. (1998). Phases of word learning: Implications for instruction with delayed and disabled readers. *Reading and Writing Quarterly, Overcoming Learning Difficulties, 14,* 135–163.

Ellis Weismer, S., Murray-Branch, J., & Miller, J. (1994). A prospective longitudinal study of language development in late talkers. *Journal of Speech, Language, and Hearing Research, 37,* 852–867.

Ekelman, B. L., Fitzpatrick, S., Vail, J., Woods, D., Sloan-Brown, N., Sopko, M., Hunter, C., Warstler, B., & Minich, N. (2004). *Kindergarten study year 2: Phonological awareness instruction and reading growth.* Paper presented at the Annual convention of the American Speech-Language-Hearing Association, Philadelphia.

Englert, C. S., Raphael, T. E., Anderson, L. M., Anthony, H. M., Fear, K. L., & Gregg, S. L. (1988). A case for writing intervention: Strategies for writing informational text. *Learning Disabilities Focus, 3*(2), 98–113.

English, K. (2002). Psychosocial aspects of hearing impairment and counseling basics. In R . L. Schow & M. A. Nerbonne (Eds.), *Introduction to audiologic rehabilitation.* (4th ed.; pp. 225–246). Boston: Allyn and Bacon.

Erber, N. (1982). *Auditory training.* Washington, DC: Alexander Graham Bell Association for the Deaf.

Fagundes, D. D., Haynes, W. O., Haak, N. J., & Moran, M. J. (1998). Task variability effects on the language test performance of southern lower socioeconomic class African American and Caucasian 5-year-olds. *Language, Speech, and Hearing Services in Schools, 29,* 148–157.

Farber, J. G., & Klein, E. R. (1999). Classroom-based assessment of a collaborative intervention program for kindergarten and first-grade students. *Language, Speech, and Hearing Services in Schools, 30,* 83–91.

Feinberg, M. (1997). The effects of medications on swallowing. In B. C. Sonies (Ed.), *Dysphagia: A continuum of care.* Gaithersburg, MD: Aspen.

Felsenfeld, S. (1997). Epidemiology and genetics of stuttering. In R. F. Curlee & G. M. Siegel (Eds.), *Nature and treatment of stuttering: New directions* (2nd ed., pp. 3–23). Boston: Allyn and Bacon.

Fey, M. E. (1986). *Language intervention with young children.* San Diego: College-Hill.

Fey, M. E., Long, S. H., & Finestack, L. H. (2003). Ten principles of grammar facilitation for children with specific language impairment. *American Journal of Speech-Language Pathology, 12,* 3–15.

Felsenfeld, S., Kirk, K. M., Zhu, G., Statham, D. J., Neale, M. C., & Martin, N. G. (2000). A study of genetic and environmental etiology of stuttering in a selected twin sample. *Behavior Genetics, 30*(5), 359–366.

Flax, J. F., Realpe-Bonilla, T., Hirsch, L. S., Brzustowicz, L. M., Bartlett, C. W., & Tallal, P. (2003). Specific language impairment in families: Evidence for co-occurrence with reading impairments. *Journal of Speech, Language, and Hearing Research, 46,* 530–543.

Fleming, J., & Forester, B. (1997). Infusing language enhancement into reading curriculum for disadvantaged adolescents. *Language, Speech, and Hearing Services in Schools, 28,* 177–180.

Flipsen, P. (2003). Articulation rate and speech-sound normalization failure. *Journal of Speech, Language, and Hearing Research, 46,* 724–737.

Fluharty, N. B. (2000). *Fluharty Preschool Speech and Language Screening Test,* 2nd edition. Austin, TX: Pro-Ed.

Fosnot, S. (1993). Research design for examining treatment efficacy in fluency disorders. *Journal of Fluency Disorders, 18,* 221–251.

Fowler, G. (1982). Developing comprehension skills in primary students through the use of story frames. *Reading Teacher, 36,* 176–179.

Fox, L. E., & Rau, M. T. (2001). Augmentative and alternative communication for adults following glossectomy and laryngectomy surgery. *Augmentative and Alternative Communication, 17,* 161–166.

Foy, J. G., & Mann, V. (2003). Home literacy environment and phonological awareness in preschool children: Differential effects for rhyme and phoneme awareness. *Applied Psycholinguistics, 24,* 59–88.

Frome Loeb, D., & Leonard, L. B. (1991). Subject case marking and verb morphology in normally developing and specifically language-impaired children. *Journal of Speech and Hearing Research, 34,* 340–346.

Fuchs, D., Fuchs, L. S., Thompson, A., Otaiba, S. A., Yen, L., Yang, N. J., Braun, N., & O'Connor, N. E. (2001). Is reading important in reading-readiness programs? A randomized field trial with teachers as program implementers. *Journal of Educational Psychology, 93,* 251–267.

Furia, C. L, Kowalski, L. P., Latorre, M. R., et al. (2001). Speech intelligibility after glossectomy and speech rehabilitation. *Archives of Otolaryngology—Head and Neck Surgery, 127,* 877–883.

Gaeth, J. H. (1948). *A study of phonemic regression in relation to hearing loss.* Unpublished doctoral dissertation, Northwestern University, Evanston, IL.

Garcia, J. M., Cannito, M. P., & Dagenais, P. A. (2000). Hand gestures: Perspectives and preliminary implications for adults with acquired dysarthria. *American Journal of Speech-Language Pathology, 9,* 107–115.

Gelb, A. B., Medeiros, L. J., Chen, Y. Y., Weiss, L. M., & Weidner, N. (1997). Hodgkin's disease of the esophagus. *American Journal of Clinical Pathology, 108*(5), 593–598.

Gelfer, M. P. (1996). *Survey of communication disorders: A social and behavioral perspective.* New York: McGraw-Hill.

Gerber, A., & Klein, E. R. (2004). *Teacher/tutor assisted literacy learning in the primary grades, a speech-language approach to early reading: T. A. L. L. while small.* Paper presented at the Annual Convention of the American Speech-Language-Hearing Association, Philadelphia.

German, D. J., & Simon, E. (1991). Analysis of children's word-finding skills in discourse. *Journal of Speech and Hearing Research, 34,* 309–316.

Geschwind, N., & Galaburda, A. (1985). Cerebral lateralization, biological mechanisms, associations and pathology: I. A hypothesis and a program for research. *Archives of Neurology, 42,* 428–459.

Gibbs, D. P., & Cooper, E. B. (1989). Prevalence of communication disorders in students with learning disabilities. *Journal of Learning Disabilities, 22,* 60–63.

Gierut, J. A. (1998). Treatment efficacy: Functional phonological disorders in children. *Journal of Speech, Language, and Hearing Research, 41*(1), S85–S100.

Gillam, R. B. (1999). Computer-assisted language intervention using Fast For Word: Theoretical and empirical considerations for clinical decision making. *Language, Speech, and Hearing Services in Schools, 30,* 363–370.

Gillam, R. B., & Gorman, B. K. (2004). Language and discourse contributions to word recognition and text interpretation. In E. R. Silliman & L. C. Wilkinson (Eds.), *Language and literacy learning in schools* (pp. 63–97). New York: Guilford.

Gillon, G. T. (2000). The efficacy of phonological awareness intervention for children with spoken language impairment. *Language, Speech, and Hearing Services in Schools, 31,* 126–141.

Girolametto, L., Hoaken, L., Weitzman, E., & van Lieshout, R. (2000). Patterns of adult-child linguistic interaction in integrated day care groups. *Language, Speech, and Hearing Services in Schools, 31,* 155–168.

Girolametto, L., Weitzman, E., Wiigs, M., & Steig Pearce, P. (1999). The relationship between maternal language measures and language development in toddlers with expressive vocabulary delays. *American Journal of Speech-Language Pathology, 8,* 364–374.

Glennen, S. (1997). Introduction to augmentative and alternative communication. In S. Glennen & D. DeCoste (Eds.), *Handbook of augmentative and alternative Communication* (p. 3–19). San Diego, CA: Singular Publishing Group.

Glennen, S., & Calculator, S. (1985). Training functional communication board use: A pragmatic approach. *Augmentative and Alternative Communication, 1,* 134–145.

Glennen, S. L., & DeCoste, C. (1997). *Handbook of augmentative communication.* San Diego, CA: Singular.

Golder, C., & Coirier, P. (1994). Argumentative text writing: Developmental trends. *Discourse Processes, 18,* 187–210.

Golding-Kushner, K. (1995). Treatment of articulation and resonance disorders associated with cleft palate and VPI. In R. J. Shprintzen & J. Bardach (Eds.), *Cleft palate speech management: A multidisciplinary approach.* St. Louis, MO: Mosby.

Goldman, R., & Fristoe, M. (2000). *Goldman-Fristoe*

test of articulation-Second edition (GFTA-2). Circle Pines, MN: American Guidance Service.

Goldstein, B. A. (2004). From the editor. *Language, Speech, and Hearing Services in Schools, 35*(3), 199.

Goodglass, H., & Kaplan, E. (1983a). *The Boston diagnostic aphasia examination.* Philadelphia: Lea & Febiger.

Goodglass, H., & Kaplan, E. (1983b). *Boston naming test.* Philadelphia: Lea & Febiger.

Goswami, U. C. (1988) Children's use of analogy in learning to spell. *British Journal of Developmental Psychology, 6,* 1–22.

Gottwald, S., & Starkweather, W. C. (1995). Fluency intervention for preschoolers and their families in the public schools. *Language, Speech, and Hearing Services in Schools, 26,* 117–126.

Grabb, W. C., Rosenstein, S. W., & Bzoch, K. R. (1971). *Cleft lip and palate: Surgical, dental, and speech aspects.* Boston: Little, Brown.

Graham, S. (1999). Handwriting and spelling instruction for students with learning disabilities: A review. *Learning Disability Quarterly, 22,* 78–98.

Graham, S., & Freeman, S. (1986). Strategy training and teacher- vs. student-controlled study conditions: Effects on LD students' performance. *Learning Disability Quarterly, 9,* 15–22.

Graham, S., & Harris, K. R. (1996). Addressing problems in attention, memory, and executive functioning: An example from self-regulated strategy development. In G. Reid Lyon & N. A. Krasnegor (Eds.), *Attention, memory, and executive function* (pp. 349–365). Baltimore, MD: Paul H. Brookes.

Graham, S., & Harris, K. R. (1997). Self-regulation and writing: Where do we go from here? *Contemporary Educational Psychology, 22,* 102–114.

Graham, S., & Harris, K. R. (1999). Assessment and intervention in overcoming writing difficulties: An illustration from the self-regulation strategy development model. *Language, Speech, and Hearing Services in Schools, 30*(3), 255–264.

Graham, S., Harris, K., & Loynachan, C. (1994). The spelling for writing list. *Journal of Learning Disability, 27,* 210–217.

Graham, S., Harris, K., MacArthur, C. A., & Schwartz, S. S. (1991). Writing and writing instruction for students with learning disabilities: A review of a program of research. *Learning Disability Quarterly, 14,* 89–114.

Gravel, J. S., & Wallace, I. F. (1999). Language, speech, and educational outcomes of otitis media. *Journal of Otolaryngology, 27* (Suppl. 2), 17–25.

Graves, A., Montague, M., & Wong, Y. (1990). The effects of procedural facilitation on the composition of learning disabled students. *Learning Disabilities Research, 5,* 88–93.

Gray, S. (2004). Word learning by preschoolers with specific language impairment: Predictors and poor learners. *Journal of Speech, Language, and Hearing Research, 47,* 1117–1132.

Gray, S., Plante, E., Vance, R., & Henrichsen, M. (1999). The diagnostic accuracy of four vocabulary tests administered to preschool-age children. *Language, Speech, and Hearing Services in Schools, 30,* 196–206.

Gray, S. D., Titze, I. R., & Lusk, R. P. (1987). Electron microscopy of hyperphonated canine vocal cords. *Journal of Voice, 1,* 109–115.

Greenamyre, J. T., & Shoulson, I. (1994). Huntington's disease. In D. Calne (Ed.), *Neurodegenerative diseases* (pp. 685–704). Philadelphia: W. B. Saunders.

Greenberg, D., Ehri, L., & Perin, D. (1997). Are word reading processes the same or different in adult literacy students and 3rd–5th graders matched for reading level? *Journal of Educational Psychology, 89,* 262–275.

Greene, J. F. (1996). Psycholinguistic assessment: The clinical base for identity of dyslexia. *Topics in Language Disorders 16*(2), 45–72.

Greenhalgh, K. S., & Strong, C. J. (2001). Literate language features in spoken narratives of children with typical language and children with language impairments. *Language, Speech, and Hearing Services in Schools, 32,* 114–126.

Gregory, R. L. (1981). *Mind in science.* New York: Cambridge University Press.

Grice, H. (1975). Logic and conversation. In D. Davidson & G. Harmon (Eds.), *The logic of grammar.* Encino, CA: Dickenson Press.

Grice, S. J., Halit, H., Farroni, T., Baron-Cohen, S., Bolton, P., & Johnson, M. H. (2005). Neural correlates of eye-gaze detection in young children with autism. *Cortex, 41,* 327–341.

Griffith, P. (1991). Phonemic awareness helps first graders invent spellings and third graders remember correct spelling. *Journal of Reading Behavior, 23,* 215–233.

Grosz, J. (1989). The development and family services unit. In P. B. Kozlowski, D. A. Snider, P. M. Victze, & H. M. Wisniewski (Eds.), *Proceedings of the Conference on Brain and Behavior in Pediatric HIV Infection* (pp. 115–125). New York: Karger.

Grunwell, P. (1985). *PACS: Phonological assessment of child speech.* San Diego, CA: College-Hill.

Grunwell, P. (1987). *Clinical phonology* (2nd ed.). London: Chapman & Hall.

Grunwell, P. (Ed.). (1993). *Analysing cleft palate speech.* London: Whurr.

Guitar, B. (1998). *Stuttering: An integrated approach to its nature and treatment.* (2nd ed.). Baltimore, MD: Williams and Wilkins.

Gummersall, D. M., & Strong, C. J. (1999). Assessment of complex sentence production in a narrative context. *Language, Speech, and Hearing Services in Schools, 30,* 152–164.

Gumperz, J. J. (1972). Introduction. In J. J. Gumperz & D. Hymes, *Directions in sociolinguistics: The ethnography of communication.* New York: Holt, Rinehart, & Winston.

Gumperz, J. J., & Hymes, D. (1972). *Directions in sociolinguistics: The ethnography of communication.* New York: Holt, Rinehart and Winston.

Gurd, J. M., Bessell, N., Watson, I., & Coleman, J. (1998). Motor speech vs. digit control in Parkinson's disease: A cognitive neuropsychology investigation. *Clinical Linguistics and Phonetics, 12,* 357–378.

Gutierrez-Clellan, V. F. (1999). Language choice in intervention with bilingual children. *American Journal of Speech-Language Pathology, 8,* 291–302.

Gutierrez-Clellan, V. F., Restrepo, M. A., Bedore, L., Peña, E., & Anderson, R. (2000). Language sample analysis in Spanish-speaking children: Methodological considerations. *Language, Speech, and Hearing Services in Schools, 31,* 88–98.

Haberfellner, H., Schwartz, S., & Gisel, E. G. (2001). Feeding skills and growth after one year of intraoral therapy in moderately dysphagic children with cerebral palsy. *Dysphagia, 16,* 83–96.

Hadley, P. A. (1998). Language sampling protocols for eliciting text-level discourse. *Language, Speech, and Hearing Services in Schools, 29,* 132–147.

Hadley, P. A., Simmerman, A., Long, M., & Luna, M. (2000). Facilitating language development in inner-city children: Experimental evaluation of a collaborative classroom-based intervention. *Language, Speech, and Hearing Services in Schools, 31,* 280–295.

Hagan, C., & Malkamus, D. (1979, November). *Interaction strategies for language disorders secondary to head trauma.* Paper presented at the annual convention of the American Speech-Language-Hearing Association, Atlanta.

Hall, J. W., & Grose, J. H. (1993). The effect of otitis media with effusion on the masking-level difference and the auditory brainstem response. *Journal of Speech and Hearing Research, 36,* 210–217.

Hall, P. K., Jordan, L. S., & Robin, D. A. (1993). *Developmental apraxia of speech: Theory and clinical practice.* Austin, TX: Pro-Ed.

Hambly, C., & Riddle, L. (2002, April). *Phonological awareness training for school-age children.* Paper presented at the annual convention of the New York State Speech-Language-Hearing Association, Rochester.

Hanson, M. L. (1994). Oral myofunctional disorders and articulatory patterns. In J. Bernthal & N. Bankson (Eds.), *Child phonology: Characteristics, assessment, and intervention with special populations* (pp. 29–53). New York: Thieme Medical Publishers.

Hardy, E., & Robinson, N. M. (1993). *Swallowing disorders treatment manual.* Bisbee, AZ: Imaginart.

Hardy, J. C. (1983). *Cerebral palsy.* Englewood Cliffs, NJ: Prentice-Hall.

Harris, K. R., & Graham, S. (1996). Improving learning disabled students' composition skills: Self-control strategy training. *Learning Disability Quarterly, 8,* 27–36.

Hart, K. I., Fujiki, M., Brinton, B., & Hart, C. H. (2004). The relationship between social behavior and severity of language impairment. *Journal of Speech, Language, and Hearing Research, 47,* 647–662.

Haynes, S. (1985). Developmental apraxia of speech: Symptoms and treatment. In D. F. Johns (Ed.), *Clinical management of neurogenic communicative disorders* (2nd ed., pp. 259–266). Boston: Little, Brown.

Haynes, W. O., & Pindzola, R. H. (1998). *Diagnosis and evaluation in speech pathology* (5th ed.). Boston: Allyn and Bacon.

Healy, J. M. (1982). The enigma of hyperlexia. *Reading Research Quarterly, 7,* 319–328.

Hebert, L. E., Scherr, P. A., Bienias, J. L., Bennett, D. A., & Evans, D. A. (2003). Alzheimer disease in the US population: Prevalence estimates using the 2000 census. *Archives of Neurology, 60*(8), 1119–1122.

Hegde, M. N. (1993). *Treatment procedures in communicative disorders* (2nd ed.). Austin, TX: Pro-Ed.

Heiss, W. D., Kessler, J., Thiel, A., Ghaemi, M., & Karbe, H. (1999). Differential capacity of left and right hemisphere areas for compensation of poststroke aphasia. *Annals of Neurology, 45,* 430–438.

Helm-Estabrooks, N., & Albert, M. C. (1991). *Manual of aphasia therapy.* Austin, TX: Pro-Ed.

Henderson, E. H. (1990). *Teaching spelling* (2nd ed.). Boston: Houghton Mifflin.

Hewlett, N. (1990). The processes of speech production and speech development. In P. Grunwell (Ed.), *Developmental speech disorders: Clinical issues and practical implications.* Edinburgh: Churchill Livingstone.

Hicks, C. B., Tharpe, A. M., & Ashmead, D. H. (2000). Behavioral auditory assessment of young infants: Methodologic limitations or natural lack of auditory responsiveness? *American Journal of Audiology, 9,* 124–130.

Hiss, S., Strauss, M., Treole, K., Stuart, A., & Boutilier, S. (2004). Effect of age, gender, bolus volume, bolus viscosity, and gustation on swallowing apnea onset relative to lingual bolus propulsion onset in normal adults. *Journal of Speech, Language, and Hearing Research, 47,* 572–583.

Hodson, B. (1985). *Computerized analysis of phonological processes: Version 1.0* (Apple II Series Computer Program). Danville, IL: Interstate.

Hodson, B. (1986). *The assessment of phonological processes—Revised.* Danville, IL: Interstate.

Hodson, B., & Paden, E. (1991). *Targeting intelligible speech: A phonological approach to remediation* (2nd ed.). Austin, TX: Pro-Ed.

Hogan, T., & Catts, H. W. (2004). *Phonological awareness test items: Lexical and phonological characteristics affect performance.* Paper presented at the Annual Convention of the American Speech-Language-Hearing Association, Philadelphia.

Holland, A., & Fridriksson, J. (2001). Aphasia management during the early phases of recovery following stroke. *American Journal of Speech-Language Pathology, 10*(1), 19–28.

Holland, A. L. (1980). *Communication abilities in daily living: A test of functional communication for adults.* Baltimore: University Park Press.

Hollien, H. (1987). Old voices: What do we really know about them? *Journal of Voice, 1,* 2–17.

Hood, L. J. (1998). *Clinical applications of the auditory brainstem response.* San Diego: Singular.

Hopper, T. (2005, November 8). Assessment and treatment of cognitive-communication disorders in individuals with dementia. *The ASHA Leader, 10*(15), 10–11.

Horn, E. (1954). *Teaching spelling.* Washington, DC: American Education Research Association.

Howell, J., & Dean, E. (1994). *Treating phonological disorders in children: Metaphon—theory to practice* (2nd ed.). London: Whurr.

Howell, P. (2004). Assessment of some contemporary theories of stuttering that apply to spontaneous speech. *Contemporary Issues in Communication Science and Disorders, 31,* 69–79. 123–140.

http://www.alz.org/AboutAD/Statistics.asp. Alzheimer's Association. Accessed October 22, 2005; updated 2005.

http://www.cdc.gov/doc.do/id/0900f3ec800101e8. Centers for Disease Control and Prevention. Accessed October 22, 2005; updated September 12, 2003.

http://www.cdc.gov/nchs/data/factsheets/Parkinsons.pdf. National Center for Health Statistics, Centers for Disease Control and Prevention. Accessed October 22, 2005; updated 1999.

http://www.ninds.nih.gov/disorders/aphasia/aphasia.htm. (2005). National Institute of Neurological Disorders and Stroke, National Institute of Health. Accessed October 22, 2005; updated February 9, 2005.

http://www.ninds.nih.gov/disorders/parkinsons_disease/parkinsons_disease_backgrounder.htm. National Institute of Neurological Disorders and Stroke, National Institute of Health. Accessed October 22, 2005; updated October 18, 2004.

http://www.strokecenter.org/pat/stats.htm. The Internet Stroke Center. Accessde October 22, 2005; updated 2005.

Huaqing Qi, C., & Kaiser, A. P. (2004). Problem behaviors of low income children with language delays: An observation study. *Journal of Speech, Language, and Hearing Research, 47,* 595–609.

Hughes, M., & Searle, D. (1997). *The violet E and other tricky sounds: Learning to spell from kindergarten to grade 6.* York, ME: Stenhouse.

Hunt-Berg, M. (2001). Gestures in development: Implications for early intervention in AAC. *American Speech-Language Hearing Association Special Interest Division 1, Language Learning and Education Newsletter, 8*(1), 5–8.

Hunter, L., Pring, T., & Martin, S. (1991). The use of strategies to increase speech intelligibility in cerebral palsy: An experimental evaluation. *British Journal of Disorders of Communication, 26,* 163–174.

Hurst, M., & Cooper, G. (1983). Employer attitudes towards stuttering. *Journal of Fluency Disorders, 8,* 1–12

Hustad, K. C., & Beukelman, D. R. (2001). Effects of linguistic cues and stimulus cohesion on intelligibility of severely dysarthric speech. *Journal of Speech, Language, and Hearing Research, 44,* 497–510.

Hustad, K. C., & Cahill, M. A. (2003). Effects of presentation mode and repeated familiarization on intelligibility of dysarthric speech. *American Journal of Speech-Language Pathology, 12,* 198–208.

Hustad, K. C., Jones, T., & Dailey, S. (2003). Implementing speech supplementation strategies: Effects on intelligibility and speech rate of individuals with chronic severe dysarthria. *Journal of Speech, Language, and Hearing Research, 46,* 462–474.

Hutchinson, J., & Marquardt, T. P. (1997). Functional treatment approaches to memory impairment following brain injury. *Topics in Language Disorders, 18*(1), 45–57.

Iacono, T., Carter, M., & Hook, J. (1998). Identification of intentional communication in students with severe and multiple disabilities. *Augmentative and Alternative Communication, 14*, 102–114.

Iglesias, A., & Goldstein, B. (1998). Language and dialectical variations. In J. E. Bernthal & N. W. Bankson (Eds.), *Articulation and phonological disorders* (4th ed.). Boston: Allyn and Bacon.

Ingham, R. J. (1990). Research on stuttering treatment for adults and adolescents who stutter: A perspective on how to overcome the malaise. In J. Cooper (Ed.), *Research needs in stuttering: Roadblocks and future directions* (ASHA Reports 18, pp. 91–97). Rockville, MD: American Speech-Language-Hearing Association.

Ingham, R. J., & Cordes, A. K. (1997). Self-measurement and evaluating stuttering treatment efficacy. In R. F. Curlee & G. M. Siegel (Eds.), *Nature and treatment of stuttering: New directions* (2nd ed., pp. 413–437). Boston: Allyn and Bacon.

Ingram, K., Bunta, F., & Ingram, D. (2004). Digital data collection and analysis: Application for clinical practice. *Language, Speech, and Hearing Services in Schools, 35*, 112–121.

Ingham, R. J., Ingham, J. C., Finn, P., & Fox, P. T. (2003). Towards a functional neural systems model of developmental stuttering. *Journal of Fluency Disorders, 28*, 297–318.

Izumikawa, M., Minoda, R., Kawamoto, K., Abrashkin, K. A., Swiderski, D. L., Dolan, D. F., et al. (2005). Auditory hair cell replacement and hearing improvement by *Atoh1* gene therapy in deaf mammals. *Nature Medicine, 11*, 271–276.

Jacobs, B. J., & Thompson, C. K. (2000). Cross-modality generalization effects of training noncanonical sentence comprehension and production in agrammatic aphasia. *Journal of Speech, Language, and Hearing Research, 43*, 5–20.

Jelm, J. M. (1994). Treatment of feeding and swallowing disorders in children: An overview. In L. R. Cherney (Ed.), *Clinical management of dysphagia in adults and children.* Gaithersburg, MD: Aspen.

Jewett, D. L., Romano, M. N., & Williston, J. S. (1970). Human auditory evoked potentials: Possible brain stem components detected on the scalp. *Science, 167*, 1517–1518.

Johns Hopkins. (2000). Help when it's hard to swallow. *Johns Hopkins Medical Letter, Health.after 50, 11*(12), 6–7.

Johnston, B. T., Colcher, A., Li, Q., et al. (2001). Repetitive proximal esophageal contractions: A new manometric finding and a possible link between Parkinson's disease and achalasia. *Dysphagia, 16*, 186–189.

Johnston, J. R. (2001). An alternative MLU calculation: Magnitude and variability of effects. *Journal of Speech, Language, and Hearing Research, 44*, 156–164.

Johnston, P. H., & Winograd, P. N. (1985). Passive failure in reading. *Journal of Reading Behavior, 4*, 156–164.

Joint Committee on Infant Hearing. (2000). Year 2000 Position Statement: Principles and guidelines for early hearing detection and intervention programs. *American Journal of Audiology, 9*, 9–29.

Justice, L. M., & Ezell, H. K. (2002). Use of storybook reading to increase print awareness in at-risk children. *American Journal of Speech-Language Pathology, 11*, 17–29.

Justice, L. M., & Kaderavek, J. N. (2004). Embedded-explicit emergent literacy intervention I: Background and description of approach. *Language, Speech, and Hearing Services in Schools, 35*, 201–211.

Kaderavek, J. N., & Justice, L. M. (2004). Embedded-explicit emergent literacy intervention II: Goal selection and implementation in the early childhood classroom. *Language, Speech, and Hearing Services in Schools, 35*, 212–228.

Kaderavek, J. N., & Sulzby, E. (1998). Parent-child joint book reading: An observational protocol for young children. *American Journal of Speech-Language Pathology, 7*(1), 33–47.

Kagan, A., Black, S. E., Duchan, J. F., Simmons-Mackie, N., & Square, N. (2001). Training volunteers as conversation partners using "Supporting conversation for adults with aphasia" (SCA): A controlled trial. *Journal of Speech, Language, and Hearing Research, 44*, 624–638.

Kahane, J. (1982). Anatomy and physiology of the organs of the peripheral speech mechanism. In N. Lass, L. McReynolds, J. Northern, & D. Yoder (Eds.), *Speech, language and hearing* (Vol. I, pp. 109–155). Philadelphia, PA: Saunders.

Kamhi, A. (1998). Trying to make sense of developmental language disorders. *Language, Speech, and Hearing Services in Schools, 29*, 35–44.

Kamhi, A. G. (2003). The role of the SLP in improving reading fluency. *The ASHA Leader, 8*(7), 6–8.

Kamhi, A. G., & Catts, H. W. (2002). The language basis of reading: Implications for classification and treatment of children with reading disabilities. In K. G. Butler & E. R. Silliman (Eds.), *Speaking, read-*

ing, and writing in children with language learning disabilities, *New paradigms in research and practice* (pp. 45–72). Mahwah, NJ: Erlbaum.

Kamhi, A. G., & Catts, H. W. (2005). Language and reading: Convergences and divergences. In H. W. Catts & A. G. Kamhi (Eds.), *Language and reading disabilities* (2nd ed.; pp. 1–25). Boston: Allyn and Bacon.

Kamhi, A. G., Gentry, B., Mauer, D., & Gholson, B. (1990). Analogical learning and transfer in language-impaired children. *Journal of Speech and Hearing Disorders, 55,* 140–148.

Kamhi, A. G., & Hinton, L. N. (2000). Explaining individual differences in spelling ability. *Topics in Language Disorders, 20*(3), 37.

Karagiannis, A., Stainback, W., & Stainback, S. (1996). Historical overview of inclusion. In S. Stainback & W. Stainback (Eds.), *Inclusion: A guide for educators.* Baltimore: Paul H. Brookes.

Katz, R. C., & Wertz, R. T. (1997). The efficacy of computer-provided reading treatment for chronic aphasic adults. *Journal of Speech, Language, and Hearing Research, 40,* 493–507.

Katz, W. F. (2003). From basic research in speech science to answers in speech-language pathology. *The ASHA Leader, 8*(1), 6–7, 20.

Katz, W. F., Bharadwaj, S. V., & Carstens, B. (1999). Electromagnetic articulography treatment for an adult with Broca's aphasia and apraxia of speech. *Journal of Speech, Language, and Hearing Research, 42,* 1355–1366.

Kavé, G., & Levy, Y. (2003). Morphology in picture descriptions provided by persons with Alzheimer's disease. *Journal of Speech, Language, and Hearing Research, 46,* 341–352.

Kay-Raining Bird, E., & Chapman, R. S. (1994). Sequential recall in individuals with Down syndrome. *Journal of Speech and Learning Research, 37,* 1369–1380.

Kearns, K. P., & Simmons, N. N. (1988). Motor speech disorders: The dysarthrias and apraxia of speech. In N. J. Lass, L. V. McReynolds, & D. E. Yoder (Eds.), *Handbook of speech-language pathology and audiology* (pp. 592–621). Burlington, Ontario, Canada: B. D. Decker.

Kemker, F. J. (1995). Audiologic management of patients with cleft palate and related disorders. In K. R. Bzoch (Ed.), *Communicative disorders related to cleft lip and palate* (4th ed.; pp. 245–260). Austin, TX: Pro-Ed.

Kemp, D. T. (1978). Stimulated acoustic emissions from within the human auditory system. *Journal of the Acoustical Society of America, 64,* 1386–1391.

Kemper, T. (1984). Neuroanatomical and neuropathological changes in normal aging and in dementia. In M. L. Albert (Ed.), *Clinical neurology of aging.* New York: Oxford University Press.

Kent, R. D. (1997). *The speech sciences.* San Diego, CA: Singular Publishing Group.

Kent, R. D., Duffy, J. R., Slama, A., Kent, J. F., & Clift, A. (2001). Clinicoanatomic studies in dysarthria: Review, critique, and directions for research. *Journal of Speech, Language, and Hearing Research, 44,* 535–551.

Kent, R. D., Kent, J. F., Duffy, J. R., Thomas, J. E., Weismer, G., & Stuntebeck, S. (2000). Ataxic dysarthria. *Journal of Speech, Language, and Hearing Research, 43,* 1275–1289.

Kent, R. D., & Rosenbek, J. C. (1983). Acoustic patterns of apraxia of speech. *Journal of Speech and Hearing Research, 26,* 231–249.

Kertesz, A., & McCabe, P. (1982). *Western Aphasia Battery.* New York: Grune & Stratton.

Kertesz, A., & McCabe, P. (1997). Recovery patterns and prognosis in aphasia. *Brain, 100,* 100–118.

Kessels, R. P. C. (2003). Patients' memory for medical information. *Journal of Royal Society of Medicine 96,* 219–222.

Khan, L. M., & Lewis, N. P. (2002). *Khan-Lewis Phonological Analysis-2 (KLPA-2).* Circle Pines, MN: American Guidance Service.

Kidd, K. (1984). Stuttering as a genetic disorder. In R. F. Curlee & W. H. Perkins (Eds.), *Nature and treatment of stuttering: New directions* (pp. 149–169). Boston: Allyn and Bacon.

Kiernan, B., Snow, D., Swisher, L., & Vance, R. (1997). Another look at nonverbal rule induction in children with specific language impairment: Testing a flexible reconceptualization hypothesis. *Journal of Speech and Hearing Research, 40,* 75–82.

Kintsch, W. (1998). *Comprehension: A paradigm for cognition.* New York: Cambridge University Press.

Kirshner, H. S. (1995). *Handbook of neurological speech and language disorders.* New York: Marcel Dekker.

Klasner, E. R., & Yorkston, K. M. (2001). Linguistic and cognitive supplementation strategies as augmentative and alternative communication techniques in Huntington's disease: Case study. *Augmentative and Alternative Communication, 17,* 154–160.

Klee, T., Schaffer, M., May, S., Membrino, I., & Mougey, K. (1989). A comparison of the age-MLU relationship in normal and specifically language impaired preschool children. *Journal of Speech and Hearing Disorders, 54,* 226–233.

Klein, H. B. (1997). *Clinical implications of nonlinear*

phonological theory: An introduction. Paper presented at the New York State Speech-Language-Hearing Association Annual Convention, Buffalo.

Klein, K. (1995). *Aphasia community group manual.* New York: National Aphasia Association.

Kochkin, S. (2001). MarkeTrak VI: The VA and direct mail sales spark growth in hearing aid market. *The Hearing Review, 8*(12), 16–24, 63–65.

Koo, E., & Price, D. (1993). The neurobiology of dementia. In P. Whitehouse (Ed.), *Dementia* (pp. 55–91). Philadelphia: F. A. Davis.

Kratcoski, A. M. (1998). Guidelines for using portfolios in assessment and evaluation. *Language, Speech, and Hearing Services in Schools, 29,* 3–10.

Kraus, J. F. (1993). Epidemiologic features of head injury. In P. R. Cooper (Ed.), *Head injury* (3rd ed.). Baltimore: Williams and Wilkins.

Kroll, B. M. (1981). Developmental relationships between speaking and writing. In B. M. Kroll & R. J. Vann (Eds.), *Exploring speaking-writing relationships: Connections and contrasts* (pp. 32–54). Champaign, IL: National Council of Teachers of English.

Kully, D., & Langevin, M. (2005). Evidence-based practice in fluency disorders. *The ASHA Leader, 10*(14), 10–11, 23.

Kummer, A. W. (2001). *Cleft palate and craniofacial anomalies: The effects on speech and resonance.* San Diego, CA: Singular Thomson Learning.

Laguaite, J. K. (1972). Adult voice screening. *Journal of Speech and Hearing Disorders, 37,* 147–151.

Langmore, S. E., Terpenning, M. S., Schork, A., Chen, Y., Murray, J. T., Lopatin, D., & Loesche, W. J. (1998). Predictors of aspiration pneumonia: How important is dysphagia? *Dysphagia, 13*(2), 69–81.

La Paro, K. M., Justice, L., Skibbe, L. E., & Pianta, R. C. (2004). Relations among maternal, child, and demographic factors and the persistence of preschool language impairment. *American Journal of Speech-Language Pathology, 13,* 291–303.

Lapko, L., & Bankson, N. (1975). Relationship between auditory discrimination, articulation stimulability and consistency of misarticulation. *Perceptual and Motor Skills, 40,* 171–177.

Larson, V. L., & McKinley, N. L. (1998). Characteristics of adolescents' conversation: A longitudinal study. *Clinical Linguistics and Phonetics, 12,* 183–203.

Lasker, J. P., & Bedrosian, J. L. (2000). Acceptance of AAC by adults with acquired disorders. In D. Beukelman, K. Yorkston, & J. Reichle (Eds.), *Augmentative communication for adults with neurogenic and neuromuscular disabilities* (pp. 107–136). Baltimore, MD: Paul H. Brookes.

Lasker, J. P., & Bedrosian, J. L. (2001). Promoting acceptance of augmentative and alternative communication by adults with acquired communication disorders. *Augmentative and Alternative Communication, 17,* 141–153.

Lau, C., & Kusnierczyk, I. (2001). Quantitative evaluation of infant's nonnutritive and nutritive sucking. *Dysphagia, 16,* 58–67.

Le Blanc, E. M., & Cisneros, G. J. (1995). The dynamics of speech and orthodontic management in cleft lip and palate. In R. J. Shprintzen & J. Bardach (Eds.), *Cleft palate speech management: A multidisciplinary approach.* St. Louis, MO: Mosby.

Leblanc, R. (1996). Familial cerebral aneurysms. *Stroke, 27,* 1050–1054.

Leder, S. B., Sasaki, C. T., & Burrell, M. I. (1998). Fiberoptic endoscopic evaluation of dysphagia to identify silent aspiration. *Dysphagia, 13*(1), 19–21.

Lennox, C., & Siegel, L. S. (1996). The development of phonological rules and visual strategies in average and poor spellers. *Journal of Experimental Child Psychology, 62,* 60–83.

Leonard, R. J. (1994). Characteristics of speech in speakers with oral/oral pharyngeal ablation. In J. Bernthal & N. Bankson (Eds.), *Child phonology: Characteristics, assessment, and intervention with special populations* (pp. 54–78). New York: Thieme Medical Publishers.

Lesar, S. (1992). Prenatal cocaine exposure: The challenge to education. *Infant-Toddler Intervention: The Transdisciplinary Journal, 2*(1), 37–52.

Levine, M. (1987). *Developmental variation and learning disorders.* Cambridge, MA: Educators Publishing Service.

Lewis, B. A., O'Donnell, B., Freebairn, L. A., & Taylor, H. G. (1998). Spoken language and written expression—interplay of delays. *American Journal of Speech-Language Pathology, 7*(3), 77–84.

Light, J. (1989). Toward a definition of communication competence for individuals using augmentative and alternative communication systems. *Augmentative and Alternative Communication, 5,* 137–144.

Light, J. (1997). "Let's go star fishing": Reflections on the contexts of language learning for children who use aided AAC. *Augmentative and Alternative Communication, 13,* 158–171.

Light, J., Beukelman, D., & Reichle, J. (2003). *Communicative competence for individuals who use AAC: From research to effective practice.* Baltimore, MD: Paul H. Brookes.

Light, J., Dattilo, J., English, J., Gutierrez, L., & Hartz, J. (1992). Instructing facilitators to support the communication of people who use augmentative communication systems. *Journal of Speech and Hearing Research, 35,* 865–875.

Light, J., & Lindsay, P. (1991). Cognitive science and augmentative and alternative communication. *Augmentative and Alternative Communication, 7,* 186–203.

Lim, S. H., Lieu, P. K., Phua, S. Y., et al. (2001). Accuracy of bedside clinical methods compared with fiberoptic endoscopic examination of swallowing (FEES) in determining the risk of aspiration in acute stroke patients. *Dysphagia, 16,* 1–6.

Lincoln, M., & Onslow, M. (1997). Long-term outcome of early intervention for stuttering. *American Journal of Speech-Language Pathology, 6,* 51–58.

Lippke, B. A., Dickey, S., Selmar, J., & Soder, A. L. (1997). *Photo articulation test-3.* Austin, TX: Pro-Ed.

Lloyd, L. L. (1985). Comments on terminology. *Augmentative and Alternative Communication, 1,* 95–97.

Lloyd, L. L. Fuller, D., & Arvidson, H. (1997). *Augmentative and alternative communication: A handbook of principles and practices.* Boston: Allyn and Bacon.

Logemann, J. A. (1994). Evaluation and treatment of swallowing disorders. *American Journal of Speech-Language Pathology, 3*(3), 41–44.

Logemann, J. A. (1996). Screening, diagnosis, and management of neurogenic dysphagia. *Seminars in Neurology, 16*(4), 319–327.

Logemann, J. A. (1997). Structural and functional aspects of normal and disordered swallowing. In C. T. Ferrand & R. L. Bloom (Eds.), *Introduction to organic and neurogenic disorders of communication: Current scope of practice.* Boston: Allyn and Bacon.

Logemann, J. A. (1998). *Evaluation and treatment of swallowing disorders* (2nd ed.). Austin, TX: Pro-Ed.

Lonsbury-Martin, B. L. (2005). Otoacoustic emissions: Where are we today? *ASHA Leader, 10,* 6–7, 19.

Lord, C. (1988). Enhancing communication in adolescents with autism. *Topics in Language Disorders, 9*(1), 72–81.

Lotze, M. (1995). Nursing assessment and management. In S. R. Rosenthal, J. J. Sheppard, & M. Lotze (Eds.), *Dysphagia and the child with developmental disabilities: Medical, clinical, and family interventions.* San Diego, CA: Singular.

Love, R. J. (1992). *Childhood motor speech disability.* New York: Macmillan.

Lubinski, R., & Masters, M. G. (2001). Special populations, special settings: New and expanding frontiers. In R. Lubinski & C. Frattali (Eds.), *Professional issues in speech-language pathology and audiology* (2nd ed.). San Diego: Singular.

Lubker, B. B. (1997). Language learning disorders in children with chronic health conditions: Epidemiologic perspectives. *American Speech-Language-Hearing Association, Special Interest Divisions, Language Learning and Education, 4*(1), 2–5.

Lund, N., & Duchan, J. (1993). *Assessing children's language in naturalistic contexts* (3rd ed.). Englewood Cliffs, NJ: Prentice-Hall.

Lyon, G. R., Shaywitz, S. E., & Shaywitz, B. A. (2003). Defining dyslexia, comorbidity, teachers' knowledge of language and reading: A definition of dyslexia. *Annals of Dyslexia, 53,* 1.

MacArthur, C. A. (1999). Word processing with speech synthesis and word prediction: Effects on the dialogue journal writing of students with learning disabilities. *Learning Disability Quarterly, 21,* 1–16.

MacArthur, C. A. (2000). New tools for writing: Assistive technology for students with writing difficulties. *Topics in Language Disorders, 20*(4), 85–104.

MacArthur, C. A., & Graham, S. (1987). Learning disabled students composing under three methods of text production: Handwriting, word processing, and dictation. *Journal of Special Education, 21,* 22–42.

MacArthur, C. A., Graham, S., Haynes, J. A., & DeLaPaz, S. (1996). Spelling checkers and students with learning disabilities: Performance comparisons and impact on spelling. *Journal of Special Education, 30,* 35–57.

MacArthur, C. A., Graham, S., Schwartz, S. S., & Schafer, W. (1995). Evaluation of a writing instruction model that integrated a process approach, strategy instruction, and word processing. *Learning Disability Quarterly, 18,* 278–291.

MacDonald, C. C. (1992). Perinatal cocaine exposure: Predictor of an endangered generation. *Infant-Toddler Intervention: The Transdisciplinary Journal, 2*(1), 1–12.

Mackay, L. E., Bernstein, B. A., Chapman, P. E., Morgan, A. S., & Milazzo, L. S. (1992). Early intervention in severe head injury: Long-term benefits of a formalized program. *Archives of Physical Medicine and Rehabilitation, 73,* 635–641.

MacLachlan, B. G., & Chapman, R. S. (1988). Communication breakdowns in normal and language-learning-disabled children's conversation and narration. *Journal of Speech and Hearing Disorders, 53,* 2–9.

Magaziner, J., German, P., Itkin Zimmerman, S.,

Hebel, J. R., Burton, L., Bruber-Baldini, A. L., May, C., & Kittner, S. (2000). The prevalence of dementia in a statewide sample of new nursing home admissions aged 65 and older: Diagnosis by expert panel. *The Gerontologist, 40,* 663–672.

Mallette, B. (1994). *The effects of fetal alcohol syndrome on children.* Workshop presented at Buffalo Hearing and Speech Center, Buffalo, NY.

Mann, G., & Hankey, G. J. (2001). Initial clinical and demographic predictors of swallowing impairment following acute stroke. *Dysphagia, 16,* 205–216.

Mann, W., & Lane, J. (1991). *Assistive technology for persons with disabilities: The role of occupational therapy.* Rockville, MD: American Occupational Therapy Association.

Margolis, R. H. (2004). What do your patients remember? *Hearing Journal, 57,* 10–17.

Markel, N., Meisels, M., & Houck, J. (1964). Judging personality from voice quality. *Journal of Abnormal Social Psychology, 69,* 458–463.

Marshall, R. C. (1997). Aphasia treatment in the early postonset period: Managing our resources effectively. *American Journal of Speech-Language Pathology, 6*(1), 5–11.

Martin, B. J. (1994). Treatment of dysphagia in adults. In L. R. Cherney (Ed.), *Clinical management of dysphagia in adults and children.* Gaithersburg, MD: Aspen.

Martin, B. J., & Corlew, M. M. (1990). The incidence of communication disorders in dysphagic patients. *Journal of Speech and Hearing Disorders, 55*(1), 28–32.

Martin, F. N. (1994). *Introduction to audiology* (5th ed.). Englewood Cliffs, NJ: Prentice-Hall.

Martin, F. N., & Clark, J. G. (2003). *Introduction to audiology* (8th ed.). Boston: Allyn and Bacon.

Martin, R. E., Neary, M. A., Diamant, N. E. (1997). Dysphagia following anterior cervical spine surgery. *Dysphagia, 12*(1), 2–10.

Marton, K., & Schwartz, R. G. (2003). Working memory capacity and language processes in children with specific language impairment. *Journal of Speech, Language, and Hearing Research, 46,* 1138–1153.

Marvin, C. A., & Wright, D. (1997). Literacy socialization in the homes of preschool children. *Language, Speech, and Hearing Services in Schools, 28,* 154–163.

Masterson, J. J., & Apel, K. (2000). Spelling assessment: Charting a path to optimal intervention. *Topics in Language Disorders, 20*(3), 50–65.

Masterson, J. J., & Crede, L. A. (1999). Learning to spell: Implications for assessment and intervention. *Language, Speech, and Hearing Services in Schools, 30,* 243–354.

Masterson, J. J., & Pagan, F. (1993). *Interactive system for phonological analysis: Version 1.0* (Macintosh Computer Program). San Antonio, TX: The Psychological Corporation.

Max, L., & Caruso, A. J. (1997). Contemporary techniques for establishing fluency in the treatment of adults who stutter. *Contemporary Issues in Communication Science and Disorders, 24,* 45–52.

McCarthy, J., & Light, J. (2001). Instructional effectiveness of an integrated theatre arts program for children using augmentative and alternative communication and their nondisabled peers: Preliminary study. *Augmentative and Alternative Communication, 17,* 88–98.

McDonald, E. T. (1964). *Articulation testing and treatment: A sensory-motor approach.* Pittsburgh: Stanwix House.

McDowell, F. H., & Cederbaum, J. M. (1988). The extrapyramidal system and disorders of movement. In R. J. Joynt (Ed.), *Clinical neurology* (vol. 3). Philadelphia: J. B. Lippincott.

McFadden, T. U. (1998). Sounds and stories: Teaching phonemic awareness in interactions around text. *American Journal of Speech-Language Pathology, 7*(2), 5–13.

McFadden, T. U., & Gillam, R. B. (1996). An examination of the quality of narratives produced by children with language disorders. *Language, Speech, and Hearing Services in Schools, 27,* 48–56.

McGregor, K. K. (2000). The development and enhancement of narrative skills in a preschool classroom: Toward a solution to clinician-client mismatch. *American Journal of Speech-Language Pathology, 9,* 55–71.

McKinlay, W. W., Brooks, D. N., Bond, M. R., Martinage, D. P., & Marshall, M. M. (1981). The short-term outcome of severe blunt head injury as reported by the relatives of the injured person. *Journal of Neurology, Neurosurgery, and Psychiatry, 44,* 527–533.

McNaughton, D., Hughes, C., & Ofiesh, N. (1997). Proofreading for students with learning disabilities: Integrating computer use and strategic use. *Learning Disabilities Research and Practice, 12,* 16–28.

McNaughton, D., Light, J., & Groszyk, L. (2001). "Don't give up": Employment experiences of individuals with amyotrophic lateral sclerosis who use augmentative and alternative communication. *Augmentative and Alternative Communication, 17,* 179–195.

McWilliams, B. J., Morris, H. L., & Shelton, R. L. (1990). *Cleft palate speech* (2nd ed.). Philadelphia: B. C. Decker.

Meilijson, S. R., Kasher, A., & Elizur, A. (2004). Language performance in chronic schizophrenia: A pragmatic approach. *Journal of Speech, Language, and Hearing Research, 47,* 695–713.

Mentis, M., Briggs-Whittaker, J., & Gramigna, G. D. (1995). Discourse topic management in senile dementia of the Alzheimer's type. *Journal of Speech and Hearing Research, 38,* 1054–1066.

Mentis, M., & Lundgren, K. (1995). Effects of prenatal exposure to cocaine and associated risk factors on language development. *Journal of Speech and Hearing Research, 38,* 1303–1318.

Merrell, A. W., & Plante, E. (1997). Norm-referenced test interpretation in the diagnostic process. *Language, Speech, and Hearing Services in Schools, 28,* 50–58.

Metsala, J. L., & Walley, A. C. (1998). Spoken vocabulary growth and the segmental restructuring of lexical representations: Precursors to phonemic awareness and early reading ability. In J. L. Metsala & L. C. Ehri (Eds.), *Word recognition n beginning literacy* (pp. 89–120). Mahway, NJ: Lawrence Erlbaum associates.

Meyers, P. S. (1999). *Right hemisphere damage.* San Diego: Singular.

Miccio, A. W., & Elbert, M. (1996). Enhancing stimulability: A treatment program. *Journal of Communication Disorders, 29,* 335–351.

Miller, C. A., Kail, R., Leonard, L. B., & Tomblin, J. B. (2001). Speed of processing in children with specific language impairment. *Journal of Speech, Language, and Hearing Research, 44,* 416–433.

Miller, J. F. (1981). *Assessing language production in children: Experimental procedures.* Baltimore: University Park Press.

Miller, J. F., Chapman, R., & MacKenzie, H. (1981). Individual differences in the language acquisition of mentally retarded children. *Proceedings from the Second Wisconsin Symposium on Research in Child Language.* Madison: University of Wisconsin.

Miller, L. (1993, January). Testing and the creation of disorder. *American Journal of Speech Language Pathology, 2,* 13–16.

Miniutti, A. (1991). Language deficiencies in inner-city children with learning and behavioral problems. *Language, Speech, and Hearing Services in Schools, 22,* 31–38.

Moats, L. (1995). *Spelling development, disability, and instruction.* Baltimore, MD: York Press.

Montague, M., Graves, A., & Leavell, A. (1991). Planning procedural facilitation, and narrative composition of junior high students with learning disabilities. *Learning Disabilities Research and Practice, 6,* 219–224.

Moeller, M. P. (2001). Intervention and outcomes for young children who are deaf and hard of hearing and their families. In E. Kurtzer-White & D. Luterman (Eds.), *Early childhood deafness* (pp. 109–138). Baltimore: York Press.

Morgan, D. L., & Guilford, A. M. (1984). *Adolescent Language Screening Test.* Austin, TX: Pro-Ed.

Mullins, T. (2004). Depression in older adults with hearing loss. *ASHA Leader, 21,* 12–13, 27.

Murray, L. L. (2000). Spoken language production in Huntington's and Parkinson's diseases. *Journal of Speech, Language, and Hearing Research, 43,* 1350–1366.

Murray, L. L., Holland, A. L., & Beson, P. M. (1997). Auditory processing in individuals with mild aphasia: A study of resource allocation. *Journal of Speech, Language, and Hearing Research, 40,* 792–808.

Murray, L. L., Holland, A. L., & Beson, P. M. (1998). Spoken language of individuals with mild fluent aphasia under focused and divided-attention conditions. *Journal of Speech, Language, and Hearing Research, 41,* 213–225.

Naremore, R. C. (2001). *Narrative frameworks and early literacy.* Seminar presented for Rochester Hearing and Speech Center and Nazareth College, Rochester, NY.

Nathan, L., Stackhouse, J., Goulandris, N., & Snowling, M. J. (2004). The development of early literacy skills among children with speech difficulties: A test of the "critical age hypothesis." *Journal of Speech, Language, and Hearing Research, 47,* 377–391.

Nation, K., & Hulme, C. (1997). Phonemic segmentation, not onset-rime segmentation, predicts early reading and spelling skills. *Reading Research Quarterly, 32,* 154–167.

Nation, K., & Norbury, C. F. (2005). Why reading comprehension fails: Insights into developmental disorders. *Topics in Language Disorders, 25*(1), 21–32.

National Dissemination Center for Children with Disabilities. (2003, October). *Deafness and hearing loss. Disability fact sheet,* No. 3. Washington, DC: Author.

National Joint Committee on Learning Disabilities. (1991). Learning disabilities: Issues on definition (A position paper). *Asha, 33* (Suppl. 5), 18–20.

National Reading Panel. (2000). *National Reading Panel Progress Report.* Bethesda, MD: Author.

Neilson, M., & Andrews, G. (1993). Intensive fluency training of chronic stutterers. In R. F. Curlee (Ed.), *Stuttering and related disorders of fluency* (pp. 139–165). New York: Thieme Medical Publishers.

Nelson, N. W. (1994). Curriculum-based language assessment and intervention across grades. In G. P. Wallach & K. G. Butler (Eds.), *Language learning disabilities in school-age children and adolescents* (pp. 104–131). Boston: Allyn and Bacon.

Nelson, N. W. (1998). *Childhood language disorders in context: Infancy through adolescence,* (2nd ed.). Boston: Allyn and Bacon.

Nelson, N. W., & Van Meter, A. M. (2002). Assessing curriculum-based reading and writing samples. *Topics in Language Disorders, 22*(2), 35–59.

Newell, A. F., Booth, L., Arnott, J., & Beattie, W. (1992). Increasing literacy levels by the use of linguistic prediction. *Child Language Teaching and Therapy, 8,* 138–187.

Nijland, L., Maassen, B., & van der Meulen, S. (2003). Evidence of motor programming deficits in children diagnosed with DAS. *Journal of Speech, Language, and Hearing Research, 46,* 437–450.

Nilsson, H., Ekberg, O., Olsson, R., & Hindfelt, B. (1998). Dysphagia in stroke: A prospective study of quantitative aspects of swallowing in dysphagic patients. *Dysphagia, 13*(1), 32–38.

Nippold, M. (2000). Language development during the adolescent years: Aspects of pragmatics, syntax, and semantics. *Topics in Language Disorders, 20*(2), 15–28.

Nippold, M. A., Ward-Lonergan, J. M., & Fanning, J. L. (2005). Persuasive writing in children, adolescents, and adults: A study of syntactic, semantic, and pragmatic development. *Language, Speech, and Hearing Service in Schools, 36,* 125–138.

Occupational Safety and Health Administration (OSHA). (1983). Occupational noise exposure: Hearing conservation amendment: Final rule. *Federal Register, 46,* 9776–9784.

Odderson, M. D., Keaton, J. C., & McKenna, B. S. (1995). Swallow management in patients on an acute stroke pathway: Quality is cost effective. *Archives of Physical Medicine and Rehabilitation, 76*(12), 1130–1133.

Oetting, J. B., & Morohov, J. E. (1997). Past-tense marking by children with and without specific language impairment. *Journal of Speech, Language, and Hearing Research, 40,* 62–74.

Olivier, C., Hecker, L., Klucken, J., & Westby, C. (2000). Language: The embedded curriculum in postsecondary education. *Topics in Language Disorders, 21*(1) 15–29.

Oller, J. W., Kim, K., & Choe, Y. (2001). Can instructions to nonverbal tests be given in pantomime? Additional applications of a general theory of signs. *Semiotica, 133,* 15–44.

Olmsted, D. (1971). *Out of the mouth of babes.* The Hague: Mouton.

Olswang, L., Bain, B., & Johnson, G. (1990). Using dynamic assessment with children with language disorders. In S. Warren & J. Reichle (Eds.), *Causes and effects of communication and language intervention.* Baltimore, MD: Paul H. Brookes.

Olswang, L. B., Rodriguez, B., & Timler, G. (1998). Recommending intervention for toddlers with specific language learning difficulties: We may not have all the answers, but we know a lot. *American Journal of Speech-Language Pathology, 7*(1), 23–32.

O'Neil-Pirozzi, T. M. (2003). Language functioning of residents in family homeless shelters. *American Journal of Speech-Language Pathology, 12,* 229–242.

Oram, J., Fine, J., Okamoto, C., & Tannock, R. (1999). Assessing the language of children with attention deficit hyperactivity disorder. *American Journal of Speech-Language Pathology, 8,* 72–80.

Orange, J. B., Lubinsky, R. B., & Higginbotham, D. J. (1996). Conversational repair by individuals with dementia of the Alzheimer's type. *Journal of Speech, Language, and Hearing Research, 39,* 881–895.

Ors, M., Ryding, E., Lindgren, M., Gustafsson, P., Blennow, G., & Rosén, I. (2005). SPECT findings in children with specific language impairment. *Cortex, 41,* 316–326.

Orsolini, M., Sechi, E., et al. (2001). Nature of phonological delay in children with specific language impairment. *International Journal of Language and Communication Disorders, 36,* 63–90.

Owen, A. J., Dromi, E., & Leonard, L. B. (2001). The phonology-morphology interface in the speech of Hebrew-speaking children with specific language impairment. *Journal of Communication Disorders, 34,* 323–337.

Owens, R. E., Jr. (2004). *Language disorders: A functional approach to assessment and intervention* (4th ed.). Boston: Allyn and Bacon.

Owens, R. E. (2005). *Language development: An introduction* (6th ed.). Boston, Allyn and Bacon.

Owens, R. M. (2001). A brief SETI chronology. [Online]. http://www.setileague.org/general/history.htm

Pannabacker, M. (2004). Velopharyngeal incompetence: The need for speech standards. *American Journal of Speech-Language Pathology, 13,* 195–201.

Paratore, J. R. (1995). Assessing literacy: Establishing

common standards in portfolio assessment. *Topics in Language Disorders, 16*(1), 67–82.

Patterson, J. L. (2000). Observed and reported expressive vocabulary and word combinations in bilingual toddlers. *Journal of Speech, Language, and Hearing Research, 43,* 121–128.

Paul, R. (1991). Outcomes of early expressive language delay. *Journal of Childhood Communication Disorders, 15,* 7–14.

Paul, R. (1995). *Language disorders from infancy through adolescence: Assessment and intervention.* St. Louis: Mosby.

Paul-Brown, D., & Goldberg, L. R. (2001). Current policies and new directions for speech-language pathology assistants. *Language, Speech, and Hearing Services in Schools, 32,* 4–17.

Peña, E., Iglesias, A., Lidz, C. S. (2001). Reducing test bias through dynamic assessment of children's word learning ability. *American Journal of Speech-Language Pathology, 10,* 138–154.

Peña, E. D., & Quinn, R. (1997). Task familiarity: Effects on the test performance of Puerto Rican and African American children. *Language, Speech and Hearing Services in Schools, 28,* 323–332.

Perez, I., Smithard, D. G., Davies, H., & Kaira, L. (1998). Pharmacological treatment of dysphagia in stroke. *Dysphagia, 13*(1), 12–16.

Perkins, W. (1992). *Stuttering prevented.* San Diego, CA: Singular Publishing Group.

Peterson-Falzone, S. J., Hardin-Jones, M. A., & Karnell, M. P. (2001). *Cleft palate speech* (3rd ed.). St. Louis, MO: Mosby.

Peterson-Falzone, S. J., & Imagire, R. (1997). Basic genetic concepts in cranialfacial anomalies. In K. R. Bzoch (Ed.), *Communicative disorders related to cleft lip and palate* (4th ed.). Austin, TX: Pro-Ed.

Piché, L., & Reichle, J. (1991). Teaching scanning selection techniques. In J. Reichle, J. York, & J. Sigafoos (Eds.), *Implementing augmentative and alternative communication: Strategies for learners with severe disabilities* (p. 257–274). Baltimore, MD: Paul H. Brookes.

Pimental, P. A., & Kingsbury, N. A. (1989). *Mini inventory of right brain injury.* Austin, TX: Pro-Ed.

Pinker, S. (1995). *The language instinct: How the mind creates language.* New York: Harper Perennial.

Poggi, S. (2003, Spring). Facing the challenge to use scientifically based research in schools. *NCREL's Learning Point,* 4–7.

Porch, B. E. (1981). *Porch index of communicative ability* (3rd ed.). Palo Alto, CA: Consulting Psychologists Press.

Postma, A., & Kolk, H. H. J. (1993). The covert repair hypothesis: Prearticulatory repair processes in normal and stuttered disfluencies. *Journal of Speech and Hearing Research, 36,* 472–487.

Poyatos, F. (1983). *New perspectives in nonverbal communication: Studies in cultural anthropology, social psychology, linguistics, literature and semiotics.* Oxford, England: Pergamon Press.

Prather, E., Hedrick, D., & Kern, C. (1975). Articulation development in children aged two to four years. *Journal of Speech and Hearing Disorders, 40,* 179–191.

Prelock, P. A. (2000). Prologue: Multiple perspectives for determining the roles of speech-language pathologists in inclusionary classrooms. *Language, Speech, and Hearing Services in Schools, 31,* 213–218.

Prelock, P. A., Beatson, J., Bitner, B., Broder, C., & Ducker, A. (2003). Interdisciplinary assessment of young children with autism spectrum disorder. *Language, Speech, and Hearing Services in Schools, 34,* 194–202.

Pressley, M., & Hilden, K. (2004). Toward more ambitious comprehension instruction. In E. R. Silliman & L. C. Wilkinson (Eds.), *Language and literacy learning in schools* (pp. 151–174). New York: Guilford.

Prieve, B. A., & Fitzgerald, T. S. (2002). Otoacoustic emissions. In J. Katz (Ed.), *Handbook of clinical audiology* (5th ed., pp. 440–466). Philadelphia: Lippincott Williams and Wilkins.

Prins, D., Hubbard, C. P., & Krause, M. (1991). Syllabic stress and the occurrence of stuttering. *Journal of Speech and Hearing Research, 34,* 1011–1016.

Prontnicki, J. (1995). Presentation: Symptomatology and etiology of dysphasia. In S. R. Rosenthal, J. J. Sheppard, & M. Lotze (Eds.), *Dysphagia and the child with developmental disabilities: Medical, clinical, and family interventions.* San Diego, CA: Singular.

Pugh, S., & Klecan-Aker, J. S. (2004). *Effects of phonological awareness training on students with learning disabilities.* Paper presented at the annual convention of the American Speech-Language-Hearing Association, Philadelphia.

Quist, R., & Lloyd, L. (1997). Principles and uses of technology. In L. Lloyd, D. Fuller, & H. Arvidson (Eds.), *Augmentative and alternative communication: A handbook of principles and practices* (p. 107–126). Boston: Allyn and Bacon.

Raffaelli, M., & Duckett, E. (1989). "We were just talking . . .": Conversation in early adolescence. *Journal of Youth and Adolescence, 18,* 567–582.

Rainforth, B., York, J., & MacDonald, C. (1992). *Collaborative teams for students with severe disabilities:*

Integrating therapy and educational services. Baltimore: Paul H. Brookes.

Ramig, L. (1986). Acoustic analysis of phonation in patients with Huntington's disease. *Annals of Otology, Rhinology, and Laryngology, 95,* 288–293.

Ramig, L. (1994). Voice disorders. In F. Minifie (Ed.), *Introduction to communication sciences and disorders* (pp. 481–520). San Diego, CA: Singular Publishing Group.

Ramig, L. (2002). The joy of research. *The ASHA Leader, 7*(8), 6–7, 19.

Ramig, L., & Ringel, R. (1983). Effects of physiologic aging on selected acoustic characteristics of voice. *Journal of Speech and Hearing Research, 26,* 22–30.

Ramig, L., & Verdolini, K. (1998). Treatment efficacy: Voice disorders. *Journal of Speech-Language-Hearing Research, 41,* S101–S116.

Redmond, S. M. (2003). Children's production of the affix -ed in past tense and past participle contexts. *Journal of Speech, Language, and Hearing Research, 46,* 1095–1109.

Redmond, S. M., & Rice, M. L. (2001). Detection of irregular verb violations by children with and without SLI. *Journal of Speech, Language, and Hearing Research, 44,* 655–669.

Reichle, J., Halle, J. W., & Drasgow, E. (1998). Implementing augmentative communication systems. In A. Wetherby, S. Warren, & J. Reichle (Eds.), *Transitions in prelinguistic communication* (pp. 417–436). Baltimore: Paul H. Brookes.

Rescorla, L., & Alley, A. (2001). Validation of the Language Development Survey (LDS): A parent report tool for identifying language delay in toddlers. *Journal of Speech, Language, and Hearing Research, 44,* 434–445.

Reynolds, M. E., & Jefferson, L. (2000). Natural and synthetic speech comprehension: Comparison of children from two age groups. *Augmentative and Alternative Communication, 16,* 174–182.

Rhea, P. (1997). Facilitating transitions in language development in children who use AAC. *Augmentative and Alternative Communication, 13,* 141–148.

Rice, M. L., Cleave, P. L., & Oetting, J. B. (2000). The use of syntactic cues in lexical acquisition by children with SLI. *Journal of Speech, Language, and Hearing Research, 34,* 582–594.

Rieber, R. W., & Wollock, J. (1977). The historical roots of the theory and therapy of stuttering. *Journal of Communication Disorders, 10,* 3–24.

Riley, G., & Riley, J. (1981). *Stuttering prediction instrument for young children.* Tigard, OR: C. C. Publications.

Ringo, C. C., & Dietrich, S. (1995). Neurogenic stuttering: An analysis and critique. *Journal of Medical Speech-Language Pathology, 2,* 111–122.

Riski, J. E. (1995). Secondary surgical procedures to correct postoperative velopharyngeal incompetencies found after primary palatoplasties. In K. R. Bzoch (Ed.), *Communicative disorders related to cleft lip and palate,* (4th ed.; pp. 121–152). Austin, TX: Pro-Ed.

Rittle-Johnson, B., & Siegler, R. S. (1999). Learning to spell: Variability, choice, and change in children's strategy use. *Child Development, 70,* 332–348.

Ritvo, E. R., & Freeman, B. J. (1978). National Society for Autistic Children definition of the syndrome of autism. *Journal of Autism and Childhood Schizophrenia, 8,* 162–167.

Robey, R. R. (1994). The efficacy of treatment for aphasic persons: A meta-analysis. *Brain and Language, 47,* 585–608.

Robey, R. R. (1998). A meta-analysis of clinical outcomes in the treatment of aphasia. *Journal of Speech, Language, and Hearing Research, 41,* 172–187.

Rogers, B. (1996). Neurodevelopmental presentation of dysphasia. *Seminars in Speech Language Pathology, 17*(4), 269–281.

Rogers, B., Arvedson, J., Buck, G., et al. (1994). Characteristics of dysphagia in children with cerebral palsy. *Dysphagia, 9*(1), 69–73.

Romski, M. A., & Sevcik, R. A. (1996). *Breaking the speech barrier: Language development through augmented means.* Baltimore: Brookes.

Rosenbek, J. C., & LaPointe, L. L. (1985). The dysarthrias: Description, diagnosis, and treatment. In D. F. Johns (Ed.), *Clinical management of neurogenic communication disorders* (pp. 97–152). Boston: Little, Brown.

Rosenbek, J. C., LaPointe, L. L., & Wertz, R. T. (1989). *Aphasia: A clinical approach.* Austin, TX: Pro-Ed.

Rosenfeld, S. J. (1999). EDLAW, LLC, Section 504 and IDEA: Basic similarities and differences. [Online] http://www.edlaw.net/service/504idea.html

Rosenfeld-Johnson, S., & Manning, D. (1997, August 4). Preventing oral-motor problems in Down syndrome. *Advance for Speech-Language-Pathologists,* 20.

Rosenfeld, D. (1991). Pharmacologic approaches to speech motor disorders. In D. Vogel & M. Cannito (Eds.), *Treating disordered speech motor control.* Austin, TX: Pro-Ed.

Rosenthal, S. R., Sheppard, J. J., & Lotze, M. (1995). *Dysphagia and the child with developmental disabili-*

ties: *Medical, clinical, and family interventions.* San Diego, CA: Singular.

Ross, K. B., & Wertz, R. T. (2003). Discriminative validity of selected measures of differentiating normal from aphasic performance. *American Journal of Speech-Language Pathology, 12,* 312–319.

Roth, F. P. (2000). Narrative writing: Development and teaching with children with writing difficulties. *Topics in Language Disorders, 20* (4), 15–28.

Roth, F. P. (2004). Word recognition assessment framework. In C. A. Stone, E. R. Silliman, B. J. Ehren, & K. Apel (Eds.), *Handbook of language and literacy: Development and disorders* (pp. 461–480). New York: Guilford.

Roth, F. P., Spekman, N. J., & Fye, E. C. (1991, November). *Written syntactic patterns of stories produced by learning disabled students.* Paper presented at the Annual Convention of the American Speech-Language-Hearing Association, Atlanta, GA.

Rowland, C., & Schweigert, P. (1989). Tangible symbols: Symbolic communication for individuals with multisensory impairments. *Augmentative and Alternative Communication, 5,* 226–234.

Rowland, C., & Schweigert, P. (2000). Tangible symbols, tangible outcomes. *Augmentative and Alternative Communication, 16,* 61–78.

Roy, N. (2005). Teachers with voice disorders: Recent clinical trials research. *The ASHA Leader, 10,* 8–9, 11.

Roy, N, Merrill, R. M., Thibeault, S., Parsa, R. A., Gray, S. D., & Smith, E. M. (2004). Prevalence of voice disorders in teachers and the general population. *Journal of Speech, Language, and Hearing Research, 47,* 281–293.

Runte, C., Lawerino, M., Dirksen, D., et al. (2001). The influence of maxillary central incisor position in complete dentures on /s/ sound production. *The Journal of Prosthetic Dentistry, 85,* 485–495.

Russell, N. (1993). Educational considerations in traumatic brain injury: The role of the speech-language pathologist. *Language, Speech, and Hearing Services in Schools, 24,* 67–75.

Ryan, B. P. (1974). *Programmed therapy for stuttering children and adults.* Springfield, IL: Charles C. Thomas.

Ryan, B. P., & Van Kirk Ryan, B. (1983). Programmed stuttering therapy for children: Comparisons of four established programs. *Journal of Fluency Disorders, 8,* 291–321.

Ryan, B. P., & Van Kirk Ryan, B. (1995). Programmed stuttering treatment for children: Comparisons of two established programs through transfer, main-tenance, and follow-up. *Journal of Speech and Hearing Research, 38,* 61–75.

Sackett, D. L., Straus, S. E., Richardson, W. S., Rosenberg, W., & Haynes, R. B. (2000). *Evidence-based medicine:How to practise and teach EBM* (2nd ed.). Edinburgh, Scotland, UK: Churchill Livingstone.

Saint-Exupéry, A. de (1968). *The little prince.* New York: Harcourt Brace.

Sameroff, A., & Fiese, B. (1990). Transactional regulation and early intervention. In S. Meisels & J. Shonkoff (Eds.), *Early intervention: A handbook of theory, practice, and analysis.* New York: Cambridge University Press.

Sanders, E. (1972). When are speech sounds learned? *Journal of Speech and Hearing Disorders, 37,* 55–63.

Sanders, L. D., & Neville, H. J. (2000). Lexical, syntactic, and stress-pattern cues for speech segmentation. *Journal of Speech, Language, and Hearing Research, 43,* 1301–1321.

Sanford, A. J., & Garrod, S. M. (1998). The role of scenario mapping in text comprehension. *Discourse Processes, 26,* 159–190.

Sapienza, C. M., Ruddy, B. H., & Baker, S. (2004). Laryngeal structure and function in the pediatric larynx: Clinical applications. *Language, Speech, and Hearing Services in Schools, 35,* 299–307.

Sarno, M. T. (1969). *Functional Communication Profile.* Rehabilitation Monographs 42. New York: New York University Medical Center.

Sarno, M. T., Buonaguro, A., & Levita, E. (1986). Characteristics of verbal impairment in closed head injury. *Archives of Physical Medicine and Rehabilitation, 67,* 400.

Scarborough, H., Wyckoff, J., & Davidson, R. (1986). A reconsideration of the relationship between age and mean utterance length. *Journal of Speech and Hearing Research, 29,* 394–399.

Schlosser, R. W., (2004). Evidence-based practice in ACC: 10 points to consider. *The ASHA Leader, 9*(12), 6–7, 10.

Schow, R. L., & Nerbonne, M. A. (2002). *Introduction to audiologic rehabilitation* (4th ed.). Boston: Allyn and Bacon.

Schraeder, T., Quinn, M., Stockman, I. J., & Miller, J. (1999). Authentic assessment as an approach to preschool speech-language screening. *American Journal of Speech-Language Pathology, 8,* 195–200.

Schreibman, L. (1988). *Developmental clinical psychology and psychiatry. Vol. 15: Autism.* Newbury Park, CA: Sage.

Schuell, H. (1972). *The Minnesota test for the differential diagnosis of aphasia.* Minneapolis: University of Minnesota Press.

Schwartz, H. (1993). Adolescents who stutter. *Journal of Fluency Disorders, 18,* 291–321.

Schwarz, S. M., Corredor, J., Fisher-Medina, J., et al. (2001). Diagnosis and treatment of feeding disorders in children with developmental disabilities. *Pediatrics, 108,* 671–676.

Scott, A. (1998). NICE and easy. *Advance for Speech-Language Pathologists and Audiologists, 8*(24), 16–17.

Scott, C. M. (1999) Learning to write. In H. W. Catts & A. G. Kamhi (Eds.), *Language and reading disabilities* (pp. 224–258). Boston: Allyn and Bacon.

Scott, C. M. (2000). Principles and methods of spelling instruction: Applications for poor spellers. *Topics in Language Disorder, 20*(3), 66–82.

Scott, C. M., & Windsor, J. (2000). General language performance measures in spoken and written narrative and expository discourse of school-age children with language learning disabilities. *Journal of Speech, Language, and Hearing Research, 43,* 324–339

Seagle, M. B. (1997). Primary surgical correction of cleft palate. In K. R. Bzoch (Ed.), *Communicative disorders related to cleft lip and palate* (4th ed.; pp. 115–120). Austin, TX: Pro-Ed.

Segebart DeThorne, L., & Watkins, R. V. (2001). Listeners' perceptions of language use in children. *Language, Speech, and Hearing Services in Schools, 32,* 142–148.

Selley, W. G., Parrott, L. C., Lethbridge, P. C., et al. (2001). Objective measures of dysphagia complexity in children related to suckle feeding histories, gestational ages, and classification of their cerebral palsy. *Dysphagia, 16,* 200–207.

Seung, H., & Chapman, R. (2000). Digit span in individuals with Down syndrome and in typically developing children: Temporal aspects. *Journal of Speech, Language, and Hearing Research, 43,* 609–620.

Shadden, B. B., & Toner, M. A. (Eds.). (1997). *Aging and communication: For clinicians by clinicians.* Austin, TX: Pro-Ed.

Shapiro, L., Swinney, D., & Borsky, S. (1998). Online examination of language performance in normal and neurologically impaired adults. *American Journal of Speech-Language Pathology, 7*(1), 49–60.

Shaw, G. Y., & Searl, J. P. (2001). Botulinum toxin treatment for cricopharyngeal dysfunction. *Dysphagia, 16,* 161–167.

Shekim, L. (1990). Dementia. In L. L. LaPointe (Ed.), *Aphasia and related neurogenic language disorders* (pp. 210–220). New York: Thieme Medical Publishers.

Shekim, L., & LaPointe, L. L. (1984, February). *Production of discourse in patients with Alzheimer's dementia.* Paper presented at the International Neuropsychology Society meeting, Houston.

Sheppard, J. J. (1991). Managing dysphagia in mentally retarded adults. *Dysphagia, 6*(2), 83–87.

Sheppard, J. J. (1995). Clinical evaluation and treatment. In S. R. Rosenthal, J. J., Sheppard, & M. Lotze (Eds.), *Dysphagia and the child with developmental disabilities: Medical, clinical, and family interventions.* San Diego, CA: Singular.

Shipley, K. G., & McAfee, J. G. (1998). *Assessment in speech-language pathology: A resource manual* (2nd ed.). San Diego, CA: Singular Publishing Group.

Shipp, T., Qi, Y., Huntley, R., & Hollien, H. (1992). Acoustic and temporal correlates of perceived age. *Journal of Voice, 6*(3), 211–216.

Shprintzen, R. J. (1995). A new perspective on clefting. In R. J. Shprintzen & J. Bardach (Eds.), *Cleft palate speech management: A multidisciplinary approach.* St. Louis, MO: Mosby.

Shprintzen, R. J., & Goldberg, R. (1995). The genetics of clefting and associated syndromes. In R. J. Shprintzen & J. Bardach (Eds.), *Cleft palate speech management: A multidisciplinary approach.* St. Louis, MO: Mosby.

Shprintzen, R. J., McCall, G. M., Skolnick, L. (1975). A new therapeutic technique for the treatment of velopharyngeal incompetence. *Journal of Speech and Hearing Disorders, 40,* 69–83.

Shriberg, L. D., Austin, D., Lewis, B. A., & McSweeney, J. L., & Wilson, D. L. (1997). The percentage of consonants correct (PCC) metric: Extensions and reliability data. *Journal of Speech, Language, and Hearing Research, 40*(4), 708–722.

Shriberg, L. D., & Kent, R. D. (1995). *Clinical phonetics* (2nd ed.). Boston: Allyn and Bacon.

Shriberg, L. D., & Kwiatkowski, J. (1994). Developmental phonological disorders. I: A clinical profile. *Journal of Speech and Hearing Research, 37,* 1100–1126.

Shugart, Y. Y., Mundorff, J., Kilshaw, J., Doheny, K., Doan, B., Wanyee, J., Green, E. D., & Drayna, D. (2004). Results of a genome-wide linkage scan for stuttering. *American Journal of Medical Genetics Part A, 124*(2), 133–135.

Sigafoos, J. (2000). Creating opportunities for augmentative and alternative communication: Strategies for involving people with developmental disabilities. *Augmentative and Alternative Communication, 16,* 183–190.

Silliman, E. R., & Wilkinson, L. C. (2004). Collaboration for language and literacy learning. In E. R.

Silliman & L. C. Wilkinson (Eds.), *Language and literacy learning in schools* (pp. 3–38). New York: Guilford.

Silverman, F. H. (1995). *Communication for the speechless* (3rd. ed.). Boston: Allyn and Bacon.

Simmons-Mackie, N. N., & Damico, J. S. (1996). The contribution of discourse markers to communicative competence. *American Journal of Speech-Language Pathology, 5*(1), 37–43.

Simmons-Mackie, N., Damico, J. S., & Damico, H. L. (1999). A qualitative study of feedback in aphasia treatment. *American Journal of Speech-Language Pathology, 8,* 218–230.

Singer, B. D., & Bashir, A. S. (2004). EmPOWER, A strategy of teaching students with language learning disabilities how to write expository text. In E. R. Silliman & L. C. Wilkinson (Eds.), *Language and literacy learning in schools* (pp. 239–272). New York: Guilford.

Singh, R., Cohen, S. N., & Krupp, R. (1996). Racial differences in cerebrovascular disease. *Neurology, 46*(Suppl. 2), A440–A441.

Small, J. A., Gutman, G., Makela, S., & Hillhouse, B. (2003). Effectiveness of communication strategies used by caregivers of persons with Alzheimer's disease during activities of daily living. *Journal of Speech, Language, and Hearing Research, 46,* 353–367.

Small, J. A., & Perry, J. (2005). Do you remember? How caregivers question their spouses who have Alzheimer's disease and the impact on communication. *Journal of Speech, Language, and Hearing Research, 48*(1), 125–136.

Small, L. H. (1999). *Fundamentals of phonetics: A practical guide for students.* Boston: Allyn and Bacon.

Smith, T. L., Pearson, M. L., Wilcox, K. R., Cruz, C., Lancaster, M. V., Robinson-Dunn, B., et al. (1998). Emergence of vancomycin resistance in *Staphylococcus aureus. New England Journal of Medicine, 340,* 493–501.

Snow, C. E., Scarborough, H. S., & Burns, M. S. (1999). What speech-language pathologists need to know about early reading. *Topics in Language Disorders, 20*(1), 48–58.

Snowling, M., & Frith, U. (1986). Comprehension in "hyperlexic" readers. *Journal of Experimental Child Psychology, 42,* 392–415.

Sohlberg, M., & Mateer, C. (1989). *Introduction to cognitive rehabilitation: Theory and practice.* New York: Guilford Press.

Sohlberg, M. M., Mateer, C. A., & Stuss, D. T. (1993). Contemporary approaches to the management of executive control dysfunction. *Journal of Head Trauma Rehabilitation, 8,* 45–58.

Solomon, N. P., McKee, A. S., Larson, K. J., Nawrocki, M. D., Tuite, P. J., Eriksen, S., Low, W. C., & Maxwell, R. E. (2000). Effects of pallidal stimulation on speech in three men with severe Parkinson's disease. *American Journal of Speech-Language Pathology, 9,* 241–256.

Solomon, N. P., Robin, D. A., & Luschei, E. S. (2000). Strength, endurance, and stability of the tongue and hand in Parkinson's disease. *Journal of Speech, Language, and Hearing Research, 43,* 256–267.

Sommers, R. K., & Caruso, A. J. (1995). Inservice training in speech-language pathology: Are we meeting the needs for fluency training? *American Journal of Speech-Language Pathology, 4*(3), 22–28.

Sonies, B. C. (1997). Evaluation and treatment of speech and swallowing disorders associated with myopathies. *Current Opinion in Rheumatology, 9*(6), 486–495.

Sonies, B. C., & Frattali, C. M. (1997). Critical decisions regarding service delivery across the health care continuum. In B. C. Sonies (Ed.), *Dysphagia: A continuum of care.* Gaithersburg, MD: Aspen.

Soto, G., Muller, E., Hunt, P., & Goetz, L. (2001). Critical issues in the inclusion of students who use augmentative and alternative communication: An educational team perspective. *Augmentative and Alternative Communication, 17,* 62–72.

Sparks, R. W., Helm, N., & Albert, M. (1974). Aphasia rehabilitation resulting from melodic intonation therapy. *Cortex, 10,* 303–316.

Sparks, R. W., & Holland, A. L. (1976). Method: Melodic intonation therapy for aphasia. *Journal of Speech and Hearing Disorders, 41,* 287–297.

Spiegel, B., Benjamin, B. J., & Spiegel, S. (1993). One method to increase spontaneous use of an assistive communication device: A case study. *Augmentative and Alternative Communication, 9,* 111–117.

Stach, B. A., Spretnjak, M. I., & Jerger, J. (1990). The prevalence of central presbycusis in a clinical population. *Journal of the American Academy of Audiology, 2,* 109–115.

Stanovich, K. (1986). "Matthew effects" in reading: Some consequences of individual differences in acquisition of literacy. *Reading Research Quarterly, 4,* 360–407.

Stanovich, K., Cunningham, A., & Crammer, B. (1984). Assessing phonological awareness in kindergarten: Issues of task comparability. *Journal of Experimental Child Psychology, 38,* 175–190.

Starch, S., & Falltrick, E. (1990). The importance of

home evaluation for brain injured clients: A team approach. *Cognitive Rehabilitation, 8,* 28–32.

Starkweather, W. (1987). *Fluency and stuttering.* Englewood Cliffs, NJ: Prentice-Hall.

Starkweather, W. (1997). Therapy for younger children. In R. F. Curlee & G. M. Siegel (Eds.), *Nature and treatment of stuttering: New directions* (2nd ed., pp. 143–166). Boston: Allyn and Bacon.

Stecker, N. A. (1998). Overview and update of central auditory processing disorders. In M. G. Masters, N. A. Stecker, & J. Katz (Eds.), *Central auditory processing disorders: Mostly management.* Boston: Allyn and Bacon.

Steele, C., & van Lieshout, P. (2005). Does barium influence tongue behaviors during swallowing? *American Journal of Speech-Language Pathology, 14,* 27–39.

Steele, C. M., Greenwood, C., Ens, I., et al. (1997). Mealtime difficulties in a home for the aged: Not just dysphagia. *Dysphagia, 12*(1), 43–51.

Stinneford, J. G., Keshavarzian, A., Nemchausky, B. A., Doria, M. I., & Durkin, M. (1993). Esophagitis and esophageal motor abnormalities in patients with chronic spinal cord injuries. *Paraplegia, 31*(6), 384–392.

Stoel-Gammon, C., & Dunn, C. (1985). *Normal and disordered phonology in children.* Austin, TX: Pro-Ed.

Strand, E. A., & McCauley, R. (1997, November). *Differential diagnosis of phonological impairment and developmental apraxia of speech.* Paper presented at the American Speech-Language-Hearing Association Annual Convention, Boston, MA.

Strange, W., & Broen, P. (1980). Perception and production of approximant consonants by 3-year-olds: A first study. In G. Yeni-Komshian, J. Kavanaugh, & C. A. Ferguson (Eds.), *Child phonology: Vol. 2. Perception.* New York: Academic Press.

Straus, D., Cable, W., & Shavelle, R. (1999). Causes of excess mortality in cerebral palsy. *Developmental Medicine and Child Neurology, 41,* 580–585.

Stredler-Brown, A., & Johnson, D. C. (2003). Functional auditory performance indicators: An integrated approach to auditory development. [Online] http://www.cde.state.co.us/cdesped/SpecificDisabilityHearing.htm

Tanner, D. C. (1980). Loss and grief: Implications for the speech-language pathologist and audiologist. *Asha, 22,* 916–928.

Tattershall, S. (2004). *SLPs contributing to and learning within the writing process.* Paper presented at the Annual Convention of the American Speech-Language-Hearing Association, Philadelphia.

Templeton, S. (2003). The spelling/meaning connection. *Voices from the Middle, 10*(3), 56–57.

Templeton, S. (2004). Instructional approaches to spelling: The window on students' word knowledge in reading and writing. In E. R. Silliman & L. C. Wilkinson (Eds.), *Language and literacy learning in schools* (pp. 273–291). New York: Guilford.

Thal, D., Jackson-Maldonado, D., & Acosta, D. (2000). Validity of a parent-report measure of vocabulary and grammar for Spanish-speaking toddlers. *Journal of Speech, Language, and Hearing Research, 43,* 1087–1100.

Thomas, C., Englert, C. S., & Morsink, C. (1984). Modifying the classroom program in language. In C. V. Morsink (Ed.), *Teaching special needs students in regular classrooms* (pp. 239–276). Boston: Little, Brown.

Thomas, L. (1979). *The medusa and the snail: More notes of a biology watcher.* New York: Viking.

Thompson, C. K. (1988). Articulation disorders in children with neurological pathology. In N. J. Lass, L. V. McReynolds, & D. E. Yoder (Eds.), *Handbook of speech-language pathology and audiology* (pp. 548–590). Burlington, Ontario, Canada: B. D. Decker.

Thompson, C. K., Shapiro, L. P., Kiran, S., & Sobecks, J. (2003). The role of syntactic complexity in treatment of sentence deficits in agrammatic aphasia: The Complexity Account of Treatment Efficacy (CATE). *Journal of Speech, Language, and Hearing Research, 46,* 591–607.

Tierney, L. M., Jr. (1993). *Current medical diagnosis and treatment, 1994.* Los Altos, CA: Appleton & Lange.

Tierney, L. M., Jr., McPhee, S. J., & Papadakis, M. A. (2000). *Current medical diagnosis and treatment* (39th ed.). New York: Lange Medical Books/McGraw-Hill.

Titze, I. R. (1994). *Principles of voice production.* Englewood Cliffs, NJ: Prentice-Hall.

Tjaden, K. (2000). A preliminary study of factors influending perception of articulatory rate in Parkinson's disease. *Journal of Speech, Language, and Hearing Research, 43,* 997–1010.

Tjaden, K., & Turner, G. (2000). Segmental timing in amyotropic lateral sclerosis. *Journal of Speech, Language, and Hearing Research, 43,* 683–696.

Tomes, L. A., Kuehn, D. P., & Peterson-Falzone, S. J. (1995). Behavioral treatments of velopharyngeal impairment. In K. R. Bzoch (Ed.), *Communicative disorders related to cleft lip and palate* (4th ed.; pp. 529–562). Austin, TX: Pro-Ed.

Tolchinsky-Landsmann, L., & Levin, I. (1985). Writing in preschoolers: An age related analysis. *Applied Psycholinguistics, 6,* 319–339.

Tomblin, J. B., Zhang, X., Buckwalter, P., & O'Brien, M. (2003). The stability of primary language disorder: Four years after kindergarten diagnosis. *Journal of Speech, Language, and Hearing Research, 46,* 1283–1296.

Tompkins, C. A. (1995). *Right hemisphere communication disorders: Theory and management.* San Diego: Singular.

Tompkins, C. A., Baumgaertner, A., Lehman, M. T., & Fassbinder, W. (2000). Mechanisms of discourse comprehension impairment after right hemisphere brain damage: Suppression of lexical ambiguity resolution. *Journal of Speech, Language, and Hearing Research, 43,* 62–78.

Toner, M. A. (1997). Targeting dysphagia in the elderly: Prevention, assessment, and intervention. In B. B. Shadden & M. A. Toner (Eds.), *Aging and communication: For clinicians by clinicians.* Austin, TX: Pro-Ed.

Torgesen, J. K. (1980). Conceptual and educational implications of the use of efficient task strategies by learning disabled children. *Journal of Learning Disabilities, 13,* 19–26.

Torgesen, J. K. (2005). Recent discoveries from research on remedial interventions for children with dyslexia. In M. Snowling & C. Hulme (Eds.), *The science of reading: A handbook* (pp. 521–537). Oxford, UK: Blackwell.

Torgesen, J. K., al Otaiba, S., & Grek, M. L. (2005). Assessment and instruction for phonemic awareness and word recognition skills. In H. W. Catts & A. G. Kamhi (Eds.), *Language and reading disabilities* (2nd ed.; pp. 127–156). Boston: Allyn and Bacon.

Towey, M., Whitcomb, J., & Bray, C. (2004). *Print-sound-story-talk, a successful early reading first program.* Paper presented at the Annual Convention of the American Speech-Language-Hearing Association, Philadelphia.

Treiman, R. (1993). *Beginning to spell.* New York: Oxford University Press.

Treiman, R. (1997). Spelling in normal children and dyslexics. In B. Blachman (Ed.), *Foundations of reading acquisition and dyslexia: Implications for early intervention* (pp. 191–218). Mahwah, NJ: Lawrence Erlbaum Associates.

Treiman, R., & Cassar, M. (1997). Spelling acquisition in English. In C. A. Perfetti, L. Rieben, & M. Fayol (Eds.), *Learning to spell: Research, theory, and practice across languages* (pp. 61–80). Mahwah, NJ: Lawrence Erlbaum Associates.

Troia, G. A., Graham, S., & Harris, K. R. (1999) Teach-ing students with learning disabilities to mindfully plan when writing. *Exceptional Children, 65,* 235–252.

Tye-Murray, N. (2004). *Foundations of aural rehabilitation: Children, adults, and their family members.* 2nd ed. Clifton Park, N. Y: Delmar Learning.

Tyler, A., & Watterson, K. (1991). Effects of phonological versus language intervention in preschoolers with both phonological and language impairment. *Child Language Teaching and Therapy, 7,* 141–160.

Tyler, A. A., Lewis, K. E., & Welch, C. M. (2003). Predictors of phonological change following intervention. *American Journal of Speech-Language Pathology, 12,* 289–298.

Ukrainetz, T. A., Harpell, S., Walsh, C., & Coyle, C. (2000). A preliminary investigation of dynamic assessment with Native American kindergarteners. *Language, Speech, and Hearing Services in Schools, 31,* 142–154.

U. S. Census Bureau. (1997). Americans with disabilities: 1997. [Online] http://www. census.gov/hhes/www/disable/sipp/ disabl97/asc97.html

U. S. Department of Justice, Civil Rights Division, Disability Rights Section. (2000). A Guide to Disability Rights Laws. [Online] http://www.usdoj.gov/crt/ada/cguide.htm

Vace, N. N. (1987). Word processor versus handwriting: A comparative study of writing samples produced by mildly mentally handicapped students. *Exceptional Children, 54,* 156–165.

Vallecorsa, A. L., & Garriss, E. (1990). Story composition skills or middle-grade students with learning disabilitles. *Exceptional Children, 57,* 48–54.

Vanderheiden, G. (1984). High and low technology approaches in the development of communication systems for severely physically handicapped persons. *Exceptional Education Quarterly, 4*(4), 40–56.

Van Kleeck, A. (1995). Emphasizing form and meaning separately in prereading and early reading instruction. *Topics in Language Disorders, 16*(1), 27–49.

Van Meter, A. M., Nelson, N. W., & Ansell, P. (2004). *Developing spelling and vocabulary skills in curriculum writing activities.* Paper presented at the Annual Convention of the American Speech-Language-Hearing Association, Philadelphia.

Van Riper, C. (1982). *The nature of stuttering.* Englewood Cliffs, NJ: Prentice-Hall.

Van Riper, C. (1992). *The nature of stuttering* (2nd ed.). Prospect Heights, IL: Waveland Press.

Van Riper, C., & Erickson, R. (1996). *Speech correction:*

An introduction to speech pathology and audiology (9th ed.). Englewood Cliffs, NJ: Prentice-Hall.

Varnhagen, C. K., McCallum, M., & Burstow, M. (1997). Is children's spelling naturally stage-like? *Reading and Writing: An Interdisciplinary Journal, 9,* 451–481.

Vaughn, S., & Klingner, J. (2004). Teaching reading comprehension to student with learning disabilities. In C. A. Stone, E. R. Silliman, B. J. Ehren, & K. Apel (Eds.), *Handbook of language and literacy: Development and disorders* (pp. 541–555). New York: Guilford.

Venezky, R. L. (1999). *The American way of spelling: The structure and origins of American English orthography.* New York: Guilford.

Venkatagiri, H. S. (2000). Efficient keyboard layouts for sequential access in augmentative and alternative communication. *Augmentative and Alternative Communication, 16,* 126–134.

Wagner, R. K., Torgesen, J. K., & Rashotte, C. A. (1999). *Comprehensive test of phonological processing (CTOPP).* Austin, TX: Pro-Ed.

Wallach, G. P., & Butler, K. G. (1995). Language learning disabilities: Moving in from the edge. *Topics in Language Disorders, 16*(1), 1–26.

Waltzman, S. B., & Cohen, N. L. (1998). Cochlear implantation in children younger than 2 years old. *American Journal of Otology, 19,* 1083–1087.

Wambaugh, J., & Bain, B. (2002). Make research methods an integral part of your clinical practice. *The ASHA Leader, 7*(21), 1, 10–13.

Warburton, E., Price, C. J., Swinburn, K., & Wise, R. J. (1999). Mechanisms of recovery from aphasia: Evidence of positron emission tomography studies.*Journal of Neurology, Neurosurgery, and Psychiatry, 66,* 155–161.

Waterman, E. T., Koltai, P. J., Downey, J. C., & Cacace, A. T. (1992). Swallowing disorders in a population of children with cerebral palsy. *International Journal of Pediatric Otorhinolaryngology, 24*(1), 63–71.

Watson, B. C., & Freeman, F. J. (1997). Brain imaging contributions. In R. F. Curlee & G. M. Siegel (Eds.), *Nature and treatment of stuttering: New directions* (2nd ed., pp. 143–166). Boston: Allyn and Bacon.

Weiner, F. (2000). *Diagnostic report writer, 2000.* West Bloomfield, MI: Parrot Software.

Weinstein, B. (1994). Presbycusis. In J. Katz (Ed.), *Handbook of clinical audiology* (4th ed., pp. 568–584). Baltimore, MD: Williams and Wilkins.

Weismer, S. E., Evans, J., & Hesketh, L. J. (1999). An examination of verbal working memory capacity in children with specific language impairment. *Journal of Speech, Language, and Hearing Research, 23,* 1234–1248.

Weismer, S. E., & Hesketh, L. J. (1996). Lexical learning by children with specific language impairment: Effects of linguistic input presented at varying speaking rates. *Journal of Speech and Learning Research, 39,* 177–190.

Weismer, S. E., Tomblin, J. B., Zhang, X., Buckwalter, P., Gaura Chynoweth, J., & Jones, M. (2000). Nonword repetition performance in school-age chidren with and without language impairment. *Journal of Speech, Language, and Hearing Research, 43,* 865–878.

Wellman, H. (1985). The origins of metacognition. In D. Forest-Pressley, G. MacKinnon, & T. Waller (Eds.), *Metacognition, cognition, and human performance* (pp. 1–31). New York: Academic Press.

Wells, G. (1985). *Language development in the preschool years.* New York: Cambridge University Press.

Wertz, R. T. (1985). Neuropathologies of speech and language: An introduction to patient management. In D. F. Johns (Ed.), *Clinical management of neurogenic communicative disorders* (2nd ed.). Boston: Little, Brown.

Wertz, R. T., LaPointe, L. L., & Rosenbek, J. C. (1991). *Apraxia of speech in adults: The disorder and its management.* San Diego, CA: Singular Publishing Group.

Westby, C. E. (1997). There's more to passing than knowing the answers. *Language, Speech, and Hearing Services in Schools, 28,* 244–287.

Westby, C. E. (2004). A language perspective on executive functioning, metacognition, and self-regulation in reading. In C. A. Stone, E. R. Silliman, B. J. Ehren, & K. Apel (Eds.), *Handbook of language and literacy: Development and disorders* (pp. 398–427). New York: Guilford.

Westby, C. E. (2005). Assessing and remediating text comprehension problems. In H. W. Catts & A. G. Kamhi (Eds.), *Language and reading disabilities* (2nd ed.; pp. 157–232). Boston: Allyn and Bacon.

Whitehurst, G. J., & Lonigan, C. J. (2001). Emergent readers: Development from prereaders to readers. In S. B. Neuman & D. K. Dickinson (Eds.), *Handbook of early literacy research* (pp. 11–29). New York: Guilford.

Whitmire, K. A. (2000). Adolescence as a developmental phase: A tutorial. *Topics in Language Disorders, 20*(2), 1–14.

Wiig, E. H., Zureich, P. Z., & Chan, H. H. (2000). A clinical rationale for assessing rapid automatized naming with language disorders. *Journal of Learning Disabilities, 33,* 359–374.

Wilcox, K., & Morris, S. (1999). *Children's speech intelligibility measure.* San Antonio, TX: Psychological Corporation.

Williams, J. P. (1998). Improving the comprehension of disabled readers. *Annals of Dyslexia, 48,* 213–218.

Willot, J. F. (1996). Anatomic and physiologic aging: A behavioral neuroscience perspective. *Journal of the American Academy of Audiology, 7,* 141–151.

Wilson, D. (1987). *Voice problems in children* (3rd ed.). Baltimore, MD: Williams and Wilkins.

Wilson, W. R. (1994). Sudden sensorineural hearing loss. In G. M. English (Ed.), *Otolaryngology.* Philadelphia: Lippicott.

Windsor, J., & Hwang, M. (1999). Testing the generalized slowing hypothesis in specific language impairment. *Journal of Speech, Language, and Hearing Research, 42,* 1205–1218.

Windsor, J., Scott, C. M., & Street, C. K. (2000). Verb and noun morphology in the spoken and written language of children with language learning disabilities. *Journal of Speech, Language, and Hearing Research, 43,* 1322–1336.

Wingate, M. E. (1969). Sound and pattern in "artificial" fluency. *Journal of Speech and Hearing Research, 12,* 677–686.

Wingate, M. E. (1970). Effect on stuttering of changes in audition. *Journal of Speech and Hearing Research, 13,* 861–873.

Winograd, P. N., & Niquette, G. (1988), Assessing learned helplessness in poor readers. *Topics in Language Disorders, 8*(3), 38–55.

Witzel, M. A. (1995). Communicative impairment associated with clefting. In R. J. Shprintzen & J. Bardach (Eds.), *Cleft palate speech management: A multidisciplinary approach.* St. Louis, MO: Mosby.

Wixson, K., Bosky, A., Yochum, M., & Alvermann, D. (1984). An interview for assessing students' perceptions of classroom reading tasks. *The Reading Teacher, 37,* 346–352.

Wolk, S., & Schildroth, A. N. (1986). Deaf children and speech intelligibility: A national study. In A. N. Schildroth & M. A. Karchmer (Eds.), *Deaf children in America* (pp. 139–159). San Diego: College-Hill.

Wong, B. Y. (2000). Writing strategies instruction for expository essays for adolescents with and without learning disabilities. *Topics in Language Disorders, 20*(4), 244.

Wong, B. Y., Butler, D. L., Ficzere, S. A., & Kuperis, S. (1996). Teaching low achievers and students with learning disabilities to plan, write, and revise opinion essays. *Journal of Learning Disabilities, 29*(2), 197–212.

Wood, P., & Emick-Herring, B. (1997). Dysphagia: A screening tool for stroke patients. *Journal of Neuroscientific Nursing, 29*(5), 325–329.

Woods, E. K. (1995). The influence of posture and positioning on oral motor development and dysphagia. In S. R. Rosenthal, J. J. Sheppard, & M. Lotze (Eds.), *Dysphagia and the child with developmental disabilities: Medical, clinical, and family interventions.* San Diego, CA: Singular Publishing Group.

Wooi, M., Scott, A., & Perry, A. (2001). Teaching speech pathology students the interpretation of videofluoroscopic swallowing studies. *Dysphagia, 16,* 32–39.

Xue, S. A., & Hao, G. J. (2003). Changes in the human vocal tract due to aging and the acoustic correlates of speech production: A pilot study. *Journal of Speech, Language, and Hearing Research, 46,* 689–701.

Yairi, E. (1981). Disfluencies of normally speaking 2-year-old children. *Journal of Speech and Hearing Research, 24,* 301–307.

Yairi, E. (1982). Longitudinal studies of disfluencies in 2-year-old children. *Journal of Speech and Hearing Research, 25,* 402–404.

Yairi, E. (1983). The onset of stuttering in 2- and 3-year-old children: A preliminary report. *Journal of Speech and Hearing Disorders, 48,* 171–177.

Yairi, E. (2004). The formative years of stuttering: A changing portrait. *Contemporary Issues in Communication Science and Disorders, 31,* 92–104.

Yairi, E., & Ambrose, N. (1992a). A longitudinal study of children: A preliminary report. *Journal of Speech and Hearing Research, 35,* 755–760.

Yairi, E., & Ambrose, N. (1992b). Onset of stuttering in preschool children: Selected factors. *Journal of Speech and Hearing Research, 35,* 782–788.

Yairi, E., & Ambrose, N. (2004). Stuttering: Recent developments and future directions. *The ASHA Leader, 18,* 4–5, 14–15.

Yairi, E., Ambrose, N., & Nierman, B. (1993). The early months of stuttering: A developmental study. *Journal of Speech and Hearing Research, 36,* 521–528.

Yairi, E., Watkins, R., Ambrose, N., et al. (2001). What is stuttering? (Letter to the editor). *Journal of Speech, Language, and Hearing Research, 44,* 585–592.

Yang, M. T., Ko, F. T., Cheng, N. Y., et al. (1996). Clinical experience of esophageal ulcers and esophagitis in AIDS patients. *Kao Hsiung I Hsueh Ko Hsueh Tsa Chih, 12*(11), 624–629.

Yaruss, J. S. (1997). Clinical measurement of stuttering behaviors. *Contemporary Issues in Communication Science and Disorders, 24,* 33–44.

Yavas, M. (1998). *Phonology: Development and disorders.* San Diego: Singular Publishing Group.

Yavas, M., & Goldstein, B. (1998). Phonological assessment and treatment of bilingual speakers. *American Journal of Speech-Language Pathology, 7*(2), 49–60.

Ylvisaker, M. (1994). Collaboration in assessment and intervention after TBI. *Topics in Language Disorders, 15*(1), 1–81.

Ylvisaker, M., & DeBonis, D. (2000). Executive function impairment in adolescence: TBI and ADHD. *Topics in Language Disorders, 20*(2), 29–57.

Ylvisaker, M., & Feeney, T. (1995). Traumatic brain injury in adolescence: Assessment and reintegration. *Seminars in Speech and Language, 16,* 32–44.

Ylvisaker, M., & Szekeres, S. F. (1989). Executive and metacognitive impairments in head injured children and adults. *Topics in Language Disorders, 9*(2), 34–49.

Ylvisaker, M., Szekeres, S. F., & Feeney, T. (1998). Cognitive rehabilitation: Executive functions. In M. Ylvisaker (Ed.), *Traumatic brain injury rehabilitation: Children and adolescents* (pp. 221–269). Boston: Butterworth-Heinemann.

Yoder, D., & Munson, L. (1995). The social correlates of co-ordinated attention to adults and objects in mother-infant interaction. *First Language, 15,* 219–230.

Yont, K. M., Hewitt, L. E., & Miccio, A. W. (2000). A coding system for describing conversational breakdowns in preschool children. *American Journal of SpeechLanguage Pathology, 9,* 300–309.

Yopp, H. K. (1988). The validity and reliability of phonemic awareness tests. *Reading Research Quarterly, 23,* 159–177.

Yorkston, K. M., Beukelman, D. R., & Bell, K. R. (1988). *Clinical management of dysarthric speakers.* Boston: College Hill Press.

Yorkston, K., & Beukelman, D. (2004). Dysarthria: Tools for clinical decision-making. *The ASHA Leader, 9,* 4–21.

Yorkston, K., Honsinger, M., Dowden, P., & Marriner, N. (1989). Vocabulary selection: A case report. *Augmentative and Alternative Communication, 5*(2), 101–108.

Yorkston, K. M., Miller, R. M., & Strand, E. A. (1995). *Management of speech and swallowing disorders in degenerative disease.* Tucson, AZ: Communication Skill Builders.

Yorkston, K. M., Smith, E., & Beukelman, D. R. (1990). Extended communication samples of augmentative communicators: I. A comparison of individualized versus standard single-word vocabularies. *Journal of Speech and Hearing Disorders, 55,* 217–224.

Yorkston, K. M., Strand, E. A., Miller, R. M., Hillel, A., & Smith, K. (1993). Speech deterioration in amyotrophic lateral sclerosis: Implications for the timing of intervention. *Journal of Medical Speech-Language Pathology, 1,* 35–46.

Yoshinaga-Itano, C., Sedley, A. L., Coulter, D. K., & Mehl, A. L. (1998). Language of early and later identified children with hearing loss. *Pediatrics, 102,* 1161–1171.

Zangari, C. (2001). Helping families gain acceptance of AAC strategies. *American Speech-Language Hearing Association Special Interest Division 1, Language Learning and Education Newsletter, 8*(1), 14–17.

Zangari, C., & Kangas, K. A. (1997). Intervention principles and procedures, In L. L. Lloyd, D. R. Fuller, & H. H. Arvidson (Eds.), *Augmentative and alternative communication: A handbook of principles and practices.* Boston: Allyn and Bacon.

Zantal-Wiener, K. (1988). Preschool services for children with handicaps. ERIC Digest #450. ERIC Clearinghouse on Handicapped and Gifted Children, Reston, VA.

Zemlin, W. R. (1998). *Speech and hearing sciences: Anatomy and physiology* (4th ed.). Boston: Allyn and Bacon.

Zeuschner, R. (1997). *Communicating today* (2nd ed.). Boston: Allyn and Bacon.

Zhang, Y., Brooks, D. W., Fields, T., & Redelfs, M. (1995). Quality of writing by elementary students with learning disabilities. *Journal of Research on Computing in Education, 27,* 483–499.

Zitnay, G. A. (1995). Foreword. In D. G. Stein, S. Brailowsky, & B. Will (Eds.), *Brain repair* (pp. v–vi). New York: Oxford University Press.

Author Index

Subject Index